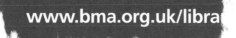

OXFORD MEDICAL PUBLICATIONS

Oxford Desk Reference
Cardiology

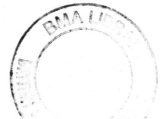

Oxford Desk Reference
Cardiology

Edited by

Hung-Fat Tse

Cardiology Division, Department of Medicine,
Queen Mary Hospital,
The University of Hong Kong, China

Gregory Y.H. Lip

University of Birmingham Centre for Cardiovascular Sciences,
City Hospital, Birmingham, UK

Andrew J. Stewart Coats

University of East Anglia,
Norwich, UK

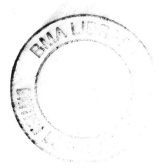

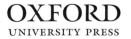

OXFORD
UNIVERSITY PRESS

OXFORD
UNIVERSITY PRESS

Great Clarendon Street, Oxford OX2 6DP

Oxford University Press is a department of the University of Oxford.
It furthers the University's objective of excellence in research, scholarship,
and education by publishing worldwide in

Oxford New York

Athens Auckland Bangkok Bogotá Buenos Aires Cape Town
Chennai Dar es Salaam Delhi Florence Hong Kong Istanbul Karachi
Kolkata Kuala Lumpur Madrid Melbourne Mexico City Mumbai Nairobi
Paris São Paulo Shanghai Singapore Taipei Tokyo Toronto Warsaw

with associated companies in Berlin Ibadan

Oxford is a registered trade mark of Oxford University Press
in the UK and in certain other countries

Published in the United States
by Oxford University Press Inc., New York

British Library Cataloguing in Publication Data

Data available

Library of Congress Cataloguing in Publication Data

Data available

ISBN 978-0-19-956809-3

10 9 8 7 6 5 4 3 2 1

Typeset in GillHandbook
by Glyph International, Bangalore, India
Printed in Great Britain
on acid-free paper by
CPI Antony Rowe, Chippenham, Wiltshire

Contents

Detailed contents

List of abbreviations

α	alpha		CLI	critical limb ischaemia
β	beta		CMR	cardiac magnetic imaging
AAA	abdominal aortic aneurysm		COC	combined oral contraceptive
AAD	anti-arrhythmic drug		COPD	chronic obstructive pulmonary disorder
ABP	ambulatory blood pressure		CPAP	continuous positive airway pressure
ACD	acute coronary syndrome		CPB	cardiopulmonary bypass
ACEI	angiotensin-converting enzyme inhibitor		CPEX	cardiopulmonary exercise testing
ACS	acute coronary syndrome		CR	controlled release
ACTH	adrenocorticotropic hormone		CrCl	creatine clearance
ADP	adenosine diphosphate		CRP	C-reactive protein
ADR	adverse drug reaction		CRT	cardiac resynchronization therapy
AED	automated external defibrillator		CS	cardiogenic shock
AF	atrial fibrillation		CSA	cross-sectional area
AHA	American Heart Association		CSM	carotid sinus massage
AHF	acute heart failure		CSS	carotid sinus syndrome
ALS	advanced life support		CSX	cardiac syndrome X
ANP	atrial natriuretic peptide		CT	computed tomography
AR	aortic regurgitation		CTO	chronic total occlusion
ARB	angiotensin receptor blocker		CTPH	chronic thromboembolic pulmonary hypertension
ARF	acute rheumatic fever			
ARVD	arrhythmogenic right ventricular dysplasia		CVA	cerebrovascular accident
ASA	atrial septal aneurysm		CVS	cardiovascular system
ASD	atrial septal defect		DAPT	dual antiplatelet therapy
AST	aspartate aminotransferase		DASH	dietary approaches to stop hypertension
AUC	area under the curve		DBP	diastolic blood pressure
AVNRT	atrioventricular nodal re-entry tachycardia		DC	direct current
AVR	aortic valve replacement		DCCV	direct current cardioversion
AVRT	atrioventricular tachycardia		DCM	dilated cardiomyopathy
BAV	bicuspid aortic valve		DE	delayed enhancement
BBB	bundle branch block		DES	drug eluting stent
BLS	basic life support		DRL	dose of radiation limit
BM	bone marrow		DTI	direct thrombin inhibitor
BMS	bare metal stent		DVT	deep vein thrombosis
BP	blood pressure		ECG	electrocardiogram
BrS	Brugada syndrome		ED	emergency department
BSA	body surface area		EDV	end-diastolic volume
CABG	coronary artery bypass graft		EDWT	end-diastolic wall thickness
CABS	coronary artery bypass surgery		EECP	enhanced external counterpulsation
CACS	coronary calcium score		EEG	electroencephalography
CAD	coronary artery disease		EF	ejection fraction
CBF	coronary blood flow		eGFR	estimated glomerular filtration rate
CCB	calcium channel blocker		EMB	endomyocardial biopsy
CCU	coronary care unit		EPD	embolic protection device
CER	cardiac event recorder		EPS	electrophysiological study
CETP	cholesterol transfer protein		EROA	effective regurgitant orifice area
CHB	complete heart block		ESC	European Society of Cardiology
CHD	coronary heart disease		ESR	erythrocyte sedimentation rate
CIN	contrast-induced nephropathy		ESV	end-systolic volume
CK	creatine kinase		FAF	familial atrial fibrillation

FBC	full blood count		MI	myocardial infarction
FDG	18F-fluorodeoxygluclose		MMR	maternal mortality rate
FFR	fractional flow reserve		MPA	microscopic polyangiitis
GC	guide catheter		MR	mitral regurgitation
GCA	giant cell arteritis		MRA	magnetic resonance angiography
GCM	giant cell myocarditis		MRI	magnetic resonance imaging
GI	gastrointestinal		NS	mitral stenosis
GP	glycoprotein		MV	mitral valve
GTN	glyceryl trinitrate		MVA	mitral valve area
HCM	hypertrophic cardiomyopathy		Na	sodium
HDL	high-density lipoprotein		NEAD	non-epileptic attack disorder
H-FABP	heart-type fatty acid binding protein		NICE	National Institute for Health and Clinical Excellence
HIV	human immunodeficiency virus			
HOT	home oxygen therapy		NO	nitric oxide
HSP	Henoch-Schönlein pupura		NSAID	non-steroidal anti-inflammatory drug
IABP	intra-aortic balloon pump		NSTEMI	non-ST-segment elevation myocardial infarction
IAST	inappropriate sinus tachycardia			
IC	intracoronary		NTG	nitroglycerin
ICD	implantable cardioverter defibrillator		NYHA	New York Heart Association
ICH	intracerebral haemorrhage		OM	obtuse marginal
ICS	intercostal space		OR	odds ratio
ICU	intensive care unit		OSA	obstructive sleep apnoea
IE	infective endocarditis		OTC	over the counter
IHD	ischaemic heart disease		OTW	over the wire
IL	interleukin		PA	posteroanterior
ILR	implantable loop recorder		PAC	plasma aldosterone concentration
IMA	ischaemia modified albumin		PAD	peripheral arterial disease
INR	international normalized ratio		PAH	pulmonary arterial hypertension
IPF	idiopathic pulmonary fibrosis		PAPP-A	pregnancy-associated plasma protein A
IV	intravenous		PCI	percutaneous coronary intervention
IVRT	isovolumetric relaxation time		PE	pulmonary embolism
IVS	interventricular septum		PET	positron emission tomography
IVST	interventricular septum thickness		PFO	patent foramen ovale
JVP	jugular venous pulsation		PISA	proximal isovelocity surface area
LBBB	left bundle branch block		PMI	point of maximal impulse
LA	left atrium		POP	progestogen-only pill
LAD	left anterior descending		POTS	postural orthostatic tachycardia syndrome
LAO	left anterior oblique		PPH	primary pulmonary hypertension
LAVI	left atrial volume index		PRA	plasma renin activity
LDH	lactate dehydrogenase		PT	prothrombin time
LDL	low-density lipoprotein		PTT	partial thromboplastin time
LL	left leg		PWT	posterior wall thickness
LMWH	low-molecular-weight heparin		pVO2	peak oxygen consumption
LV	left ventricle		QoL	quality of life
LVEDD	left ventricular end-diastolic diameter		RA	right arm
LVEF	left ventricular ejection fraction		RAO	right anterior oblique
LVH	left ventricular hypertrophy		RBBB	right bundle branch block
LVM	left ventricular mass		RCA	right coronary artery
LVSED	left ventricular end-systolic diameter		RCM	restrictive cardiomyopathy
MAC	monitored anaesthetic care		RCT	randomized controlled trial
MACE	major adverse cardiovascular event		RER	respiratory exchange ratio
MCCT	multislice coronary computed tomography		RFA	radiofrequency ablation
MDCT	multidetector row computed tomography		ROC	receiver operating characteristic
MEN	multiple endocrine neoplasia		RV	right ventricle

RVOT	right ventricular outflow tract		TEE	transoesophageal echocardiogram
SARS	severe acute respiratory distress syndrome		TGA	transposition of the great arteries
			TIA	transient ischaemic attack
SBE	subcutaneous infective endocarditis		T-LOC	transient loss of consciousness
SCD	sudden cardiac death		TNF	tumour necrosis factor
SCr	serum creatinine		TOE	transoesophagela echocardiography
SDB	sleep disordered breathing		TOF	tetralogy of Fallot
SIRS	systemic inflammatory response syndrome		TR	tricuspid regurgitation
			TV	tricuspid valve
SLE	systemic lupus erythematosus		UA	unstable angina
SND	sino-atrial nodal dysfunction		U+E	urea and electrolytes
SPB	systolic blood pressure		UFH	unfractionated heparin
SPECT	single-photon emission computed tomography		VCD	vascular closure device
			VCO2	carbon dioxide production
SSRI	selective serotonin reuptake inhibitor		VF	ventricular fibrillation
STEMI	ST-segment elevation myocardial infarction		VKA	vitamin K antagonist
			V/Q	ventilation/perfusion
SVG	saphenous vein graft		VSD	ventricular septal defect
SVT	supraventricular tachycardia		VT	ventricular tachycardia
T2DM	type 2 diabetes mellitus		WBC	white blood cell
TA	Takayasu's arteritis		WCT	wide complex tachycardia
TAA	thoracic aortic aneurysm		WG	Wegener's granulomatosis
TAPSF	tricuspid annular plane systolic excursion		WHO	World Health Organization
TB	tuberculosis		WPW	Wolff-Parkinson-White syndrome
TCA	tricyclic antidepressant		XL	extended release
TDI	tissue Doppler imaging			
TdP	torsades de pointes			

List of contributors

Walter Ageno
Department of Clinical Medicine, University of Insubria,
Varese, Italy

Manuel J. Antunes
Department of Cardiothoracic Surgery,
University of Coimbra, Portugal

Paul W. Armstrong
University of Alberta, Edmonton, Alberta, Canada

Sameer Ather
Department of Medicine, Baylor College of Medicine,
Houston, USA

George L. Bakris
University of Chicago Pritzker School of Medicine,
Chicago, USA

Ragavendra R. Baliga
Ohio State University Hospital East, Columbus,
and The Ohio State University, USA

Jeroen J. Bax
Department of Cardiology, Leiden University Medical
Center, The Netherlands

David Benditt
University of Minnesota Cardiac Arrhythmia Center,
Minneapolis, USA

Karen Blair
Department of Health, Wellbeing and Family
Canterbury Christchurch University-Medway Campus,
Chatham Maritime, Kent, UK

Rutger J. van Bommel
Department of Cardiology, Leiden University Medical
Center, The Netherlands

Philipp Bonhoeffer
Cardiac Catheter Laboratory, Great Ormond Street
Hospital for Children, London, UK

Robert S. Bonser
Department of Cardiothoracic Surgery, Queen Elizabeth
Hospital, Edgbaston, Birmingham, UK

Michele Brignole
Ospedale Tilgullio, Lavagna, Italy

Alida Caforio
Department of Cardiological, Thoracic and Vascular
Sciences, University of Padua, Italy

John L. Caplin
Hull and East Yorkshire Hospitals NHS Trust, Castle Hill
Hospital, Hull, UK

Thierry P. Carrel
Director and Head of Cardiovascular Surgery,
Swiss Cardiovascular Centre, Division of Cardiovascular
Surgery, University Hospital of Bern, Switzerland

David Carruthers
City Hospital, Sandwell and West Birmingham Hospitals
Trust, Birmingham, UK

Stefan Cash
Department of Child Health,
Birmingham City University, UK

John B. Chambers
Guy's and St Thomas' Hospitals, London, UK

Bernard M.Y. Cheung
Division of Clinical Pharmacology and Therapeutics,
Department of Medicine, University of Hong Kong, China

Andrew L. Clark
Hull York Medical School in the University of Hull,
Castle Hill Hospital, UK

John G.F. Cleland
Hull York Medical School, University of Hull,
East Riding of Yorkshire, UK

Andrew J. Stewart Coats
University of East Anglia, Norwich, UK

Louise Coats
Freeman Hospital, Newcastle upon Tyne, UK

Derek T. Connelly
Glasgow Royal Infirmary and Golden Jubilee National
Hospital, UK

Filippo Crea
Department of Cardiovascular Medicine,
Catholic University of the Sacred Heart, Rome, Italy

L. Ceri Davies
Barts and the London NHS Trust, UK

Diego F. Davila
Instituto de Investigaciones Cardiovasculares,
Universidad de Los Andes, Venezuela

François Delahaye
Cardiology A Unit, Hôpital Louis Pradel, Bron Cedex,
France

Victoria Delgado
Department of Cardiology, Leiden University Medical
Center, The Netherlands

Mario C. Deng
Columbia University Medical Center, New York, USA

Francesco Dentali
Department of Clinical Medicine, University of Insubria,
Varese, Italy

W. Florian Dick
Swiss Cardiovascular Centre, Division of Cardiovascular
Surgery, University and University Hospital of Bern,
Switzerland

Michael Donnally
Division of Cardiovascular Medicine, The Ohio State University Medical Center, Columbus, Ohio

Vamsidhar Dronavalli
Department of Cardiovascular Medicine, University of Birmingham

Kim A. Eagle
Cardiovascular Center, University of Michigan Health System, Ann Arbor, USA

Lars Eckardt
Department of Cardiology and Angiology University Hospital Münster, Germany

Perry Elliot
Department of Cardiovascular Medicine, UCL Medical School, London, UK

Judith Ellis MBE
Faculty of Health & Social Care, London South Bank University, UK

Gerasimos Filippatos
Heart Failure Unit, Department of Cardiology, Athens University Hospital Attikon, Greece

Adam P. Fitzpatrick
Manchester Heart Centre MRI, UK

Lee A. Fleisher
Department of Anesthesiology and Critical Care, Hospital of the University of Pennsylvania, Philadelphia, USA

Keith A.A. Fox
Centre for Cardiovascular Science, Edinburgh, UK

Michael Frenneaux
Institute of Medical Sciences, University of Aberdeen, UK

Matteo Galli
Department of Clinical Medicine, University of Insubria, Varese, Italy

Naveen Garg
Department of Cardiology, Sanjay Gandhi Post Graduate Institute of Medical Sciences, Lucknow, India

Scott Garg
Department of Cardio-Vascular-Respiratory Medicine, University of Hull, UK

M.A. Gatzoulis
National Heart and Lung Institute, Imperial College of Science and Medicine, London, UK

Jacob George
Centre for Cardiovascular & Lung Biology, University of Dundee, UK

Tony Gershlick
University Hospitals of Leicester, UK

Ehud Grossman,
The Chaim Sheba Medical Center, Tel Hashomer, Israel and
Sackler faculty of medicine, Tel Aviv University, Israel

Peter Groves
University Hospital of Wales, Cardiff, UK

Sampath Gunda
Department of Medicine, Cardiovascular Division, Section of Vascular Medicine, University of Pennsylvania, USA

Stephan von Haehling
Applied Cachexia Research, Department of Cardiology, Charité Medical School, Berlin, Germany

Jo-Jo Hai
Cardiology Division, Department of Medicine, Queen Mary Hospital, The University of Hong Kong, Hong Kong

David Hare
Austin Health and Northern Health, University of Melbourne, Australia

James Harrison
Imperial College Healthcare NHS Trust, London, UK

Benji Heran
Research Fellow (Cochrane Heart Group), Health Services Research and Peninsula Clinical Trials Unit, Peninsula College of Medicine & Dentistry, University of Exeter, UK

Steven M. Hollenberg
Robert Wood Johnson Medical School, University of Medicine and Dentistry of New Jersey and
Coronary Care Unit, Cooper University Hospital, Camden, USA

Shunichi Homma
Columbia University Medical Center, New York, USA

Ross Hunter
Cardiology Research Department, Barts and The London NHS Trust, St Bartholomew's Hospital, London, UK

Syed Ahmed Hussain
Department of Medicine, Cardiovascular Division, Section of Vascular Medicine, University of Pennsylvania, USA

Graham Jackson
Guys and St Thomas Hospitals, London, UK

Elizabeth Justice
City Hospital, Sandwell and West Birmingham Hospitals Trust, Birmingham, UK

Paulus Kirchhof
Department of Cardiology and Angiology, IZKF Münster, AFNET, University Hospital Münster, Germany

K. von Klemperer
Adult Congenital Heart Centre and Centre for Pulmonary Hypertension, Royal Brompton Hospital, London, UK

Bradley P. Knight
Bluhm Cardiovascular Institute of Northwestern, Feinberg School of Medicine, Northwestern University, Chicago, USA

Lucia J.M. Kroft
Department of Radiology, Leiden University Medical
Center, The Netherlands

Uwe Kühl
Medical Clinic II, Department of Cardiology and
Pneumology, University Medicine Berlin, Germany

Elena Ladich
CVPath Institute, Inc, Gaithersburg, USA

Seema Lalani
Department of Molecular and Human Genetics,
Baylor College of Medicine, Houston, USA

Gaetano Lanza
Department of Cardiovascular Medicine,
Catholic University of the Sacred Heart, Rome, Italy

Chu-Pak Lau
Cardiology Division, Department of Medicine,
Queen Mary Hospital, The University of Hong Kong,
Hong Kong

Wai-Ting Nicola Lee
Scottish Pulmonary Vascular Unit, Golden Jubilee
National Hospital, Glasgow, UK

Gregory Y.H. Lip
University of Birmingham, Centre for Cardiovascular
Sciences, City Hospital, Birmingham, UK

Robert J. MacFadyen
University of Birmingham, Centre for Cardiovascular
Sciences, City Hospital, Birmingham, UK

Gillian Manning
School of Graduate Entry Medicine & Health,
University of Nottingham, UK

Francisco Marín
Cardiology Department, Hospital Universitario Virgen de
la Arrixaca, Murci, Spain

Thomas H. Marwick
Center for Cardiovascular Imaging, Cleveland Clinic,
Ohio, USA

Gerald Maurer
Division of Cardiology, Medical University of Vienna,
Austria

Franz H. Messerli
Columbia University College of Physicians and Surgeons,
Division of Cardiology, St. Luke's-Roosevelt Hospital,
New York, USA

Evy Micieli
Department of Clinical Medicine, University of Insubria,
Varese, Italy

Emile R. Mohler
Department of Medicine, Cardiovascular Division,
Section of Vascular Medicine,
University of Pennsylvania, USA

Gerold Mönnig
Department of Cardiology and Angiology
University Hospital Münster, Germany

John Morgan
Wessex Cardiac Centre,
Southampton University Hospital, UK

Angel Moya
Val d'Hebron Hospital, Barcelona, Spain

Christopher Munsch
Yorkshire Heart Centre, Leeds General Infirmary, UK

Sunil Nadar
Heart of England NHS Trust, Birmingham, UK

Jerry Nolan
Royal United Hospital, Bath, UK

Raymond Oliva
University of Chicago Pritzker School of Medicine,
Chicago, USA

John T. Parissis
University of Athens and Attikon General Hospital,
Heart Failure Clinic and Second Cardiology Department,
Athens, Greece

Andrew Peacock
Scottish Pulmonary Vascular Unit, Regional Heart and
Lung Centre, Golden Jubilee National Hospital,
Glasgow, UK

Jill Pell
University of Glasgow, Centre of Population Health
Sciences, Glasgow, UK

John Pepper
Imperial College, Royal Brompton Hospital, London

Sanjiv Petkar
Central Manchester and Manchester Children's University
Hospitals NHS Trust, UK

Henry Purcell
Royal Brompton Hospital, London, UK

Bernard Prendergast
John Radcliffe Hospital, Oxford, UK

Giovanni V. Riva
Welsh Ambulance Service NHS Trust,
South East Region, Wales

Giuseppe M.C. Rosano
Department of Medical Science, IRCCS San Raffaele,
Roma, Italy

John Sanderson
Department of Cardiology, University Hospital of
North Staffordshire NHS Trust, City General Hospital,
Stoke-on-Trent

Luca Santini
Division of Cardiology, Policlinico Tor Vergata,
University of Rome, Italy

Massimo Santini
Division of Cardiology, Policlinico Tor Vergata,
University of Rome, Italy

Michael Schachter
Imperial College London (National Heart and Lung
Institute and International Centre for Circulatory Health),
St Mary's Hospital, London, UK

Richard Schilling
Cardiology Research Department, Barts and
The London NHS Trust, St Bartholomew's Hospital,
London, UK

Joanne D. Schuijf
Department of Cardiology, Leiden University
Medical Center, The Netherlands

Heinz-Peter Schultheiss
Department of Cardiology and Pneumology,
University Medicine Berlin, Germany

Victor Serebruany
Division of Neurology, Johns Hopkins University,
Baltimore, USA

Patrick Serruys
Thoraxcentre, Erasmus Medical Centre, Rotterdam,
The Netherlands

Melchior Seyfarth
Universität Witten-Herdecke, HELIOS Klinikum
Wuppertal/Herzzentrum, Wuppertal, Germany

Dipak Shah
University of Chicago, Chicago, USA

Chung Wah David Siu
Cardiology Division, Department of Medicine,
The University of Hong Kong, Queen Mary Hospital,
Hong Kong

Hannah Solomon
Royal Cornwall Hospital Treliske, Cornwall, UK

Simon Stewart
Preventative Health, Baker IDI Heart and Diabetes
Institute, Melbourne, Australia

Allan D. Struthers
University of Dundee, Ninewells Hospital & Medical
School, UK

Alessandro Squizzato
Department of Clinical Medicine,
University of Insubria, Varese, Italy

Richard Sutton
St Mary's Hospital, Imperial College and Imperial
Healthcare NHS Trust, London, UK

Yu-ting Tan
Department of Cardiovascular Medicine,
University of Birmingham, Birmingham, United Kingdom

Rod Taylor
Health Services Research and Peninsula Clinical Trials
Unit, Peninsula College of Medicine & Dentistry,
University of Exeter, UK

G. Neil Thomas
School of Health and Population Sciences,
The University of Birmingham, Edgbaston, UK

David R. Thompson
Cardiovascular Research Centre, Australian Catholic
University/University of Melbourne, Australia

Sara Thorne
Queen Elizabeth Hospital, Birmingham, UK

Adam Timmis
Department of Cardiology, London Chest Hospital, UK

Michael C. Tjandrawidjaja
University of Alberta, Edmonton, Alberta, Canada

Hung-Fat Tse
Cardiology Division, Department of Medicine,
Li Ka Shing Faculty of Medicine, The University of
Hong Kong, Hong Kong

Marco R. Di Tullio
Columbia University Medical Center, New York, USA

Kristina Wasmer
Department of Cardiology and Angiology University
Hospital Münster, Germany

Xander H.T. Wehrens
Department of Molecular Physiology and Biophysics, and
Medicine, Baylor College of Medicine
Houston, USA

Frans Van de Werf
University of Leuven, University Hospital Gasthuisberg,
Belgium

Stephen Westaby
Oxford Heart Center, John Radcliffe Hospital, Oxford, UK

Harvey White
Green Lane Cardiovascular Services, Cardiovascular
Research Unit, Auckland City Hospital, Auckland,
New Zealand

Petr Widimsky
Cardiocenter, University Hospital Vinohrady, 3rd Medical
School, Charles University, Prague, Czech Republic

Anthony S. Wierzbicki
King's College, London and
Guy's & St Thomas' Hospitals, London, UK

Robert George Wilcox
Department of Cardiovascular Medicine,
Nottingham University Hospitals NHS Trust, UK

Lynne Williams
College of Medical and Dental Sciences,
University of Birmingham, UK

Joanna Wykrzykowska
MD, Boston, USA

Renu Virmani
CVPath Institute, Inc, Gaithersburg, USA

Han B. Xiao
Homerton University Hospital, London, UK

Yee Guan Yap
Prince Court Medical Centre, Kuala Lumpur, Malaysia

Kai-Hang Yiu
Cardiology Division, Department of Medicine, Queen
Mary Hospital, The University of Hong Kong, Hong Kong

Yuen-Fung Yiu
Cardiology Division, Department of Medicine,
Queen Mary Hospital, The University of Hong Kong,
Hong Kong

Mehmood Zeb
Wessex Cardiac Centre, Southampton University
Hospital, UK

Chapter 1

Introduction

Cardiac history and examination

Accurate history taking and clinical examination is the bedrock of successful diagnosis and treatment. The twin errors of missing a crucial diagnosis or over-investigating and/or over-treating a patient are some of the most serious errors a cardiologist can make.

History taking

History taking will determine the eventual diagnosis in more than two-thirds of unselected cases. Crucially it is also the means of detecting where serious heart disease is unlikely and expensive unnecessary investigation and concern to the patient can be avoided.

The referral letter

Crucial features

- Who is it from? Does the referring doctor know the patient or his/her family well, and hence does he/she have insight into their past medical and family history, their history of similar complaints in the past and their likelihood to complain of minor symptoms. Knowledge of these features will indicate how much one can depend on the information given. A clear history given by a reliable medical source may allow some testing to be organized before the first consultation and/or the urgency of the appointment to be determined.
- Does it give reliable evidence of previous specialist investigation or diagnoses which can be used to fast-track the patient to a more advanced stage of diagnostic testing?

The background history

Who gives it?

Sometimes even for an adult patient the history may need to come from a friend or relative instead of the patient, i.e. where there are language difficulties or there is an involved carer. In these cases it is important to also ask, if possible, the patient directly as the answers to such questions as 'How bad is the pain or breathlessness?' may be quite revealingly different between the patient and the carer.

Crucial features

- Past medical history: you should seek information on previous operations, significant medical illnesses (those that have for example required admission to hospital) and regular medication (prescription and over the counter) both cardiac and non-cardiac. This helps set the tone of the consultation and makes you aware of the background health and medical experiences of the patient.
- Family history: this needs to cover known inherited conditions, such as certain cardiomyopathies, arrhythmias, connective tissue diseases and hyperlipidaemias as well as giving an overall cardiac risk estimate for the patient. It is useful to ask for the cause of death and age at death for all first-degree relatives who have died as well as specifically asking for family members who have suffered heart attack, stroke, diabetes, thyroid disease, high blood pressure (BP) or abnormal blood lipids requiring treatment.
- Medication history and allergies: necessary for assessing drug-induced problems as well as for planning potential therapy.
- Social history: knowledge of the degree of local support and social circumstances will be useful for planning assessment and treatment options. Also include occupational history for particular risks such as asbestos exposure, exercise habit, overseas travel for rarer infections, IV drug use in the past as risk factor for infective endocarditis.
- Drug and alcohol use: may be important for cardiomyopathies, risks of infective endocarditis and as an exacerbating factor for hypertension and angina.

The symptom history

The series of questions depends on the initial complaint. Features which need to be determined are time of onset, progression, precipitating and relieving factors, associated features. It is important to ask about other cardiac symptoms even if they were not the presenting symptom.

Specific symptoms (see also specific sections in Chapter 2)

- Chest pain: onset, precipitating factors, predictability, duration, location, radiation of pain, detailed description (burning, crushing, pressing, sharp, dull?), intensity (using a scale out of 10 is helpful).
- Dyspnoea: relate to activities of daily life that patients are familiar with, such as stair climbing, dressing, getting out of chair; determine onset, progression, predictability, precipitating or relieving factors; associated features such as chest pain, palpitations, dizziness, wheeze, cough.
- Palpitation: ask patient to tap it out as the fastest way to determine, rate, regularity, etc.; ask about date of onset, progression, frequency, duration, precipitating and relieving factors, e.g. relationship to alcohol, exercise, coffee, or tea.
- Syncope: try to differentiate between syncope preceded by dizziness (suggesting hypotension) and unexpected drop attacks (suggesting Stokes–Adams attacks), and syncope with muscle or neurological symptoms (epilepsy) that was precipitated by head or neck movements (vertebro-basilar insufficiency).
- Oedema: ask how long it has been occurring, what it is associated with (e.g. diet, menstrual cycle).

Clinical examination

Although there is a standard minimum examination for a proper cardiovascular assessment, further detailed examination may be indicated if the history raises particular diagnostic possibilities, such as certain provocation tests to diagnose some congenital heart lesions or arrhythmias or hypertrophic cardiomyopathy for an outflow tract murmur. Reference is made to the specific chapters for individual cardiac disorders for these specialist clinical examinations for specific conditions.

Observation

Crucial features

- State of nutrition: for cachexia as end-stage of heart failure or as risk factor for nutritional cardiomyopathies and obesity for metabolic syndrome.
- Skin colour: jaundice in liver congestion, paleness of anaemia, slate grey of haemochromatosis, central cyanosis in right to left heart shunt associated congenital heart disease.
- Nails: clubbing in some congenital heart disease, subacute infective endocarditis (SBE), koilonychia in iron deficiency, splinter haemorrhages in SBE.

- Palms: erythema in liver disease.
- Nodding head of severe aortic regurgitation.
- Observation of jugular venous pulsation (JVP): for heart failure, pulmonary hypertension, tricuspid regurgitation. 'A' waves are increased in pulmonary hypertension and tricuspid stenosis. Giant 'A' waves (Cannon waves) are seen in atrioventricular dissociation or occasionally when right ventricular (RV) paced. 'V' waves increased in tricuspid regurgitation. 'X' descent is steep in cardiac tamponade. 'Y' descent is abrupt in effective poor RV compliance (e.g. restrictive myopathy or constrictive pericarditis).
- Observation of breathing (at rest on an getting undressed and onto bed): for undue use of accessory breathing muscles, respiratory rate and pattern (Cheyne–Stokes or periodic breathing common in heart failure).
- Chest wall: visible cardiac pulsation indicating cardiac enlargement, RV heave of RV hypertrophy/failure.

Palpation

Crucial features

- Pulse: feel at radial for rhythm, rate symmetrical nature on both sides and for radio-femoral delay (indicative of coarctation). Feel at carotid and/or brachial for character, e.g. collapsing (see Chapter 7.6, Aortic regurgitation), slow rising (see Chapter 7.7, Aortic stenosis).
- Chest wall: for respiratory expansion (?symmetrical, if not unilateral lung disease likely), for apex beat and character (displaced in left ventricular hypertrophy (LVH), left ventricular (LV) enlargement, tapping in mitral stenosis; see Chapter 7.4, Mitral stenosis), for RV heave in right heart overload, e.g. right to left shunt, pulmonary hypertension.
- Over heart: effectively indicate a high-intensity heart murmur.
- Oedema detection: look for pitting oedema at ankles, or sacrum if bed bound.
- Liver edge for hepatic congestion of right heart failure.
- Spleen edge palpable if enlarged.
- Feel for enlarged ballotable kidneys in polycystic disease.

Percussion

- To detect pulmonary effusion, cardiac enlargement or pneumothorax and differential diagnosis for chest pain and dyspnoea.

Auscultation

Where to listen

- Listen over arteries for bruits and shunts.
- Chest wall: listen in aortic, mitral pulmonary and tricuspid areas for best determination of murmurs. Use augmentation strategies, e.g. ask patient to breathe out and stop while leaning forward to accentuate aortic murmurs.
- Over lungs for signs of congestion (crackles which do not clear with coughing) as opposed to infection (crackles which may clear after coughing), pericardial effusion (may have scratchy rubbing sound, like walking on dry snow) or pulmonary effusion (diminished breath sounds).
- Back of chest for collateral vessels in coarctation.

Heart murmurs (see Fig. 1.1.1)

- Murmurs can be graded by intensity (on a six-point scale) and described in terms of location over the heart, timing in the cardiac cycle, intensity over time, nature, e.g. crescendo, decrescendo, or crescendo-decrescendo, and

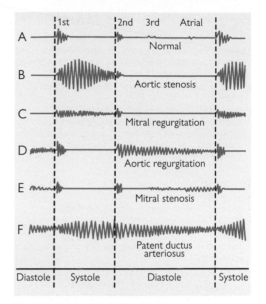

Fig. 1.1.1 Murmurs. See also Plate 1.

radiation of the murmur, pitch (high pitch best heard by diaphragm, low by bell) and quality (such as blowing, harsh, rumbling or musical).

- Ejection systolic murmur: in aortic area, accentuated by leaning forward, late crescendo murmur, can have soft A2: aortic stenosis. Differential includes dynamic left ventricular outflow tract murmur in hypertrophic cardiomyopathy more obvious after Valsalva manoeuvre, late systolic murmur; in pulmonary area louder on inspiration: pulmonary stenosis.
- Pansystolic murmur: can be mitral regurgitation (louder on expiration), tricuspid regurgitation (louder on inspiration or ventricular septal defect (usually harsh sound).
- Holosystolic (or machinery murmur loudest upper left sternal edge indicative of patent ductus).
- Early diastolic murmur: loudest in aortic area on expiration with collapsing pulse = aortic regurgitation.
- Mid-systolic murmur in mitral area or with late diastolic augmentation if in sinus rhythm and louder if patient lies of left side—mitral stenosis (may have associated opening snap), on right sternal edge if augmented by inspiration if right atrial enlargement suspected by electrocardiogram (ECG) or JVP characteristics might be tricuspid stenosis.
- Late systolic (seagull cry quality): suggests mitral valve prolapse
- Manoeuvres to augment murmurs: squatting increases afterload and can increase the intensity of mitral valve prolapse murmur; inspiration makes second pulmonary sound later and can accentuate right heart murmurs, Valsalva makes LV cavity smaller and can accentuate LV outflow tract murmurs, exercise increases blood flow therefore useful to make quiet murmurs, e.g. mitral stenosis louder; positioning on the left to make left-sided murmurs louder.

Heart sounds

- S1 and S2—are the first and second sounds normal? Second sound is split into A2 and P2; loud P2 indicates pulmonary hypertension, absent A2 in severe aortic stenosis.

- A2 usually occurs before P2. Widely split S2 may indicate right bundle branch block or secundum atrial septal defect (fixed splitting which does not vary as usual with inspiration/expiration cycle).
- Reverse split S2 may indicate left bundle branch block (LBBB).
- Extra heart sounds (or gallop rhythm): if rhythm like 'Kentucky' = S3 may occur in young people who are nervous because of high flow or due to increased filling pressure in LV failure, if like 'Tennessee' = S4 often means volume overload or LV failure, if both = summation gallop.

Other sounds
- Opening snap: in mitral stenosis.
- Mid-systolic click: suggests mitral valve prolapse.
- Diastolic knock: at time of S3 but louder, and more thudding, indicates non-compliant, constricting pericardium.
- Pericardial rub: like walking on dry snow, suggests pericarditis.

Other measurements

Blood pressure
- Should be measured with patient supine (and standing and measure postural drop, less than 10 mmHg is normal).
- Patient should be rested and BP should be measured at least three times to take average reading because of high variability.
- Semi-automated machines are accurate and patient self-monitoring (or 24-hour BP monitoring can give lower values because of 'white coat' effect).
- Pulsus paradoxus: if BP on inspiration is more than 10 mmHg lower than on expiration can indicate cardiac tamponade, constrictive pericarditis, severe asthma, chronic obstructive pulmonary disease, restrictive cardiomyopathy or pulmonary embolism.

Special manoeuvres

See also previous sections.
- Valsalva manoeuvre: to detect hypertrophic cardiomyopathy (HCM)-related outflow tract murmur.
- Squatting: increases afterload and reduces venous return; reduces outflow tract murmur of HCM and augments murmurs of aortic regurgitation, aortic stenosis, mitral valve prolapse, and mitral regurgitation and diastolic murmur of mitral stenosis.
- Dilators such as amyl nitrite: decreases afterload and increases outflow tract murmur of HCM.

Electrocardiogram

Electrocardiogram (ECG) is the most commonly performed investigation in cardiovascular medicine. Almost all patients will have an ECG at hospitalization. It may help to diagnose life-threatening emergencies (e.g. acute coronary syndrome), guide subsequent management, and monitor the disease progression. Therefore, it is important for every physician to understand the principle and interpretation of ECG.

Electrical properties of the heart
- The sinoatrial node initiates atrial depolarization.
- Impulse propagates to the atrioventricular node and is then conducted to the ventricles via the bundle of His and then Purkinje fibres.
- The bundle of His is divided into the left and right bundle branch. The left bundle branch further divides into the anterior and posterior hemifascicles.
- During cardiac depolarization and repolarization, electro-ionic changes that take place in the myocardial cells can be recorded on the body surface by electrodes. An ECG is recorded from two or more electrodes.
- A depolarization wave moving towards the positive electrode will be shown as a upward (positive) deflection in the ECG, while a depolarization wave moving away from the positive electrode will result in a downward (negative) deflection.
- The resultant waveform displayed is the vector sum of all depolarization and repolarization potentials of all cardiomyocytes.

Basic concepts
Calibrations
- The ECG is recorded at a rate of 25 mm/s.
- The paper consists of big squares of 5-mm width, each big square is made up of 5 × 5 small squares of 1-mm width.

- Horizontally, each small square is equivalent to 0.04 s and each big square 0.2 s.
- Vertically, each small square is equivalent to 0.1 mV and each big square is equivalent to 0.5 mV.

Leads
- A standard ECG should consist of a total of 12 leads: six standard (limb) leads and six chest leads.
- By comparing specific electrodes, each lead 'views' the heart from a different angle and creates a different electrical picture of the heart.
- The positions for placing electrodes are listed in Table 1.2.1.
- Anatomically, leads can be grouped by the cardiac structures which they look at (Table 1.2.2).

Components
A number of deflections should be present in most leads of a standard ECG. They are called waves and were named arbitrarily as P, Q, R, S, T, and U. They represent different parts of electrical conduction in a cardiac cycle.
- P wave: the result of atrial depolarization
- QRS complex: collectively includes the Q, R, and S waves and represents the electrical activity in ventricular depolarization. The three waves are not always present
- Q wave: any initial negative deflection
- R wave: any positive deflection
- S wave: any negative deflection following R wave
- T wave: represents ventricular repolarization
- U wave: origin is unclear, may represent repolarization of the mid-myocardial cells
- PR interval: from the beginning of the P wave to the beginning of the QRS complex. Represents the conduction through the atrioventricular node and the His–Purkinje system.

Table 1.2.1 Location of electrodes and lead connections for a standard 12-lead ECG

Lead	Positive input	Negative input
I	LA	RA
II	LL	RA
III	LL	LA
aVR	RA	LA plus LL
aVL	LA	RA plus LL
aVF	LL	LA plus RA
V1	Right sternal margin, 4th ICS	Average of (LA+RA+LL)
V2	Left sternal margin, 4th ICS	Average of (LA+RA+LL)
V3	Midway between V2 and V4	Average of (LA+RA+LL)
V4	Left midclavicular line, 5th ICS	Average of (LA+RA+LL)
V5	Left anterior axillary line 5th ICS	Average of (LA+RA+LL)
V6	Left midaxillary line, 5th ICS	Average of (LA+RA+LL)

ICS, intercostal space; LA, left arm; LL, left leg; RA, right arm.

Table 1.2.2 Anatomical relations of leads in a 12-lead ECG

Leads	Represented cardiac structures
II, III, aVF	Inferior surface of the heart
V1–V2	The right ventricle
V3–V4	The septum and anterior wall of left ventricle
I, aVL, V5–V6	The lateral surface of the heart
V1 and aVR	The right atrium and cavity of left ventricle

- ST segment: between the end of the QRS complex and onset of T wave. Represents the period between end of ventricular depolarization and the beginning of repolarization.
- QT interval: from onset of QRS to end of T wave. Represents the total time taken for ventricular depolarization and repolarization.

Interpretation of an ECG

Rate
- The rate in a normal individual should be less than 100 bpm and greater than 60 bpm (or 50 bpm during sleep).
- A rate that is too fast is termed tachycardia. A rate that is too slow is termed bradycardia.
- If the QRS complexes are regular, the rate can be calculated as 300/number of large squares between two consecutive R waves. For example, if there are four large squares in between two R waves, the rate is 300/4 = 75 bpm.
- If the rhythm is irregular, rate can be calculated as 6 times number of R waves in 10 s (the usual duration of a standard ECG).

Rhythm
- Rhythm refer to the part of the heart that is controlling the activation sequence.
- 'Sinus rhythm' is a term used when the rhythm is originated from the sinoatrial node and conducted to the ventricles.
- The P wave should be positive in I, II, aVF, V2–V6; positive or biphasic (+/−) in III and V1; positive of biphasic (−/+) in aVL, negative in aVR.

Cardiac axis
- The cardiac axis represents the direction of the vector sum of ventricular depolarization.
- The angle that lead I views the heart is used as the reference point 0°.
- The normal axis should be located between −30° and +90°. An axis lying beyond −30° is termed left axis deviation and that lying beyond +90° is termed right axis deviation.
- Lead I, II, and aVF can be used to determine the cardiac axis. In an ECG with a normal axis, the QRS complex in leads I and II should be positive while that in aVF can be positive or negative.

P wave
- P waves are best seen at leads II and V1.
- The first half represents the right atrium while the later half represents the left atrium.

- P waves should be upright in most leads except aVR and are commonly biphasic (+/−) in V1.
- A normal P wave should have duration of less than 0.12 s and amplitude less than 0.3 mV.
- Abnormalities of P waves may signify disease in the atria.

PR interval
- The normal duration of the PR segment is 3–5 small squares (0.12–0.20 s).
- A long or changing PR interval may be signs of diseases in the conducting system. A short PR interval may represent pre-excitation.
- Horizontally, each small square is equivalent to 0.04 s and each big square 0.2 s.
- The PR segment (between the P wave and the QRS complex) should be isoelectrical. It may also be depressed in pathological conditions, e.g. pericarditis.

QRS complex
- The duration in the lead with widest QRS complex should not exceed 0.12 s.
- Q waves in leads I, aVL, V5, and V6 can be normal, resulting from septal depolarization. The width of these septal Q waves should be less than 1 small square and the depth less than 1 small square wide and 25% of corresponding R wave amplitude.
- The height of R wave should increase from V1 to V6 but remain <25 mm in V5 and V6 in normal circumstances.
- The depth of S wave is greatest in the right chest leads but should not exceed 30 mm.

ST segment and T wave
- The ST segment should be isoelectrical in a normal ECG.
- Elevation or depression of the ST segment has a large variety of causes, including normal variant, cardiac ischaemia or infarct, pericarditis, etc.
- Normal T wave is asymmetrical. The height is commonly greater than one-eighth but less than two-thirds of the corresponding R wave amplitude.
- T wave is positive in all leads except aVR. Inversion of T wave may be a sign of myocardial ischaemia or secondary to other ECG changes, e.g. left ventricular hypertrophy.

QT interval
- QT interval should not exceed 0.44 s in male and 0.46 s in female. Prolonged QT interval is associated with increased risk of ventricular arrhythmia and sudden death.
- QT interval lengths when the heart rate decreases. Therefore, several formulas are used to calculate the QT interval corrected for heart rate (QTc).
- Fridericia's correction: QTc = QT/RR interval$^{1/3}$.
- Bazett's correction: QTc = QT/RR interval$^{1/2}$.
- We should be careful not to mistake a prominent U wave as a T wave and calculate a falsely prolonged QT interval.

Common abnormalities on ECG
Atrial enlargement (dilatation or hypertrophy)
- Left atrial enlargement: a late second peak in P wave in lead II, a large late negative deflection in P wave in lead V1.
- Right atrial enlargement: P wave height in lead II increase.

Ventricular enlargement
- Left ventricular enlargement: height of R wave in V5 or V6 plus depth of S wave in V1 >35 mm, or amplitude of R wave in V5 or V6 >25 mm.
- Right ventricular enlargement: right axis deviation, dominant R wave in V1, or R wave in V1 >7 mm.

Acute coronary syndrome (ACS)
- The evolution of ECG appearance in a complete coronary occlusion follows a specific sequence:
  1 hyperacute T wave: 5–30 minutes
  2 ST segment elevation: within hours
  3 loss or R wave height and development of pathological Q waves: 12–24 hours
  4 resolution of ST segment and inversion of T wave: up to weeks.
- ACS can be classified into ST segment elevation ACS (STE-ACS) and non-ST segment elevation ACS (NSTE-ACS). Fibrinolytic treatment is indicated in only patients with STE-ACS. Early treatment may prevent the development of a pathological Q wave.
- In STE-ACS, there is elevation of ST segment for more than 2 mm in V1 to V3 and more than 1 mm in other leads and ST segment is present in more than two anatomically contagious leads.
- In NSTE-ACS, the ST segment can be depressed. Other changes including T wave inversion or flattening may also be seen.
- Left bundle branch block makes interpretation of the ST segment difficult. However, in a patient with a previously normal ECG, a new-onset left bundle branch block is one of the diagnostic criteria for STE-ACS.

Pericarditis
- Often no change in ECG.
- Occasionally extensive concave upwards ST elevation in most leads, reflecting myocardial injury.
- Depression of the PR interval may also be seen.

Pulmonary embolism
- Often sinus tachycardia is the only ECG finding.
- In case of a large pulmonary embolus, acute right ventricular dilatation may occur and produce the classic S1,

Q3, T3 pattern: an S wave in lead I, and a Q wave and T wave inversion in lead III.
- Accompanied changes may include right bundle branch block and right axis deviation.

Tachyarrhythmias
- Classified as wide QRS complex tachycardia and narrow QRS complex tachycardia by whether the duration of QRS complex is prolonged.
- Narrow complex tachycardia is usually due to supraventricular tachycardia or junctional tachycardia. Wide complex tachycardia is usually of ventricular origin with the exception of supraventricular tachycardia with bundle branch block and atrial tachycardia with pre-excitation.

Atrioventricular blocks
- First-degree block: PR interval prolonged to >0.2 s.
- Second-degree block.
- Mobitz type I block: PR interval is initially normal but progressively lengthens until a P wave is not followed by a QRS complex and the whole cycle repeats (Wenckebach phenomenon).
- Mobitz type II block: intermittent failure of conduction of P waves, with constant PR interval.
- Third-degree block: complete failure of P wave conduction and the atrial and ventricular contraction are completely independent.
- First-degree and Mobitz type I block maybe found in normal individuals. Left atrial enlargement: a late second peak in P wave in lead II, a large late negative deflection in P wave in lead V1.

Further reading

Hampton JR. *The ECG made easy*, 7th edn. Edinburgh: Churchill Livingstone, 2008.

Meek S, Morris F. ABC of clinical electrocardiography. Introduction. I-Leads, rate, rhythm, and cardiac axis. *BMJ* 2002;**324**:415–8.

Meek S, Morris F. ABC of clinical electrocardiography. Introduction. II-Basic terminology. *BMJ* 2002;**324**:470–3.

de Luna AB, Batchvarov VN, Malik M. The morphology of the electrocardiogram. In: Camm AJ, Luscher TF, eds. *The ESC Textbook of Cardiovascular Medicine*. Malden–Oxford–Carlton: Blackwell, 2006.

Exercise testing

Exercise testing is an ubiquitous, cheap, and safe test, which is central to the assessment of cardiac patients. It has the potential to provide diagnostic and prognostic information.

While conventional exercise testing requires an electro-cardiogram (ECG) machine, treadmill (or exercise bike) and blood pressure (BP) monitoring, the procedure can be complicated (with the introduction of a metabolic cart) to assess metabolic exercise capacity or simplified to measure the 6-minute walk distance.

The disadvantages of exercise testing are the numerous contraindications to exercise, the difficulty in interpreting abnormal resting ECGs, and also some recent evidence that exercise testing has little incremental value over routine clinical assessment in patients in a Rapid Access Chest Pain environment (Sekhri et al. 2008).

The test

Exercise testing is most commonly performed with a treadmill that gradually increases in speed and gradient every 2–3 minutes. The Bruce protocol has been widely adopted but has been modified for patients unable to manage the treadmill speed and for those post myocardial infarction. There are other gentle treadmill exercise protocols such as the Naughton.

In those unable to exercise on a treadmill, a bicycle ergometer can be used with a gradual increase in workload (e.g. 10- or 25-W increments).

Supervision of exercise tests is normally performed by appropriately trained physiologists or nurses, but physicians should be present for high-risk patients. Resuscitation equipment must always be available in the exercise room.

Patients can be asked to withhold medication (especially beta-blockers) prior to testing. The need for this will depend on the clinical reason for the test (e.g. diagnostic, symptomatic assessment, vocational assessment).

All patients should undergo a history and examination before exercise testing to ensure there are no significant contraindications.

During the test, there is continuous 12-lead ECG monitoring and frequent BP measurements are taken.

Indications

- Diagnosis of ischaemic heart disease (IHD)
- Evaluation of arrhythmias
- Assessment of exertional symptoms
- Risk stratification post myocardial infarct
- Risk stratification in patients with hypertrophic cardiomyopathy
- Diagnostic and prognostic assessment in heart failure
- Vocational assessment.

Contraindications

- Unstable ischaemic heart disease
- Fever/acute viral illness
- Myocarditis
- Severe aortic stenosis
- Aortic dissection
- Uncontrolled hypertension (>200/120)
- Overt heart failure
- Deep vein thrombosis
- Inability to exercise.

Safety

Exercise testing is generally considered extremely safe, but the potential for complications will depend to a certain extent on the population being tested. The rate of complications in a population with little coronary artery disease is around 0.8 in 10 000 tests. In contrast, the rate of complications in a population with malignant ventricular arrhythmias can be as high as 23 in 10 000 tests.

Stopping the test

Ideally, an exercise test should last around 9 minutes with the aim of a diagnostic test being to reach the target heart rate (85% of 220 (210 for women) minus the patient age). The development of significant ECG changes (severe ST depression, ST elevation and arrhythmias), severe symptoms (both cardiological and neurological), or changes in BP (a fall of >20 mmHg or hypertension) should lead to early termination of the test. ECG and BP monitoring needs to be continued after the end of exercise as abnormalities may occur at this stage.

Interpretation

ECG changes

There are a number of normal ECG changes that can occur during exercise. They include an increase in P wave height, a decrease in R wave height, and depression of the J point (the point of inflection at the junction of the S wave and ST segment) with an accompanying up-sloping ST segment.

By convention, ST segment shift is measured 60–80 ms after the J point (depending on heart rate), relative to the isoelectric baseline.

Abnormal ECG changes are horizontal or down-sloping ST depression of >1 mm and ST elevation of >1 mm. T wave changes such as inversion (or reversion) that occur during exercise are non-specific and do not carry the same significance as ST segment shifts.

ECG interpretation is difficult in the presence of an abnormal resting ECG (e.g. left bundle branch block, ST depression, digoxin use) and for the diagnosis of IHD, other diagnostic techniques are recommended.

Diagnosis

For the diagnosis of IHD, exercise testing has a sensitivity of 78% and a specificity of 70%. However, the ability to successfully interpret the results of exercise tests relies on an understanding of Bayes theorem. This theory has been used to relate the predictive ability of a diagnostic test to the pre-test probability of a patient actually having the disease.

As an example, a patient with a pre-test probability of IHD of 90% who has 2-mm ST segment depression during exercise testing has a post-test probability of IHD of 99%. A patient in a low pre-test group (5% probability of IHD) with the same exercise test findings will have a post-test probability of only 50%. The group in which exercise testing is most useful is those patients with an intermediate probability of IHD. Using the same exercise test results as before, a 30% pre-test probability jumps to 90% (Rifkin and Hood 1977).

Risk assessment

After myocardial infarction (not in those who have received percutaneous coronary intervention), exercise test predictors of adverse outcome include ST segment depression >1 mm, particularly if at a low level of exercise, or in the presence of compensated heart failure; functional capacity <5 METs (metabolic equivalent); inadequate BP response (peak systolic BP <110 mmHg or <30 mmHg rise from resting level).

In patients with hypertrophic cardiomyopathy a hypotensive or flat BP response to exercise is considered a risk factor for sudden death in patients under the age of 40 years.

Vocational testing

In the UK, holders of vocational licences with cardiovascular disease need to satisfy certain exercise test criteria on a regular basis (every 3 years). The requirements for IHD are to reach the end of Stage III of the Bruce protocol without significant symptoms or ECG changes while remaining off anti-anginal medication for at least 48 hours.

Full details can be found at www.dvla.org.

Screening exercise tests may also be required for amateur and professional pilots.

Cardiopulmonary exercise testing (CPEX)

The addition of a metabolic cart (measuring ventilation, oxygen and carbon dioxide concentrations) to standard exercise testing equipment allows for metabolic exercise testing. The most useful values obtained are peak oxygen consumption (pVO_2), carbon dioxide production (VCO_2), the ratio between VCO_2 and VO_2 (respiratory exchange ratio, RER) and the gradient of the line relating ventilation to VCO_2 (VE/VCO_2 slope).

Patients with heart failure typically have a low pVO_2 (with an RER >1) and a high VE/VCO_2 slope. Patients with respiratory disease may show a low VO_2 (but with an RER <1, indicating termination of exercise before limitation of aerobic exercise capacity), a high VE/VCO_2 slope and desaturation.

A pVO_2 <14 mL/kg/min has been used as a cut-off to identify patients who may benefit from cardiac transplantation.

Both pVO_2 and VE/VCO_2 slopes are among the most powerful prognostic markers in ambulant patients with chronic heart failure.

CPEX testing can also been used in the anaesthetic preassessment of patients undergoing major surgery to predict their postoperative requirements.

6-minute walk test

Patients are asked to walk as far as they can (at their own pace) for 6 minutes and the total distance covered is measured. The test has reasonable reproducibility, correlates with pVO_2 and has prognostic value in heart failure.

Its ease and low cost make it an attractive test and a number of recent device trials in heart failure have used it as a study endpoint.

References

Rifkin R, Hood W. Bayesian analysis of electrocardiographic exercise stress testing. *N Engl J Med* 1977;**297**:264.

Sekhri N, Feder G, Junghans C, *et al.* Incremental prognostic value of the exercise electrocardiogram in the initial assessment of patients with suspected angina: cohort study. *BMJ* 2008;**337**:a2240.

Echocardiography

Echocardiography is the most widely used imaging modality for diagnosis and risk stratification of patients with cardiovascular diseases. Technical advances throughout the last 50 years have yielded multiple echocardiographic methodologies that allow for exact characterization of anatomy and function of the heart.

Echocardiographic techniques

Table 1.4.1 summarizes the main echocardiographic methodologies used in the routine clinical practice and the clinical applications.

M-mode echocardiography

This methodology displays the motion of cardiac structures at a high temporal resolution (1000–3000 Hz). The ultrasound beam transmitted from the transducer is reflected by the cardiac structures along one single scan line. The reflected ultrasound is received back by the transducer and registered as reflective interfaces. The location and strength of these reflective interfaces displayed over time result in the M-mode images (Fig. 1.4.1a). The main clinical applications are linear measurements of cardiac chambers and the identification of rapid brief motion, such as systolic anterior motion of the mitral valve.

Two-dimensional echocardiography

Two-dimensional echocardiography (2D) displays the cardiac anatomy in real time, by scanning along series of lines spanning at 90° (Fig. 1.4.1b). The main clinical applications are characterization of cardiac anatomy, cardiac chamber quantification, and evaluation of the anatomy and morphology of valvular structures.

Doppler echocardiography

Doppler echocardiography permits the evaluation of cardiac haemodynamics and blood flow. This technique converts the changes in the frequency of the transmitted ultrasound *(Doppler shift)* into flow velocities using the Doppler equation. When an ultrasound beam with known frequency is transmitted to the heart, the red blood cells reflect the ultrasound at a different frequency, depending on the direction of the blood flow: the frequency increases when the blood flow is directed towards the transducer and decreases when the blood flow moves away from the transducer. Spectral Doppler interrogation can be performed with two different methods: continuous wave or pulsed wave. In continuous wave Doppler imaging, the transducer transmits and receives the ultrasound signal

Table 1.4.1 Echocardiographic techniques and main clinical applications

Echocardiography technique	Clinical application
M-mode	Linear measurements of cardiac chambers and aorta
	Detection of rapid brief movement of cardiac structures (i.e. systolic anterior mitral movement in hypertrophic cardiomyopathy)
2D echocardiography	Linear/volumetric measurements of cardiac chambers
	Linear measurements of the aorta
	Anatomic characterization of cardiac valves
Doppler echocardiography	Cardiac homodynamic and blood flow assessment
Continuous wave	Mean and peak transvalvular gradients
Pulsed wave	LV diastolic function
	Aortic and pulmonary valve area estimation
	Assessment of intracardiac shunts
Colour Doppler imaging	Valvular heart disease (stenotic or regurgitant lesions)
	Assessment of intracardiac shunts
Colour Doppler M-mode	LV diastolic function
	Aortic valve regurgitation
Tissue Doppler imaging	Assessment of myocardial motion
Pulsed wave	LV diastolic function
Colour-coded TDI	LV mechanics assessment (velocity, displacement, strain)
	LV dyssynchrony assessment
Contrast echocardiography	Detection of right-to-left intracardiac shunts
Agitated serum	Volumetric measurements of cardiac chambers
Microbubbles	Evaluation of wall motion
	Detection of intracardiac mass
	Myocardial perfusion assessment
3D-echocardiography	Volumetric measurements of cardiac chambers
	Anatomic characterization of cardiac valves
	Cardiac interventions (to guide atrial septal defect closure, transcatheter valve implantations ...)

LV, left ventricular; TDI, tissue Doppler imaging.

continuously (Fig. 1.4.1c). This technique permits the identification of the highest velocity along the ultrasound path, without indicating where exactly that velocity occurs. In pulsed wave Doppler imaging, the transducer transmits a short burst of ultrasounds at a known rate *(repetition frequency)* and receives the ultrasounds reflected by the red blood cells moving across a determined location *(sample volume)* (Fig. 1.4.1d). The velocity of the blood flow can be measured at any location within the cardiac anatomy. The calculation of the maximum velocity by this method is limited by the Nyquist frequency limit. When the frequency shift is higher than the Nyquist frequency limit, aliasing phenomenon occurs, resulting in misrepresentation of the velocity.

Colour flow imaging or *colour-Doppler imaging* is a variation of pulsed Doppler echocardiography that displays the velocity and direction of the blood flow in different colours, superimposed on real-time 2D images (Fig. 1.4.1e). Colour-Doppler imaging permits the simultaneous interrogation of multiple regions within an area of interest. The frequency shift of each region is encoded with different colours, depending on the velocity, the direction, and the turbulence of the flow. Conventionally, when the flow moves away from the transducer, the resultant negative velocity is encoded in shades of blue, whereas the flow directed towards the transducer (positive velocities) is encoded in shades of red. The intensity of the shade of the primary colour is related to the velocity of the flow: the higher the velocity is, the lighter is the shade of the colour within the Nyquist frequency limit. Aliasing phenomenon can also occur and the flow may be encoded in its opposite colour. In case of turbulent flow, there is substantial variation in flow velocity and direction, being encoded in shades of yellow or green. Besides the limitations of the pulsed Doppler echocardiography, colour-Doppler imaging has a lower temporal resolution than 2D echocardiography (15–30 Hz). With *colour-Doppler M-mode imaging*, pulsed Doppler interrogation is performed along a single scan line. The Doppler shift is first recorded and then it is colour encoded and superimposed on the M-mode image, providing high temporal resolution data on timing and direction of flow events (Fig. 1.4.1f). This technique is typically used to assess the left ventricular (LV) inflow pattern and to evaluate the severity of the aortic regurgitation.

The main clinical applications of Doppler echocardiography are assessment of LV systolic and diastolic function, valvular heart disease, and intracardiac shunts.

Tissue Doppler imaging

Tissue Doppler imaging (TDI) evaluates the motion of myocardial tissue. The myocardium has a lower frequency shift (lower velocity) and higher amplitude (more intense reflector of the ultrasound) than red blood cells. Therefore, instrumentation filters are set to exclude the high velocities

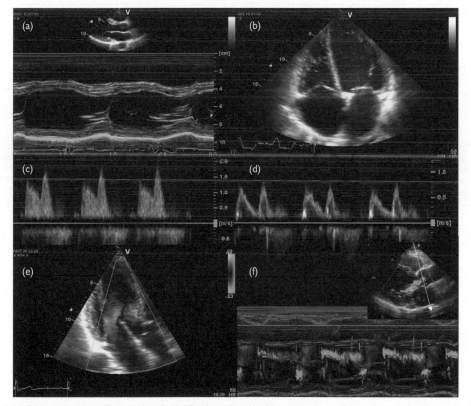

Fig. 1.4.1 Echocardiographic techniques. M-mode (a), 2D echocardiography (b), continuous wave Doppler (c), pulsed wave Doppler (d), colour Doppler imaging (e) and colour Doppler M-mode (f). See also Plate 2.

of the blood flow and to record only the low velocities of the myocardium. TDI calculates myocardial velocities by spectral pulsed wave TDI or colour-coding of the 2D image. Pulsed wave TDI records the velocities from one single region (Fig. 1.4.2a). Colour-encoded TDI collects the Doppler signal for each depth and ultrasound beam (Fig. 1.4.2b). Colour-encoded TDI uses traditional blue–red encoding for direction of motion: red for motion towards the transducer and blue for motion away from the transducer.

The fundamental parameter obtained with TDI is myocardial velocity. By integrating the velocity over time, myocardial displacement can be calculated (Fig. 1.4.2c). Either velocity or displacement can overestimate or underestimate the active component of myocardial function, since these parameters are strongly influenced by tethering or translational motion. Strain and strain rate, more complex derivatives of velocity, evaluate the active deformation of the myocardium, reflecting more closely the myocardial contractility. Strain is calculated as the percentage change in length during myocardial contraction or relaxation and strain rate is calculated as the difference between two velocities, normalized to the distance between them. The measurement of colour-coded Doppler-derived strain or strain rate is affected by the insonation angle of the ultrasound beam.

Two-dimensional strain imaging

This imaging technique permits myocardial deformation assessment. On conventional grey-scale 2D images, this methodology identifies natural acoustic markers (so-called *speckles*) equally distributed within the myocardial wall. Tracking the speckles throughout the cardiac cycle,

myocardial motion can be evaluated and strain can be derived (Fig. 1.4.3). This technique is not affected by the insonation angle and permits the evaluation of multidirectional strain (in the longitudinal, circumferential and radial directions). LV twist, a novel parameter of LV global performance, can also be evaluated.

Contrast echocardiography

Contrast echocardiography is used to detect the presence of right-to-left intracardiac shunts (i.e. patent foramen ovale), to improve the Doppler signal from the right-sided cardiac chambers and to improve the definition of the LV endocardial border, yielding a better quantification of LV size and function. In addition, myocardial perfusion can be assessed (relevant for the management of patients with coronary artery disease). Current contrast agents are listed below.

- Agitated saline: the bubbles enhance only the right-sided cardiac chambers and do not pass through the pulmonary circulation. When a right-to-left intracardiac shunt exists, the bubbles appear in the left atrium immediately after they reach the right atrium. When an intrapulmonary shunt (i.e. hepatopulmonary syndrome) is present, the bubbles enhance the left atrium several cardiac cycles after right atrial opacification.

- Microbubbles of a high-molecular-weight gas, encapsulated in a shell of lipids or proteins: permit the opacification of the left-sided cardiac chambers and the assessment of myocardial perfusion. With a low ultrasound acoustic power (mechanical index 0.4–0.5) the microbubbles are not destroyed and remain in the LV, improving the endocardial border detection (Fig. 1.4.4a).

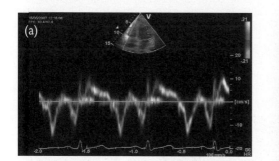
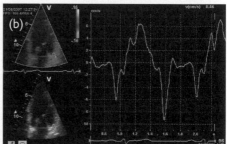

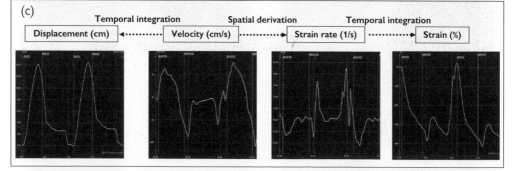

Fig. 1.4.2 Tissue Doppler imaging (TDI). Pulsed wave tissue Doppler (a) and colour-coded TDI (b). (c) From colour-coded TDI, several parameters of left ventricular mechanics can be measured: velocity, displacement, strain rate and strain. See also Plate 3.

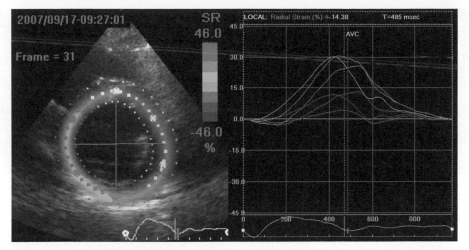

Fig. 1.4.3 Two-dimensional speckle tracking imaging. By applying this echocardiographic technique to mid-ventricular parasternal short-axis view of the left ventricle, myocardial strain can be measured. The example illustrates the measurement of radial strain (myocardial thickening). See also Plate 4.

With high mechanical index (>1.5), the microbubbles are destroyed and perfuse the myocardium. Those areas with normal perfusion appear as enhanced myocardium, whereas those areas with impaired perfusion appear as dark or patchy areas (Fig. 1.4.4b). In stress echocardiography, the use of myocardial contrast perfusion imaging may result in higher sensitivity for the detection of myocardial ischemia.

Three-dimensional echocardiography

Current matrix-array transducers (more than 3000 imaging elements) provide live 3D volume-rendered images or two or three simultaneous orthogonal planes. The 3D data acquisition modes include:

- real-time mode or narrow-angle mode: displays a pyramidal data set of 50° × 30° (Fig. 1.4.5a)

- zoom mode: displays a small, magnified pyramidal data set of 30° × 30° at a high resolution (Fig. 1.4.5b).
- wide-angle mode: includes a large cardiac volume in a pyramidal data set of 90° × 90° (Fig. 1.4.5c). This acquisition mode requires electrocardiographic gating as data set is compiled by merging four narrower pyramidal sub-volumes acquired over four consecutive beats.

The acquired 3D data set is post-processed to visualize the cardiac structures within the pyramid. The main clinical applications of real-time 3D echocardiography are cardiac chamber quantitation, assessment of valvular heart disease, and congenital heart disease. In addition, real-time 3D echocardiography is a valuable imaging tool to guide cardiac interventions (surgical valve repair, transcatheter valve implantation, septal atrial defect closure).

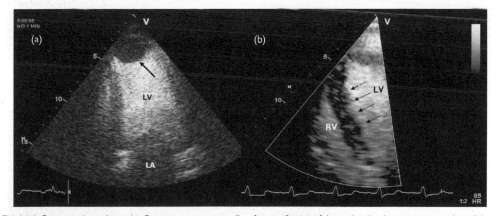

Fig. 1.4.4 Contrast echocardiography. Current contrast agents allow for opacification of the cardiac chambers, improving endocardial border detection and identification of intracardiac mass (a, apical thrombus). By increasing the mechanical index, myocardial perfusion can be assessed (b, example of a patient with septal myocardial infarction; the arrows indicate the large perfusion defect). LA, left atrium; LV, left ventricle; RV, right ventricle. See also Plate 5.

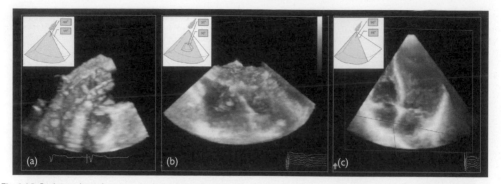

Fig. 1.4.5 Real-time three-dimensional echocardiography acquisition modes: (a) real-time mode or narrow-angle mode, that displays the cardiac structures in real-time within a narrow sector (50° × 30°); (b) zoom mode, that displays a smaller, magnified pyramidal dataset (30°×30°) with a high resolution; wide-angle mode (c) includes a large cardiac volume in a pyramidal data set of 90° × 90°. (Adapted with permission from Hung J et al. J Am Soc Echocardiogr 2007). See also Plate 6.

Clinical applications

Quantitation of the left ventricle

LV dimensions and global systolic function have important clinical and prognostic implications and are key for the clinical management of patients with cardiovascular disease.

LV diameters and thickness of the septal and posterior walls are usually measured on 2D targeted M-mode images acquired at the parasternal long-axis view. These linear parameters should be measured at the LV minor axis (approximately at the tips of the mitral valve) (Figure 1.4.6a). To obtain reliable measurements, the M-mode cursor should be aligned perpendicularly to the long axis of the left ventricle. Alternatively, LV dimensions can be measured from 2D parasternal short-axis images using direct 2D measurements.

LV volumes are usually measured at the apical two- and four-chamber views. The endocardial boundaries are manually traced, excluding the papillary muscles. This tracing should be performed at end-systole (the frame preceding mitral valve opening or the frame of the cardiac cycle with the smallest cardiac dimension) and end-diastole (frame following mitral valve closure or the frame of the cardiac cycle with the largest cardiac dimension).

Left ventricular mass (LVM) is calculated from linear measurements of the left ventricle performed on 2D targeted M-mode: LVM = 0.8 × (1.04[(LVEDD + PWT + IVST)^3 – (LVEDD)^3]) + 0.6, where LVEDD is LV end-diastolic diameter, PWT is posterior wall thickness and IVST is the interventricular septum thickness.

LV systolic function can be assessed with linear or volumetric measurements. The most representative parameter of LV systolic function is LV ejection fraction. Teichholz' method calculates the LV ejection fraction from linear measurements obtained at 2D targeted M-mode recordings. However, in patients with distorted geometries of the left ventricle, the accuracy of this method is reduced. The Biplane method of discs (modified Simpson's method) calculates the LV ejection fraction by volumetric measurement of the end-diastolic (EDV) and end-systolic (ESV) volumes: LV ejection fraction = (EDV – ESV)/EDV × 100 (Fig. 1.4.6b). This method is currently the recommended

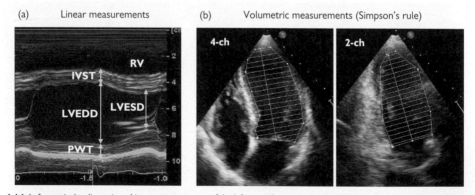

(a)   Linear measurements   (b)   Volumetric measurements (Simpson's rule)

Fig. 1.4.6 Left ventricular dimensions. Linear measurements of the left ventricle are usually obtained from long-axis parasternal M-mode recordings (a). Biplane Simpson's rule is the preferred method to measure left ventricular volumes and ejection fraction (b): the endocardial border of the left ventricle is traced on the apical four- and two-chamber views at the end-diastolic and end-systolic frames. IVST, interventricular septum thickness; LVEDD, left ventricular end-diastolic diameter; LVESD, left ventricular end-systolic diameter; PWT, posterior wall thickness; RV, right ventricle. See also Plate 7.

method to assess LV volumes and systolic function. LV systolic function can be expressed also in terms of midwall fractional shortening or stroke volume. Midwall fractional shortening reflects the intrinsic contractility of the LV and is calculated with mathematical models that compute this parameter from linear measurements obtained at 2D targeted M-mode recordings. Stroke volume is the volume of blood ejected by the LV at each cardiac cycle and can be calculated by subtracting the end-systolic volume from the end-diastolic volume. When significant mitral regurgitation exists, the regurgitant volume should be subtracted to obtain the volume ejected through the LV outflow tract. With Doppler echocardiography, stroke volume can be calculated by the product of the cross-sectional area of the LV outflow tract and the time velocity integral at the LV outflow tract.

Table 1.4.2 summarizes the reference values for LV measurements.

Quantitation of the right ventricle (RV)

The RV has a complex spatial disposition and structure. Accurate evaluation of the RV requires multiple echocardiographic views. The assessment of the RV dimensions comprises the measurement of the thickness of the RV free wall on M-mode or 2D images acquired from the subcostal view and the mid-cavity, basal and longitudinal diameters on the apical four-chamber view (Fig.1.4.7a). In addition, linear measurements of the RV outflow tract are

usually performed at 2D parasternal short-axis views, proximal to the pulmonary valve (Figure 1.4.7b). Quantitative assessment of RV function comprises:
- Tricuspid annular plane systolic excursion (TAPSE): obtained from 2D targeted M-mode of the apical four-chamber view. Normal excursion of the tricuspid annular plane towards the apex is 1.5–2.0 cm.
- Right ventricular fractional area change: calculated by tracing the endocardial border at the apical four-chamber view in end-systole and end-diastole.
- Table 1.4.2. summarizes the reference values for RV measurements.

Left and right atrial dimensions
The assessment of left atrial dimensions includes:
- Anteroposterior diameter measured at parasternal long-axis M-mode recordings.
- Left atrial volume (preferred over linear measurements), calculated with the biplane area–length formula: $8(A_1)(A_2)/3\pi(L)$, where A_1 and A_2 are the planimetred areas of the left atrium obtained at the apical two- and four-chamber views and L represents the left atrial long-axis length.
- Right atrial dimensions are usually measured from the apical four-chamber view. The minor axis dimension and the volume based on single plane area–length formula are the standard measurements to quantitate the right atrium.

Table 1.4.2 Reference limits of cardiac chambers dimensions (adapted with permission from Lang RM *et al. J Am Soc Echocardiograph* 2005)

		Reference range	
		Women	**Men**
LV measurements	LV EDD (cm)	3.9–5.3	4.2–5.9
	IVST (cm)	0.6–0.9	0.6–1.0
	PWT (cm)	0.6–0.9	0.6–1.0
	LV mass index (g/m²)	43–95	49–115
	Biplane LV EDV (mL)	56–104	67–155
	Biplane LV ESV (mL)	19–49	22–58
	Biplane LV EF (%)	≥55	≥55
	Endocardial fractional shortening (%)	27–45	25–43
RV measurements	Diameters (cm)		
	Basal	2.0–2.8	
	Midventricular	2.7–3.3	
	Longitudinal	7.1–7.9	
	RVOT	2.5–2.9	
	TAPSE	>1.5	
	Fractional area change	32–60%	
LA measurements	Anteroposterior diameter (cm)	2.7–3.8	3.0–4.0
	LA indexed volume (ml/m²)	22 ± 6	22 ± 6
RA measurements	Minor axis dimension (cm)	2.9–4.5	

EDD, end diastolic diameter; EDV, end-diastolic volume; EF, ejection fraction; ESV, end-systolic volume; IVST, interventricular septum thickness; LA, left atrial; LV, left ventricular; PWT, posterior wall thickness; RA, right atrial; RV, right ventricular; RVOT, right ventricular outflow tract; TAPSE, tricuspid annular plane systolic excursion.

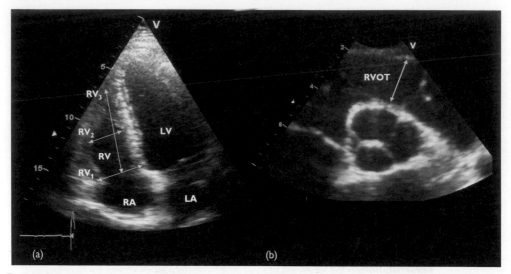

Fig. 1.4.7 Right ventricular dimensions. Linear dimensions of the right ventricle are measured at the apical four-chamber view (a), including the basal (RV$_1$), mid-ventricular (RV$_2$), and longitudinal (RV$_3$) diameters. From parasternal short-axis view at the level of the aortic valve, the diameter of the right ventricular outflow tract can be measured (b). LA, left atrium; LV, left ventricle; RA, right atrium; RV, right ventricle; RVOT, right ventricular outflow tract. See also Plate 8.

Table 1.4.2. summarizes the reference values for left and right atrial measurements.

Evaluation of the aorta

Echocardiographic evaluation of the aorta includes the assessment of:

- Aortic root and proximal ascending aorta: linear measurements are performed either at M-mode recordings or on 2D images at the parasternal long-axis views and include diameters of the aortic valve annulus, sinuses of Valsalva, sinotubular junction and ascending aorta (Fig. 1.4.8). These measurements should be performed at those views that show the largest diameter of the aortic root.
- Aortic arch: visualized from the suprasternal view, the linear dimensions can be calculated from 2D imaging. Blood flow through the aorta can be assessed with Doppler imaging (i.e. to rule out aortic coarctation).
- Thoracic descending aorta: evaluated with two-dimensional transoesophageal echocardiography, acquiring short-axis (0°) and long-axis (90°) images of the aorta.

Evaluation of inferior vena cava

The echocardiographic assessment of the inferior vena cava provides useful information on right atrial pressure. Linear dimensions can be measured from 2D images or M-mode recordings at the subcostal view. In addition, the collapse of the vessel during inspiration should be assessed. A dilated inferior vena cava without inspiratory collapse indicates markedly elevated right atrial pressures.

Valvular heart disease

Echocardiography provides comprehensive information on the structure, anatomy, function, and haemodynamics of the cardiac valves. On the basis of this information, clinical decision-making as well as timing of surgical intervention are taken.

The assessment of the severity of stenotic or regurgitant valve disease relies mostly on Doppler echocardiography.

Stenotic valve lesions

- Assessment of transvalvular gradients: the continuous wave Doppler cursor should be aligned as parallel as possible to the stenotic jet. By modified Bernoulli equation, the maximum velocity is transformed into maximum pressure gradient: $\Delta P = 4v^2$. By tracing the Doppler spectral velocity recordings, the average of the instantaneous gradients over the ejection period is calculated, yielding the mean pressure gradient.
- Assessment of the effective valvular area: the area of the stenotic orifice is usually calculated by continuity equation for aortic valve stenosis, or pressure half-time method for mitral stenosis (Fig. 1.4.9).

Regurgitant valve lesions

- Assessment of the severity of the regurgitant valve lesions can be performed by measuring the regurgitant volume, regurgitant fraction and effective regurgitant orifice area.
- Proximal isovelocity surface area (PISA): this method is recommended to calculate the regurgitant volume. When blood flow converges towards the regurgitant orifice, its velocity increases and forms concentric hemispheric shells of increasing velocities. With colour Doppler, the hemispheres can be identified and the flow rate through the regurgitant orifice can be calculated as the product of the surface area of the hemisphere ($2\pi \times r^2$) and the aliasing velocity (V_a) (determined by the Nyquist limit) (Fig. 1.4.10). Assuming that the maximal PISA radius occurs at the peak regurgitant flow (V_{max}), the maximal effective regurgitant orifice area is derived from: $6.28 \times r^2 \times V_a/V_{max}$. The regurgitant volume can be calculated as the product of the effective orifice area and the velocity time integral of the regurgitant jet.

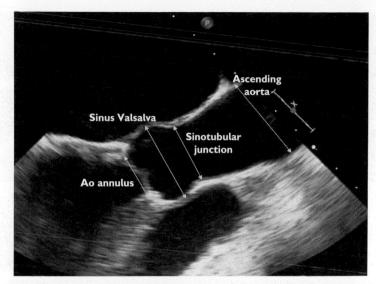

Fig. 1.4.8 Aortic dimensions. Linear dimensions of the aortic root includes the diameters of the aortic annulus, sinus of Valsalva, sinotubular junction, and ascending aorta. See also Plate 9.

The PISA method may underestimate the severity of those regurgitant valve lesions with extremely eccentric jets.

Assessment of aortic valve stenosis
- Anatomy of the valve (tricuspid/bicuspid) and degree of valvular calcification: from the 2D parasternal short-axis view at the level of the aortic valve.

- Peak and mean transvalvular gradients: with continuous wave Doppler echocardiography.

- Aortic effective valve area estimation by the continuity equation, taken into account the cross-sectional area of the LV outflow tract, velocity–time integral of the flow at the LV outflow tract and at the stenotic orifice.

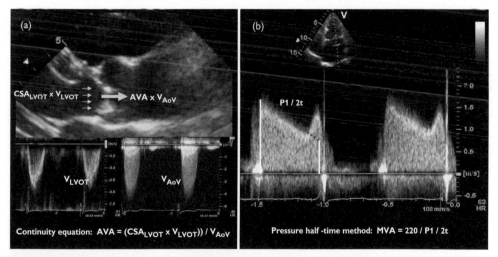

Fig. 1.4.9 Estimation of the effective valvular area. The continuity equation (a) states that the flow passing through a stenotic orifice is equal to the flow proximal to the stenosis. Flow is equal to the product of velocity and cross-sectional area (CSA). Therefore, at a known CSA of the LV outflow tract (LVOT) and flow velocity at that location (by pulsed wave Doppler) and velocity through the aortic valve (continuous wave Doppler), aortic valve area can be obtained. To evaluate mitral stenosis, pressure half-time method (b) yields accurate estimations of the mitral valve area (MVA). The formula expresses the time needed to reduce by 30% the peak stenotic velocity. See also Plate 10.

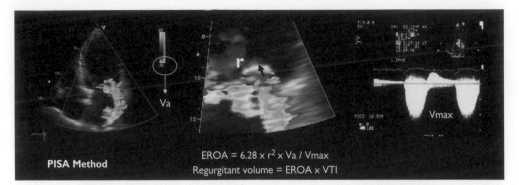

Fig. 1.4.10 Estimation of the regurgitant volume by the PISA method. By colour Doppler echocardiography, the regurgitant flow is evaluated. The Nyquist limit is adjusted to clearly visualize the different velocity hemispheric surfaces that the flow forms when converges towards the regurgitant orifice. The effective regurgitant orifice area (EROA) is calculated by the product of the area of the hemisphere and the aliasing velocity (Va), given by the Nyquist limit, and divided by the maximal velocity of the regurgitant flow (Vmax). The regurgitant volume can be then calculated as the product of the EROA and the velocity time integral of the regurgitant flow. See also Plate 11.

Assessment of mitral valve stenosis
- Anatomy and morphology assessment: 2D echocardiography typically demonstrates thickened mitral leaflets and subvalvular apparatus, with varying degrees of calcification and restrictive motion of one or both leaflets with typical 'hockey-stick' appearance.
- Peak and mean transvalvular gradients: calculated by continuous wave Doppler through the stenotic orifice.
- Mitral valve area: calculated by planimetry on 2D parasternal short-axis view at the level of the tips of the leaflets or by pressure half time method on continuous wave Doppler recordings of the transmitral velocity. This method has been extensively validated and can be reliably used in clinical decision making.

Assessment of aortic valve regurgitation
- Assessment of the underlying structural abnormalities on 2D echocardiography: congenital valvular disease, endocarditis, degenerative valve disease, dilatation of the ascending aorta or aortic dissection.

- The severity of the regurgitant aortic valve disease is usually assessed with the following methods:
  - Measurement of the width of the regurgitant jet at its origin relative to the dimension of the LV outflow tract on M-mode colour-Doppler applied to parasternal long-axis view.
  - Measurement of the pressure half-time at the continuous wave Doppler recordings of the regurgitant jet. The pressure half-time indicates the pressure difference between the aorta and the left ventricle. In severe aortic regurgitation the pressure half-time becomes shorter, indicating the rapid increase of LV diastolic pressure and rapid decrease in aortic pressure (Figure 1.4.11a).
  - Measurement of the vena contracta (the narrower neck of the colour flow region at the level of the aortic valve) (Fig. 1.4.11b).
  - Measurement of regurgitant volume and orifice regurgitant area by the PISA method.

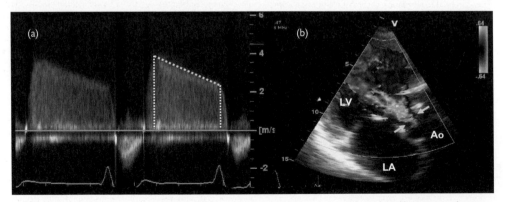

Fig. 1.4.11 Evaluation of aortic regurgitation severity. The severity of the aortic regurgitation can be evaluated by measuring the pressure half-time of the continuous wave Doppler recordings of the regurgitant jet (a) or the measurement of the vena contracta at the level of the aortic valve on color-Doppler image (arrows, b). Ao, aorta; LA, left atrium; LV, left ventricle. See also Plate 12.

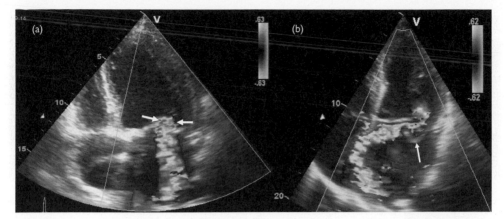

Fig. 1.4.12 Evaluation of mitral valve regurgitation. Colour-Doppler imaging displays the direction of the regurgitant jet and yields clues to define the underlying mechanism of the lesion: in functional mitral valve regurgitation, left ventricular remodelling and dilatation of the mitral annulus result in tethering of the mitral leaflets and coaptation failure and a central regurgitant jet is usually observed (a). In contrast, mitral valve prolapse is characterized by anatomically abnormal mitral valve (i.e. prominent flail leaflets) showing eccentric regurgitant jets, impinging on the wall of the left atrium (coanda effect). (b) The white arrow shows the prolapse of the posterior mitral leaflet and, consequently, the regurgitant jet is directed towards the interatrial septum. See also Plate 13.

Assessment of mitral valve regurgitation

- Assessment of the underlying structural abnormalities on 2D or 3D echocardiography: congenital heart disease (mitral clefts), mitral valve prolapse (Barlow disease), rheumatic valve disease, rupture of one of the papillary muscles (acute myocardial infarction), or dilatation of the mitral annulus and failing left ventricle (functional mitral regurgitation) (Fig. 1.4.12).
- The severity of the regurgitant mitral valve disease is usually assessed with the following methods:
  - Semiquantitative assessment of the color-flow area of the regurgitant jet relative to the area of the left atrium.
  - Measurement of the vena contracta.
  - Measurement of the regurgitant volume and the effective regurgitant orifice area by the PISA method.

Assessment of tricuspid valve regurgitation

- Mild tricuspid regurgitation is common and the maximum velocity of the regurgitant jet obtained on continuous wave Doppler recordings is used to calculate the right ventricular pressure.
- Assessment of the underlying causes: congenital heart disease, rheumatic heart disease, carcinoid or drug therapies, or increased pulmonary pressure secondary to increased LV pressures.
- The severity of the tricuspid valve regurgitation is usually assessed with the following methods:
  - Assessment of the regurgitant jet area on colour-Doppler imaging.
  - Late systolic concave pattern of the continuous wave Doppler recordings of the regurgitant jet.
  - Late systolic flow reversal in the hepatic veins on pulsed wave Doppler recordings.
  - Measurement of the vena contracta.
  - Calculation of the regurgitant volume and effective regurgitant orifice area by the PISA method.

Diastolic function

The assessment of LV diastolic function should be included in the routine echocardiographic examinations. Diastolic dysfunction is an early marker of several heart diseases and its presence determines poor prognosis. The echocardiographic evaluation of the LV filling pattern includes:

- Assessment of transmitral flow: the assessment of the transmitral flow is performed with pulsed wave Doppler echocardiography at the apical four-chamber view. The sample volume is placed between the tips of the mitral valve during diastole. From the spectral mitral velocity recordings, the following diastolic parameters can be measured: early (E) and late (A) diastolic filling velocities, E/A ratio and deceleration time of the E-wave (DT). By placing the sample volume at an intermediate position between the mitral and the aortic valve, the isovolumetric relaxation time (IVRT; time between the closure of the aortic valve and the opening of the mitral valve) can be measured. Diastolic function can be classified according to the transmitral inflow profile in normal, impaired relaxation, pseudo-normal, and restrictive, representing a progressive worsening of diastolic function. However, these parameters are highly loading dependent and are not interpretable when sinus tachycardia, atrial fibrillation, or conduction system diseases coexist.
- Pulmonary venous flow: the assessment of the pulmonary venous flow is performed with pulsed wave Doppler echocardiography at the apical four-chamber view. Colour-Doppler imaging helps to place the sample volume at the right upper pulmonary vein. From the spectral pulmonary venous velocity recordings, the forward systolic (S) and diastolic (D) velocities into the left atrium can be measured. In addition, the backward late diastolic wave (Ar), corresponding to atrial contraction, can be detected. The S/D ratio and the relationship between the Ar-wave and the A-wave duration (Ar − A difference) are the most commonly used parameters.

Table 1.4.3 Left ventricular diastolic function assessment by echocardiography (adapted with permission from Lester SJ et al. *J Am Coll Cardiol* 2008). See also Plate 14.

	Normal	Mild (Grade 1)	Moderate (Grade 2)	Severe (Grade 3)	Severe (Grade 4)
Pulsed wave mitral inflow					
E/A	0.9–1.5	<0.9	0.9–1.5	>2.0	>2.5
DT (ms)	160–240	>240	160–240	<160	<130
IVRT (ms)	70–90	>90	<90	<70	<70
Tissue Doppler imaging					
e'(cm/s)	≥10	<10	<8	<5	<5
E/e'	1–14	≥15	≥15	≥20	≥25
Mitral inflow propagation					
Vp (cm/s)	≥50	<50	<50	<50	<50
E/Vp	≤1.5	>1.5	>1.5	>1.5	>1.5
Pulmonary vein flow	S≥D	S>>D	S<D	S<<D	S<<D
Indexed LA volume (ml/m²)	22±6	>28	>28	>35	>40

E/A = the ratio of the early (E) and atrial (A) components of the mitral inflow spectral velocity recording; e', tissue Doppler early diastolic velocity; D, pulmonary vein diastolic forward flow velocity; DT, deceleration time; IVRT, isovolumetric relaxation time; LA, left atrial; S, pulmonary vein systolic forward velocity; Vp, mitral inflow propagation velocity.

- Mitral inflow propagation velocity: with colour-Doppler imaging, an early inflow velocity across the mitral valve from the apical four-chamber view can be identified. By aligning the M-mode cursor in the centre of the brightest inflow velocity, a recording of a colour M-mode of the inflow jet can be obtained. Flow propagation velocity is measured as the slope of the first aliasing velocity during early LV filling. This parameter is related to the suction force of the left ventricle (attributed to the LV restoring forces and relaxation).
- Tissue Doppler annular early and late diastolic velocities. The measurement of mitral annular velocities is performed with pulsed wave TDI at the apical four-chamber view. The sample volume should be placed at 1 cm within the septal and the lateral insertion sites of the mitral leaflets. From the spectral recordings, the systolic velocity *(Sm)* and the early *(Em, Ea, E', e')* and the late *(Am, A', a')* velocities can be measured. In addition, the *E/e'* ratio can be derived, being an accurate estimate of LV filling pressures.
- Left atrial volume: the measurement of the left atrial volume reflects the chronicity of diastolic dysfunction.
- Table 1.4.3 summarizes the normal values of the aforementioned parameters and displays the diastolic function grade.

Further reading

Amundsen BH, Helle-Valle T, Edvardsen T, *et al.* Noninvasive myocardial strain measurement by speckle tracking echocardiography: validation against sonomicrometry and tagged magnetic resonance imaging. *J Am Coll Cardiol* 2006;**47**:789–93.

Bursi F, Weston SA, Redfield MM, *et al.* Systolic and diastolic heart failure in the community. *JAMA* 2006;**296**:2209–16.

Cohen JL, Cheirif J, Segar DS, *et al.* Improved left ventricular endocardial border delineation and opacification with OPTISON (FS069), a new echocardiographic contrast agent. Results of a phase III Multicenter Trial. *J Am Coll Cardiol* 1998;**32**:746–52.

Hung J, Lang R, Flachskampf F, *et al.* 3D echocardiography: a review of the current status and future directions. *J Am Soc Echocardiogr* 2007;**20**:213–33.

Lang RM, Bierig M, Devereux RB, *et al.* Recommendations for chamber quantification: a report from the American Society of Echocardiography's Guidelines and Standards Committee and the Chamber Quantification Writing Group, developed in conjunction with the European Association of Echocardiography, a branch of the European Society of Cardiology. *J Am Soc Echocardiogr* 2005;**18**:1440–63.

Lester SJ, Tajik AJ, Nishimura RA, Oh JK, Khandheria BK, Seward JB. Unlocking the mysteries of diastolic function: deciphering the Rosetta Stone 10 years later. *J Am Coll Cardiol* 2008;**51**:679–89.

Nagueh SF, Appleton CP, Gillebert TC, *et al.* Recommendations for the evaluation of LV diastolic function by echocardiography. *J Am Soc Echocardiogr* 2009;**22**:107–33.

Quinones MA, Otto CM, Stoddard M, *et al.* Recommendations for quantification of Doppler echocardiography: a report from the Doppler Quantification Task Force of the Nomenclature and Standards Committee of the American Society of Echocardiography. *J Am Soc Echocardiogr* 2002;**15**:167–84.

Sutherland GR, Di SG, Claus P, *et al.* Strain and strain rate imaging: a new clinical approach to quantifying regional myocardial function. *J Am Soc Echocardiogr* 2004;**17**:788–802.

Zoghbi WA, Enriquez-Sarano M, Foster E, *et al.* Recommendations for evaluation of the severity of native valvular regurgitation with two-dimensional and Doppler echocardiography. *J Am Soc Echocardiogr* 2003;**16**:777–802.

Non-invasive cardiac imaging

In addition to echocardiography several other non-invasive cardiovascular imaging modalities are available:
1 Nuclear imaging, including single-photon emission computed tomography (SPECT) and positron emission tomography (PET).
2 Multidetector row computed tomography (MDCT).
3 Magnetic resonance imaging (MRI).

These modalities have a wide range of cardiovascular applications including the assessment of coronary artery disease (CAD), left ventricular (LV) function, viability and valvular heart disease.

Choice of a particular technique depends on technical aspects as well as local availability and expertise.

Diagnosis and prognosis of CAD

Hallmarks non-invasive evaluation of CAD
Basically, two approaches are available for non-invasive evaluation of CAD.

Functional testing for ischaemia
Traditionally functional techniques are applied to detect the presence of ischaemia as an indirect marker for CAD. For this purpose, imaging of myocardial perfusion or wall motion is performed during stress (physical exercise or pharmacological stress) and rest. Reversible abnormalities (abnormalities during stress but normal images during rest) indicate the presence of ischaemia. Irreversible abnormalities (abnormalities during stress and persisting in rest) indicate the presence of scar tissue.

Anatomical testing for atherosclerosis
More recently, anatomical imaging techniques have become available. These techniques evaluate the presence of atherosclerosis and degree of luminal narrowing in the coronary arteries directly.

Nuclear imaging
- Myocardial perfusion is assessed with radionuclide tracers: thallium-201, technetium-99m sestamibi, or technetium-99m tetrofosmin.
- A large body of evidence is available supporting a high accuracy for detecting significant CAD.
- In addition, extensive data show that a normal nuclear study is associated with excellent prognosis (annual event rate <1%) while event rates are substantially higher (>5%) in the presence of an abnormal study.
- With the introduction of electrocardiogram (ECG) gating, simultaneous assessment of left ventricular ejection fraction (LVEF) and wall motion has become possible, improving diagnostic certainty.
- In addition to perfusion defects, reduction in LVEF, ECG changes during stress and transient ischaemic dilation of the ventricle are highly suggestive of CAD.
- For imaging with PET, nitrogen-13 ammonia and rubidium-82 are the most commonly used tracers, but also O-15-labelled water can be used.
- PET offers the advantage of higher spatial resolution, allowing identification of subendocardial perfusion defects.
- In addition, PET allows absolute quantification of myocardial blood flow and systematic use of attenuation correction.
- Limitations of PET include higher costs and limited availability.

MRI
- A truly non-invasive technique that uses magnetism to obtain high-resolution images.
- Both myocardial perfusion and wall motion can be assessed during rest and pharmacological stress to detect CAD.
- For perfusion imaging five to eight slices in the short-axis orientation are imaged during the first pass of a bolus of a gadolinium-based MR contrast agent. Similarly, images in the short-axis orientation are obtained for imaging of wall motion.
- Although less robust than MDCT, the technique may potentially also allow non-invasive angiography.
- Advantages of MRI include the high resolution allowing differentiation of subendocardial perfusion defects as well as its versatility.
- Limitations include the relatively long acquisition times, restricted availability while patients with metallic implants or claustrophobia cannot be imaged.
- The information obtained with MRI on wall motion and perfusion may be valuable for prognostication, although only limited data are currently available.

MDCT
- Relatively new technique that allows non-invasive direct visualization of coronary anatomy with high spatial resolution.
- Coronary calcium score (CACS) can be obtained with non-contrast-enhanced images and provides an estimate of total atherosclerotic plaque burden.
- For non-invasive angiography (CTA), images are acquired in a single breath-hold during the administration of a bolus of iodinated contrast agent while gated to the ECG.
- During CTA the presence of luminal stenosis can be assessed with high diagnostic accuracy compared with invasive coronary angiography.
- The technique has a high negative predictive value, indicating that the technique may be particularly useful to rule out CAD with high diagnostic certainty.
- Limitations of CTA include the fact that image quality and accuracy are reduced in patients with irregular heart rates or extensive coronary calcifications. Also the technique is associated with a high radiation dose, although recent developments have resulted in substantial dose reduction. Finally, no information on the presence of ischaemia is obtained.
- In addition to luminal narrowing, CTA can provide some information on plaque composition by differentiating between lesions that are non-calcified, calcified, or a combination of the two.
- Numerous studies support the prognostic value of CACS to refine risk stratification, particularly in patients classified as being at intermediate risk.
- Initial prognostic data obtained with CTA suggest that also the information obtained by CTA may enhance risk stratification.

Hybrid imaging
- Recently, hybrid imaging modalities such as PET-CT, SPECT-CT, or even MRI-CT have become available.
- These modalities allow co-registration of anatomical landmarks with physiological data and may improve diagnostic accuracy and patient management.

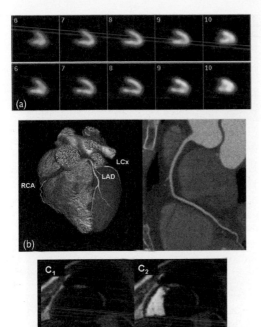

Fig. 1.5.1 Examples of the different imaging modalities to detect coronary artery disease. (a) Myocardial perfusion imaging with SPECT; vertical long-axis reconstructions during adenosine stress (top) and rest (bottom) show normal myocardial perfusion. (b) Non-invasive coronary angiography with 320-slice MDCT: (left) a 3D volume-rendered reconstruction showing the left anterior descending coronary artery (LAD), left circumflex coronary artery (LCx) and right coronary artery (RCA) is provided; (right) a curved multiplanar reconstruction of the RCA showing a normal coronary artery without stenosis. (c) Myocardial perfusion imaging with magnetic resonance imaging: (1–4) consecutive images in the short-axis orientation showing the arrival of a bolus of gadolinium contrast in the myocardium. Normal homogeneous enhancement is visible in 4. See also Plate 15.

Image examples of the individual techniques are provided in Fig. 1.5.1.

Evaluation of resting ejection fraction and wall motion

LVEF is a major determinant of outcome. Assessment of LV dimensions and LVEF therefore is an important component of any cardiac examination. In addition, information on regional wall motion is frequently needed. For this purpose, the standardized 17-segment approach is commonly used to divide the myocardium and classify segments as showing normokinetic, hypokinetic, akinetic, or dyskinetic wall motion patterns.

Nuclear imaging
- The introduction of technetium-based perfusion tracers has resulted in images with sufficient count density to allow gating of the images to the ECG.
- As a result, wall motion, wall thickening, and LVEF can be evaluated in addition to myocardial perfusion.
- With the use of dedicated software, high accuracies have been observed, particularly for 16-frame gating, in the assessment of LVEF. However, eight-frame gating may slightly underestimate LVEF.
- The addition of information on LVEF and wall motion to perfusion data has been shown to improve both diagnostic accuracy and prognostication.

MRI
- MRI can be regarded as the standard of reference investigation for evaluating left and right ventricular function. Approximately 8–12 slices in the short-axis orientation are needed for covering the ventricle. LV volumes and EF are calculated using the Simpson's method.
- Global ventricular function (i.e. ventricular volumes, stroke volume, and EF), and ventricular mass can be obtained after post-processing (Fig. 1.5.2).
- Regional LV function can be quantified by wall thickness and wall thickening analysis by using the centreline method showing the size, extent, and severity of regional ventricular dysfunction.
- However, for practical reasons, regional wall function is frequently assessed by visual estimation of wall motion and thickening.

LV ejection fraction was calculated at 26% with an EDV of 204 mL. LV mass was 87 g.

MDCT
- When images are acquired using retrospective gating, the same data set as used for non-invasive angiography can be used for assessment of global and regional LV function. For this purpose, the obtained images are reformatted in the short-axis orientation and LV volumes and EF are calculated similar to MRI.
- Good correlations have been observed with MRI or 2D echocardiography.
- However, because of the lower temporal resolution of multislice computed tomography, LVEF is frequently slightly underestimated.
- Also evaluation of more subtle wall motion abnormalities remains difficult and accuracy is highest for the identification of either normal or a/dyskinetic myocardium.

Evaluation of viability

A large proportion of patients with chronic CAD develop heart failure. Although revascularization can improve long-term prognosis, not all patients show improvement in function or symptoms. In addition, mortality in the perioperative period is high. Accordingly, it is important to select only patients with myocardium that has the potential to recover to justify the high risks of surgery.

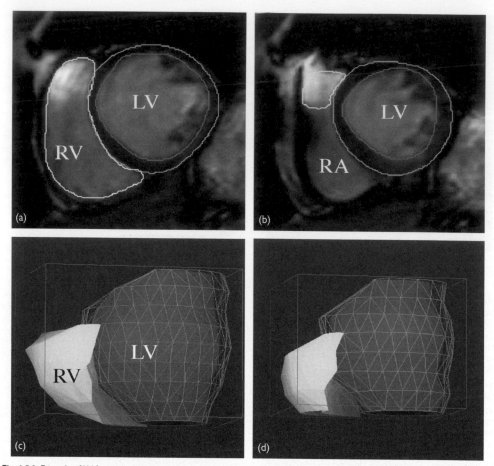

Fig. 1.5.2 Example of LV function assessment with magnetic resonance imaging in a patient with dilated cardiomyopathy using dedicated software (MASS software package (Medis, Leiden, The Netherlands). (a, b) Short-axis mid-ventricular end-diastolic (ED) and end-systolic (ES) images after drawing of the epi- and endocardial LV contours. (c, d) are graphical 3D representations of the ED and ES volumes of the LV and the right ventricle (RV). See also Plate 16.

Thus, non-invasive assessment of myocardial viability may guide patient management. Several techniques have been developed that rely on different markers, as specified in Table 1.5.1, to identify viable tissue.

Nuclear imaging
Nuclear imaging is frequently applied to identify viable myocardium. Several approaches are available.

PET or SPECT with 18F-fluorodeoxyglucose (FDG)
This is the most frequently applied technique that relies on glucose uptake in areas with reduced perfusion as an indicator of viability. Thus a 'mismatch' between the perfusion and FDG images indicates viability, whereas a 'match' (both reduced perfusion and glucose uptake) indicates scar tissue.

SPECT with thallium-201
Viability imaging with thallium-201 is based on the fact that while early uptake of the tracer reflects perfusion, late uptake (redistribution imaging 3–4 hours after injection) indicates cell membrane integrity. In general, two protocols can be applied. Rest redistribution imaging provides information

on viability whereas the stress redistribution reinjection protocol also provides information on ischaemia.

SPECT with technetium-99m-labelled tracers
The uptake and retention of these tracers are dependent on perfusion, cell membrane integrity, and mitochondrial function and thus reflect viability. The most commonly used viability criterion is the percentage of tracer uptake (generally >50–60%) in dysfunctional segments. Use of nitrates enhances accuracy.

MRI

Low-dose dobutamine MRI
Infusion of low-dose dobutamine (5–10 µg/kg/min) has been demonstrated to increase contractility (contractile reserve) in dysfunctional but viable myocardium. In general assessment contractile reserve has reduced sensitivity for viability in the setting of severe resting dysfunction, as with exhausted coronary flow reserve any inotropic stimulation may result in ischaemia rather than contractile improvement.

Table 1.5.1 Characteristics of dysfunctional but viable myocardium for the various imaging modalities

Technique	Characteristics of viability
Nuclear imaging	
PET or SPECT with ^{18}F-FDG	Glucose use
SPECT with [201]Tl	Perfusion and cell membrane integrity
SPECT with ^{99m}Tc-labeled tracers	Perfusion, cell membrane integrity, and mitochondrial intactness
MRI	
Low-dose dobutamine infusion	Contractile reserve
End diastolic wall thickness	Thickness >6 mm
Delayed enhancement	Absence of (transmural) hyperenhancement
MSCT	
End diastolic wall thickness	Thickness >6 mm
Delayed enhancement	Absence of (transmural) hyperenhancement

Adapted with permission from Schinkel AF, Poldermans D, Elhendy A, Bax JJ. Assessment of myocardial viability in patients with heart failure. *J Nucl Med* 2007; 48:1135–1146.

Wall thickness

Evaluation of end-diastolic wall thickness (EDWT) may also provide information on viability and segments with an EDWT <5.5 mm are unlikely to show recovery of function after revascularization. However, recovery in segments with an EDWT ≥5.5 mm is uncertain since non-transmural infarction can be present.

Delayed enhancement

Delayed enhancement MRI after administration of gadolinium-based contrast agents is currently an accepted method for assessing myocardial viability (Fig. 1.5.3). With an inversion recovery pulse, a heavily T_1 weighted image is obtained at an appropriate time delay after contrast administration that maximizes the contrast between the injured and normal myocardium. In irreversibly injured myocardium, the contrast agent accumulates, resulting in 'hyperenhanced' or 'delayed enhanced' tissue. Non-enhancing myocardium consists of living myocytes and is viable.

A strong inverse relationship between the transmural extent of delayed enhancement and the likelihood of improvement of contractility after revascularization has been found. Several studies have shown that in the presence of <50% transmural enhancement LV function improvement can be expected. In contrast, the likelihood for functional improvement reduces with increasing transmural enhancement and recovery is unlikely when >75% of the LV wall contains scar tissue.

MDCT

The value of MDCT in assessing myocardial viability is currently under investigation. EDWT can be assessed similar to MRI. Left ventricular hypoperfusion early after administration of contrast agents is also shown to reflect scar tissue. Moreover, experimental and clinical studies have shown that delayed-enhancement MDCT shows enhancement patterns similar to that of MRI. Three major factors that hamper using MDCT for identifying scar tissue in general practice are the contrast-to-noise ratio that is a factor four to seven times lower for MDCT than MRI, the relative high-dose iodinated contrast agent that is needed for good delineation of scar tissue, and the radiation dose associated with MDCT.

Evaluation of cardiac valves

Non-invasive imaging plays an important role in the assessment of valvular heart disease. For accurate diagnosis of the severity of valve disease and subsequent management decisions, the imaging modality should provide information regarding valve morphology, valve function, and cardiac function.

The principally used techniques for evaluation of valvular heart disease are echocardiography and MRI while no role currently exists for nuclear imaging techniques. In contrast, the potential of MDCT for cardiac valve is under investigation. Although this technique may not provide absolute measures of flow, detailed information on morphology and even function can be obtained.

MRI

- MRI is a useful technique for the evaluation of patients with valvular heart disease.
- Morphologic and functional information can be obtained by using bright-blood cine MRI sequences.
- Phase-contrast (velocity-encoded) MRI is used for quantifying flow measures such as blood flow volume or maximum velocity.
- Systolic and diastolic function parameters can be obtained. Valve stenosis can be estimated by measuring the maximum peak velocity across the valve and applying the modified Bernoulli equation $\Delta P = 4V^2$, in which ΔP is the pressure gradient in mmHg and V is the peak velocity in m/s.
- Valve regurgitation can be quantified as a direct measure in ml by producing a time–volume curve by using 2D one-directional acquisitions; regurgitation can be expressed as a percentage by dividing the backward flow

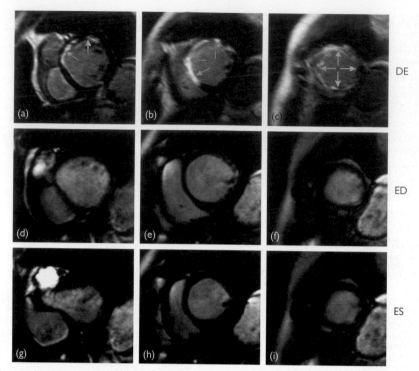

DE

ED

ES

Fig. 1.5.3 Imaging of myocardial viability with MRI. In the upper row the delayed enhancement (DE) images clearly depict the extent of scar tissue (i.e. infarction). Note the approximately 50% transmural subendocardial delayed enhancement in the anteroseptal/anterior segments at the base (arrows, a). At midventricular level, transmural septal enhancement and approximately 75% transmural enhancement is present in the anterior and anterolateral segments (arrows, b). All apical segments are enhanced (arrows, c), with parts of the inferior segment spared. The corresponding end-diastolic images (ED; d–f) and end-systolic images (ES; g–i) show ventricular function at rest. Note poor wall thickening in delayed enhancement areas representing scar tissue.

by the forward flow, for the pulmonary valve and aortic valve.

- However, quantifying regurgitation across the mitral and tricuspid valves, which may occur as complication in ischaemic heart disease, is hampered by inaccuracies due to valve motion throughout the cardiac cycle.
- 3D measures may provide improved accuracy for estimating regurgitation across these atrioventricular valves by adaptation of the reformation plane to the valve plane throughout the cardiac cycle and by correction for the direction of the regurgitation jet.

MDCT

- Recent investigations have shown the feasibility of MDCT to evaluate mitral and aortic valve anatomy and function.

- The leaflet or cusp motion can be evaluated in cine loop using multiphase data sets obtained during ECG gating.
- On diastolic images the valve apparatus including thickness of the leaflets, apposition point, commissures, and annulus is accurately depicted.
- The degree of calcification of the leaflets can be easily assessed (Fig. 1.5.4) and is a strong risk factor for disease progression and ad verse outcome.
- In addition aortic and mitral valve areas can be measured while to some extent assessment of aortic or mitral regurgitation may be feasible.
- The opportunity to non-invasively visualize valvular anatomy and surrounding structures may become of particular interest in the setting of percutaneous valve repair or replacement techniques.

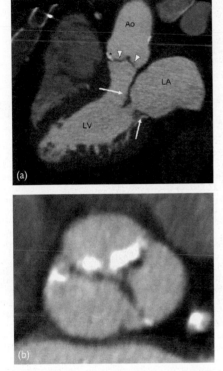

Fig. 1.5.4 Visualization of the valvular anatomy with MDCT.
(a) Oblique view. Mitral (arrows) and aortic valves (arrowheads)
are clearly visible, including the presence of some calcification of
the aortic leaflet and annulus. (b) Cross-sectional image showing
a calcified aortic valve in more detail (valvular calcifications
indicated by black arrows). Ao, aorta; LA, left atrium,
LV, left ventricle.

Further reading

Cerqueira MD, Weissman NJ, Dilsizian V, et al. Standardized myocardial segmentation and nomenclature for tomographic imaging
of the heart. A statement for healthcare professionals from the
cardiac imaging committee of the counsil on clinical cardiology of
the American Heart Association. *Circulation* 2002;**105**:539–42.

Chen JJ, Jeudy J, Thorn EM, et al. Computed tomography assessment of valvular morphology, function, and disease. *J Cardiovasc
Comput Tomogr* 2009;**3**:S47–S56.

Cury RC, Nieman K, Shapiro MD, Nasir K, Brady TJ. Comprehensive
cardiac CT study: evaluation of coronary arteries, left ventricular
function, and myocardial perfusion: is it possible?. *J Nucl Cardiol*
2007;**14** :229–243.

Di Carli MF, Dorbala S, Curillova Z et al. Relationship between CT
coronary angiography and stress perfusion imaging in patients
with suspected ischemic heart disease assessed by integrated
PET-CT imaging. *J Nucl Cardiol* 2007;**14**:799–809.

Kim RJ, Wu E, Rafael A, et al. The use of contrast-enhanced magnetic resonance imaging to identify reversible myocardial dysfunction. *N Engl J Med* 2000;**343**:1445–53.

Pattynama PM, de Roos A, Van der Wall EE, Van Voorthuisen AE.
Evaluation of cardiac function with magnetic resonance imaging.
Am Heart J 1994; **128**:595–607.

Schinkel AF, Poldermans D, Elhendy A, Bax JJ. Assessment of
myocardial viability in patients with heart failure. *J Nucl Med*
2007;**48**:1135–46.

Sciagra R, Leoncini M. Gated single-photon emission computed
tomography. The present-day 'one-stop-shop' for cardiac imaging.
Q J Nucl Med Mol Imaging 2005;**49**:19–29.

Schuijf JD, Poldermans D, Shaw LJ, et al. Diagnostic and prognostic
value of non-invasive imaging in known or suspected coronary
artery disease. *Eur J Nucl Med Mol Imaging* 2006; **33**:93–104.

Underwood SR, Anagnostopoulos C, Cerqueira M, et al. Myocardial
perfusion scintigraphy: the evidence. *Eur J Nucl Med Mol Imaging*
2004; **31**:261–91.

Coronary angiography

History tells us that in 1714 Stephen Hales opened the carotid artery of a horse, inserted a brass tube, and measured the pressure of the blood. This was a careful, scientific experiment demonstrating that the heart exerts pressure in order to pump blood; however, another result of the experiment was that, sadly, the horse died. Some 130 years later, in 1844, the French physiologist Bernard first coined the term 'cardiac catheterization'. Although he used catheters to record intracardiac pressures in animals it wasn't until some 80 years later that the first cardiac catheterization was undertaken in man. In 1929 Dr Werner Forsmann in Eberswald, Germany inserted a urinary catheter into his own left brachial vein, threaded it until it would progress no further, made his way to the X-ray department of his hospital and took an X-ray to show the catheter in his right atrium. He was dismissed from the hospital, but was subsequently made professor in another. The definitive breakthrough came in 1958 when Mason Sones in the USA accidentally undertook the first selective diagnostic coronary angiogram. Sones catheters, which had no shape but were 'shaped' *in situ* (against the aortic sinus), were used until the early 1990s being replaced with pre-shaped catheters—again some named after their designers/inventors—Amplatz and Judkins became standard catheters and with the advent of specific catheters for coronary angioplasty—subsequently the Voda, EBU (Extra-Back-Up), Hockeystick, and Right Back Up, and more recently the 3D right designed by Masa Kahn from Belfast.

The advent of selective coronary angiography was the turning point in the development of our understanding of the natural history and progression of ischaemic heart disease—being able to actually see a 'significant' stenosis and correlate this with the patient's symptoms and non-invasive investigations was a major breakthrough. At the same time coronary artery bypass grafting was an evolving therapy. The possibility of identifying the flow-limiting lesion(s), and being able to relieve anginal symptoms and improve prognosis by bypassing these lesions with harvested veins and internal mammary arteries led to major changes in the management and development of therapeutic modalities for coronary artery disease. Vogues for alternative approaches to enable access to the arterial system such as the use of the radial approach appeared in the mid-1990s, being driven by Kiemeneij and others; this approach has recently had a resurgence, and is likely to become the access site of choice with its reduced bleeding complication compared with the femoral route, early mobilization and patient preference (de Bono 1999). It is almost a return to the early days of angiography when all cardiac catheterizations were undertaken with Sones catheters via a brachial artery cut down—learning again all the previously learnt lessons of catheter engagement via tortuous arm vessels.

Indications

Coronary angiography remains the gold standard for understanding the potential management options for a patient with symptoms of angina, despite the rapid advance of multislice computed tomography and cardiac magnetic resonance. Since angiography is an invasive procedure it is mandatory that there is an appropriate, full, and sound pre-angiography clinical assessment and patient work-up, including the taking of a complete history, especially documenting the presence of risk factors such as:

- Hypertension
- Previous stroke
- Acute myocardial infarction
- The presence of diabetes (especially noting if the patient is taking oral diabetic medication such as metformin)
- A history of dye and other allergies
- Any bleeding tendencies need careful documenting.

If the patient presents with chest pain it is important to document the likelihood that that is due to coronary disease. This means that prior to angiography, to all intents and purposes all patients should undergo some form of non-invasive imaging to document evidence of ischaemia. For those who are mobile this will normally be an exercise stress test which has a 75% positive predictive value for the presence of coronary disease. For those with equivocal exercise tests, uninterpretable electrocardiograms (e.g. left bundle branch block, atrial fibrillation), or who are unable to exercise, the choice lies between the single-photon emission computed tomography (SPECT), the stress echocardiogram, or perfusion magnetic imaging. Each has its supporters—SPECT is less operator dependent and is a very good screening test, but exposes the patient to radiation and generally tends to be radiologist interpreted rather than having cardiological involvement. Stress echocardiography avoids radiation exposure but is operator dependent—magnetic resonance imaging is excellent for myocardial viability but not everywhere has perfusion options and if generic equipment is being used availability may be limited.

Informed consent

Coronary angiography is in general terms a safe procedure and is routinely undertaken as a day case procedure, not infrequently in mobile catheter laboratories, and provides important information for revascularization options. In the UK in particular there has been a significant increase in the number of new catheter laboratories set up in District General cardiology with 90 new laboratories funded by New Opportunities Funding since 2003, and this together with changes through formalization in junior doctor training has led to many more patients being considered for angiography and more importantly undergoing the procedure locally.

Overall coronary angiography has a low associated mortality (0.07%) (de Bono 1999) and low arterial risk (<0.25%), especially if small-diameter catheters are used from the femoral route (O'Sullivan et al. 1990). Although patients and operators are exposed to radiation risk, this is generally lower than other imaging procedures such as SPECT and computed tomography (CT) imaging, and can be considered acceptable for patient and staff during a single diagnostic procedure, even when undertaken by non-physician staff (Boulton et al. 1997). Increasing numbers of units are training non-medical staff to undertake coronary angiography (currently approximately five units in the UK). The fact that more patients have access to the procedure means it has become even more embedded into the management algorithm of those with suspected coronary artery disease (CAD). The ease of being able to undertake multiple procedures in a session together with increased generic working of catheter laboratory staff has led to increased efficiency.

Informed consent requires that the patient truly understands the procedure and the risks associated with it. In many centres this is ensured by providing written information often incorporated into the consent form, with care in particular being taken when the patient's first language is not English.

In general terms patients can be informed there is about a 1 in 1000 risk of death, acute myocardial infarction, or stroke occurring during and after procedure. The femoral arterial risk although low may be the factor delaying hospital discharge and this together with the patients' understanding of increased earlier post-procedure mobility has led to the increase in popularity of the radial approach (Jolly et al. 2009). Spasm, dissection, and negotiation of tortuous vasculature to access the ascending aorta need however to be considered and for both approaches documented, adequate training is mandatory.

The technique

For both the femoral and the radial approach general patient preparation is the same. Bloods should be drawn to provide full blood count and urea and electrolytes; if the case is being undertaken as a day case then these should be taken in a pre-admission clinic run by nurses. Such clinics have become popular in the UK and provide the patient with excellent preparation and information provided by experienced nurses with time to sit and chat to the patient. Informed consent can be obtained in such pre-admission clinics and prescriptions for required new medication, such as clopidogrel when the case is planned as a catheter query proceed onto angioplasty, can be written.

On admission, groins are shaved and the Allen's test performed in those undergoing the radial approach to ensure that there is more than just the radial artery as a blood supply to the hand.

Tips and tricks: ensure that the puncture in the femoral artery is high enough to avoid the femoral bifurcation using the Seldinger technique. In general the first catheters to use tend to be the Judkins 5 or 6 French. Whether one approaches the left or the right coronary artery first is a matter of personal preference—in general I always engage the left coronary first. If the Judkins distal end curls back into its out of body shape while in the aortic root, it is too small and the next size up (Judkins 4 to Judkins 5) is required. If the catheter sits below the left coronary ostia then the catheter is too big as may occur with small ladies with narrow aortic arches—is such cases a 3.5 Judkins should be considered. Many don't exchange catheters over a 180 cm 0.35 J wire, but you only need to have been halfway through a case once and had to abandon because of an aortic bifurcation problem to lead you to exchange over a wire routinely. Any wires used for access must be wiped clean and stored on the trolley in heparinized saline. Prior to engagement of the left coronary the manifold syringe should be drawn back so that blood enters the manifold, to ensure there is no clot or air in the catheter; once happy a test shot into the aortic root should be undertaken. Once engaged the pressure trace should be checked for normality and a test shot should establish that there is flush back into the aortic root. For acquisition, use only a small volume of dye (2–3 mL) injected at a moderate rate but ensure full filling of the artery. Although standard views were originally derived to allow for appropriate

targeting for coronary bypass grafts, the world has moved on and with coronary angioplasty now being the dominant reperfusion therapy it is important the views are taken to allow for important decisions to be made about the appropriateness and feasibility of this procedure. Thus with the following views panning should not be so quick as to miss important evaluation of the lesion itself (surgeons in general are only interested in the normality of the distal artery where they will place their graft, percutaneous interventions are more interested in the lesion itself) but at the same time if there is an occluded vessel (i.e. if you see retrograde collateral filling) then it is essential to plan to follow the retrograde filling until it ends to see whether antegrade angioplasty is going to be possible if the vessel needs opening.

When engaging the right coronary artery, be aware of pressure drop—it may mean you have engaged the conus branch and a standard injection here could result in an episode of ventricular tachycardia.

The 'standard views' should be modified and the following sequence in my personal opinion should be the starting views. All areas of interest should be appropriately centred. There is never really a 'set' view but start with a set of views such as below and adjust as you go if the acquisition is not going to demonstrate the lesion fully; it is essential to get all the information at one sitting.

Left coronary evaluation standard views

Initial left anterior oblique (LAO) 35–50° with cranial 25–30° (to assess the course of the left anterior artery and the relationship of the diagonal; if the projection is not steep (towards LAO) enough the spine will restrict the view of the left anterior descending (LAD) diagonal bifurcation. For the LAD left cranial assessment there should be a 'triangle' between the diaphragm, the spine, and the triangular, wedge X-ray filter, with the LAD sitting in the middle, remembering that the whole vessel will move down once the patient breathes in.

To assess the circumflex, the LAO, caudal ('spider view' 35° and 25°), will tell a good deal about the circumflex and its branches. I then further assess the circumflex artery using the shallow right anterior oblique (RAO) caudal (10° and 15°). This view will tend to highlight any lesions in the obtuse marginal branches.

To further assess the LAD/diagonal the next view I undertake is the RAO or posteroanterior (PA) (35°) cranial 25° (adjustments will need to made and depend on the patients anatomy); in this view the LAD and its distal integrity will be best highlighted. It should be noted that in this view the imaging is best with the patient breathing and holding their breath out rather than on inspiration as per the other views.

For the right coronary artery an R Judkins 4 or a Williams catheter is probably the best first choice. In terms of views, a straight LAO (35° or 50°) suffices for the initial view but sometimes some degree of caudal tilt (10–15°) will allow better visualization of the distal right coronary artery free from diaphragmatic overlap. Occasionally a PA caudal is required to show best the distal RCA.

An RAO view with either cranial or caudal tilt, 10° or 15° (depending on the patient's anatomy), will be required to fully assess the mid-body of the RCA.

The important issue is that these are a guide to the views most likely to show the coronary arteries and any lesions, but are flexible without exposing the patient to too much excess radiation; if you cannot quite see a lesion then change the angle slightly or until you can; it can be very frustrating for an interventionist to be asked for an opinion on a film and not to fully see what really is going on.

Post procedure from femoral approach vascular closure devices are now commonly used to allow early mobilization. There should be a well-documented programme of training in the hospital if such devices are to be used.

For the radial artery appropriate artery compression devices should be used.

All hospitals should have written protocols for post-procedure assessment per hospital discharge that should be aimed for as day cases. Audit of complications is mandatory.

Radiation protection issues

Training in and adherence to Ionizing Radiation Medical Exposure (IRMER) Regulations is an essential component of safe catheter laboratory practice. Full protective equipment and radiation dosimeters should be worn at all times. Dose of radiation limits (DRLs) are set by the local radiation protection officer for each invasive procedure, and although relative rather than absolute, do provide important guidance for practice. Radiation exposure to the patient should be kept as low as reasonably possible while gathering adequate information. Patients receiving high X-ray doses (i.e. >15 Gy) in a single procedure or undergoing repeated exposure should be monitored for deterministic effects (e.g. skin erythema or necrosis). The following influence (increase) the effective radiation dose:

- Extreme intensifier angulation away from the sagittal plane, especially extreme caudal and steep LAO projection (Table 1.6.1) (Pristipino 2008)
- Patient size (especially abdominal obesity)
- Inverse distance from intensifier to patient (image gap)
- Inadequate main-beam focusing (collimation)
- Unnecessary screening (e.g. during gantry movement or non-critical manoeuvres)
- Inadequate use of radiation protection equipment (e.g. lead eye shields or under-table skirts)
- Use of the radial access route (Kuon 2004).

Coronary anomalies

There are three issues that need consideration when addressing anomalous origin of the coronary artery: first, what the variations are and how commonly they are each likely to be found during coronary angiography; what is the clinical significance; and, for the purposes of this section, what are the practical steps to take when, during what starts as a routine angiogram a particular coronary artery is not where it should be, when standard procedures, technique and catheters are utilized. When using coronary angiography the various variations were found with a prevalence of around 1% in a large study of over 100 000 patients (Yamanaka and Hobbs 1990). Whether the anomalous origins are of clinical significance in themselves (as opposed to the anomalous artery having an atheromatous flow limiting lesion) is less clear. Some suggest (Loukas et al. 2009) that not all the noted variations are clinically significant, and unless detected as part of an ancillary investigation, even those anomalies that supposedly can cause sudden death, may produce no symptoms at any stage. If this is true it may therefore be difficult to be sure what the true prevalence is.

Defining the anomalous coronary artery is also interestingly difficult. The descriptive for one of the figures in the Luokas (2009) article states 'As the concept used for description in the normal heart depends on the origin of the coronary arteries themselves, it is inappropriate to use the notation of right and left coronary aortic sinuses when there is anomalous sinus origin of one of the arteries. According to Leiden convention a new system for categorization of the coronary arterial patterns has been developed. The system works by the observer considering him or herself as positioned in the sinus of the aorta farthest from the pulmonary trunk (i.e. at the back of the heart

Table 1.6.1 Time-adjusted radiation exposure (mGy × cm²/s) to an Alderson-Rando phantom in dependency on tube angulation.* From Pristipino C (2008) with permission from Oxford University Press

	RAO										PA	LAO									
	100°	90°	80°	70°	60°	50°	40°	30°	20°	10°	0°	10°	20°	30°	40°	50°	60°	70°	80°	90°	100°
Cranial																					
40°						43	54	44	47	50	57	71	80								
30°	94	89	58	33	31	32	31	29	25	23	19	29	34	46	67	75	84	82	106	111	133
20°	53	49	34	29	25	24	24	19	18	18	17	22	25	28	34	43	49	51	52	79	85
10°	35	33	28	26	23	22	19	17	14	14	13	17	20	35	24	31	38	35	36	39	48
PA																					
0°	30	31	27	26	24	23	16	13	12	12	13	16	17	19	19	30	31	29	27	28	29
Caudal																					
10°	37	47	46	44	32	30	21	16	13	12	12	18	18	21	24	38	42	43	33	28	30
20°	50	70	81	69	66	41	28	21	15	15	15	20	23	23	31	49	61	63	55	41	39
30°	83	102	108	84	78	44	25	23	18	22	23	32	31	34	34	55	81	98	94	89	58
40°						80	33	24	36	40	49	51	55	57							

* **Boldface** characters indicate range of typically used tube angulations.
LAO = left anterior oblique; PA = posteroanterior; RAO = right anterior oblique.

facing forward), the two sinuses adjacent to the pulmonary trunk being the ones, almost without exception, which give rise to the coronary arteries. When these sinuses are viewed from the non-adjacent sinus, with the observer standing upright, one of the sinuses is always to the right hand of the observer, and the other to the left hand. The right hand sinus, which is known as sinus 1 among the surgical community, gives rise, in the normal heart, to the right coronary artery. The other adjacent sinus, to the left hand of the observer, is known as sinus 2, and normally gives rise to the main stem of the left coronary artery. Using the convention of sinus 1 and sinus 2, therefore, it is always possible to account accurately for anomalous sinus origin of one or more of the three major coronary arteries'.

The real issue is what to do if routine technique fails to demonstrate a coronary artery where it normally should be. Frequently the best thing is to take an Amplatz-shaped catheter and sweep with small injections to see if the origin can be identified and then to carefully try and engage the catheter. Alternatively, as the anomalous right coronary artery mostly comes off anterior, it may be worth taking the image intensifier to a much more LAO/lateral projection and then aim the normal diagnostic catheter anteriorly. Be aware of the circumflex starting from the ostium of the RCA. Knowing when to give up is part of normal training. Having said that, the anomalous left coronary artery may take either a septal, anterior interarterial (between the pulmonary and aortic vessels) or posterior course. The anomalous RCA tends to course interarterially. The option at one time if the coronary artery was not where it was supposed to be and could not be found selectively was to perform aortic arch angiography to see if one could get an idea where the origins were and then try to selectively engage again, but unless one is clear that the only option is coronary angioplasty (and details of the disease especially if it is likely to be distal are thus mandatory) then coronary CT is a good option for assessing the proximal segments and the course of the anomalous coronary arteries.

Coronary angiography remains the gold standard in the assessment of patients with suspected CAD and plays an important part in the timely delivery of revascularization therapies. While recent expansion in the availability of coronary angiography is welcomed, the importance of adequate training, delivery of diagnostic, safely acquired images, and continued awareness of the potential for serious complications is paramount.

References

de Bono D. Investigation and management of stable angina: revised guidelines 1998. Joint Working Party of the British Cardiac Society and Royal College of Physicians of London. *Heart* 1999;**81**:546–55.

Boulton BD, Bashir Y, Ormerod OJ, *et al.* Cardiac catheterisation performed by a clinical nurse specialist. *Heart* 1997;**78**:194–7.

Jolly SS, Amlani S, Hamon M, *et al.* Radial versus femoral access for coronary angiography or intervention and the impact on major bleeding and ischemic events: a systematic review and meta-analysis of randomized trials [Review]. *Am Heart J* 2009;**157**:132–40.

Kuon E. Identification of less-irradiating tube angulations in invasive cardiology. *JACC* 2004;**44**:7:1420–8.

Loukas M, Groat C, Khangura R, *et al.* The normal and abnormal anatomy of the coronary arteries. *Clin Anat* 2009;**22**:114–28.

O'Sullivan JJ, McDonald K, Crean PA, *et al.* Cardiac catheterisation with 5 French catheters. *Br Heart J.* 1990;**64**:211–3.

Pristipino C. Radial artery catheterization and radiological exposure. *Eur Heart J* 2000;**29**:2316–7.

Yamanaka O, Hobbs RE. Coronary artery anomalies in 126,595 patients undergoing coronary arteriography. *Cathet Cardiovasc Diagn* 1990;**21**:28–40.

Biomarkers in cardiovascular diseases

Definition

The Biomarker Definitions Working Group (2001) has recently suggested to define a biomarker as 'a characteristic that is objectively measured and evaluated as an indicator of normal biological processes, pathogenic processes or pharmacologic responses to a therapeutic intervention'. According to this definition, biomarkers include but are not limited to laboratory-based imaging (e.g. ultrasonography, computed tomography), electrocardiographic (e.g. the QT interval in the surface electrocardiogram), and genetic markers. Height, weight, or blood pressure are other valid examples. This chapter is restricted to laboratory-based markers used in cardiovascular diseases.

Classification

Biomarkers can be classified according to their application in clinical practice. Natural history markers are biomarkers used in measuring disease predisposition, severity, or outcome. Drug activity markers reflect the response to therapy or drug treatment; they demonstrate proof of concept, and are used to establish dose regimens and for the optimization of combination therapies. Biomarkers also serve as surrogate markers. Surrogate literally means 'substitute'. In a setting in which the alteration of a biomarker by a given treatment that has direct effects on health, the biomarker serves as a surrogate marker for the clinical benefit. There is, however, no guarantee for a direct relationship between the biomarker and the clinical effect. Surrogate markers are used either when the clinical endpoint is undesired (e.g. stroke, death) or when the number of expected clinical events during the trial is very small. Typical examples include cholesterol (as a surrogate endpoint for 'death from heart disease') or blood pressure (surrogate endpoint for 'stroke').

The ideal biomarker

Laboratory-based biomarkers need to fulfil a number of criteria and performance characteristics to be used in clinical practice. An ideal biomarker should have high sensitivity, specificity, reproducibility, and stability. Furthermore, it should have low biovariability and should be independent of clinical and demographic characteristics (e.g. age, gender, body weight, kidney function, presence of hepatic injury). Its method of analysis should be rapid, simple, accurate, and inexpensive. The preferred method of analysis is a point-of-care (bedside) test.

The diagnostic performance of a biomarker is typically assessed using a receiver operating characteristic (ROC) curve, which provides a graphical description of the sensitivity and specificity of the test. The area under the curve (AUC) is a measure of test performance (Bloom 2003). Values above 0.7 indicate that the test is useful in clinical practice, but values above 0.85 would normally be expected. Excellent performance is indicated by a value of 0.9 or greater, and a value of 1.0 indicates perfection (Collinson and Gaze 2007).

Biomarkers of cardiac ischaemia and necrosis

The rupture or erosion of an atherosclerotic plaque leads to the development of an acute coronary syndrome. It is now understood that a sequence of events follows plaque formation and destabilization. These events include ischaemia, infarction (cardiac necrosis), and repair/remodelling (Collinson and Gaze 2007). Although biomarker research in cardiology was initially mostly concerned with the search for an ideal marker of myocyte necrosis, markers are now available for all three phases.

Biomarkers of reversible ischaemia are still used only in an experimental setting. Such markers include plasma choline, unbound free fatty acids, ischaemia modified albumin (IMA), pregnancy-associated plasma protein A (PAPP-A) and several others. Biomarkers that indicate cardiac necrosis have received tremendous research endeavours in recent decades (Table 1.7.2). The list of potential pitfalls of such a marker is long. Thus, it should not be present in tissues other than cardiac myocytes, and it should differentiate reversible from irreversible cardiac injury (Christenson and Azzazy 2006). The onset of release should be shortly after the onset of necrosis, and the release should be in direct proportion to the extent of necrosis (i.e. infarct size). Furthermore, the detectability of such a marker should persist for hours to days after the acute event. Finally, biomarker clearance should be predictable. Several markers had been suggested, were used for some time in the past, and were later abandoned because more recent developments came closer to fulfilling the criteria of an ideal biomarker. Aspartate aminotransferase (AST), for example, was one of the first markers of myocardial necrosis; measurements were performed as early as the 1950s. However, AST is not specific for myocardial tissues, and its measurement—routinely performed with activity assays—is no longer recommended. The same holds true for lactate dehydrogenase (LDH), whose serum levels were used until the 1980s to diagnose myocardial infarction.

Unfortunately, no single biomarker has as yet fulfilled all the criteria outlined above. Over the last decade, the troponins have emerged as coming closest to this ideal, and the advent of commercial test kits has led to changing the guidelines on the diagnosis and treatment of acute coronary syndromes and myocardial infarction (Van de Werf et al. 2003; Bassand et al. 2007). The development of tests for troponin analysis started in 1979. Cardiac troponins are expressed only in the heart, and their levels become detectable only when myocardial damage is present. The available test kits are able to detect damage to the myocardium of approximately 1 g or higher, but so called high-sensitivity or third-generation troponin tests are currently being developed. In cardiac muscle, the troponin complex consists of three proteins, troponin T, troponin I, and troponin C, that mediate muscle contraction. Since the troponins are structural components of the myocyte, their release kinetics are relatively slow, requiring 4–6 hours to become detectable in serum after the initial event. It is now acknowledged that troponin assessment provides diagnostic and prognostic insight, and initial studies reported that elevated levels of troponin T were associated with an increased rate of major adverse cardiovascular events. Although an assay for the measurement of troponin T is currently available from one manufacturer only, assays for troponin I measurement are supplied from a vast array of providers. Thus, reference limits for troponin I vary.

Total creatine kinase (CK) activity in the blood stream is the cumulative activity of three of its isoenzymes. CK activity is highest in skeletal muscle, cardiac myocytes, and brain, but is also present in the small intestine, tongue, diaphragm, uterus, and prostate. High serum CK values are present after myocardial or skeletal muscle necrosis and trauma, but also after extreme exercise. CK is a dimer consisting of two subunits designated B and M. The homodimers CK-BB and CK-MM are present primarily in brain and skeletal muscle, respectively. The myocardium is the only tissue that contains large concentrations and large proportions of the heterodimer CK-MB the percentage of CK-MB is about 1.1% of the total CK activity in healthy subjects, but rises to 20% in patients with significant myocardial disease (e.g. aortic stenosis, coronary artery disease). Current guidelines recommend the use of CK-MB but not that of total CK activity for the assessment of myocardial infarction. CK-MB assessment became standard in the 1970s. Myoglobin is the earliest of all available markers, but it lacks specificity for the myocardium; heart-type fatty acid binding protein (H-FABP) is not yet in routine use.

Biomarkers of haemodynamic stress

Volume overload as seen in patients with heart failure is associated with myocardial wall stretch. The physiological response of the body is natriuresis and diuresis, both of which are mediated through the action of natriuretic peptides. The release of atrial natriuretic peptide (ANP) from the cardiac atria, for example, is triggered by atrial wall stretch or atrial distension due to volume expansion ('stretch-secretion coupling'). B-type natriuretic peptide (BNP) is mostly released from ventricles in response to volume overload. Since natriuretic peptides also reduce the activity of the renin–angiotensin–aldosterone system, these peptides can be viewed as opponents of the physiological abnormalities of heart failure.

The natriuretic peptides form a group of structurally similar but genetically distinct peptide hormones. ANP was originally discovered in 1979. BNP was originally termed brain natriuretic peptide, as it was first discovered in 1988 in pig brain. It was later renamed to B-type natriuretic peptide when it became clear that the cardiac ventricles are its principal site of synthesis. A third member of the group is C-type natriuretic peptide (CNP). All natriuretic peptides are secreted as prohormones (e.g. proANP and proBNP), which are then cleaved into an inactive N-terminal fragment (e.g. NT-proANP and NT-proBNP) and the respective active hormone (e.g. ANP and BNP). The plasma half lives of ANP and BNP are 2–3 minutes each, but those of their N-terminal fragments are considerably longer. Thus, NT-proBNP plasma concentrations are higher than those of BNP.

Test kits for BNP are available from a vast array of different manufacturers. An assay for NT-proBNP is available from one manufacturer only. A test that uses an antibody against the mid-region of NT-proANP (MR-proANP) was recently shown to have similar diagnostic and prognostic value like BNP and NT-proBNP (von Haehling 2007). Overall, the plasma levels of natriuretic peptides have been used to ascertain the diagnosis of heart failure, to guide therapeutic decisions, and to assess the patients' prognosis (Braunwald 2008). Natriuretic peptide testing is recommend by current heart failure guidelines (Dickstein et al.

2008). Recent data, however, support the view that the prognostic utility of the novel biomarker midregional pro-adrenomedullin is better than that of BNP or NT-proBNP (Braunwald 2008).

Since heart failure is regarded as a multisystem disorder, a large number of other plasma biomarkers have been researched in recent years (Torbicki et al. 2008). These include neurohormones (e.g. noradrenalin, renin, angiotensin II, endothelin-1), inflammatory markers (e.g. tumour necrosis factor-α and its soluble receptors, interleukin 6), the above-mentioned markers of myocardial injury (e.g. cardiac troponin I or T, H-FABP), and many more (e.g. chromogranin, growth differentiation factor 15). However, none of them is currently part of a routine diagnostic workup.

Multimarker strategies

Several groups of workers have recently advocated testing of more than one biomarker for diagnostic and prognostic assessments. In particular, the detection of myocardial necrosis calls for the combination of a rapid early-rise marker in conjunction with a marker that offers high sensitivity and specificity. This could be the combination of myoglobin, CK-MB, and cardiac troponin assessment (Morrow 2009). The additional measurement of the acute-phase reactant C-reactive protein yields further prognostic information in patients with acute coronary syndromes. Patients with heart failure may also require testing not only for a natriuretic peptide, but also for C-reactive protein, a cardiac troponin, and potentially MR-proADM in order to accurately assess the patients' risk of adverse events. Likewise, current guidelines on pulmonary embolism recommend simultaneous testing of D-dimer and cardiac troponin I or T (Torbicki et al. 2008). It should, however, always be kept in mind that no biomarker will ever replace the experience and knowledge of a well-trained clinician.

References

Bassand JP, Hamm CW, Ardissino D, et al. Task Force for Diagnosis and Treatment of Non-ST-Segment Elevation Acute Coronary Syndromes of European Society of Cardiology. Guidelines for the diagnosis and treatment of non-ST-segment elevation acute coronary syndromes. Eur Heart J 2007;**28**:1598 660.

Biomarkers Definitions Working Group. Biomarkers and surrogate endpoints: preferred definitions and conceptual framework. Clin Pharmacol Ther 2001;**69**:89–95.

Bloom JC. Biomarkers in clinical drug development: definitions and disciplines. In: Bloom JC, Dean RA, eds. Biomarkers in clinical drug development. New York: Marcel Dekker, 2003: pp. 1–10.

Braunwald E. Biomarkers in heart failure. N Engl J Med 2000;**358**:2148–59.

Christenson RH, Azzazy HM. Biomarkers of myocardial necrosis: past, present, and future. In: Morrow DA, eds. Cardiovascular biomarkers: pathophysiology and disease management. Totowa: Humana Press, 2006: pp. 3–25.

Collinson PO, Gaze DC. Biomarkers of cardiovascular damage and dysfunction: an overview. Heart Lung Circ 2007;**16** (Suppl 3):S71–S82.

Dickstein K, Cohen-Solal A, Filippatos G, et al., for the Task Force for Diagnosis and Treatment of Acute and Chronic Heart Failure 2008 of the European Society of Cardiology. ESC Guidelines for the diagnosis and treatment of acute and chronic heart failure 2008: developed in collaboration with the Heart Failure Association of the ESC (HFA) and endorsed by the European Society of Intensive Care Medicine (ESICM). Eur Heart J 2008;**29**:2388–442.

Morrow DA. A multimarker approach to evaluation of patients with acute coronary syndromes. In: Morrow DA, ed. *Cardiovascular biomarkers: pathophysiology and disease management*. Totowa: Humana Press, 2009: pp. 545–558.

Torbicki A, Perrier A, Konstantinides S, *et al*. Task Force for the Diagnosis and Management of Acute Pulmonary Embolism of the European Society of Cardiology. Guidelines on the diagnosis and management of acute pulmonary embolism. *Eur Heart J* 2008;**29**:2276–315.

Van de Werf F, Ardissino D, Betriu A, *et al*., Task Force on the Management of Acute Myocardial Infarction of the European Society of Cardiology. Management of acute myocardial infarction in patients presenting with ST-segment elevation. *Eur Heart J* 2003;**24**:28–66.

von Haehling S, Jankowska EA, Morgenthaler NG, *et al*. Comparison of midregional pro-atrial natriuretic peptide with N-terminal pro-B-type natriuretic peptide in predicting survival in patients with chronic heart failure. *J Am Coll Cardiol* 2007;**50**:1973–80.

Chapter 2

Clinical presentations

Chest pain

Chest pain is an extremely common symptom accounting for about 5% of Accident and Emergency visits and 40% of emergency hospital admissions. There are many possible causes emanating from any of the musculoskeletal structures of the thoracocervical spine and rib cage, the intrathoracic organs, and the upper abdominal viscera:

- Musculoskeletal
  - Cervical or thoracic disc prolapse, malignancy, infection, and inflammatory disease
  - Inflammation of the rotator cuff of the shoulder
  - Traumatic or pathological vertebral or rib fractures
  - Perichondritis of the costochondral junctions (Tietze's disease)
  - Pre-vesicular pain of herpes zoster
  - Coxsackie B virus infection of the intercostal muscles (Bornholm disease)
  - Bone marrow infiltrations, sickle cell anaemia
  - As part of functional syndrome with elements of anxiety and depression (Da Costa syndrome).
- Pulmonary
  - Pleurisy, pneumonia, pneumothorax, embolism
  - Carcinoma of the lung, pleura, lymph nodes
  - Pleural effusion
  - Pulmonary hypertension.
- Cardiovascular
  - Acute myocardial ischaemia
  - Progressive coronary atherosclerosis
  - Coronary artery thrombus, rarely embolus
  - Coronary artery spasm—spontaneous (Prinzmetal's angina), drug induced (cocaine, amphetamines)
  - Coronary artery dissection—peripartum
  - Coronary artery anomalies, vasculitis
  - Left ventricular apical ballooning (Tako-Tsubo) syndrome
  - Secondary to a tachyarrhythmia, anaemia, hypoxia, sepsis, thyrotoxicosis, aortic stenosis, chest wall irradiation
  - Pericarditis, myocarditis, pericardial effusion
  - Hypertrophic cardiomyopathy, mitral valve prolapse
  - Aortic aneurysm, dissection, intramural haematoma.

Oesophageal
- Spasm, acid reflux, Mallory–Weiss tear, carcinoma.

Upper abdominal
- Peptic ulceration, pancreatitis, cholecystitis
- Subdiaphragmatic disease
- Hepatic congestion secondary to congestive cardiac failure or tricuspid incompetence.

Acute chest pain

Many of the above causes of chest pain may present with a chronic course accompanied by diagnostically helpful additional symptoms and clinical signs. Acute chest pain, however, should be treated as a medical emergency necessitating both a prompt recognition by the patient of its potential dangers and an urgent response by the acute medical services. Pre-hospital assessment is optimally provided by medical or paramedical ambulance personnel adequately equipped and trained in chest pain assessment, electrocardiogram (ECG) recording and interpretation, the administration of thrombolytic and antiplatelet drugs,

defibrillation, and the emergency relief of a tension pneumothorax.

After urgent attention of the **a**irway, **b**reathing, and **c**irculation, assessment should focus on the three most serious causes to **die** from—acute aortic **d**issection, myocardial **i**schaemia, and pulmonary **e**mbolism.

Clinical assessment

History: key points
- Location, radiation and nature of the pain
- Time of onset—crucial for later decisions on reperfusion therapy
- Any past history of ischaemic heart disease or interventional procedures—where and when?
- Any significant co-morbidities—pulmonary disease, diabetes, hypertension, rheumatological or haematological problems, including thrombophillia
- Any significant occupational exposure, smoking, alcohol consumption
- Any recent pyrexial illnesses
- Current drug treatment.

Examination: key points
- Airway, breathing, circulation.
- Quick general review—anaemia, icterus, thyroid status, nails, nodes, skin, mouth, palate, central cyanosis.
- Examine all pulses—may be the only clue to an aortic dissection.
- Pulse rhythm and volume: clubbing.
- Blood pressure, jugular venous pressure, peripheral oedema, vein salvage scars.
- Movement of the chest wall, sternotomy and thoracotomy scars, local joint or muscle tenderness, rashes, bruises, lymph nodes.
- Position of the apex beat and trachea: any abnormal characteristics to the left and right ventricular impulses?
- Percussion and auscultation of the lungs, e.g. excessive breathlessness in the presence of unremarkable chest signs suggests a substantial pulmonary embolus.
- Auscultation of the heart: left ventricular (LV) systolic murmurs (mitral regurgitation, ventricular septal defect, obstructive hypertrophic cardiomyopathy, aortic stenosis). Aortic diastolic murmur—think of aortic dissection.
- Abdominal examination.
- Musculoskeletal and neurological examination as dictated by the history and physical findings thus far.
- Associated symptoms—nausea, vomiting, pallor, sweating, fear.

Investigations

- 12-lead ECG supplemented by right ventricular and posterior leads if the recording is 'normal'.
- Venous blood sample for a marker of myocardial necrosis (preferably troponin T or I), creatinine for current renal function and some drug dosing, full blood count, lipids, and others as suggested by the history and examination, e.g. D-dimer, thyroxine, liver function tests, amylase, thrombophillia screen, baseline viral titres, 'rheumatological' antibodies.
- Arterial blood gases and pH.
- Chest X-ray.

- Computed tomography (CT) pulmonary angiogram.
- CT thorax if pulmonary embolism or dissection of the aorta suspected.
- Echocardiogram for pericardial effusion, right and left ventricular function, valve or other intracardiac lesions, including thrombus, myxoma, and vegetations.
- Plain abdominal X-ray and upper abdominal ultrasound as suggested by the history and clinical signs.
- Other investigations, e.g. spinal magnetic resonance imaging (MRI) in conjunction with appropriate specialist advice.

Management

Management will obviously be directed by the presumed diagnosis, e.g. of a tension pneumothorax, pleural effusion, acute pancreatitis, etc., but for 'the big three' intrathoracic problems (dissection, ischaemia, embolism) the principles of treatment are discussed below.

- Dissection of the aorta–should be discussed with a cardiothoracic surgeon. Those involving the ascending aorta are treated by urgent surgery if possible, whereas involvement of or limited to the descending aorta are treated by hypotensive rate slowing drugs, such as beta-blockers and diltiazem. For descending dissections there is growing interest and expertise in endovascular stent placement.
- Ischaemia of the myocardium in association with ST segment elevation in regional leads of the electrocardiogram or presumed new left bundle branch block usually represents complete occlusion of a major epicardial coronary artery. Treatment must start urgently with aspirin, clopidogrel, a heparin and either a thrombolytic drug or primary percutaneous coronary intervention (PCI) plus stent according to local availability and expertise. In patients presenting early, markers of myocardial necrosis may not yet be elevated but this must not delay treatment.

Ischaemia in association with ST segment depression or T-wave inversion usually represents non-occlusive coronary thrombus, which do not respond to thrombolytic therapy. As with ST elevation ischaemia, treatment includes aspirin, clopidogrel, and a heparin. Glycoprotein IIb/IIIa receptor blockers may also be administered or their use confirmed to the interventional catheter laboratory. Alternative anticoagulants such as fondaparimux (an antifactor X drug) and bivalirudin (an antithrombin) will be discussed elsewhere. Reperfusion, usually with PCI and stent, is the current treatment strategy, although the optimum timing for interventional treatment is not yet settled. What is agreed, is that patients with continuing pain, hypotension, and fluctuating ECG changes should proceed to intervention as soon as possible. There are various risk assessment scores which may aid decision-making, such as the TIMI risk score (Table 2.1.1):

Variables on admission—one point each:
- Age >65
- Prior coronary stenosis > 50%
- ST segment deviation on ECG at presentation
- At least 2 original events in prior 24 hours
- Use of aspirin in prior 7 days
- At least three risk factors for coronary artery disease (family history, male, hypertension, diabetes, hyperlipidaemia, smoking, obesity)
- Elevated serum cardiac markers.

In both ST and non-ST elevation syndromes adequate pain relief may require intra-venous morphine plus an antiemetic.

Table 2.1.1 The TIMI risk score

Score	% 14-day death, new or recurrent MI, urgent revascularization	Risk
0–1	5	low
2	8	low
3	13	medium
4	20	medium
5	26	high
6–7	40	high

Treatment with a beta-blocker and IV nitrate will also help. In the absence of contraindications beta-blockers are up-titrated and given indefinitely. Naïve patients are also started on an angiotensin converting enzyme inhibitor and a statin for indefinite secondary prophylactic treatment.

Interpreting an elevated troponin

Troponin is a component of muscle contractile apparatus and is composed of three subunits (TnT, TnI and TnC), of which TnT and I are cardiac muscle specific. They are usually not detected in the blood of healthy people, but they leach out of the cell when membrane integrity is compromised, e.g. due to hypoxia, ischaemia, sepsis. After an episode of myocardial ischaemia detectable levels may not appear for up to 12 hours, so an initially undetectable level does not equate to no myocyte death and repeats up to 12 hours from symptom onset are essential for correct and safe diagnosis. Levels may remain detectable for 14 days and thus offer diagnostic help for events that occurred several days before presentation, but make the diagnosis of re-infarction difficult unless frequent estimates are performed.

Although indicative of myocyte necrosis, elevated troponins do not indicate the reason for the event, although most occur in the context of acute ischaemia secondary to complete or partial thrombotic coronary artery occlusion. However, there are many conditions in which elevated troponins have been detected, which can complicate a clinical presentation:
- Acute ischaemic coronary syndromes
- Acute pulmonary oedema
- Myopericarditis
- Apical ballooning syndrome (Tako-Tsubo)
- Cardiac contusion, cardioversion, ablative therapy
- Cardiac infiltration—amyloid, haemochromatosis, sarcoid, scleroderma
- Cardiotoxic drugs—adriamycin, 5-fluorouracil, herceptin, snake venom
- Excessive tachycardia (even exercise induced) or bradycardia
- Dissection of the aorta
- Pulmonary embolism
- Hypertensive crisis
- Hypothyroidism
- Renal failure
- Subarachnoid haemorrhage
- Sepsis, severe burns, rhabdomyolysis.

Dyspnoea

The sensation of breathlessness is almost universal in humans and is obviously not pathological per se. Dyspnoea is an uncomfortable awareness of the process of breathing and is an extremely common symptom of many forms of heart disease. Differentiating cardiac from other causes of dyspnoea is a vital part of assessing the breathless patient. The commonest cardiac cause of dyspnoea is heart failure, although cardiac conditions can cause breathlessness. Although the central mechanisms underlying the perception of dyspnoea are still disputed, it is worth considering the pathophysiology of dyspnoea in acute and chronic heart failure separately.

Acute heart failure

Acute heart failure is more or less synonymous with acute pulmonary oedema. The mechanism by which dyspnoea arises is:
- Some initial cardiac insult causes an acute decrease in left ventricular function;
- In order for peripheral blood flow to be maintained, the left ventricular filling pressure rises, thus increasing cardiac output by the Frank–Starling mechanism;
- The rise in left ventricular filling pressure (LVEDP) is transmitted to the left atrium, and, in turn, the pulmonary veins and the pulmonary capillaries;
- Within the pulmonary capillaries, fluid is normally retained intravascularly because colloid osmotic pressure exceeds the hydrostatic pressure tending to force fluid out of the vessels;
- As the LVEDP rises to maintain cardiac output, it will eventually exceed the colloid osmotic pressure and fluid will start to transude into the lung interstitium and then the alveoli (Fig. 2.2.1);
- When the rate of fluid accumulation exceeds the rate at which the pulmonary lymphatics can remove it, the airspaces fill with fluid and pulmonary oedema develops;

- As the airspaces fill, gas exchange becomes impaired and the patient becomes hypoxic;
- The lungs become stiff and shifting air in and out becomes progressively more difficult and as a consequence the work of breathing.

Clinical picture

The breathlessness of acute heart failure is very dramatic and exceptionally distressing. The clinical picture is of a very frightened patient who is often (correctly) convinced that he or she is dying. The patient:
- Is extremely breathless and may not be able to speak more than a word or two at a time;
- Has to sit up or forward (and may succumb if forced to lie flat for medical procedures such as central line insertion);
- May produce quantities of pink, frothy sputum and occasionally frank haemoptysis;
- Is pale and sweaty, with poorly perfused peripheries due to sympathetic nervous system activation;
- Often wheezes.

There is usually a precipitant for acute pulmonary oedema, and so the features of, for example, acute myocardial infarction or acute arrhythmia may also be present.

Differential diagnosis (see also Table 2.2.1)

Breathlessness due to florid pulmonary oedema is usually straightforward to diagnose, but it may be confused with pulmonary disease, particularly when less severe.

Pulmonary embolus can present with similarly severe breathlessness and cardiovascular collapse. Any haemoptysis tends not to be pink and frothy. The typical crackles of pulmonary oedema are absent.

Exacerbation of chronic airways disease is commonly confused with pulmonary oedema and it is common to see patients treated for both conditions simultaneously. Patients with predominant lung disease tend not to be

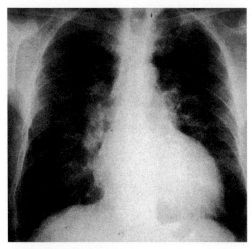

Fig. 2.2.1 Chest X-ray of patient developing pulmonary oedema. The heart is enlarged, there is venous congestion, and there are interstitial lines clearly seen at the periphery, particularly of the right lung.

Table 2.2.1 A differential diagnosis of chronic breathlessness

	Examples
Physiological	Normal
	Obesity, fitness, sarcopaenia
Psychogenic	Hyperventilation
Chest wall disease	Muscular dystrophy
	Kyphoscoliosis
Lung disease	Chronic obstructive pulmonary disease
	Asthma
	Pleural effusion
Pulmonary vascular disease	Primary pulmonary hypertension
	Pulmonary emboli
Cardiac	Heart failure
	Angina equivalent
	Arrhythmia
	Chronotropic incompetence
Anaemia	

affected so much by posture, and tend to have prominent wheezing and sputum production.

Non-cardiac pulmonary oedema including high altitude pulmonary oedema and pulmonary oedema following transfusion may occur in the absence of cardiac injury.

Many other pulmonary diseases cause breathlessness, but their clinical course and pictures make differentiating from acute pulmonary oedema straightforward.

Variants of acute heart failure

A similar pathophysiological explanation underlies cardiac dyspnoea in other situations:

Angina

● Need not be experienced as pain or chest discomfort and patients may describe breathlessness. The mechanism is presumably an acute rise in left ventricular end-diastolic pressure due to ischaemia. The typical patient describes the breathlessness as being associated with a tight sensation and occasionally wheeze.

Orthopnoea

● Happens when the patient is recumbent: venous return increases but cannot be dealt with by the failing left ventricle. Sitting up leads to rapid relief of symptoms. The *nocturnal cough* of patients with heart failure has a similar mechanism: the transient rise in left ventricular pressure results in transient increase in lung stiffness and consequent cough.

Paroxysmal nocturnal dyspnoea

● Can be very alarming and in contrast to orthopnoea can last for half an hour or so. Typically, a patient is woken a few hours into sleep with transient acute pulmonary oedema. The mechanism is presumed to be increased intrathoracic blood volume with possible ischaemia.

Chronic heart failure

Chronic heart failure is defined by the presence of symptoms in a patient with objective evidence of cardiac dysfunction. The cardinal symptoms are, of course, breathlessness, particularly on exertion, and fatigue. The clinical severity of chronic heart failure is often graded using the New York Heart Association (NYHA) classification:

● NYHA I: breathlessness only on maximal exertion. Normal or near-normal exercise capacity
● NYHA II: breathlessness on moderate exertion with reduced exercise capacity
● NYHA III: breathlessness on minor exertion and greatly reduced exercise capacity
● NYHA IV: breathlessness at rest. The patient is usually bed- or chair-bound.

The mechanisms underlying breathlessness in chronic heart failure are uncertain.

Measuring breathlessness

It is notoriously difficult to measure a subjective symptom. Approaches include using linear scales, such as the Borg scale, where patients are asked to rate their breathlessness on a scale between 1 and 10 (or 1 and 20 in some versions), or more complex questionnaires. Many are disease specific, and no single tool adequately covers all the dimensions of breathlessness. Even though it appears very simple to use, the time-hallowed NYHA classification system gives different results depending upon whether the patient or his or her physician is responsible for the scoring.

Exercise testing

Exercise testing is invaluable for exploring the pathophysiology of breathlessness. Many different exercise protocols have been used.

Incremental tests to exhaustion give an index of maximal exercise capacity. They are artificial as they don't represent 'real life' activity well.

Fixed work load tests with the 6-minute walk test being the most widely used. They don't give maximal exercise capacity, but reflect real life better.

With metabolic gas exchange measurements, maximal tests allow derivation of peak oxygen consumption (VO_2) and the slope of the ventilation—carbon dioxide production (VE/VCO_2) relation. Patients with chronic heart failure have a reduced peak VO_2 and increase in the VE/VCO_2 slope (in other words, for a given increase in carbon dioxide production, patients have a greater increase in ventilation than do normal subjects.

Haemodynamic model

The breathlessness of chronic heart failure might come about by mechanisms similar to those of acute heart failure: exercise is accompanied by a rise in filling pressure to maintain cardiac output, resulting in an increase in lung water, impaired gas exchange, and stiff lungs; breathlessness follows. The sensation of fatigue in the haemodynamic model is explained by the inability of the failing heart to perfuse the exercising muscle adequately.

However, against the haemodynamic model are some perplexing observations:

● There is no relation between any measure of resting left ventricular function and exercise capacity: indeed, some patients with exceptionally poor left ventricular function have apparently normal exercise capacity.
● Exercise responses of patients with fatigue as their predominant limiting symptom are identical to those with breathlessness.
● Peak exertion is not limited by cardiac output. If additional arm exercise is imposed on a patient with chronic heart failure performing maximal leg exercise, oxygen consumption (and cardiac output) increases further.
● Arterial blood gas levels are normal during exercise, including at peak exertion. Indeed, many patients at peak have a higher arterial oxygen and lower carbon dioxide tension than normal.
● Acute changes in cardiac function by, for example, positive inotropic drug therapy or even heart transplantation, do not improve exercise capacity or reduce the VE/VCO_2 slope.

The lungs in chronic heart failure

There is some abnormality of lung function on spirometric testing in approximately two-thirds of patients with chronic heart failure, although the defects are rarely severe. In addition, many patients have abnormalities of gas transfer. However, the normal blood gases militate against gas transfer being the cause of breathlessness; in addition, patients with chronic heart failure stop exercise during incremental tests long before they reach their potential maximal voluntary ventilation.

Ventilation—perfusion (V/Q) mismatching might be responsible for breathlessness. Components of potential V/Q mismatching include *dead space*, that is areas of lung ventilated, but underperfused with blood (V/Q ratio >1), and *shunt*, that is areas perfused but not adequately ventilated

(V/Q ratio <1). The relation between ventilation and carbon dioxide production is governed by the equation:

$$VE/VCO_2 = 863/PaCO_2 \times (1 - VD/VT)$$

where 863 is a constant, $PaCO_2$ is arterial CO_2 tension and VD/VT is the proportion of tidal volume occupied by dead space. Given that $PaCO_2$ is normal or low, there must be an increase in dead space to explain the increase in VE/VCO_2 slope.

Although V/Q mismatch is often quoted as being the cause for the increase in VE/VCO_2 slope, it is difficult to know what the biological signal causing the increase might be. The normal arterial blood gases suggest that shunt cannot be a prominent component, and how an increase in dead space might be sensed is not clear.

Control of ventilation during exercise

Multiple interlocking signals drive the increase in ventilation with exercise. At the onset of exercise, for example, central command anticipates the need for more ventilation so that the arterial CO_2 tension falls due to relative 'hyperventilation'.

Chemoreflexes are mediated by two sets of chemosensors: the peripheral chemoreceptors are in the carotid bodies near the bifurcation of the common carotid arteries, and the central chemoreceptors in the brain.

The chemoreflexes can be tested by controlling altering inspired gases. Hypoxic drive is measured by measuring ventilation as it increases relative to falling arterial oxygen saturation during 100% nitrogen breathing (mainly a measure of peripheral chemoreflex sensitivity); and carbon dioxide sensitivity is measured by either single breath carbon dioxide inhalation (testing peripheral sensitivity) or carbon dioxide rebreathing (testing central responses to hypercapnia).

Patients with chronic heart failure commonly have a greater than normal response to hypoxia, and this increase in chemosensitivity is closely related to the increase in the VE/VCO_2 slope. Suppressing chemoreflex sensitivity (using dihydrocodeine) results in a reduction in the VE/VCO_2 slope and reduction in the sensation of breathlessness, together with a small increase in peak exercise capacity.

Skeletal muscle, ventilation, and breathlessness

A second reflex input into the control of ventilation during exercise comes from the exercising muscle itself. Receptors sensitive to muscle work (ergoreceptors) transmit via the lateral spinothalamic tract to the central nervous system via non- and poorly myelinated nerve fibres. Stimulation of these fibres results in ventilation, but also results in sympathetic activation and parasympathetic withdrawal.

The skeletal muscle of patients with chronic heart failure is abnormal. It:

• Is decreased in bulk
• Is not as strong as normal
• Fatigues more easily than normal muscle
• Is histologically abnormal with a shift away from type I, oxidative fibres towards type II fast twitch glycolytic fibres with reduced oxidative enzyme levels
• Has abnormal mitochondrial structure, and the mitochondria have reduced levels of enzymes of the Krebs cycle and in the oxidative chain
• Has abnormal metabolism with more rapid depletion of phosphocreatine and early acidosis than normal.

It is easy to envisage how these changes to working muscle might lead to the sensation of fatigue, and involvement of respiratory muscles might contribute to the sensation of breathlessness.

A more profound link is via the ergoreflex. In normal subjects, increased ergoreflex activation increases the VE/VCO_2 slope and the ergoreflex is more active than normal in patients with chronic heart failure.

The ergoreflex can be measured in experiments using cuffs inflated around an exercising limb at peak exercise. The manoeuvre traps the metabolic products of exercise in the muscle. In normal subjects, this leads to prolonged post-exercise hyperventilation. The effect is greater in patients with heart failure (Fig. 2.2.2). The increase in ergoreflex activation correlates closely with both decreased exercise capacity and with increase in the VE/VCO_2 slope.

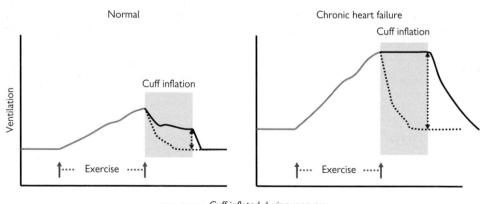

Fig. 2.2.2 Measuring the ergoreflex. When a cuff is inflated (shaded area) at peak exercise around the exercising limb, the ventilatory response to exercise persists into recovery. The effect is more marked in patients with heart failure. With permission from Wolters Kluwer Health.

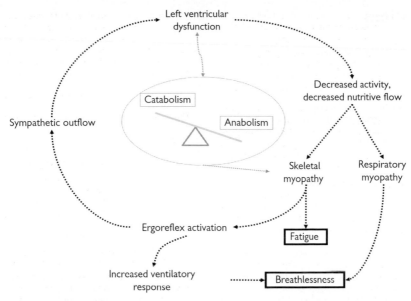

Fig. 2.2.3 Outline of the muscle hypothesis.

The muscle hypothesis

A unifying schema to explain the symptoms of chronic heart failure is the 'muscle hypothesis'. Chronic heart failure causes abnormal skeletal muscle. In turn, this leads to enhanced ergoreflex activity and an increase in the VE/VCO$_2$; the result is both fatigue and breathlessness on exertion (Fig. 2.2.3).

The origin of the skeletal muscle myopathy remains unclear. Possible contributing factors include:

• Disuse as patients with heart failure perform less and less exercise and become detrained;

• Impaired nutritive flow to the skeletal muscle, perhaps due to the increased peripheral vasoconstriction of chronic heart failure;

• A myopathy induced by imbalance between catabolic and anabolic factors. Such imbalance is common in the heart failure syndrome, and characterized by, for example, insulin and growth hormone resistance.

Implications

The muscle hypothesis as an explanation for the symptoms of patients with chronic heart failure is important as it suggests that treatments aimed at improving skeletal muscle function might improve patients' symptoms. Approaches include exercise training and using anabolic agents for selected patients.

Further reading

Bausewein C, Farquhar M, Booth S, et al. Measurement of breathlessness in advanced disease: a systematic review. *Respir Med* 2007;**101**:399–410.

Clark AL, Poole-Wilson PA, Coats AJS. Exercise limitation in chronic heart failure: The central role of the periphery. *J Am Coll Cardiol* 1996;**28**:1092–102.

Goode KM, Nabb S, Cleland JG, Clark AL. A comparison of patient and physician-rated New York Heart Association class in a community-based heart failure clinic. *J Card Fail* 2008;**14**:379–87.

Olsson LG, Swedberg K, Clark AL, et al. Six minute corridor walk test as an outcome measure for the assessment of treatment in randomized, blinded intervention trials of chronic heart failure: a systematic review. *Eur Heart J* 2005;**26**:778–93.

Pang PS, Cleland JG, Teerlink JR, et al., Acute Heart Failure Syndromes International Working Group. A proposal to standardize dyspnoea measurement in clinical trials of acute heart failure syndromes: the need for a uniform approach. *Eur Heart J* 2008;**29**:816–24.

Palpitations

Palpations are defined as the sensation of a rapid, forceful, or irregular heartbeat. Palpations can have numerous cardiac and non-cardiac causes (Table 2.3.1). Although palpitations many times are benign, ominous symptoms include syncope or presyncope, especially in individuals with a structurally abnormal heart. A patient who presents with palpitations requires a careful, systematic evaluation (Figure 2.3.1). The two most important objectives are to determine whether the palpitations are a warning sign of significant underlying heart disease and to obtain a recording of the heart rhythm at the moment of the palpitations. If the clinical diagnosis cannot be made by history, physical examination, and resting electrocardiogram (ECG), then ambulatory monitoring with a Holter monitor or cardiac event recorder (CER) should be considered. If symptoms continue with the diagnosis still in question and an arrhythmic cause suspected, invasive electrophysiological study (EPS) can be performed. Depending on the cause of the palpitations and the presence or absence of structural heart disease, a range of treatments can be considered: watchful waiting, medications, catheter ablation, or device therapy (pacemaker and implantable cardioverter defibrillator (ICD)).

Among the various causes listed in Table 2.3.1, the two most frequent causes are cardiac and psychiatric, with a prevalence of approximately 40% and 30% respectively. The remaining causes are classified as miscellaneous and include recreational drugs and endocrine disorders. Interestingly, those who present to an emergency room are more likely to have a cardiac cause of their palpitations whereas those who present in an ambulatory setting are more likely to have a psychiatric cause. Independent predictors of a cardiac cause of palpitations include being male, history of heart disease, palpitations lasting greater than 5 minutes, and a description of the palpitations as irregular. The aetiology of palpitations is not established in ~20% of patients.

Clinical approach

History
Clues during the history that may suggest a diagnosis are listed in Table 2.3.2.

Table 2.3.1 Common causes of palpitations

Arrhythmias	ST, AF, AFL, SVT, PACs, PVCs, VT
Psychiatric	Anxiety disorder, panic attacks
Drugs	Caffeine, cocaine, alcohol, tobacco, beta-agonists, certain over-the-counter medications
Cardiac (non-arrhythmia)	Valvular disease, mitral valve prolapse, pacemaker-mediated tachycardia
Extracardiac	Anaemia, hyperthyroidism, pheochromocytoma, pregnancy, pulmonary disease, hyperventilation

ST, sinus tachycardia; AF, atrial fibrillation; AFL, atrial flutter; SVT, supraventricular tachycardia; PACs, premature atrial contractions; PVCs, premature ventricular contractions; VT, ventricular tachycardia.

- Other questions to ask when taking a history: cardiac conditions, psychiatric disease, medications, stimulants, recreational drugs, endocrine or pulmonary conditions, family history of arrhythmias or sudden cardiac death
- Syncope is a worrisome sign and should prompt a rapid evaluation for ventricular tachycardia and structural heart disease.

Examination
Clues during the physical examination (Table 2.3.3).

- It is important to discern if there are signs of structural heart disease on physical examination. This is critical in determining the likelihood that the palpitations are of a more benign versus malignant nature and how quickly therapy needs to be instituted.

Testing
1 Baseline 12-lead ECG: Table 2.3.4.
2 Electrocardiographic recording of rhythm during symptoms (Table 2.3.5).
  - Holter: if there are episodes at least daily, a Holter can capture the arrhythmia and correlate with the patient's symptoms at that point in time.
  - Cardiac event recorder (CER): if palpitations are random and infrequent a CER can be used to record the rhythm during palpitations. Usually a patient has to press a button when they occur and this stored loop can then be wirelessly transmitted. Newer CERs are available which self-trigger and transmit once a certain threshold heart rate is met.
  - Implantable loop recorder (ILR): implantation of an ILR should be considered when the suspicion is high that there is an arrhythmic aetiology for the palpitations and long-term external monitoring has been unable to capture an episode of palpitations. It is a device which is implanted in the subcutaneous tissue and can be interrogated like a pacemaker.
3 Echocardiogram: an echocardiogram helps to evaluate for structural heart disease (i.e. reduced left ventricular function, hypertrophic cardiomyopathy (HCM), left atrial enlargement (LAE)). If further characterization of the heart is required a cardiac MRI can provide more detail (arrhythmogenic right ventricular dysplasia (ARVD)).
4 Electrophysiologic study (EPS): An invasive evaluation with intracardiac catheters used to pace and record and induce the clinical arrhythmia.
5 Labs: thyroid function test (evaluate thyroid status), haemoglobin (if anaemia is suspected), possible toxicology screen
6 Exercise testing to evaluate for ischemia or exercise-induced arrhythmias.

Management
- For the patients with a documented arrhythmia and structural heart disease medical management can be tried initially. If AFL becomes difficult to manage and appears isthmus dependent, an ablative approach can be considered as first-line therapy. Also, if there is a high burden of PVCs and monomorphic VT that appears amenable to ablation this can be attempted. For these patients it is crucial to manage their underlying cardiac

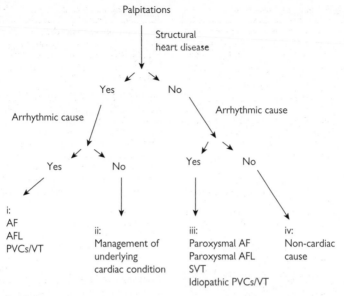

Fig. 2.3.1 Evaluation of palpitations.

Table 2.3.2 Historical causes

Historical features	Possible causes
Rapid fluttering	ST, SVT, AF, AFL, VT
Flip-flopping	PVCs and PACs
Intermittent forceful beats	PVCs
Irregular pounding in neck	AV dissociation: PVCs, VT, CHB
Regular pounding in neck (frog sign)	SVT (suggestive of AVNRT)
Young age of onset	SVT
Sudden onset	AVNRT, AVRT, VT
Gradual onset	AT, ST
Response to vagal manoeuvres, positional changes	AVNRT, AVRT
Syncope	VT, SVT, CHB
Occur at night in bed	PACs, PVCs, AF
Occur during exercise	SVT, AF, VT (structurally normal heart)

CHB, complete heart block; AVNRT, AV nodal re-entrant tachycardia; AVRT, atrioventricular re-entrant tachycardia; AT, atrial tachycardia.

Table 2.3.3 Examination clues

Exam findings	Possible causes
Irregular rhythm	AF, AFL (palpitations with rapid rate)
Harsh systolic murmur	VT (HCM)
Mid-systolic click	Mitral valve prolapse
Friction rub	Pericarditis
Heart failure (MR, displaced PMI, increased JVP, S3)	PVCs, VT
Hyperthyroid features	ST

HCM, hypertrophic cardiomyopathy; MR, mitral regurgitation; PMI, point of maximal impulse; JVP, jugular venous pulsation.

Table 2.3.4 Clues on the baseline ECG

ECG findings	Possible causes
Delta wave, short PR	AVRT
Q waves, LBBB, RBBB	VT, PVCs
LBBB PVCs (superior axis)	RVOT PVCs, RVOT VT
Prolonged QT	TdP, LQT
Increased septal R waves	HCM
Inverted T waves V1–V2, epsilon wave, RBBB	ARVD
Coved or saddleback type ST elevation V1–V3	Brugada
LAE, PACs	Atrial fibrillation
Bradycardia	PVCs

RBBB, right bundle branch block; RVOT, right ventricular outflow tract; TdP, torsades de pointes; LQT, long QT syndromes; ARVD, arrhythmogenic right ventricular dysplasia; LAE, left atrial enlargement.

Table 2.3.5 ECG characteristics of tachycardia

Tachycardia characteristics	Possible causes
Initiates with PAC and long PR interval	AVNRT, AVRT
Wide complex tachycardia	VT, SVT with aberrancy
Terminates with AV block	AVNRT, AVRT
AV dissociation, capture or fusion beats, negative concordance	VT
Irregularly irregular	AF
Saw-toothed pattern of atrial activity	AFL
Pseudo R' in V1 or S wave in AVF	AVNRT
Long RP tachycardia	Atypical AVNRT, AVRT, AT

pathology. If the ejection fraction is less than 35% an ICD should strongly be considered for primary prevention of sudden cardiac death.

• If palpitations are found to have a benign arrhythmic aetiology and are not bothersome to the patient one may elect to avoid medications. If the patient is experiencing bothersome palpitations from a supraventricular tachycardia such as atrial fibrillation medications may be tried with rate or rhythm-controlling agents. However, if these arrhythmias are recurrent, symptomatic, or if medications are not desired or are contraindicated catheter ablation should strongly be considered.

• Non-cardiac causes: lifestyle changes as well as stopping an offending agent are advised. Also the underlying medical condition should be treated. If a mental illness is suspected a referral to a psychiatrist should strongly be considered.

Further reading

Abbott A. Diagnostic approach to palpitations. *Am Fam Physician* 2005;**71**:743–50.

Brugada P, Andries E, Gursoy S, Brugada J. Investigation of palpitations. *Lancet* 1993;**341**:1254–8.

Fox DJ, Tischenko A, Krahn AD, *et al.* Supraventricular tachycardia: diagnosis and management. *Mayo Clin Proc* 2008;**83**:1400–11.

Weber B, Kapoor W. Evaluation and outcomes of patients with palpitations. *Am J Med* 1996;**100**:138–48.

Zimetbaum P, Josephson M. Evaluation of patients with palpitations. *N Engl J Med* 1998;**338**:1369–73.

Syncope

Definition

Syncope is a transient loss of consciousness (T-LOC) due to transient global cerebral hypoperfusion characterized by rapid onset, short duration and spontaneous complete recovery. See Fig. 2.4.1 for the clinical approach.

Epidemiology and aetiology (Table 2.4.1)

Syncope is common in the general population but only a small fraction of patients with syncope seek medical attention. Reflex syncope is the most frequent aetiology, especially in the young. Syncope secondary to cardiovascular disease is the second most common cause, with higher frequencies being observed in emergency presentations, mainly in older subjects and in settings orientated towards cardiology. Syncope secondary to orthostatic hypotension (OH) is rare in people under 40 years and is frequent in very old people.

Prognosis and quality of life

Structural heart disease is the major risk factor for sudden cardiac death (SCD) and overall mortality in syncope. The number of episodes of syncope during life and during the previous year are strong predictors of recurrence. Mortality is high in elderly people, although primarily determined by the severity of the underlying disease. Recurrent syncope is seriously prejudicial to quality of life.

Table 2.4.1 Classification of syncope

Reflex (neurally mediated) syncope

Vasovagal
Situational
Carotid sinus syndrome
Atypical forms without apparent triggers and/or atypical presentation

Orthostatic hypotension

Primary autonomic failure
Secondary autonomic failure
Drug induced
Volume depletion

Cardiovascular

Arrhythmia
Structural cardiovascular disease

Initial evaluation (Fig. 2.4.2)

The initial evaluation of a patient presenting with T-LOC consists of a careful history, physical examination, including blood pressure (BP) measurement, and standard

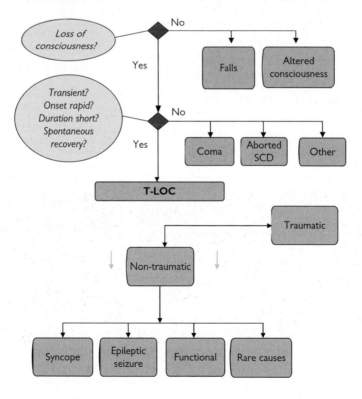

Fig. 2.4.1 Clinical approach to loss of consciousness.

electrocardiogram (ECG). Based on the findings additional examination may be indicated:
- Carotid sinus massage in patients >40 years
- Echocardiogram when there is evidence of structural heart disease
- Immediate ECG monitoring on suspicion of arrhythmic syncope
- Active standing test or head-up tilt test when syncope is prompted by upright posture or is thought to be reflex
- Other tests when T-LOC is considered not to be syncope.

The initial evaluation should answer three key questions:
1 Is the episode syncope or not?
2 Has the aetiology been determined?
3 Is there a suggestion of high risk of cardiovascular events or death?

Risk stratification (Fig. 2.4.2)

Short-term high-risk criteria requiring prompt hospitalization or intensive evaluation are listed below:
Severe structural or coronary artery disease (heart failure, low left ventricular ejection fraction or previous myocardial infarction).

Clinical or ECG features suggesting arrhythmic syncope
- Syncope during exertion or supine
- Palpitations at the time of syncope
- Bifascicular block (left bundle branch block (LBBB) or right BBB with left anterior or posterior hemiblock or QRS >120 ms)
- Sinus bradycardia (<40 bpm) or sinoatrial block in the absence of negatively chronotropic drugs or physical training

- Pre-excited QRS
- Prolonged or short QT interval
- ST elevation in ECG leads V1–3 (Brugada pattern)
- Negative T waves in right precordial leads, epsilon waves and ventricular late potentials suggesting arrhythmogenic right ventricular cardiomyopathy
- Family history of sudden death.

Important co-morbidities
- Severe anaemia
- Electrolyte disturbance.

Clinical features of syncope at initial evaluation suggesting a diagnosis

In neurally mediated (or reflex) syncope:
- Long history
- Triggered by unpleasant sights, smells, or by pain
- Prolonged standing
- Association of nausea or vomiting
- During or after a meal
- Precipitated by head rotation
- After exertion
- Post-episode fatigue.

In orthostatic hypotension:
- On standing up
- Related to commencing or increasing dosage of vasodilator medication
- Presence of autonomic neuropathy or Parkinson's disease.

In cardiac disease:
- Presence of structural heart disease
- Family history of sudden death or known channelopathy

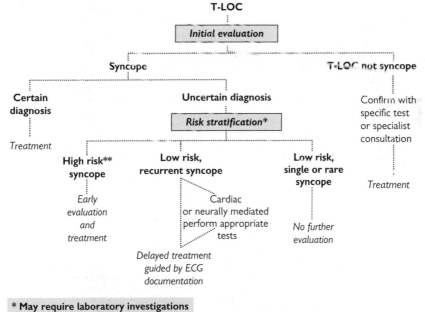

Fig. 2.4.2 Diagnostic flowchart in syncope.

- During exertion or supine
- Abnormal ECG
- Sudden palpitation leading to syncope.
- Suggestive ECG findings are:
  - Mobitz 1 second-degree atrioventricular (AV) block
  - asymptomatic sinus bradycardia <50 bpm
  - Q waves suggesting myocardial infarction.

Diagnostic criteria for syncope

Vasovagal syncope is diagnosed when syncope is precipitated by emotion, prolonged standing, dehydration and there is a typical prodrome. Situational syncope is diagnosed when it occurs in close proximity to a specific trigger such as cough, micturition, etc. Arrhythmic syncope is diagnosed when ECG criteria are present (see p. 49). Additionally, non-sustained ventricular tachycardia (VT) and evidence of pacemaker or implantable defibrillator (ICD) malfunction with cardiac pauses are also included. Cardiovascular syncope is diagnosed in the presence of acute ischaemia with or without infarction and in those with evidence of left atrial myxoma, severe aortic stenosis, pulmonary hypertension or acute aortic dissection.

Diagnostic tests useful in further evaluation of syncope

Carotid sinus massage (CSM)

Is indicated in patients with syncope >40 years but it should be avoided in those who have sustained a myocardial infarction in the last 3 months and in the presence of carotid bruits unless Doppler studies have shown no significant arterial stenosis. Carotid sinus syndrome (CSS) is diagnosed if massage causes >3 s asystole or a fall in BP >50 mmHg with reproduction of symptoms. Massage should be performed both supine and erect.

Active standing test

Is indicated in patients with severe dizziness or syncope in the first 3 minutes of adopting erect position. BP is measured repeatedly by cuff for at least 3 minutes. A diagnosis of orthostatic hypotension is made when systolic BP falls >20 mmHg or to <90 mmHg or diastolic BP falls >10 mmHg from baseline. These criteria are considered diagnostic when there are symptoms.

Tilt testing

Method: The patient is supine for 5 minutes before tilt-up (20 minutes if a vein is cannulated), then tilted head-up at 60–70° for 20 minutes (maximum 45 minutes); if no event tilt is continued for a further 15 minutes commencing with the administration of nitroglycerine 400 µg sublingually. If isoproterenol is given as an alternative to nitroglycerine, 1 µg/min is given intravenously for 5 minutes increasing by 1 µg/min to 3 µg/min in order to raise the heart rate by 25% above baseline. The end-point of the test is either syncope (positive) or conclusion of the protocol without syncope (negative).

Indications: tilt testing is employed in patients with recurrent syncope, no structural heart disease, or in those with a single episode at high risk of consequences at a future recurrence. Tilt testing is undertaken when it is considered of value to demonstrate to the patient the nature of the syncope. Tilt testing is of value in separating reflex syncope from orthostatic hypotension and from epilepsy when abnormal movements have been observed in an attack. Tilt testing is also valuable in the investigation of recurrent unexplained falls and in patients with very frequent syncope

when attacks may be psychogenic. Tilt testing is not recommended for assessment of treatment as it has been found unreliable and use of isoproterenol is contraindicated in ischaemic heart disease.

Diagnostic criteria: reflex syncope in patients without structural heart disease may be diagnosed in the presence of hypotension with or without bradycardia after >3 minutes. Stability of these parameters from tilt-up and, at the same time, the patient's usual symptoms are reproduced. OH is diagnosed when the criteria stated above are present. Negative tilt tests do not exclude reflex syncope. In patients with structural heart disease, cardiovascular causes of syncope must be excluded before a diagnosis of reflex syncope can be made from a positive tilt test. Induction of apparent syncope without fall in blood pressure or heart rate is diagnostic of psychogenic pseudosyncope.

ECG monitoring

Monitoring of the ECG should be undertaken in any patient suspected of arrhythmic syncope. The method of monitoring depends on the patient's presentation. High-risk patients require in-hospital assessment. Holter monitoring is only appropriate in patients who have frequent symptoms. An implantable loop recorder (ILR) is advised for use early in evaluation of patients with recurrent syncope unexplained by the initial evaluation. Evidence suggests that this approach yields more precise information about spontaneous attacks than that available from induced syncope on the tilt table. This includes assessment of the contribution of bradycardia to reflex syncope in older patients. External loop recorders are only an alternative to ILRs when symptoms occur at a rate of >2 per month as patient tolerance of these devices is often poor.

Diagnostic criteria: The correlation of spontaneous syncope with a documented arrhythmia is diagnostic of the patient's mechanism of syncope. In the absence of syncope ECG documentation of Mobitz 2 AV block, complete heart block, a ventricular pause of >3 seconds (except in athletes, during sleep, in presence of negatively chronotropic drugs and in rate-controlled atrial fibrillation) and rapid supra- and ventricular tachycardia. Other asymptomatic arrhythmias are not diagnostic of the mechanism of syncope including sinus bradycardia. A finding of no rhythm disturbance during syncope excludes a diagnosis of arrhythmic syncope but does not exclude syncope as this can occur due to hypotension without arrhythmia. ECG documentation of presyncope is not an accurate surrogate for syncope.

Electrophysiological study

Electrophysiological study (EPS) is only indicated in the presence of structural heart disease. The method employed depends on the findings on both initial evaluation and ECG monitoring. Diagnostic criteria are available in published guidelines (EHRA 2009).

Echocardiography

Echocardiography is valuable in the assessment of structural heart disease but only makes a diagnosis in aortic stenosis, obstructive cardiac tumours, or thrombi, pericardial tamponade, aortic dissection, and congenital abnormalities of the coronary arteries.

Exercise testing

Exercise testing is valuable in patients whose syncope occurs during or shortly after exercise. It is diagnostic when syncope is reproduced and there are rhythm disturbances and/or hypotension. It is also diagnostic, without syncope, if Mobitz 2 AV block or complete heart block is precipitated.

Psychiatric evaluation
Psychiatric evaluation is helpful in patients with frequent syncope and tilt testing has demonstrated apparent loss of consciousness without falls in blood pressure and heart rate.

Neurological evaluation
Neurological evaluation is rarely needed in patients with syncope but is recommended in patients where OH is likely to be due to autonomic failure and in those when T-LOC is suspected of not being syncope but epilepsy.

EEG and brain scans (CT or MR)
EEG and brain scans (CT or MR) are not recommended unless the loss of consciousness is suspected not to be syncope.

Treatment (Fig. 2.4.3)
Treatment—reflex syncope
The mainstays of treatment of reflex syncope are explanation and reassurance, avoidance of triggers and situations which may induce syncope, modification of any hypotensive drug regimen, use of isometric manoeuvres as physical counter-measures to combat falling blood pressure during a prodrome. In CSS with cardioinhibition, dual chamber pacing has been shown to be helpful in prevention of recurrent syncope. In reflex syncope in those >40 years documentation of severe bradycardia or asystole in a spontaneous attack (or also on tilt-testing) should prompt consideration of dual chamber pacing. Midodrine, an alpha-agonist vasoconstrictor with predominant venoconstrictive action, may be helpful in reducing reflex syncope. No other drug has any clinical trial evidence in its favour for this indication. Pacing is contraindicated in the absence of severe cardioinhibition.

Treatment—orthostatic hypotension
Triggers and precipitating situations should be avoided. Adequate hydration and salt intake must be maintained. Hypotensive medication must be modified or discontinued. Medication with fludrocortisone or midodrine is indicated if tolerated. Physical counter-measures are helpful but may be limited in effect by the lack of muscle bulk in elderly people. Abdominal binders and/or full-length support stockings may also be helpful. Sleeping in a bed, raised by >10° at the head, may help to condition the body for the upright posture as well as ameliorate nocturnal hypertension.

Treatment—cardiac arrhythmia
Pacing is indicated in sinus node disease and AV block according to the guidelines on pacing. Ablation and anti-arrhythmic drug therapy are also indicated in patients according to guidelines. Implantable cardioverter-defibrillators (ICDs) are indicated in patients with ventricular tachyarrhythmias according to guidelines for these devices.

Syncope in elderly people
The most common causes of syncope in elderly people, in descending order of frequency, are OH (often drug induced) CSS, reflex syncope, and cardiac arrhythmias. Different forms may often co-exist in the same patient.

Important points in the evaluation of syncope in elderly people:
- OH is not always reproducible (particularly medication related); assessment may have to be repeated in the morning or after spontaneous syncope.
- CSM is particularly useful in this age group.
- In reflex syncope in older patients tilt testing is safe and well tolerated with positive rates similar to those in the young. Nitroglycerine challenge may be needed. Induced syncope may be unrecognized by the patient. Prodrome may be absent.

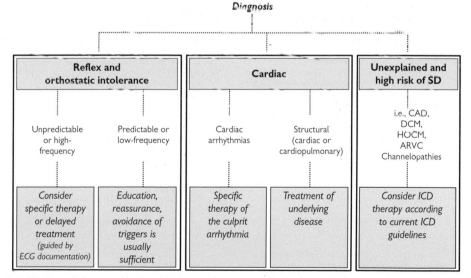

Fig. 2.4.3 Treatment of syncope.

• 24-hour ambulatory BP if fluctuation of BP is suspected (e.g. nocturnal hypertension or postprandial hypotension).
• ILR is very valuable as incidence of arrhythmias is high.
• Evaluation of mobile, independent, cognitively normal elderly subjects must be performed as for the young.

Syncope in paediatric patients

Diagnostic evaluation in paediatric patients is similar to that in adults, except that previously undiagnosed congenital anomalies and channelopathies are of greater concern. Reflex syncope represents the vast majority of the causes but in rare cases syncope is a manifestation of life-threatening arrhythmia or structural abnormality. Syncope must also be differentiated from epilepsy and psychogenic pseudosyncope, which are rare but important causes of T-LOC in this age group. Some aspects of the history should prompt cardiac evaluation:
• Family history of sudden cardiac death (<30 years), familial heart disease
• Known or suspected heart disease
• Syncope triggers: loud noise, fright, extreme emotional stress
• Syncope during exercise, including swimming
• Syncope without prodrome, while supine or sleeping or preceded by chest pain or palpitations.

Syncope management unit

Objectives: Any syncope or T-LOC facility has the following goals.
• Provide state-of-the-art guideline-based assessment of symptomatic patients in order to risk stratify them, then obtain an accurate aetiological diagnosis, advise on driving (Table 2.4.2) and assess prognosis.
• Physician(s) in the unit lead the process of comprehensive management from diagnosis to therapy and may also offer follow-up. Core tests are provided within the unit and there is preferential access to other diagnostic tests and therapies.
• Reduce hospitalizations. The majority of patients can be managed as out-patients or day-cases.
• Set standards for clinical excellence in adherence to current guidelines on syncope.

Key points for standardized care delivery:
• A structured care pathway, either delivered in a single facility or as a more multifaceted service is recommended for global assessment of patients with T-LOC.

Table 2.4.2 Syncope and driving

Diagnosis	Private drivers	Vocational drivers
Arrhythmias Medical therapy	After successful treatment established	After successful treatment established
Pacemaker implant	After 1 week	After correct function established
Catheter ablation	After successful treatment established	After long-term success confirmed
ICD implant	In general low risk restriction case-by-case	Restriction permanent
Single/mild reflex syncope	No restriction	No restriction unless occurrence during high risk activity
Recurrent/severe syncope	After symptoms controlled	Permanent restriction unless effective therapy established
Unexplained syncope	No restriction unless absence of prodrome, occurrence during driving or presence of severe structural heart disease	After diagnosis and appropriate therapy established

• Experience and training in cardiology, neurology, geriatrics, paediatrics and emergency medicine are pertinent to this facility.

Further reading

European Heart Rhythm Association (EHRA); Heart Failure Association (HFA); Heart Rhythm Society (HRS); European Society of Emergency Medicine (EuSEM); European Federation of Internal Medicine (EFIM); European Union Geriatric Medicine Society (EUGMS); American Geriatrics Society (AGS); European Neurological Society (ENS); European Federation of Autonomic Societies (EFAS); American Autonomic Society (AAS), Moya A, Sutton R, Ammirati F, et al., ESC Committee for Practice Guidelines (CPG), Vahanian A, Auricchio A, Bax J, et al. Guidelines for the diagnosis and management of syncope (version 2009): the Task Force for the Diagnosis and Management of Syncope of the European Society of Cardiology (ESC). Eur Heart J 2009;**30**:2631–71.

Oedema

Oedema (derived from the ancient Greek word 'ο δημα' meaning swelling) can be defined as excessive tissue fluid. The definition implies that the fluid excess has become visible and is causing swelling. It has been estimated that in a normal adult a litre or more of fluid can be accumulated in the tissues before any visible swelling is evident and therefore accurate measurement of the amount of excess tissue fluid is difficult. Oedema has been known to be associated with heart failure since ancient times, with Hippocrates describing a case of heart disease (which we would now recognize as heart failure with cardiac cachexia) as having the following features '... the flesh is consumed and becomes water, ... the abdomen fills with water, the feet and legs swell, the shoulders, clavicles, chest and thighs melt away ... this illness is fatal ...'. In Withering's time in eighteenth-century England foxglove extract use was described for dropsy, the common term for oedema at the time.

Of course not all oedema is heart failure and therein lies the diagnostic challenge. As oedema is excess tissue fluid we need to look at the mechanism of control of tissue fluid. Because we as humans live our waking hours mainly awake our lower limbs are subject to the hydrostatic effect of a column of fluid exerting pressure through gravity on the tissues of the lower extremities. The fact that the endothelium of the capillaries have fenestrations means that fluid can (and would) seep out and form oedema were it not normally counterbalanced by an inward pressure, which in this case is the inward colloid osmotic pressure exerted on fluid by plasma proteins too large to cross the capillary membrane and therefore 'sucking' fluid back into the capillaries. This keeps the tissues at below atmospheric pressure in health. This simplification (often referred to as Starling's law or Starling's forces) is helpful clinically to classify the causes of oedema even though the true situation is far more complicated, as the effect of venous valves, the pumping of muscular action on the tissues and lymphatic drainage all need to be taken into account (Renkin 1994). As a simple guide, tissue oedema is caused when one of the following three events occur: (1) the hydrostatic pressure in the capillaries goes up (itself either caused by increased venous pressure or increased arterial pressure

conducted through by vasodilatation); (2) the colloid osmotic pressure of the capillary blood goes down (due for example to hypoproteinaemia); or (3) the vessels themselves get excessively leaky and allow proteins to escape and reduce the osmotic pressure gradient. Examples of all three causes of oedema are seen in routine practice and the diagnostic challenge is to determine which is the most important pathophysiologically.

Types of oedema

According to a simplified Starling's law, classification of oedema may be due to increased capillary hydrostatic pressure (which itself may be mainly arterial or venous derived) to leaky capillary walls or due to hypoproteinaemia. One must also not confuse this clinical picture with lymphoedema due to damaged lymphatics (commonly caused by surgery or cancer or infection/inflammation) or other causes of tissue swelling. Oedema due to excess tissue fluid is referred to as pitting, because if a finger is pressed in it the impression lasts a few seconds (see Fig. 2.5.1) before disappearing whereas other forms of swelling do not exhibit this behaviour.

Distribution of oedema

Oedema will occur where the disturbance of Starling's forces determines it should. It is thus logical it should occur where hydrostatic forces are highest, which will be the most dependent part of the body, the legs and ankles when standing or the sacrum or eyes (with their low tissue turgor) when lying in bed. Where it is not so distributed, there may be local factors, such as local vascular obstruction (e.g. cerebral oedema) or local alterations in capillary permeability, local allergic, or histamine reaction as the cause. Thus one should seek systemic causes when the oedema is gravitationally distributed. This includes cardiac oedema. One should seek alternative explanations for other patterns of oedema distribution, and also be aware of rarer but more dangerous forms of localized oedema such as angio-oedema and certain clinical situations such as pre-eclampsia. Oedema which is not dependent (gravity related) may be due to an organ-specific cause, which should be sought where the oedema distribution is not

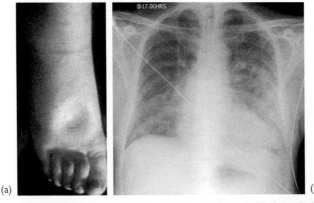

(a)   (b)

Fig. 2.5.1 The clinical picture of oedema. (a) Peripheral pitting oedema (from the *ESC Textbook of Cardiovascular Medicine*, courtesy of Oxford University Press); (b) pulmonary oedema (image courtesy of Dr Jeremy Jones, from http://commons.wikimedia.org/wiki/File:APO.jpg).

Table 2.5.1 Classification of causes of generalized pitting oedema

Increased hydrostatic pressure
Arterial: vasodilatation e.g. allergic reaction, insect bite, urticarial reaction, direct-acting vasodilator side-effects, etc.
Venous: heart failure, venous obstruction (e.g. embolus, DVT, IVC obstruction), varicose veins, venous valvular incompetence, acute renal failure, water intoxication, iatrogenic fluid overload
Capillary leakiness
Early stages of nephrotic syndrome, calcium antagonist-induced oedema, angio-oedema, pre-eclampsia
Hyproteinaemia
Nephrotic syndrome (see Kodner 2009), cirrhosis, severe malnutrition (Kwashiorkor), protein-losing enteropathy

explicable on the basis of gravitational effects. These include local inflammatory reactions (such as contact dermatitis, insect bites), cerebral oedema, perio-orbital oedema when localized (this can be gravitational when the patient has been supine for a prolonged period), scrotal oedema (when localized), or certain forms of pulmonary oedema (high altitude, neurogenic, acute respiratory distress syndrome).

Clinical picture
Oedema may be of insidious onset and hardly noticed by the patient or it may dramatically occur overnight. The onset depends on fluid and salt intake and renal excretion as well as the onset of the underlying disease process.

Differential diagnosis
The differential diagnosis of pitting oedema is of other forms of swelling which do not pit. These include tumours, lymphoedema, myxoedema, foreign bodies, fractures, effusions, and infections.

If the oedema is pitting, one should evaluate the distribution; if local only then seek a local cause; if gravitationally distributed one should seek one of the causes in Table 2.5.1. There is another condition which is cyclical in some women and occurs mostly in the years of menstruation, idiopathic cyclic oedema of women, which is a diagnosis of exclusion in patients who fit these criteria.

In assessing an oedematous patient in addition to a routine cardiac history and questions concerning the onset and clinical pattern of the oedema itself, one should ask about recent drug intake, salt and fluid and dietary habits, any history or family history of swelling, renal diseases, heart disease, relationship to periods, diurnal pattern of swelling, and symptoms of breathlessness.

Diagnostic tests for gravitational pitting oedema should include chest X-ray looking for cardiomegaly and pulmonary congestion, urinalysis, urea and electrolytes, serum protein estimation, and an echocardiogram if left ventricular dysfunction is suspected.

Treatment of oedema
One should attempt to determine the cause of the oedema as quickly as possible and treatment will be guided by the underlying cause. The following account is restricted to the management of cardiac causes of oedema.

Cardiac oedema can be treated by either improving cardiac function (such as correcting ischaemia, correcting an arrhythmia, or by revascularization or drugs that eventually improve cardiac performance such as beta blockers, but these effects are slow) or by treating the fluid retention directly, such as by diuretics, or salt and water restriction.

If the oedema is mild, a reduced salt diet can help and may be sufficient for symptom control. This diet is not easy however and nor is it side-effect free; such patients may need their electrolytes checked for abnormalities of sodium or potassium homeostasis. If drug treatment is required, the most gentle treatment is a low-dose thiazide diuretic. This would be first choice in a hypertensive patient. The alternative is to go for a loop diuretic (such as furosemide starting at a dose of 40 mg per day) to which a potassium-sparing diuretic such as amiloride can be added if needed. In resistant cases and under very careful fluid and electrolyte monitoring high doses of loop diuretics together with potassium-sparing diuretics and thiazides (in particular metolazone) may be needed, but this is a highly potent combination that should be used only under very careful specialist supervision. For a tabular description of the diuretics used to treat oedema associated with acute heart failure, see Table 6.5.6, p. 230.

Other treatment options
In end-stage heart failure or severe cardiogenic shock, oedema can be removed by ultrafiltration, and this approach is superior in terms of fluid removal to even high-dose diuretics, yet its effects on long-term outcomes or symptom status is not yet clear (Goldsmith 2010). Compression bandaging of the periphery has been used with marginal success but is not recommended. Recent experimental approaches to controlling oedema that have not yet proven effective include vasopressin antagonism and adenosine antagonism.

References

Goldsmith SR. Brandimarte F. Gheorghiade M. Congestion as a therapeutic target in acute heart failure syndromes. [Review]. *Prog Cardiovasc Dis* 2010;**52**:383–92.

Kodner C. Nephrotic syndrome in adults: diagnosis and management. *Am Fam Physician.* 2009;**80**:1129–34. Review.

Renkin EM. Cellular aspects of transvascular exchange: a 40-year perspective. *Microcirculation* 1994;**3**:157–67.

Chapter 3

Cardiac arrhythmias

Bradycardia due to conduction disturbances

Bradyarrhythmias due to atrioventricular node dysfunction

The atrioventricular (AV) node is situated subendocardialy within the atrial septum at the apex of Koch (boundaries are made by (1) the coronary sinus os, (2) the tendon of Todaro, and (3) the septal leaflet of the tricuspid valve). The AV node is less compact than the SA (sinoatrial) node but is composed of variety of cells including atrial, T cells, P cells, and conduction cells. It has autonomic nervous supply and its own arterial branch called the AV nodal artery, arising from the right coronary artery in 90% and the circumflex coronary artery in 10% of people. The node is divided into three areas known as atrionodal, central compact, and nodal His portions. These areas are important when junctional escape rhythm is required in situations when the SA node fails or when electrical activity is totally blocked to pass from atrium to ventricle in complete heart block. The atrionodal cells depolarize faster and can generate an electrical activity at 45–60 bpm with narrow QRS complexes and are responsive to autonomic nervous system and atropine. The cells of nodal His depolarize at a slower rate, can produce about 40 bpm, with wider QRS complexes, and do not respond to autonomic nervous system and atropine. The causes of AV dysfunction are given in Table 3.1.2. AV node disease can give rise to the following bradyarrhythmias:

- First-degree AV block
- Second-degree AV block
- Third-degree or complete AV block.

First-degree AV block

In first-degree AV block all the atrial impulses are conducted to ventricles but with a delay. Therefore, it is characterized by prolongation of the PR interval on the surface electrocardiogram (ECG) that exceeds 220 ms (Fig. 3.1.1). The PR interval represents passage of impulse through interatrial (10–50 ms), AV nodal (90–150 ms), and His–Purkinje (25–55 ms) conduction systems. First-degree AV block with narrow QRS complexes arise from the intra-AV nodal region in more than 85%.

Second-degree AV block

In this condition not all the atrial impulses are conducted to the ventricles. The conduction ratio is described as the ratio of P to QRS complexes, e.g. 2:1. There are two subtypes of second-degree AV block.

- Mobitz type I AV (Wenckebach) block.
- Mobitz type II AV block.

Mobitz type I AV block

This type of second-degree AV block is due to progressive delay in conducting the atrial impulse to the ventricle due to refractiveness of the AV node leading to failure of conduction. This cycle repeats itself. On surface ECG it is characterized by narrow QRS complexes and progressive lengthening of the PR interval followed by a P wave without (drop) QRS complexes (Fig. 3.1.2). The conduction ratio is usually 3:2, 4:3, or 6:5. Mobitz type I AV block is considered benign and usually does not require treatment.

Table 3.1.1 Causes of sinus node dysfunction

Medications
Beta-blockers
Rate-limiting calcium channel blockers (diltiazem, verapamil)
Digitalis (Digixin, Digitoxin)
Class I antiarrhythmic agents (flecanide, propafenone)
Class III anti-arrhythmic agents (sotalol, amiodarone)
Clonodine
Idiopathic
Normal aging
Degenerative process
Myocardial infarction or ischaemia
RCA or left CX coronary artery occlusion
Jarisch-Bezold reflex
RCA, right coronary artery
CX, circumflex coronary artery

Table 3.1.2 Causes of AV node, His Purkinje and bundle dysfunction

Drugs	Iatrogenic
Digitalis, beta-blocker, calcium channel blockers, amiodarone, sotalol	AV nodal His radiofrequency ablation
Ischaemic heart disease	Cardiac surgeries like AVR, CABS, VSD repair
Ischaemic cardiomyopathy	**Infection and infiltrative**
Acute MI	**disorders**
Idiopathic	Aortic valve endocarditis
Degenerative	Lyme disease
Calcific aortic stenosis	Chagas disease
Lev's disease (His–Purkinje fibrosis in elderly)	Amloidosis
	Sarcoidosis
Lenegre disease (His–Purkinje fibrosis in young)	Neoplasia
	Connective tissues disease
Congenital	SLE, rheumatoid arthritis
Congenital complete heart block in mothers with SLE	**Neuromuscular diseases**
	e.g. Duchene muscular dystrophy
Transposition of great arteries	

SLE, systemic lupus erythematosus; CABS, coronary artery bypass surgery; VSD, ventricular septal defect.

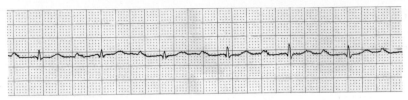

Fig. 3.1.1 Demonstrating first degree AV, block PR interval of 336 ms (>220 ms).

Mobitz type II AV block
In Mobitz type II AV block the electrical impulses fail abruptly to transmit to the ventricle. The block is usually at a lower level of the His bundle or bundle branches (broad QRS complexes). This condition represents more advanced disease in the conduction system and carries a high risk of complete failure of conduction. On surface ECG the PR interval is normal and a sudden drop in QRS complexes can be seen on a rhythm strip (Fig. 3.1.3).

2:1 AV conduction ratio represent either type I or type II AV block, as two or more consecutive PR intervals are not recorded, which makes the differentiation of type I and type II AV block difficult. However, a prolonged PR interval and narrow QRS complex favours type I AV block. Carotid sinus massage may help differentiate between the two by altering AV conduction.

Third-degree AV block or complete heart block
In complete AV block there is no transmission of atrial electrical impulse to the ventricles; if the conduction system distal to the block is capable of generating escape electrical impulses then both the atrium and the ventricle depolarize independent of each other through their respective pacemakers (Fig. 3.1.4). The atrial rate is always higher than the ventricular rate. The width of QRS complexes and the ventricular rate depends on the level of escape rhythm. The higher location in the conduction system favours a faster rate and narrower QRS complexes, which may arise at the AV junction, bundle of His, bundle branches, or distal Purkinje system.

In the context of atrial fibrillation or flutter, complete heart block can be identified by a regular slow ventricular rate and QRS widening (Figs 3.2.5 and 3.2.6). The regularity of ventricular rhythm indicates that it has not arisen from the atrial rhythm but from an independent pacemaker distal to the conduction block.

Congenital third-degree AV block
Congenital complete heart block is found in 1 out of 22 000 live births and has a close association with maternal systemic lupus erythematosus (SLE) and anti-Ro antibodies. Asymptomatic individuals may not require any treatment but patients with symptoms of syncope, presyncope, or infants with an awake heart rate <55 bpm, and prolonged QTc >460 ms require permanent pacemaker implantation.

Clinical features
First-degree AV block and second-degree AV block do not produce any symptoms and the diagnosis is usually coincidental, unless a patient develops an intermittent higher degree AV block. A third-degree AV block (complete AV block) may produce acute symptoms of cerebral hypoperfusion (dizziness, light-headedness, confusion, presyncope, or syncope) if the ventricular escape rhythm (<40 bpm) is slow and not capable of supporting the body's haemodynamic system. An escape rhythm of less than 60 bpm may cause symptoms of fatigue, breathlessness, poor exercise tolerance, and may decompensate heart failure causing poor renal perfusion and peripheral oedema.

Investigations
12-lead ECG
First-degree AV block will show a prolonged PR interval >220 ms. In second-degree Mobitz type I the 12-lead ECG will demonstrate progressive prolongation of the PR interval for a few cycles followed by a drop in QRS complexes, best seen on a rhythm strip. In Mobitz type II, a sudden drop in the QRS complex is seen, although the preceding PR interval may be normal. Third-degree AV block is seen as a complete dissociation of atrial (P waves) and ventricular (QRS complexes) activity; the morphology of QRS complexes and the ventricular rate depend on the level of origin of the ventricular escape rhythm.

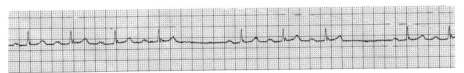

Fig. 3.1.2 Demonstrating (Wenckebach) Mobitz type 1, second degree AV block, as progressive lengthening of PR interval followed by a drop beat.

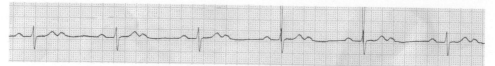

Fig. 3.1.3 Demonstrating Mobitz type 2, 2:1 second-degree AV block.

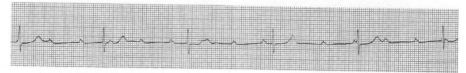

Fig. 3.1.4 Demonstrating third-degree (complete) AV block.

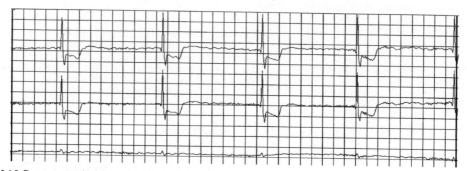

Fig. 3.1.5 Demonstrating third-degree (complete) AV block in atrial fibrillation.

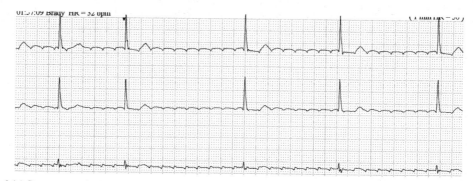

Fig. 3.1.6 Demonstrating third-degree (complete) AV block in atrial flutter.

Ambulatory ECG recoding

This may show pauses in its duration and relation to symptoms. A poor chronotrophic response and day and night variation of the heart rate or occurrence of a high degree AV block can also be seen in patients with first- or second-degree AV block. Periodic ambulatory ECG recording may be necessary in first-degree AV block to monitor progression of the disease.

Exercise tolerance test

This may show a poor, or even negative, chronotrophic response in complete AV block.

Treatment

Urgent treatment may be required in a third-degree AV block producing symptoms of cerebral hypoperfusion or haemodynamic compromise. Atropine is effective only if the escape rhythm arises from the AV nodal part of the AV node, which does respond temporarily to atropine; lower level pacemakers in the AV node, in the His or right and left bundles are less responsive to atropine. Transcutaneous pacing may be required until a temporary pacing catheter is inserted.

Permanent pacemaker implantation is required for Mobitz II, intermittent, or continuous third-degree AV block.

Benign vagotonic block

High vagal tone due to drugs (digitalis, morphine), interventions (such as endotracheal intubation/suction, nasogastric tube insertion, femoral arterial puncture), or during sleep may precipitate bradycardia, which can take the form of sinus node or AV node conduction disorder. It is important to exclude and recognize any condition inducing high vagal tone before committing to permanent pacemaker implantation.

Bundle branch block and conduction delay

The His bundle lies within the membranous part of the interventricular septum and consists of parallel conduction fibres in a collagen framework. It has no or minimal nervous supply and blood supply is by AV nodal artery and septal branches of the left anterior coronary artery. The His bundle gives rise to right and left bundle branches extending downwards into the interventricular septum and then to the left and right ventricles. The left bundle branch subdivides into the anterior and posterior divisions. The bundle branches end in the Purkinje fibres, which deliver electrical impulses to the myocardium. There is minimal or no nervous supply but extensive blood supply from all coronary arteries to the bundles and branches.

Incomplete bundle branch block or bundle branch conduction delay

This is also known as partial bundle branch block and may present as trivial widening of QRS complexes (up to 120 ms) (Fig. 3.1.7).

Complete bundle branch block

This may occur in the right or left bundles and produces QRS complexes of 120 ms (three small squares) or more. The morphology of the QRS complex depends on the side of block.

Right bundle branch block

This results in late activation of the right ventricle (moving towards the right and away from the left side) and therefore produces S waves in leads I and V6, as well as a tall late R wave in V1 (Fig. 3.1.8).

Left bundle branch block

This results in late activation of the left ventricle and produces the opposite pattern in the form of tall R waves in I and V6, and a deep S wave in V1. Left bundle branch block also produces abnormal Q waves (Fig. 3.1.9).

Hemiblock

This may occur as a complete block or a conduction delay in the anterior or posterior divisions of the left bundle. When the anterior branch is affected (left anterior hemiblock) it results in activation (depolarization) of the left ventricle from inferior to superior direction giving rise to left axis deviation (Fig. 3.1.9). In cases of posterior division block, the axis of depolarization swings in the opposite direction, from superior to inferior producing right axis deviation.

Bifasicular block

This is combination of right bundle branch block and either anterior or posterior hemiblock. If all three are blocked, it will result in complete heart block (Fig. 3.1.8).

Trifasicular block

This is a combination of bifasicular block and first-degree AV block (i.e. (1) right bundle branch block, (2) left anterior hemiblock resulting in left axis deviation, and (3) first-degree AV block (Fig. 3.1.10).

Clinical features

Conduction delay or block in one bundle branch or branches of the left bundle usually does not produce any symptoms. The diagnosis is usually coincidental. These findings show disease in the conduction system and if the patient has intermittent symptoms of cerebral hypoperfusion it increases the suspicion of high-degree conduction disease and warrants further investigation in form of ambulatory monitoring.

Investigations

12-Lead ECG

Confirm the diagnosis, mostly as a coincidental finding. If the patient is asymptomatic no further investigations may be required, although new onset left bundle branch block or intermittent right and left bundle branch block may need to be investigated with left heart catheterization to exclude significant coronary artery disease.

Treatment

For isolated conduction delay or bundle branch block usually no treatment is required. Alternating right and left bundle branch block may represent significant disease in both bundles with high risk of progression to complete AV block; therefore, a permanent pacemaker may be required.

Prognosis

Syncope is common in patients with bifasicular block but recurrent syncope is not associated with a high risk of

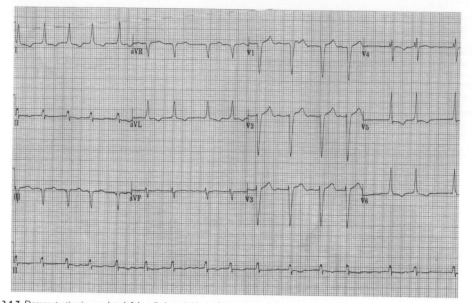

Fig. 3.1.7 Demonstrating incomplete left bundle branch block, QRS duration 118 ms.

sudden death. The rate of bifasicular block progression to complete AV block is variable and slow; however, the association of prolonged PR interval with bifasicular block carries a high risk of sudden death, not only because of bradyarrhythmias but because these patient have a high risk of malignant ventricular arrhythmias; therefore, implantation of a pacemaker may help neurological symptoms of syncope but does not improve overall survival. Development of any new symptoms of syncope or presyncope in patients with bifasicular block may warrant long-term monitoring with a loop recorder and electrophysiological investigations, although currently no factors have been identified to predict sudden death in this group.

General consideration in management of conduction abnormality and bradyarrhythmias
Myocardial infarction and AV block
Inferior myocardial infarction
The right coronary artery often supplies the AV node; therefore, inferior myocardial infarction may result in AV block, the immediate treatment of myocardial infarction in the form of thrombolysis or primary angioplasty should

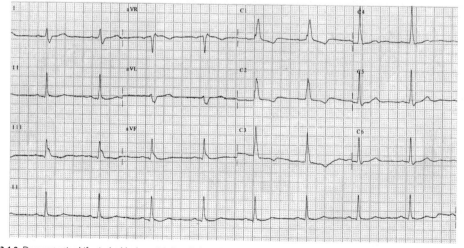

Fig. 3.1.8 Demonstrating bifascicular block, as right bundle branch block and left posterior hemiblock.

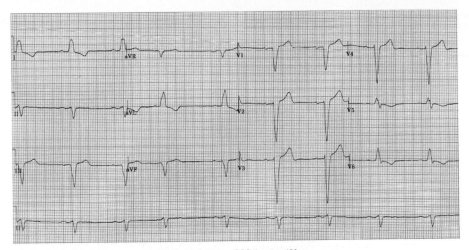

Fig. 3.1.9 Demonstrating left bundle branch and left axis deviation, QRS duration 158 ms.

not be delayed for management of AV block unless patient has haemodynamic instability. A temporary pacemaker is rarely required but should be inserted for haemodynamic instability. Often reperfusion results in restoration of normal AV conduction within 48 hours and in such situations a permanent pacemaker is not required. Occasionally, recovery of AV conduction may take over a week.

Anterior myocardial infarction
Second- and third-degree AV block in the context of anteroseptal myocardial infarction results from extensive damage to the conduction system and caries poor prognosis; therefore, insertion of a temporary transvenous pacemaker should be considered.

The insertion of a transvenous temporary pacemaker in the context of myocardial infarction caries a high risk of myocardial perforation through infarcted tissues, but if indicated it should be performed as the risk of not pacing is higher than that of perforation.

Cardiac surgery and AV block
Complete AV block is common after aortic valve replacement and certain other cardiac surgeries. Removable epicardial pacing leads are usually implanted to facilitate temporary pacing if required. If an epicardial lead fails and significant AV block develops then a transvenous temporary pacemaker is needed. The AV block may develop because of direct damage to AV nodal tissues or transient

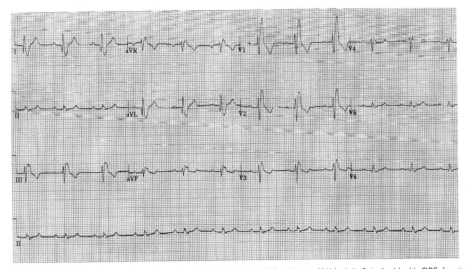

Fig. 3.1.10 Demonstrating right bundle branch, anterior hemiblock (LAD) and first-degree AV block (trifasicular block), QRS duration 170 ms.

oedema; therefore, for persistent conduction abnormality of more than a week, a permanent pacemaker is required.

Transient bradyarrhythmias

It is important to identify transient bradyarrhythmias either due to *high vagal tone, sympathetic withdrawl* and/or *rate-limiting medications* such as beta-blockers, calcium channel blockers, or other antiarrhythmic drugs. These bradyarrhythmias are seldom accompanied by symptoms of pre-syncope or frank syncope and usually do not require treatment except removal of the precipitating factor. *Vagally mediated bradyarrhythmias* can be identified by concomitant slowing of the sinus rate, changing PR intervals, atypical Wenckebach, inconstant escape rate, and ectopics. These bradyarrhythmias can be reversed or abolished by intravenous atropine.

Some vasovagal episodes (hypotension due to vasodilatation and bradycardia), also called neurocardiogenic, neurovascular syncopal syndromes, may be frequent, abrupt, and disabling, requiring treatment with medications or a permanent pacemaker.

In an acute setting drugs like theophylline and ephedrine can be used for heart rate support, or intravenous fluids for volume support may be required. In *vasovagal syndrome* left ventricular baroreceptor stimulation occurs due to vigorous contraction, which in turn leads to reflex vasodilatation; therefore, drugs with negative inotropic effects (e.g. beta-blocker, verapamil, diltiazem, disopyramide) or alpha-agonists (midodrine) can be used in management. In addition, vasovagal syndromes are centrally mediated and at times hypotension may occur without bradycardia; therefore, anticholinergic agents (e.g. serotonin reuptake inhibitors) can be useful. If all the above measures fail then a rate drop permanent pacemaker can be considered.

Commonly used *rate-limiting medications* cause bradycardia either by enhancing vagal tone (e.g. digitalis), or reducing sympathetic tone facilitation of AV conduction (e.g. beta-lockers or agents with beta-blocking properties like sotalol and propafenone), or direct action on SA and AV conduction tissues (e.g. verapamil and diltiazem). Most commonly the withdrawal of the offending drug settles the situation, but rarely, in cases of overdose or haemodynamic compromise, a transvenous temporary pacemaker may be necessary for transient support as the drugs may take several days to clear of the system. Usually a permanent pacemaker is not required. If the offending drug cannot be withdrawn due to concomitant tachyarrhythmias or angina pectoris, then a permanent pacing system may be required.

Temporary transcutaneous pacing

In patients with acute haemodynamic compromise transcutaneous pacing can be established until temporary transvenous pacemaker insertion, and is successful in 70% of cases depending on body habitus. In cases where transcutaneous pacing fails, isoprenaline (if available) can be used; immediate help from the cardiologist and ITU anaesthetist should be sought as such patient who fail to respond to atropine and transcutaneous pacing are at high risk of cardiac arrest with poor outcome.

For transcutaneous pacing, two large low impedance surface electrodes are placed on the anterior and posterior chest walls. The electrical current is delivered to the heart through the skin from a defibrillator machine with pacing facility (pacemaking generator). The transcutaneous pacing works in demand VVI mode (see Chapter 3.10), delivering a long-pacing stimulus output (duration 20–40 ms, non-programmable by operator) and high current output of more than 70 mA, adjusted by the operator to achieve ventricular capture by overcoming thoracic tissue impedance. The deflections on the surface ECG can be confused with QRS complexes; therefore, ventricular capture should be confirmed on a pacemaker generator oscilloscope (defibrillator) showing the pacer output pulse followed by the QRS complex. The rate should be kept to a minimum and sedation should be used for uncomfortable muscle twitching. If an initial successful capture is lost, fresh pads should be used.

Temporary transvenous pacing

This is always required in bradycardia with acute haemodynamic compromise, the venous access can be achieved through one of several routes (e.g. the internal jugular vein, most commonly used, subclavian vein, or femoral vein). A pacing catheter is inserted in the right ventricle by an experienced operator and connected to the pacing generator; a threshold of less than 1 mA should be achieved, and pacing at about 60 bpm at 2–3 mA output should be commenced. The temporary transvenous catheter should be exchanged every 5 days in cases where a permanent pacemaker cannot be implanted due to the presence of infection or other factors; otherwise, a permanent pacemaker should be implanted as soon as the decision in favour of a permanent pacemaker is taken, e.g. persistent bradycardia or conduction disturbance despite appropriate clearance time for offending drugs.

There are at least three types of temporary pacing catheters.

1 *The semi-rigid pacing wire or catheter* is most commonly used, has long length and can be used easily from femoral vein and has a blunt metallic end which is inserted in and attached to the endocardium in the right ventricle; it has a higher rate of displacement and risk of myocardium perforation giving rise to tamponade.

2 *The flotation temporary pacing catheter* has a balloon near the metallic end, which is inflated to facilitate insertion in to the right ventricle; it can be used by operators with less experience, and has a low risk of displacement.

3 *The active fixation right ventricular lead* is normally used in permanent pacemakers but can be extremely useful in an emergency setting to achieve stable, safe, and quick pacing for a temporary pacing system. Specially designed compatibility kits are available to connect this system with a temporary pacing generator. An operator with experience in permanent pacing is required for this method of pacing and due to its short length it cannot be inserted from femoral route.

Patients on warfarin who require transvenous temporary pacing can be a challenge. Usually the international normalized ratio (INR) is significantly high due to hepatic congestion as a consequence of poor circulation and low cardiac output. Femoral access is usually advised but patients with a prosthetic valve carry a significantly high risk of infection; therefore, where possible an internal jugular vein should be used. The INR can be corrected with fresh frozen plasma or with Beriplex. In cases where transcutaneous pacing is not successful, temporary transvenous pacing should be

Table 3.1.3 Indications for temporary cardiac pacing

AV node or sinus node dysfunction with heart rate less than 40 bpm or pauses >3 second associated with symptoms of haemodynamic compromise.
For overdrive pacing of supraventricular or ventricular arrhythmias.
Prophylactic after cardiac surgery or acute myocardial infarction to prevent high degree AV block.
To treat drug induced prolonged QT and Torsade.
To determine the site of AV block.

Indications for permanent pacemaker

AV node (second and third degree) and sinus node dysfunction with heart rate less than 40 bpm or pauses >3 seconds associated with symptoms of haemodynamic compromise.
Chronotrophic incompetence with sinus node dysfunction.
Refractory recurrent syncope with >3-second pauses or bradycardia inducible by carotid sinus massage or head up tilt test.

inserted without waiting for correction of the INR because of the high risk of death. Table 3.1.3 shows the indications for transvenous and permanent pacemakers.

Permanent pacing
Please see Chapter 3.10 for further details.

Further reading
Baine WB, Yu W, Weis KA. Trends and outcomes in the hospitalization of older Americans for cardiac conduction disorders or arrhythmias. *J Am Geriatr Soc* 1998;**49**:763–70.

Epstein AE, DiMarco JP, Ellenbogen KA, *et al*. ACC/AHA/HRS 2008 Guidelines for Device-Based Therapy of Cardiac Rhythm Abnormalities: a report of the American College of Cardiology/ American Heart Association Task Force on Practice Guidelines (Writing Committee to Revise the ACC/AHA/NASPE 2002 Guideline Update for Implantation of Cardiac Pacemakers and Antiarrhythmia Devices): developed in collaboration with the American Association for Thoracic Surgery and Society of Thoracic Surgeons. *Circulation* 2008;**117**:350–408.

Mobitz W. Über die unvollständige Störung der Erregungsüberleitung zwischen Vorhof und Kammer des menschlichen Herzens. *Z Gesamte Exp Med* 1924;**41**:180–237.

Peuch P, Groileau R, Guimond C. Incidence of different types of A-V block and their localization by His bundle recordings. In: Wellens HJJ, Lie KI, Janse MJ, eds. *The conduction system of the heart*. Philadelphia: Lea & Febiger, 1976: pp. 467–84.

Wenckebach KF. Zur Analyse der unregelmässigen Pulses. *Ztschr klin Med* 1899;**36**:181.

Paroxysmal supraventricular tachycardia

Supraventricular tachycardia (SVT) is a broad and non-specific term for an abnormal rapid heart rate (>100 bpm) originating above the ventricles. For the purposes of this chapter we will be discussing regular SVT. Palpitation due to SVT is a common reason for attendance to both emergency and outpatient departments. The overall prevalence is around 3%, although it is twice as common in women as in men. Unlike ventricular arrhythmias the majority occur in young patients without underlying heart disease. There are a variety of underlying mechanisms according to which they are classified.

Mechanisms of SVT

SVT dependent on the atrioventricular (AV) node

1 AV nodal re-entry tachycardia (AVNRT)—this is a re-entry circuit that occurs in those with dual AV nodal physiology and is contained entirely within the AV node. The impulse travels down the slow pathway and back up the fast pathway (this is true in 90%, although the circuit is reversed in around 10%). This is very common particularly in young women, and accounts for around 70% of SVT.

2 AV re-entry tachycardia (AVRT)—here the impulse travels down the AV node and back up an accessory pathway (again the reverse is true in 10% of cases). This accessory pathway may be concealed or manifest. If there is anterograde conduction in sinus rhythm then there may be a short PR interval with a slurred upstroke of the QRS complex known as a 'delta wave', in which case the patient has Wolff–Parkinson–White syndrome, or just a short PR interval, in which case they have Lown–Ganong–Levine syndrome.

3 Junctional tachycardia—where there is rapid discharging of the AV node or His bundle. This can occur in young patients with normal hearts or in association with congenital heart disease. It can also occur secondary to other problems such as digoxin toxicity.

SVT originating entirely within the atria

1 Atrial tachycardia—these can be focal (due to a focus/foci of enhanced automaticity or micro-re-entry) or macro-re-entrant. There may be an abnormal P wave visible on the electrocardiogram (ECG) during the tachycardia. This is often secondary to other medical problems such as respiratory disease and hypoxia, hypovolaemia (especially in the postoperative state), and drugs such as digoxin toxicity.

2 Inappropriate sinus node tachycardia—this is a persistent increase in sinus rate which is unrelated or out of proportion to its cause. It is common in young women and is thought to be due to abnormal automaticity of the sinus node or abnormal autonomic regulation.

3 Atrial fibrillation (AF) and atrial flutter—these have a characteristic ECG appearance and their management in some respects is different. This is covered in other chapters.

Clinical approach

History: key points

- Palpitations are the commonest symptoms.
- Typically, onset and termination are abrupt.
- Frequency and duration of symptoms.

- Chest pain is common and does not necessarily suggest concurrent coronary disease.
- Breathlessness is common.
- Dizziness is common but syncope is rare and more suggestive of ventricular arrhythmias.
- Polyuria (atrial natriuric peptide (ANP) is released due to contraction of the atria against the closed AV valves).
- Comorbidity, particularly cardiorespiratory.
- Precipitants such as alcohol, caffeine, or drugs.

Examination: key points

- Heart rate and blood pressure.
- Physical examination concentrating on cardiorespiratory system.
- An irregular pulse suggests AF, but at rates over 150 bpm this is difficult to assess.
- A variable S1 and cannon waves in the jugular venous pressure suggest ventricular tachycardia (again difficult to assess with high rates).

Acute investigations

- ECG usually shows a regular narrow complex tachycardia. A broad complex tachycardia is possible with SVT (for example with bundle branch block), but VT should always be suspected in this context.
- Attach the patient to a cardiac monitor.
- Baseline blood tests including full blood count and urea and electrolytes looking for precipitants.
- Echocardiogram at some point (when in normal rhythm) may be useful to exclude structural disease.

Initial management

In the emergency setting, priority should be given to assessing the conscious level, blood pressure, and evidence of cardiac ischaemia or heart failure. If any of these are present then the patient should be urgently cardioverted. Any reversible causes such as hypovolaemia or electrolyte disturbances should be corrected. Assuming the patient is stable and there is no correctable precipitant, the following stepwise guide is suggested.

1 After assessment the next step is vagal manoeuvres to terminate the arrhythmia (this should be done while recording a rhythm strip). There are a few options:
   - A Valsalva manoeuvre can be performed asking the patient to 'bear down'. Better results are sometimes achieved asking the patient to blow out against their thumb, or to blow the plunger out of a syringe.
   - If there are no carotid bruits, carotid sinus massage can be performed by resting the palm against the clavicle and using the thumb to apply a gentle vertical rubbing motion to the carotid pulse at the level of the thyroid cartilage for 10 seconds. If there is no response then this can be repeated on the opposite side.
   - Diving reflex—dipping the face into a bowl of ice cold water.
   - Painful pressure over the eyes is no longer used.

2 If the SVT persists the next step is adenosine:
   - First check the patient does not have uncontrolled asthma or is taking dipyridamole (which potentiates the effect of adenosine).
   - An antecubital fossa vein is ideal, as adenosine decomposes quickly.

- Warn the patient that they may feel tight chested and unwell but that it will pass quickly.
- Give a bolus of 6 mg of adenosine followed by a 20-ml flush.
- If there is no effect try again with 12 mg.

3 If adenosine fails to terminate the SVT (or if it has recurred) then an AV nodal blocking agent such as verapamil can be given IV starting at 5 mg over 2 minutes. This can be repeated twice at 5-minute intervals. One should be very cautious about this if the patient is already taking AV nodal blocking medication such as beta-blockers.

4 If the SVT persists despite the above, then an anaesthetist should be called to sedate the patient for DC cardioversion.

ECG characteristics and effect of adenosine on the different types of SVT (Table 3.2.1)

Table 3.2.1 ECG characteristics and effect of adenosine on the different types of SVT

Mechanism of SVT	ECG characteristics	Effect of vagal manoeuvres/adenosine
AVNRT	P wave absent or buried in end of QRS in V1	Termination
AVRT	Abnormal p wave sometimes visible	Termination
Atrial tachycardia	Abnormal p wave visible	Transient AV block, abnormal p waves visible
Sinus tachycardia	Normal p waves visible	Transient AV block, p waves visible
AF/atrial flutter	Irregular/flutter waves inferiorly	Transient AV block, atrial rhythm unmasked

Long-term management

For a well patient where an SVT is terminated and does not recur, discharge (after giving the patient a copy of their ECG) from the emergency department after no more than an hour is appropriate. After a first episode a patient need not be offered long-term medical treatment or ablation therapy and should be given advice regarding

Valsalva manoeuvres. If there is a history of palpitations, or previous arrhythmia, then catheter ablation is the treatment of first choice. The risk of major complications is under 1% (most of this is need for a pacemaker, and other risks such as stroke or tamponade are exceptionally rare). Where patients would prefer a trial of medical treatment as first line, oral verapamil or beta-blockers are reasonable options.

Management as an outpatient

The majority of those presenting to the outpatient department will be in sinus rhythm. If they have been referred from A&E with an ECG in SVT, then the patient should be offered catheter ablation if they feel that symptoms are interfering with their quality of life. Those with only a history of palpitations need some thought as to their mode of investigation. If there is evidence of pre-excitation on their ECG together with symptoms of palpitations, both for symptoms and to reduce the risk of sudden cardiac death, electrophysiology testing and ablation are recommended. Otherwise capturing an ECG during symptoms should be the ideal. Event and Holter monitoring may be helpful, but recording periods of less than a week are not helpful unless symptoms are very frequent. In rare cases where symptoms are classical but do not sustain for long enough to be captured on the emergency room ECG and are too infrequent to capture on event monitors then diagnostic electrophysiological study with a view to therapeutic ablation at the same procedure should be considered.

Other modes of investigation such as the implantable loop recorders are usually reserved for those with infrequent brief symptoms such as syncope.

Further reading

Blomström-Lundqvist C, Scheinman MM, Aliot EM, et al. ACC/AHA/ESC guidelines for management of patients with supraventricular arrhythmias. *Eur Heart J* 2003;**24**:1857–97 (available online: www.acc.org).

Schilling RJ. Which patient should be referred to an electrophysiologist: supraventricular tachycardia. *Heart* 2002;**87**:299–304.

Showkathali R, Earley MJ, Alzetani M, et al. Current case mix and results of catheter ablation of regular supraventricular tachycardia: are we giving unrealistic expectations to patients?. *Europace* 2000;**9**:1064–8.

Website

Resuscitation Council UK guidelines for management of tachycardias, available online: www.resus.org.uk.

Atrial flutter and fibrillation

Atrial fibrillation (AF) is the commonest occurring cardiac arrhythmia and confers a substantial mortality and morbidity from stroke, thromboembolism, heart failure, and impaired quality of life. In the majority of patients, AF can be easily recognized from the surface electrocardiogram (ECG) with the presence of rapid, irregular fibrillatory waves, and irregular ventricular response. However, there is significant overlap on the ECG appearances between AF, atrial flutter and atrial tachycardia. It is classified according to the temporal pattern of the arrhythmia (Fuster et al. 2006; National Collaborating Centre for Chronic Conditions 2006):

1 Recurrent AF: two or more episodes of AF (paroxysmal or persistent).
2 Paroxysmal AF: AF episodes terminate spontaneously within 7 days.
3 Persistent AF: AF episodes which required termination by cardioversion (electrical or pharmacological).
4 Permanent AF: AF episode which failed to cardivert or deemed inappropriate.

The incidence of AF is estimated at 0.4% of the general population and increases with age (2–5% at age 65; 9% at age 80). In Western countries, the lifetime risks for development of AF are approximately 1 in 4 for men and women at age 40 years or above (Lloyd-Jones et al. 2004). In the Framingham Heart Study, age, sex, body mass index, systolic blood pressure, treatment for hypertension, PR interval, clinically significant heart murmur, and heart failure are risk factors for AF (Schnabel et al. 2009). Nevertheless, it can also occur in about 30% of patients without underlying aetiological cause—lone AF.

The aim of assessment is to determine the patient symptomatology, the risk of thromboembolism, the presence of concomitant medical and/or cardiovascular diseases, and the occurrence of complications (thromboembolism, heart failure, tachycardia-induced cardiomyopathy).

Clinical manifestations
- Asymptomatic (1/10)
- Symptoms: palpitation (>50%), dyspnoea, malaise, dizziness, angina, polyuria
- Heart failure
- Thromboembolism (~1 in 6 strokes occurs in patients with AF).

Risk factors and underlying aetiologies to consider
Risk factors
- Age, male sex, body mass index
- Alcohol (holiday heart syndrome).

Cardiovascular diseases
- Hypertension
- Valvular heart diseases
- Ischaemic heart disease
- Cardiomyopathies, heart failure
- Congenital heart diseases
- Wolff–Parkinsonson–White (WPW) syndrome and sinus node dysfunction.

Medical illnesses
- Hyperthyroidism, diabetes mellitus, chronic obstructive lung diseases, severe infection, pulmonary embolism, postoperative (cardiac or non-cardiac).

Clinical approach
History: key points
- Risk factors
- Concomitant medical and cardiovascular illnesses
- Complications: heart failure and stroke
- Bleeding risk (? antithrombotic therapies).

Examination: key points
- To confirm the diagnosis of AF (irregularly irregular pulse, variable intensity of first heart sound and pulse deficit)
- Measure blood pressure
- Exclude structural abnormalities of the heart such as cardiomegaly, valvular heart diseases
- Signs of heart failure? (outpatient, 10–20%; inpatient, 40–50%) (Schnabel et al. 2009; Godtfredsen and Falk 2003)
- Signs of other medical illnesses, such as hyperthyroidism and lung diseases
- Presence of neurological deficits.

Special investigations
- 12-lead ECG to confirm the presence of AF, to determine the ventricular rate, PR interval prolongation and QT interval (? use of antiarrhythmic drugs, AADs) and to exclude left ventricular hypertrophy, new or old myocardial infarction, bundle branch block and WPW (delta wave).
- 24-hour ECG recording to confirm the presence of AF (if the patient is in sinus rhythm during assessment), to identify sinus node dysfunction (bradycardia–tachycardia syndrome), and to assess the rate of AF over a 24-hour period.
- Blood tests include complete blood count, thyroid and renal function tests, and cardiac markers (if myocardial infarction is suspected).
- Transthoracic echocardiogram to detect and quantify valvular diseases, left ventricular function, and the size of the left atrium.
- Transoesophageal echocardiogram (TEE) when a left atrial clot is suspected or to be excluded prior to defibrillation.
- The exercise treadmill test may be useful to evaluate underlying coronary artery disease (if suspected) and to assess rate control.

Natural history
- Within the first 24 hours, up to 70–80% of patients with new-onset AF convert back to sinus rhythm (Lip and Tse 2007).
- In patients presenting with paroxysmal AF, 3–6% of these patients develop permanent AF per year.
- The reported incidence of tachycardia-induced cardiomyopathy range from 0.9% to 25%.

- The mortality in AF is increased by 1.5- to 2.0-fold, mainly due to increased risk of thromboembolic stroke by five-fold compared with sinus rhythm (Godtfredsen and Falk 2003).

Management

- The management of patients with AF should broadly be guided by symptoms, the presence or absence of haemodynamic compromise, and associated co-morbidities (Lip and Tse 2007).
- The clinical subtypes of AF and a patient's symptomatology will also help to define the objectives of management and therapeutic strategies (Fuster *et al.* 2006; National Collaborating Centre for Chronic Conditions 2006).
- Most important, appropriate antithrombotic therapy use is mandatory, based on risk factors for stroke and thromboembolism independent of the clinical subtypes of AF.

Acute AF

- Patients who remain in AF and develop haemodynamic instability (WPW syndrome, heart failure, cardiogenic shock, and acute coronary syndrome) due to rapid ventricular rates should undergo emergency cardioversion.
- In the majority of patients with acute AF, acute ventricular rate control is required to improve haemodynamic status and relieve symptoms. The dosage, side-effects, and indications for different atrioventricular (AV) nodal blocking agents are summarized in Table 3.3.1.
- When rapid control of ventricular rate is required or oral administration of medication is not feasible, intravenous drugs are needed.
- In many acute situations, either a beta-blocker or calcium channel blocker (CCB) is the preferred agent for slowing ventricular rate. The non-dihydropyridine (or rate-limiting) CCBs, verapamil and diltiazem, prolong the AV nodal refractory period to slow AV nodal conduction, and are effective agents for ventricular rate control during AF. Since intravenous verapamil has a more potent negative inotropic and peripheral vasodilator effect, intravenous diltiazem has became a more popular drug for acute ventricular rate control during AF, especially in patients with left ventricular dysfunction and hypotension.
- Intravenous beta-blockers are also effective AV nodal blocking agents through their sympatholytic properties. They are more effective in conditions in which the rapid ventricular rate is due to heightened adrenergic tone, such as in the postoperative period. Except for esmolol, all the beta-blockers have a slower onset of action than diltiazem. However, intravenous esmolol has a very short half-life, which requires careful monitoring and titration of dosage.
- Both beta-blockers and CCBs should be used with caution in patients with hypotension or heart failure and should be started with a smaller dose and administered slowly.
- In patients with heart failure and AF, relief of pulmonary congestion by diuretics and vasodilators may aid in decreasing the heart rate. Digoxin has both negative

chronotropic and positive inotropic effects and therefore is an appropriate first-line drug in patients with heart failure and AF. Furthermore, in patients with borderline blood pressure, intravenous digoxin is a useful alternative to beta-blockers or CCBs that may cause further decrease in blood pressure. As the effect of digoxin on ventricular rate is mediated by its vagotonic effect on the AV node, the onset of action may take several hours. For the same reason, digoxin is usually ineffective during the acute setting with high catecholamines status, such as postoperative status, acute sepsis, myocardial ischaemia and pulmonary diseases.

- Both digoxin and verapamil are contraindicated for AF associated with the WPW syndrome.
- In critically ill patients with severe heart failure or hypotension in whom other agents are ineffective or contraindicated for ventricular rate control, intravenous amiodarone is an effective alternative. The most common side-effects of intravenous amiodarone include hypotension, bradycardias, and thrombophlebitis (preferable administrated via central intravenous line).
- In patients with acute AF who have no contraindications and not receiving therapeutic anticoagulation, heparin should be considered, especially initiated if medical or electrical cardioversion is planned. The patients should then receive detail assessment for the need of long-term antithrombotic therapy based on stroke risk stratification.

Recurrent and permanent AF

In paroxysmal and persistent AF, either 'rhythm-control' or 'rate-control' can be initially applied, and a significant proportion of patients will need both. The NICE guidelines suggest that a rate-control strategy should be the preferred *initial* option in the following patients:

- Those aged over 65
- Those with coronary artery disease
- Those with contraindications to AADs
- Those without congestive heart failure
- Those unsuitable for cardioversion.

In contrast, a rhythm-control strategy should be the preferred *initial* option in the following patients:

- Symptomatic patients
- Younger patients
- Patients presenting for the first time with lone AF
- AF secondary to a treated/corrected precipitant.

The categories mentioned are not mutually exclusive, and the strategy to adopt should take into account any co-morbidities, symptoms, and patient preferences.

- For rhythm-control in patients with paroxysmal AF, the objective of management is the reduction of paroxysms and the long-term maintenance of sinus rhythm, and, thus, AADs or non-pharmacological approaches, surgical and catheter based ablation procedures are used.
- In patients with persistent AF, restoration of sinus rhythm can be achieved initially by either pharmacological or electrical cardioversion.

Table 3.3.1 Drugs for control of the ventricular rate in patients with atrial fibrillation

Drug	Acute intravenous therapy (loading dose)	Chronic oral therapy	Efficacy	Comments
Calcium channel blockers				
Diltiazem	IV bolus 20 mg or 0.25 mg/kg over 2 min followed if necessary by IV 25 mg or 0.35 mg/kg 15 min later. Maintenance infusion of 5–15 mg/h	90–360 mg daily in divided doses or in slow release form	Good	Acute side-effects: heart block, worsening of heart failure and hypotension (3%). Usually well tolerated and no effect on digoxin levels Chronic side-effects: constipation and bradycardia. Useful in hypertension and coronary artery disease
Verapamil	IV 5–1 0 mg or 0.075–0.15 mg/kg over 2–3 min. Repeat 5–1 0 mg 30 min later if required. Maintenance infusion rate is not well documented	120–360 mg daily in divided doses or in slow release form	Good	Acute side-effects: heart block, worsening of heart failure and hypotension (5–10%). Synergistic with digoxin but also increases digoxin levels Chronic side-effects: constipation and bradycardia. Useful in hypertension and coronary artery disease
Beta-blockers				
Metoprolol	IV 2.5–5 mg bolus over 2 min. Repeat every 5 min up to total 15 mg	20–100 mg twice daily or in slow release form	Good	Acute side-effects: heart block, worsening of heart failure and bronchospasm and hypotension Useful in post-operative setting Long-term side-effects: fatigue and depression Useful in hypertension, heart failure and coronary artery disease
Propranolol	IV 1–5 mg (1 mg every 2 min) or 0.15 mg/kg	80–240 mg daily in divided dose or in slow release form	Good	Acute and chronic side effects as above. Useful in hypertension thyrotoxicosis and coronary artery disease
Atenolol		25–100 mg once daily in slow release form	Good	Acute and chronic side effects as above. Useful in hypertension and coronary artery disease
Esmolol	IV 0.5 mg/kg over 1 min. Repeat if necessary. Maintenance infusion 0.05mg/kg/min		Short-acting	Acute and chronic side-effects as above. Useful in post-operative setting, hypotension (20–50%) is common.
Pindolol		2.5–20 mg twice to three daily	Fair	Chronic side-effects as above, but can avoid excessive bradycardia
Carvedilol		3.125–25mg twice daily	Good	Chronic side-effects as above. Useful in hypertension, coronary artery disease and heart failure
Cardiac glycoside				
Digoxin	IV 0.25 mg every 2 h (total 1–1 .5 mg/24 h)	0.125–0.375 mg once daily	Moderate to low	Delayed onset of AV node slowing (hours). Caution for digoxin toxicity in patients with electrolytes imbalance and renal failure. Useful in patients with heart failure
Others				
Amiodarone	IV 5–7 mg/kg or 150 mg over 10 min, then 0.5 to 1 mg/min up to total 1500 mg/24 h	Oral loading dose 600–800 mg daily, maintenance 200–400 mg QD	Good	Acute side-effects: bradycardia, hypotension and thrombophlebitis. Useful in critically ill patients and hypotension Chronic side-effects (see Table 3.3.2). Useful in refractory patients and heart failure

Cardioversion

- In general, in patients with non-valvular AF and who can precisely determine the onset of <48 hours' duration, cardioversion can be safely performed after anticoagulation with heparin. In patients with AF >48 hours or in those with a higher risk of thromboembolism (valvular heart disease and prior stroke), 3 weeks of oral anticoagulation with INR ≥2.0 prior to cardioversion is recommended.
- Alternatively, a TEE to exclude atrial thrombi allows immediate cardioversion with intravenous unfractionated heparin and/or low-molecular-weight heparin cover. When the left atrial appendage cannot be adequately visualized, cardioversion should be performed after 3 weeks of therapeutic anticoagulation.
- Anticoagulation with warfarin should then be continued for a minimum of 4 weeks post cardioversion to prevent thrombi formation in the postcardioversion period. Nevertheless, current clinical practice recommends that anticoagulation should be continued lifelong in patients at high risk of thromboembolism or risk factors for AF recurrence (history of failed attempts at cardioversion, mitral valve disease, left ventricular dysfunction or an enlarged left atrium, AF >12 months, and previous recurrences of AF).
- In AF of recent onset (<48 hours), either pharmacological or electrical cardioversion can be used as the initial strategy as they have fairly similar effectiveness (~80%).
- However, for AF of longer duration, the efficacy of pharmacological cardioversion (40–50%) is lower than electrical cardioversion (monophasic, 80%; biphasic, 95%).
- Before attempted cardioversion, serum potassium should be normal, and withholding the preceding digoxin dose to avoid QT prolongation and excessive bradycardia after cardioversion.
- A number of AADs may be used for pharmacological cardioversion with variable success rates and risk of proarrhythmia (Table 3.3.2). After successful pharmacological cardioversion, the rhythm should be carefully monitored for potential ventricular tachycardias (long QT interval, heart failure) and sinus pause (tachycardia–bradycardia syndrome).
- If pharmacological cardioversion fails, external electrical cardioversion can still be performed to restore sinus rhythm. Furthermore, pre-treatment with Class Ic AADs (flecainide, propaferone) and Class III AADs (amiodarone, ibutilide, sotalol) can facilitate electrical cardioversion and prevent recurrent AF (Fuster et al. 2006; Lip and Tse 2007).
- Electrical cardioversion should be performed after 6 hours of fasting using either monophasic (200 J, 300 J, 360 J) or biphasic (70 J, 120 J, 150 J) after sedation or general anaesthesia.

Maintenance of sinus rhythm

- Some patients may not have recurrence after a single episode of AF, especially in those with clear precipitant of AF (which has been corrected/treated, e.g. hypokalaemia and infection) and no chronic form of drug therapy is needed after cardioversion.
- However, in most patients cardioverted from persistent AF, the recurrence rate is high without AAD therapy.

The efficacy of different AADs is similar, and only about 50% of patients remain in sinus rhythm, with the possible exception of amiodarone.

- Furthermore, some caution should be taken for potential adverse effects when using AADs for suppression of AF, and the choice of long-term drug depends on the underlying co-morbidities.
- Class I AADs should be avoided in patients with structural heart diseases, and the long-term adverse effects of AADs should be considered (Table 3.3.2). The risk for drug-induced Torsades de Pointes is enhanced by metabolic disturbances (hypokalaemia, hypomagnesaemia), left ventricular dysfunction, history of ventricular tachycardia, prolongation of QT interval, and relative bradycardia.
- In patients with infrequent paroxysmal AF and without structural heart diseases, a 'pill-in-the-pocket' strategy with Class IC AADs (single oral dose of propafenone 600 mg or flecainide 300 mg) could be considered in patients whom this strategy have proven safe in hospital (Lip and Tse 2007).
- Dronedarone is a derivative of amiodarone and has been recently approved for the treatment of AF. Dronedarone is superior to placebo but less efficient than amiodarone in maintaining sinus rhythm. Dronedarone appears to have improved tolerability at the expense of decreased efficacy when compared with amiodarone. In patients with AF and risk factors, dronedarone reduces cardiovascular mortality and morbidity. Dronedarone is not appropriate in patients with recently decompensated heart failure or those treated with strong CYP3A4 inhibitors or medications prolonging the QT interval.
- The use of concomitant beta-blocker, non-dihydropyridine CCBs, or digoxin is recommended to avoid rapid AV conduction in the event of atrial flutter.

Ventricular rate control

- In patients with persistent or permanent AF whom a 'rate-control' strategy is used, the objective is heart rate control of the ventricular response, and, hence, drugs or non-pharmacological approaches-AV nodal ablation and permanent pacemaker implant are used.
- The aims of chronic ventricular rate controls during AF are to relieve symptoms and to prevent tachycardia-associated cardiomyopathy. Based on the recent prospective clinical trials (Van Gelder 2010), a lenient rate control strategy (resting heart rate <110 bpm) is more easy to achieve but is associated with similar clinical benefits as a strict rate-control strategy (resting heart rate <80 bpm and exercise heart rate <110 bpm). Therefore, a target resting heart rate of <110 bpm should be achieved by using AV nodal blocking agents (verapamil and diltiazem, beta-blocker, and digoxin) administrated intravenously or orally (Table 3.3.1).
- The heart rate response on treadmill test and/or the heart rate trend during ambulatory Holter monitoring are valuable in assessing rate control in AF patients. In certain conditions, such as mitral stenosis and diastolic heart failure, even lower resting heart rate may be desirable. However, excessive blunting of the heart rate response during exercise during AF can actually lead to a decrease in exercise capacity.

Table 3.3.2 Antiarrhythmic drug therapy in atrial fibrillation

Drug	Intravenous dose	Oral dose	Cardioversion efficacy (%)	Relapse rate (%)	Useful in	Comments
Class IA						
Quinidine gluconate		Oral 0.75–1.5 g/day in divided dose	40–84	46–89	Renal failure	Vagolytic. Many side effects including diarrhea, nausea, *Tdp* and hypotension. Avoid in patients with congestive heart failure
Procainamide	IV 100 mg bolus over 2 min up to 25 mg/min to 1 g, then 2–6 mg/min	Oral 1 g, then up to 500mg 3 hourly	43–65	NA	Men, short-term therapy	*Tdp* rare. Hypotension with IV dose. Limit oral use to 6 months to reduce the risk of drug-induced lupus.
Disopyramide		Oral 100–200 mg 6 hourly. Loading dose 300 mg		46–56	Women Vagally mediated AF	Vagolytic (urinary retention, dry mouth) and negative inotropic effects. Hypotension and *Tdp*. Avoid in patients with congestive heart failure/renal failure
Class IC						
Flecainide	IV 1.5–3.0 mg/kg over 10–20 min	Oral 100–300 mg in two divided doses	67–95	19–51	Patients without heart disease. Failure of Class IA drugs	Proarrhythmia. Negative inotropic. Central nervous system effects. Increased incidence of sudden death post infarct. Avoid in patients with heart failure and coronary artery disease
Propafenone	IV 1.5–2.0 mg/kg over 10–20 min	Oral 450–900 mg in three divided doses	45–87	54–70	Patients without heart disease. Failure of Class IA drugs	Proarrhythmia. Modest negative inotropic effect. Gastrointestinal side-effect. Unknown effects post infarct.
Sotalol		po 80–240 mg bd	8–54	51–63	Coronary artery diseases Failure of Class IA or IC drug	Sinus bradycardia, AV block, negative inotropic, *Tdp* if hypokalemic. Avoid in patients with congestive heart failure
Ibutilide	1–2 mg or 0.01–0.025 mg/kg		33–63	NA	Acute therapy with short half-time (4 h)	*Tdp*. Avoid in patients with low ejection fraction and hypokalemia
Amiodarone	IV 5–7 mg/kg or 150 mg over 10 min, then 0.5–1 mg/min up to total 1500 mg/24 h	Oral loading dose 600–800 mg daily, maintenance 200–400 mg QD	17–47	37–73	Congestive heart failure. Failure of other drug. Renal failure	Many side effects including pulmonary fibrosis, gastrointestinal upset, thyroid dysfunction, eye and skin changes. *Tdp* uncommon
Dronedarone		400 mg in two divided doses	NA	35–63	Decompensated congestive heart failure, LVEF<35%	Nausea, vomiting, diarrhoea and rash. *Tdp* uncommon. Need dose adjust for renal function, body size and age

- Either beta-blockers or rate-limiting CCBs are the preferable initial choice of monotherapy for ventricular rate control in AF patients. Both classes of agents are effective for controlling heart rate during exercise.
- In AF patients with concomitant coronary artery disease, hypertension and systolic heart failure, the use of beta-blockers (e.g. carvedilol and metoprolol) may provide additional benefit.
- The non-dihydropyridine (or rate-limiting) CCBs (diltiazem, verapamil) are also effective in reducing ventricular rate. These agents are also useful in AF patients with concomitant hypertension and coronary artery disease, or with contraindication with beta-blockers, such as asthma.
- Digoxin should only be considered for use as monotherapy in sedentary and elderly patients, as it is less effective for ventricular rate control during exercise.
- If monotherapy is inadequate to control the ventricular rate, combination therapy with beta-blockers or rate-limiting CCBs with digoxin can provide better overall control of ventricular rate in chronic AF especially during exercise.
- Furthermore, in patients with systolic heart failure and AF, a combination of digoxin and beta-blockers can provide additional beneficial effect on rate control, symptoms and left ventricular function.
- In refractory patients, long-term low-dose amiodarone may be required for additional rate control. Alternative, AV nodal ablation and pacing are useful for rate control when other agents failed or contraindicated. In the setting of left ventricular systolic dysfunction, the use of biventricular pacing after AV nodal ablation should preserve or further improve left ventricular function.

References

Fuster V, Rydén LE, Asinger RW, et al. ACC/AHA/ESC guidelines for the management of patients with atrial fibrillation: a report of the American College of Cardiology/American Heart Association Task Force on Practice Guidelines and the European Society of Cardiology Committee for Practice Guidelines (Writing Committee to Revise the 2001 Guidelines for the Management of Patients With Atrial Fibrillation). J Am Coll Cardiol 2006;**48**:e149–246.

Godtfredsen J, Falk RH. Atrial fibrillation: hemodynamic and clinical features. In: editor Lip G, Godtfredsen J (eds) Cardiac arrhythmias: a clinical approach. Mosby 2003.

Lip GY, Tse HF. Management of atrial fibrillation. Lancet 2007;**370**:604-618.

Lloyd-Jones DM, Wang TJ, Leip EP, et al. Lifetime risk for development of atrial fibrillation: the Framingham Heart Study. Circulation. 2004;**110**:1042-6.

National Collaborating Centre for Chronic Conditions. Atrial fibrillation: national clinical guideline for management in primary and secondary care. London: Royal College of Physicians, 2006.

Schnabel RB, Sullivan LM, Levy D, et al., Development of a risk score for atrial fibrillation (Framingham Heart Study): a community-based cohort study. Lancet. 2009;**373**:739–745.

Van Gelder IC, Groenveld HF, Crijns HJ, et al. Lenient versus strict rate control in patients with atrial fibrillation. N Engl J Med 2010;**15**;362:1363–73.

Ventricular tachyarrhythmias

Ventricular tachycardia (VT) is an abnormal cardiac rhythm characterized by three or more consecutive beats emanating from the ventricle at a rate of ≥100 bpm (cycle length ≤600 ms). It can be classified according to duration, morphology, and haemodynamic effect as follows (Zipes *et al.* 2006):
1 Non-sustained VT: VT that spontaneously terminates within 30 s.
2 Sustained VT: VT >30 s in duration or requiring termination within 30 s due to haemodynamic compromise.
3 Monomorphic VT: VT with a single QRS morphology.
4 Polymorphic VT: VT with a changing QRS morphology at cycle lengths between 600 and 180 ms.
   • Bidirectional VT: VT with a beat-to-beat alternans (classically 180°) in the QRS frontal plane axis.
   • Torsade de Pointes (tdp): VT with peaks of the QRS complexes twisting around the isoelectric line. Typical tdp are initiated by 'short–long–short' coupling intervals whereas short coupled variants are initiated by 'normal–short' coupling interval.
5 Ventricular flutter: a regular (cycle length variability ≤30 ms) monomorphic VT at a rate of ~300 bpm (cycle length ~200 ms) with no isoelectric interval between successive QRS complexes.
6 Haemodynamic effect:
   • Haemodynamically stable: asymptomatic or associated with minimal symptoms.
   • Haemodynamically unstable: associated with symptoms of end-organ hypoperfusion.

Mechanisms

Increased automaticity
• This is seen in diseased tissue in which myocardial fibres develop abnormal phase 4 depolarizations e.g. VT early after myocardial infarction (MI).

Triggered activity
• This develops with the occurrence of early or delayed afterdepolarization that achieves activation threshold, e.g.
   • Early afterdepolarizations: polymorphic VT in long QT syndromes
   • Delayed afterdepolarizations: idiopathic VT, catecholaminergic polymorphic VT, digitalis-induced VT.

Re-entry
• A circular propagating electrical activity across tissues of differential conduction and repolarization properties. Re-entry is the most common mechanism of monomorphic VT, e.g. VT late after MI, fascicular VT.

Epidemiology

• VT is a heterogeneous group of disorders in which prevalence varies with the types of arrhythmia, underlying aetiologies, and the presence of structural heart diseases. In general, over half the patients with recurrent symptomatic VT have coronary artery disease (CAD), and those who have sustained VT are more likely to have previous MI, reduced left ventricular ejection fraction (LVEF), left ventricular aneurysm, intraventricular conduction, and other electrocardiographic (ECG) abnormalities. Major causes of VT are summarized in Table 3.4.1.

Clinical manifestations

• VT may present as follows:
   • Asymptomatic with or without ECG abnormalities
   • Palpitation
   • Chest pain, dyspnoea
   • Flushing, diaphoresis, weakness
   • Presyncope, syncope, seizure
   • Sudden cardiac arrest/sudden cardiac death.

The most common presenting symptoms of sustained VT is palpitation (57%), followed by chest pain (27%), dyspnoea (25%), presyncope (15%) and syncope (15%). The presence of chest pain, dyspnoea, and presyncope, although non-specific, may suggest haemodynamic compromise by VT.

Clinical approach of wide complex tachycardia

• Other than the exceptional cases of fascicular tachycardia, most VT manifests as wide complex tachycardia (WCT). The differential diagnoses of WCT include VT, supraventricular tachycardia (SVT) with aberrant conduction, SVT with anterograde conduction via an

Table 3.4.1 Aetiologies of VT

Ischaemic heart disease	Myocardial infarction
	Unstable angina
	Ischaemic cardiomyopathy
	Coronary spasm
	Coronary artery anomalies
Other structural heart disease	Hypertrophic cardiomyopathy
	Dilated cardiomyopathy
	Arrhythmogenic RV dysplasia
	Valvular heart disease
	Congenital heart disease
	Myocarditis
	Infiltrative cardiomyopathy
Primary electrical disease	Idiopathic VT
	Brugada syndrome
	Long QT syndrome
	Short QT syndrome
	Catecholaminergic polymorphic VT
	Sinus/atrioventicular nodal disease
Non-cardiac disease	Drug induced
	Metabolic/electrolyte disturbances
	Intracranial pathologies

accessory pathway; direct proarrhythmic effect of antiarrhythmic drugs (AADs), electrolyte abnormalities (e.g. marked hyperkalaemia), and drug toxicity (e.g. tricyclic antidepressant overdose). Ventricular pacing and artefacts can also appear as WCT and should not be mistaken as VT.

History: key points
- WCT should be assumed to be VT in patients with prior MI until proven otherwise.
- Symptoms, including those suggestive of the haemodynamic effect of the tachycardia, are not reliable for distinguishing between VT and SVT.
- Drug history should be elicited if possible (see below).

Physical examination: key points
- Signs of AV dissociation, which strongly suggest VT in the context of WCT, are only present in <50% of cases.
- The most specific sign of AV dissociation is cannon A waves in the jugular venous pressure waveform. Variable first heart sound and beat-to-beat alteration in blood pressure are suggestive but not specific for AV dissociation.
- Patients should be continuously monitored for signs of haemodynamic instability, which include hypotension, hypoperfusion, and heart failure, as their presence mandate prompt cardioversion.

12-lead ECG
- 12-lead ECG should be obtained if possible. Falsely narrow QRS complex may be generated in a single lead when a portion of the QRS vector is perpendicular to the lead axis yielding an isoelectric component.
- The following ECG criteria help differentiating VT from SVT:
  - AV dissociation: particularly in the presence of fusion or capture beats, is virtually diagnostic of VT.
  - Concordance: negative concordance in all precordial leads is specific for VT, whereas positive concordance can be due to VT originated from the posterobasal region of the left ventricle or conduction via a posterior accessory pathway.
  - Axis: northwest axis is almost always due to VT; right axis in the presence of left bundle branch block (LBBB) is also suggestive of VT.
  - QRS width: in patients with pre-existing bundle branch block or intraventricular conduction defect, a WCT with QRS that is narrower than that in sinus rhythm is always VT. QRS >140 ms in those with RBBB pattern, and QRS >160 ms in those with LBBB pattern, are also suggestive of VT.
  - V1/V2 and V6 morphology: right bundle branch block pattern: monophasic R wave, qR or Rs in V1/V2, together with QS, QR, or R/S <1 in V6, are suggestive of VT; LBBB pattern: R wave ≥30 ms, onset of R to nadir of S ≥70 ms, or notched S wave in V1/V2, together with QS or qR in V6, are suggestive of VT.
- All morphological criteria for diagnosing VT show limited sensitivity and specificity and apply only in the absence of AADs, accessory pathway, and marked electrolyte disturbance.

Management of WCT of undetermined origin: key points
- One should follow the latest guideline on advanced cardiac life-support for resuscitation of cardiac arrest due to pulseless VT.
- In patients with haemodynamically unstable WCT as evidenced by shock, hypotension, acute pulmonary oedema, or myocardial ischaemia, direct current cardioversion (DCCV) (initially at 100 J monophasic or 50 J biphasic current for monomorphic VT, high energy shock for polymorphic VT) under appropriate sedation should be performed promptly.
- IV procainamide (20–30 mg infusion till arrhythmia suppressed/hypotension develops/QRS widens ≥50% above baseline, followed by 1–4 mg/min infusion, max 17 mg/kg) is the treatment of choice for pharmacological termination of a stable WCT. IV amiodarone (150 mg over 10 minutes, followed by 1 mg/min for 6 h then 0.5 mg/min in 18 h, maximum 2.2 g/day) is preferred in patients with impaired LVEF or signs of heart failure.
- IV lidocaine (1–1.5 mg/kg bolus, with additional 0.5–0.75 mg/kg if arrhythmia not suppressed, followed by 2–4 mg/min infusion, maximum 3 mg/kg), along with IV amiodarone, are recommended as the first-line agents in patients with very poor EF.
- DCCV should be considered at any point of time especially when pharmacological treatment fails.

Acute management
DCCV should be promptly performed for VT associated with haemodynamic instability, and is reasonable as first-line treatment for all other circumstances. Advantages of DCCV include high efficacy and lack of proarrhythmic effect; the major drawbacks are the requirement of sedation and an inability to prevent recurrence. Nevertheless, DCCV should still be considered early if pharmacological cardioversion fails, or in patients who are expected to tolerate VT or AADs poorly (Table 3.4.2).

All identifiable causes and triggering factors should be removed or corrected immediately. Therapies targeting to the arrhythmic substrates (e.g. revascularization in acute MI, transvenous pacing in bradycardia-related VT, antidigitalis antibodies in digitalis toxicity) are often needed to terminate the arrhythmias and prevent their recurrences.

Treatments for specific types of arrhythmia are discussed below.

Sustained monomorphic VT
- IV procainamide is reasonable for initial treatment of stable VT.
- IV amiodarone is preferred in patients with impaired EF and signs of heart failure, and is reasonable in for VT that is unstable, refractory to DCCV, or recurrent despite other AADs.
- Transvenous pace termination may be useful for refractory or frequently recurrent VT despite other treatments.
- IV lidocaine may be considered for VT associated with acute myocardial ischaemia.

Polymorphic VT
- IV beta-blockers are recommended for recurrent polymorphic VT especially if ischaemia cannot be excluded.
- IV amiodarone is recommended for recurrent polymorphic VT in the absence of long QTc.
- Urgent coronary angiograph with a view to revascularization is recommended if ischaemia cannot be excluded.
- IV lidocaine can be considered if VT is associated with acute myocardial ischaemia.
- All reversible causes including hyperkalaemia and hypomagnesaemia should be corrected concurrently.

Torsades de Pointes
- Correct electrolyte/metabolic abnormalities and withdraw offending agents.
- Acute and long-term pacing is indicated in patients with tdp due to heart block or symptomatic bradycardia, and is reasonable in those with recurrent pace-dependent tdp. Alternatively, IV isoproterenol can be given to patients with recurrent pace-dependent tdp who do not have long QTc.
- Combined beta-blockers and pacing is a reasonable acute therapy for patients with tdp and sinus bradycardia.
- IV magnesium sulphate (2 g in 1–2 min) can be given to patients with tds and long QTc.
- IV lidocaine or oral mexiletine (loading dose 400 mg, followed by 200–400 mg 8 hourly) may be considered in patients with tdp and long QT3 syndrome.
- Maintaining plasma potassium at a level of 4.5–5 mmol/L may be beneficial.

Incessant VT and VT storm
- Both terms have been variably defined. The most commonly accepted definition of incessant VT is VT lasting for hours, and that of VT storm is two or more VT in 24 h.
- IV beta-blockers are the most effective agents for treatment of recurrent or incessant polymorphic VT. IV amiodarone/procainamide can also be considered.
- Polymorphic VT storm usually occurs with acute myocardial ischaemia, which requires beta-blockers and urgent revascularization followed by IV amiodarone/procainamide. Intra-aortic balloon counterpulsation may be useful.
- General anaesthesia, overdrive pacing, and spinal cord modulation may be considered in refractory cases.

Evaluation

Evaluation usually begins on presentation and continues after initial stabilization. The aim of evaluation is to identify the underlying causes and possible triggers, obtain information to guide patient management, and occasionally identify family members who are at risk of sudden cardiac death for primary preventive treatment.

History
- Symptoms
  - VT: enquire about the duration of illness, duration of episode, frequency of attack, haemodynamic stability, and effect on daily life; symptoms precipitated by exertion suggests catecholamine-dependent VT, while symptoms occurring with arousal is typical for long QT2 syndrome; termination with Valsalva manoeuvre is suggestive of VT due to triggered activity.
  - Underlying causes: look for evidence of CAD, heart failure, and involvement of other systems.
- Past health: ask if patients have previously diagnosed MI, CAD, myocardial diseases, arrhythmias, musculoskeletal diseases, and psychiatric illnesses.
- Drug history: specifically question about the use of AADs, tricyclic antidepressants, and diuretics; recent exposure to antibiotics, antihistamines, antifungal, and antipsychotics should be enquired in patients with polymorphic VT associated with prolonged QTc.
- Social history: cigarette smoking, alcohol consumption, and the use of illicit drugs and toxins should be explored; patients may inadvertently ingest proarrhythmic agents when drugs are given for weight reduction (e.g. amphetamine) or as an alternative treatment of cancer (e.g. caesium).
- Family history: ask if any family members have premature CAD, sudden death, heritable myocardial, musculoskeletal, or electrical diseases.

Examination
- Once the diagnosis of VT is made, physical examination should focus on the underlying aetiologies:
  - Examine the cardiovascular system for signs of isolated left/right or biventricular failure, hypertrophic cardiomyopathy, valvular or congenital heart diseases. Also look for aneurysms and signs of peripheral vascular disease that may suggest underlying CAD.
  - Full examination should be performed to look for evidence of systemic diseases with heart involvement, e.g. hepatomegaly and peripheral neuropathy in amyloidosis; lymph nodes and skin lesions in sarcoidosis.

Investigations
1 Blood tests
  - Complete blood count, electrolytes, including potassium, calcium, and magnesium levels, arterial blood gas, renal and liver function tests, cardiac enzymes, toxicology screening, and thyroid function test.
2 12-lead ECG
  - 12-lead ECGs performed both during and after abortion of arrhythmias provide important clues to the underlying aetiologies.
  - Monomorphic VT: usually related to myocardial scarring; alternative causes include idiopathic VT and arrhythmogenic RV dysplasia.
  - Polymorphic VT: usually associated with acute ischaemic events. Arrhythmogenic RV dysplasia, heritable arrhythmia syndromes, myocarditis and pre-excited atrial fibrillation may also present with polymorphic VT.
  - tdp: usually resulting from congenital/acquired long QT syndrome or profound bradycardia/pauses due to severe conduction system diseases. Acquired causes of long QTc include ingestion of QT-prolonging agents, hypokalaemia, hypomagnesaemia, hypocalcaemia, hypothermia, and hypothyroidism. Metabolic and electrolyte abnormalities more commonly precipitate arrhythmias in patients with pre-existing long QT syndrome than causing tdp themselves.

- Bidirectional VT: an uncommon form of VT often associated with digitalis toxicity. It is also seen with catacholaminergic polymorphic VT and myocarditis.
- Pathological Q waves, ST elevations/depressions, and new-onset LBBB: suggestive of prior or ongoing myocardial ischaemia.
- Severe bradycardia and type II second- or third-degree heart block: can be related to drugs, myocardial ischaemia, or conduction system diseases.
- QRS width has been shown to predict mortality in patients with impaired LVEF. Prolonged QRS may also be due to the use of AAD and tricyclic antidepressants.
- QT intervals: prolonged QTc can be congenital or acquired (see p. 76). Congenital short QT syndrome has been recently described as a cause of ventricular arrhythmias.
- Severe left ventricular hypertrophy: can be due to hypertensive heart disease or hypertrophic cardiomyopathy.
- Delta waves: suggestive of pre-excitation syndrome.
- LBBB pattern with cove-typed ST elevation over V1–V3: suggestive of Brugada syndrome.
- Epsilon waves associated with T wave inversions over V1–V3: specific for arrhythmogenic RV dysplasia.
- Low voltage of ECG complexes: may be seen with infiltrative heart diseases.

3 Workup for structural heart diseases
- All patients should have echocardiography performed for detailed assessment of cardiac chambers, valves, septa, and vessels.
- If echocardiography does not provide adequate information, computed tomography angiography and magnetic resonance imaging and radionuclide scan should be considered.

4 Workup for myocardial ischaemia
- Urgent coronary angiography with revascularization is indicated in all patients with suspected VT associated with acute myocardial ischaemia.
- Coronary angiography is useful to diagnose obstructive CAD in the moderate- to high-risk group.
- Exercise testing with or without imaging modality (e.g. exercise SPECT) and pharmacological stress testing with imaging modality (e.g. stress echocardiography) may be considered as alternatives to coronary angiography for detection of myocardial ischaemia with or without induction of arrhythmias in patients with intermediate probability CAD.
- Coronary artery anomalies should be excluded especially among young patients. High-quality computed tomography angiography may be considered in selected cases.
- The use of pharmacological provocative testing to diagnose coronary spasm remains controversial.

5 Exercise testing
- Other than detection of ischaemia, exercise testing is useful for diagnosis of catecholamine-dependent VT and assessment of treatment response to medical or ablative therapy.
- Exercise testing should be performed under close monitoring by trained personnel with intravenous beta-blockers and resuscitation equipment available.

6 Ambulatory monitoring and other ECG measurements
- Ambulatory monitoring is useful for detection of arrhythmias, ST changes, QTc changes, and measurement of T wave alternans.

- T wave alternans, heart rate variability, and baroreflex sensitivity were all found to predict sudden cardiac death among MI survivors, although their role in guiding patient management remains unclear.
- Signal averaged ECG has largely lost its predictive value among MI patients in the reperfusion era. However, it remains one of the minor diagnostic criteria for arrhythmogenic RV dysplasia.

7 Pharmacological provocative testing
- Various protocols are being used. Examples include:
  - Catecholaminergic polymorphic VT: epinephrine infusion at 0.05–0.5 µg/kg/min. Appearance of frequent polymorphic ventricular ectopies, non-sustained or sustained polymorphic VT is considered diagnostic.
  - Brugada syndrome: IV procainamide 10 mg/kg over 10 minutes or flecainide 2 mg/kg over 10 minutes. Appearance of type I Brugada ECG is considered diagnostic.

9 Electrophysiological study (EPS)
- Apart from performing with an intent of radiofrequency ablation (RFA), EPS is a useful investigative tool for the following patients:
  - History of remote MI presented with symptoms suspected to be related to VT.
  - Post MI ≥40 days, LVEF ≤40%, and non-sustained VT, to determine the need of implantable cardioverter defibrillator (ICD) therapy.
  - Syncope of undetermined cause.
  - WCT of uncertain origin.
  - Bradyarrhythmia-induced VT, for exclusion of VT/VF prior to pacemaker implantation.

10 Genetic testing
- Consider in selected patients with suspected but unconfirmed monogenic disorders
- May be useful for family screening

Long-term management
General measures
- Underlying causes should be identified and treated as appropriate.
- Patients should be educated to avoid potential triggers, including proarrhythmic agents (e.g. QT-prolonging agents in patients with long QT syndrome) and proarrhythmic situations (e.g. severe exertion in patients with catecholaminogenic polymorphic VT), and maintain a healthy lifestyle.

Pharmacological therapies
- Beta-blockers are effective in suppressing VT and were shown to reduce sudden cardiac death in both MI and heart failure patients. They work through competitive adrenergic blockade, therefore reduce myocardial ischaemia and increase electrical stability of the heart. They are also useful treatments for catecholamine-dependent arrhythmias including idiopathic VT, long QT1 and 2 syndromes, and catecholaminergic polymorphic VT.
- Although effective in suppressing VT, the overall survival benefit from chronic use of amiodarone is controversial. Sotalol also reduces arrhythmia recurrence, but was found to increase mortality among MI patients with impaired LVEF.
- Except in patients who are not candidate for ICD implantation, AADs and other beta-blockers are largely used as adjunctive therapy to reduce ICD shocks.

ICD implantation

- Recent guidelines support ICD Implantations for management of VT for the following patients:
  - survivors of sudden cardiac arrest due to haemodynamically unstable sustained VT after exclusion of completely reversible causes.
  - spontaneous sustained VT in the presence of structural heart disease.
  - syncope of undetermined origin and haemodynamically significant sustained VT induced at EPS.
- ICD implantation is reasonable even in patients who had sustained VT without structural heart disease, including those who have long QT syndrome or catecholaminergic polymorphic VT who develop sustained VT while receiving beta-blockers
- ICD implantation should also be considered in patients with non-sustained VT and hypertrophic cardiomyopathy.

Radiofrequency ablation

- RFA is the treatment of choice for idiopathic VT with a success rate exceeding 90% in those originated from the RV outflow tract. It should be considered in patients who are drug-refractory, drug-intolerant, or unwilling for long-term medications.
- Bundle branch re-entry VT, usually associated with severe cardiomyopathy, is often resistant to AADs. RFA of the right bundle branch is both curative and safe and should be offered as first-line treatment.
- EPS with an intent of RFA should be performed for patients suspected to have ventricular arrhythmias due to pre-excited atrial fibrillation.
- RFA is increasingly used as adjunctive therapy for prevention as well as treatment of frequently recurrent VT/VF in patients with ICD and cardiomyopathy. The use of the endocardial and/or epicardial ablation approach has increased the successful rate of VT ablation in those patients.

Table 3.4.2 Anti-arrhythmic agents for treatment of ventricular tachycardia

Drug	Dosage (IV)	Dosage (Oral)	Side-effects
Procainamide*	Loading: 20–30mg/min† Maintenance: 1–4mg/min Max: 17mg/kg	Loading: 800–1000mg Maintenance: 300–600mg q6h Max: 50mg/kg	*CVS:* hypotension, proarrhythmia, heart block *Blood:* cytopenias *GI:* GI upset, elevated liver enzymes *Neuro:* dizziness, drowsiness, weakness, psychosis, convulsion *Others:* lupus-like syndrome
Amiodarone	Loading: 150mg in 10 min Maintenance: 1mg/min for 6h followed by 0.5mg/min for 18h Max: 2.2g/24h	800mg to 1.6g per day in divided dose for 1–3 weeks, then tail down to 400mg per day maintenance	*CVS:* hypotension, sinus bradycardia, heart block, tdp *GI:* GI upset, deranged liver function test *Resp:* pneumonitis, pulmonary fibrosis *Skin:* photosensitivity, pigmentation *Eye:* corneal microdeposits, optic neuritis and neuropathy *Thyroid dysfunction* *Neuro:* tremor, ataxia, involuntary movement, loss of coordination, peripheral neuropathy
Lidocaine	Loading: 1–1.5mg/kg; additional 0.5–0.75mg/kg as needed. Maintenance: 2–4mg/min Max: 3mg/kg		*CVS:* hypotension, proarrhythmia, bradycardia *Neuro:* tremors, tinnitus, paresthesia and numbness, blurred vision, loss of coordination, dizziness, drowsiness, euphoria, confusion, psychosis, convulsion *Resp:* respiratory depression *GI:* GI upset *Others:* malignant hyperthermia
Sotalol*		80–160mg q12h	*CVS:* hypotension, proarrhythmia including tdp, bradycardia, heart failure *Resp:* dyspnea, asthma *CNS:* fatigue, dizziness
Mexiletine		Loading: 400mg Maintenance: 200–400mg q8h	*CVS:* proarrhythmia, chest pain *GI:* GI upset, heartburn *Neuro:* tremor, nervousness, tinnitus, paresthesia and numbness, blurred vision, loss of coordination, dizziness, drowsiness, weakness, confusion, psychosis, convulsion, short term memory loss, headache and sleep disturbance *Others:* yellowish discoloration of eye and skin

*Dosage should be adjusted for renal function.

†Till arrhythmia suppressed, hypotension develops, QRS widens ≥50% above baseline, or maximum dosage reached.

Abbreviations: CVS–cardiovascular system; GI–gastrointestinal system; neuro–neurological system; tdp–torsades de pointes; resp–respiratory system

Outcomes

Prognosis depends on the presentation, aetiology, and severity of the underlying structural heart disease. Patients who present with sudden cardiac arrest are at the highest risk. Idiopathic VT is associated with the best prognosis. Patients with VT associated with ischaemic or non-ischaemic cardiomyopathy are prone to sudden cardiac arrest. More recent studies have shown that even VT/VF that occurred within 48 hours of presentation predicted poorer 90-day survival among ST-elevated MI patients undergoing primary percutaneous coronary intervention. The prognosis of other rarities is less well studied.

References

Arshad A, Mandava A, Kamath G, Musat D. Sudden cardiac death and the role of medical therapy. *Prog Cardiovasc Dis* 2008;**50**:420–38.

Cohen TJ, Chien WW, Lurie KG, et al. Radiofrequency catheter ablation for treatment of bundle branch reentrant ventricular tachycardia: results and long-term follow-up. *J Am Coll Cardiol* 1991;**18**:1767–73.

Epstein AE, Dimarco JP, Ellenbogen KA, et al. ACC/AHA/HRS 2008 Guidelines for device-based therapy of cardiac rhythm abnormalities. *Heart Rhythm* 2008;**5**:e1–62.

Goldberger ZD, Rho RW, Page RL. Approach to the diagnosis and initial management of the stable adult patient with a wide complex tachycardia. *Am J Cardiol* 2008;**101**:1456–66.

Koplan BA, Stevenson WG. Ventricular tachycardia and sudden cardiac death. *Mayo Clin Proc* 2009;**84**:289–97.

Libby P, Bonow RO, Mann DL, Zipes DP. Specific arrhythmias: diagnosis and treatment. *Braunwald's heart disease. A textbook of cardiovascular medicine*, 8th edn. Saunders, 2008:863–931.

Mehta RH, Starr AZ, Lopes RD, et al. Incidence of and outcomes associated with ventricular tachycardia or fibrillation in patients undergoing primary percutaneous coronary intervention. *JAMA* 2009;**301**:1779–89.

Morady F, Shen EN, Bhandari A, et al. Clinical symptoms in patients with sustained ventricular tachycardia. *West J Med* 1985;**142**:341–4.

Proceedings of the 2005 International Consensus on Cardiopulmonary Resuscitation and Emergency Cardiovascular Care Science with Treatment Recommendations. *Resuscitation* 2005;**67**:157–341.

Subbiah R, Gula LJ, Klein GJ, et al. Workup of the cardiac arrest survivor: for the symposium on sudden cardiac death for progress in cardiovascular diseases. *Prog Cardiovasc Dis* 2008;**51**:195–203.

Zimetbaum PJ, Josephson ME. *Practical clinical electrophysiology*. Lippincott Williams & Wilkins 2009.

Zipes DP, Camm AJ, Borggrefe M, et al. ACC/AHA/ESC 2006 Guidelines for Management of Patients With Ventricular Arrhythmias and the Prevention of Sudden Cardiac Death: a report of the American College of Cardiology/American Heart Association Task Force and the European Society of Cardiology Committee for Practice Guidelines (writing committee to develop Guidelines for Management of Patients With Ventricular Arrhythmias and the Prevention of Sudden Cardiac Death): developed in collaboration with the European Heart Rhythm Association and the Heart Rhythm Society. *Circulation* 2006;**114**:e385–484.

Sudden cardiac death

According to the ACC/AHA/HRS definition, sudden cardiac death (SCD) is an unexpected death due to sudden cessation of cardiac activity. The term sudden cardiac arrest (SCA) is employed if the event is rapidly reversed by effective intervention (Buxton et al. 2006). Whether to include only deaths that occur within 1 hour of symptom onset remains debatable as events are usually unwitnessed and durations of symptoms are often unknown. Likewise, strictly limiting these terms to describe primary cardiac events may be impractical since cardiac arrhythmias can be the final common pathway of both cardiac and non-cardiac insults (Priori et al. 2002).

Epidemiology

The annual incidence rate of SCD as shown in prospective studies ranged from 37 to 100 per 100 000 inhabitants. The age-related incidence first peaks at infancy, and begins to increase sharply again at the age of 55 until it reaches the second peak at 75–85 years. At all ages, men are more prone to SCD than women, accounting for over 60% of all events (Chugh et al. 2008).

The major risk factors for SCD are prior myocardial infarction (MI), reduced left ventricular ejection fraction (LVEF), and history of ventricular arrhythmias. Among populations without known structural heart disease, coronary risk factors including age, male gender, smoking, hypertension, increased low-density lipoprotein cholesterol, and diabetes mellitus predispose to coronary artery disease (CAD) and therefore increase the risk SCD. Conversely, excessive alcohol intake, elevated plasma free fatty acids and C-reactive protein levels, increased heart rate, acute psychosocial stress, and positive family history were shown to be associated with SCD unrelated to CAD (Kark et al. 1995; Jouven et al. 1999, 2001; Albert et al. 2002; Priori et al. 2002; Turakhia et al. 2007).

The higher relative risk of SCD (RR 2.8) in young athletes than in non-athletes is probably due to the combined effect of underlying cardiovascular disease and intense exercise triggering arrhythmias rather than the sport activity itself. Although there is a clear male predominance in the incidence of SCD, the role of ethnicity and the risk of different diseases that predispose to SCD needed to be clarified (Borjesson et al. 2009).

Pathophysiologies

Previous studies showed that 84% of the immediate rhythms leading to SCD were ventricular fibrillation (VF) or ventricular tachycardia (VT), whereas bradyarrhythmias only accounted for 16% of all cases. A dramatic decline in the prevalence of VF to 40% and increase in pulseless electrical activity (PEA) to 25% over the past 20 years have been reported, probably resulting from the improvement in management of MI, which is the most common cause of VT/VF (Chugh et al. 2008).

Aetiologies

Over 70% of SCDs are related to acute or chronic myocardial ischaemia. Other causes include non-ischaemic structural heart disease (10–15%), primary electrical disease (5–10%), and non-cardiac disease (Chugh et al. 2008), with those non-ischaemic causes more frequently encountered among patients ≤35 years of age (Eckart et al. 2004). Major aetiologies of SCD are summarized in Table 3.5.1.

Management strategy

Management of SCA includes reversal of the event by timely resuscitation, limitation of neurological damage by optimal post-arrest care, identification of aetiologies and treatment of reversible causes, and long-term prevention of future SCD.

Resuscitation

Advanced cardiac life support should be initiated immediately after SCA is recognized. Survival from SCA depends upon the promptness to restore organized electrical activity, which is facilitated with the use of an automated external defibrillator (AED) by paramedics and bystanders. Every effort to decrease AED-associated delays is of

Table 3.5.1 Major causes of sudden cardiac death

Ischaemic heart disease	Myocardial infarction
	Unstable angina
	Ischaemic cardiomyopathy
	Coronary spasm
	Coronary artery anomalies
Non-ischaemic heart disease	Hypertrophic cardiomyopathy
	Dilated cardiomyopathy
	Arrhythmogenic RV dysplasia
	Valvular heart disease
	Congenital heart disease
	Myocarditis
	Infiltrative cardiomyopathy
	Cardiac tamponade
Primary electrical disease	Idiopathic VF
	Brugada syndrome
	Long QT syndrome
	Short QT syndrome
	Catecholaminergic polymorphic ventricular tachycardia
	Pre-excitation syndrome
	Sinus/atrioventricular nodal disease
	Chest wall trauma
Non-cardiac disease	Pulmonary embolism
	Ruptured aortic aneurysm
	Aortic dissection
	Upper airway obstruction
	Drug intoxication
	Electrolyte imbalance
	Intracranial haemorrhage

the utmost importance, and chest compressions and ventilations should be provided throughout the resuscitative process to minimize hypoxic brain damage. The role of adjunctive medications in improving patients' outcomes remains uncertain (ECC Committee 2005; Rea et al. 2010).

Post-resuscitation care

Patients who survive the initial resuscitation should be transferred to the high-dependency unit to optimize haemodynamic, respiratory, and neurological support. Patients should have their cardiac rhythms monitored and mean arterial blood pressure maintained slightly elevated to improve cerebral perfusion. Electrolyte, acid–base, and blood glucose levels should be kept normal. Sustained hypocapnia reduces cerebral blood flow and should be avoided. Both hyperthermia and seizure exacerbate cerebral ischaemia and need to be controlled. Induced hypothermia to 32–34°C by external (e.g. cooling blankets and ice bags) or more effectively internal (e.g. cold saline, endovascular cooling catheter) cooling techniques for 12–24 hours has been shown to improve both neurological outcome (RR 1.40) and mortality (RR 0.74) (ECC Committee 2005; Polderman 2008).

Evaluation

History taking, physical examinations, and investigations should focus on the following areas.
1 Assess neurological damage and potential of recovery.
2 Identify possible triggers.
3 Determine aetiologies.

This is a continuous process that should begin at the time of event recognition, as rapid correction of the underlying cause may be necessary to restore cardiac activity, and evidence for specific conditions may wane over time. Early diagnoses of MI and extracardiac causes of sudden arrest (Table 3.5.1) are particularly important as rapid implementation of specific treatment may be life-saving.

History

Often the patient is either stuporous or unable to recall the event, particularly soon after resuscitation. Information from witness, family members, and friends is therefore helpful.
1 Symptoms: antecedent symptoms immediately before arrest and prior to the event may suggest specific aetiology, e.g. exertional or resting chest pain may suggest myocardial ischaemia; poor exercise tolerance, paroxysmal nocturnal dyspnoea, and ankle oedema are clues to pre-existing heart failure, recurrent palpitation or syncope during exertion indicates adrenergic-dependent arrhythmias, etc.
2 Past medical history—apart from history of cardiac or vascular diseases, enquire whether the patient has been told to have abnormal electrocardiography (ECG).
3 Drug history: in particular, the use of antiarrhythmics, diuretics, and drugs that may prolong QT intervals. Use of over-the-counter drugs or herbal medications should also be explored.
4 Social history: cigarette smoking, alcohol consumption, ingestion of toxins, and use of recreational drugs should be specifically questioned. Patients may be exposed to thyroxine, amphetamine, or other illicit drugs unintentionally when given pills for weight reduction.

5 Family history: enquire about history of sudden death, early-onset CAD, and heritable syndromes.

Examination

1 Assess and monitor blood pressure, pulse rate and rhythm, oxygen saturation, body temperature, glucostix, and organ perfusion.
2 A careful search for the followings especially in patients presenting with PEA:
  • Upper airway obstruction: stridor, use of accessory respiratory muscles, neck swelling
  • Cardiac tamponade: congested neck veins, elevated jugular venous pressure, muffled heart sounds
  • Tension pneumothorax: hyper-resonant percussion notes with mediastinal shift to the contralateral side
  • Aortic dissection: pulse deficit, aortic regurgitation murmur
  • Aortic aneurysm: pulsatile mass
  • Pulmonary embolism: unilateral lower limb swelling, congested neck veins, elevated jugular venous pressure, loud P2
  • Most of the above signs will not be present before some return of circulation with the initial resuscitative effort, which unfortunately cannot sustain without correcting the underlying causes. High index of suspicion is therefore needed for prompt diagnosis and treatment.
3 Neurological examination should be performed to assess neurological status and look for evidence of primary intracranial pathologies (e.g. pin-point or unequal pupils, upper motor neuron signs).
4 Thorough cardiovascular examination may reveal signs of hypertrophic cardiomyopathy, valvular or congenital heart disease. Evidence of severe peripheral vascular disease may hint at coexisting coronary or aortic atherosclerotic disease.

Investigations

Blood tests
  • Complete blood count
  • Electrolytes, including potassium, calcium, and magnesium levels, renal and liver function tests, arterial blood gas and glucose levels
  • Cardiac enzymes
  • Toxicology screening
  • Thyroid function tests

ECG
  • ECGs performed both during and after abortion of the arrhythmia provide important clues to the underlying aetiology.
  • Monomorphic VT: usually related to myocardial scarring. Idiopathic VT is monomorphic but a less common cause cardiac arrest.
  • Polymorphic VT or VF: usually associated with acute ischaemic events. Other causes include Brugada syndrome, idiopathic VF, and pre-excited atrial fibrillation.
  • Torsade de pointes: a specific form of polymorphic VT, usually results from congenital or acquired long QT syndrome. Common acquired causes include the use of QT-prolonging agents, hypokalaemia, hypomagnesaemia, hypocalcaemia, hypothermia, hypothyroidism, and intracranial pathologies.

- Bidirectional VT: an uncommon form of VT often associated with digitalis toxicity. It is also seen with catacholaminergic polymorphic VT and myocarditis.
- Pathological Q waves, ST elevations/depressions, and new-onset left bundle branch block: suggestive of prior or ongoing myocardial ischaemia.
- Severe bradycardia and type II second- or third-degree heart block: related to drugs, myocardial ischaemia, and sinus or atrioventricular nodal disease.
- Prolonged or shortened QT intervals: congenital or acquired (see Torsade de Pointes).
- Severe left ventricular hypertrophy: due to hypertensive heart disease or hypertrophic cardiomyopathy.
- Delta waves: pre-excitation syndrome.
- Right bundle branch block pattern with cove-typed ST elevation over V1–V3: Brugada syndrome.
- Epsilon waves and T-wave inversions over V1–V3: arrhythmogenic right ventricular (RV) dysplasia.
- Low voltage of ECG complexes: cardiac tamponade and infiltrative heart disease.
- Electrical alternans: cardiac tamponade.
- Sinus tachycardia, p-pulmonale, S1Q3T3, right bundle branch block, and anterior ST depressions/T-wave inversions: pulmonary embolism.

Echocardiography
- LVEF is the strongest predictor of SCD (Subbiah *et al.* 2008)
- Regional wall motion abnormality along the territory of a coronary artery suggests MI
- RV dilatation, paradoxical septal movement, and McConnel sign (akinetic RV free wall and normal motion at RA apex) may be present in acute pulmonary embolism
- Dilated aortic root, aortic regurgitation, and dissection flap suggest aortic dissection
- Thickened myocardium can be due to hypertension, hypertrophic cardiomyopathy, or infiltrative heart disease
- Also look for valvular and congenital heart disease, and features suggestive of RV dysplasia
- Electrolyte and acid–base abnormalities, ECG alterations such as ST/T changes and prolonged QT interval, and impaired LVEF may be consequences of circulatory arrest, defibrillation, or induced hypothermia as opposed to being primary causes of SCA. Repeating investigations at regular intervals may sometimes be helpful.

Coronary angiography
- Urgent coronary angiography with revascularization is indicated in all patients with suspected acute myocardial ischaemia.
- The 2006 ACC/AHA/ESC guidelines suggested consideration of coronary angiography in survivors of SCA, particularly those who had an intermediate or greater probability for CAD.
- Coronary artery anomalies should be excluded, especially among young patients. High-quality computed tomography angiography may be considered in selected cases.
- The use of pharmacological provocative testing to diagnose coronary spasm is controversial.

Exercise testing (Zipes et al. 2006; Subbiah et al. 2008)
- This is recommended in unexplained cardiac arrest to unmask exercise-induced polymorphic VT in catecholaminergic polymorphic VT and QT prolongation in congenital long QT syndrome.
- Should be performed under close monitoring by trained personnel with intravenous beta-blockers and resuscitation equipment available.

Ambulatory ECG monitoring
- Less useful nowadays as most SCA survivors will have an implantable cardioverter defibrillator (ICD) inserted before discharge.

Pharmacological provocative testing
Various protocols are being used. Examples include
- Catecholaminergic polymorphic VT: Epinephrine infusion at 0.05–0.5 μg/kg/min. The appearance of frequent polymorphic ventricular ectopies, non-sustained or sustained polymorphic VT is considered diagnostic.
- Brugada syndrome: IV procainamide 10 mg/kg over 10 min or flecainide 2 mg/kg over 10 min. Appearance of type I Brugada ECG is considered diagnostic.

Cardiac magnetic resonance imaging
- This is indicated in selected patients for whom diagnoses remain uncertain after the initial evaluation.
- It is most valuable in diagnosing arrhythmogenic right ventricular dysplasia, hypertrophic cardiomyopathy, infiltrative cardiomyopathy, and acute myocarditis.

Electrophysiological studies
This is less useful in the era of secondary prevention with ICD implantation, except under the following circumstances:
- Bradyarrhythmia is presumed to be the culprit where ventricular stimulation is performed to rule out significant VT/VF prior to pacemaker implantation.
- Known or suspected accessory pathway for radiofrequency ablation to prevent recurrence.
- Performed in conjunction with radiofrequency ablation to reduce ICD shocks.

Genetic testing
- This should be considered in selected patients with suspected but unconfirmed monogenic disorders.
- It may be useful for family screening.

Prevention of recurrence
Remove reversible factors
- Treatment targeting identifiable causes should be implemented as soon as possible.
- Correct hypoxia, electrolyte and acid–base imbalances.
- Urgent coronary angiography and revascularization for acute myocardial ischaemia.
- Acute and permanent pacing for patients with bradyarrhythmia-induced torsades de pointes.
- Pericardiocentesis in cardiac tamponade.
- Thrombolytics or embolectomy in massive pulmonary embolism.

- Use of antidote, e.g. antidigitalis antibodies in digitalis toxicity; sodium injection in sodium channel blockers toxicity.
- Reimplantation of coronary artery of anomalous origin.

Avoid further triggers
- Proarrhythmic agents, e.g. QT-prolonging medications in long QT syndrome, sodium channel blockers in Brugada syndrome.
- Proarrhythmic situations, e.g. severe exertion in catecholaminogenic polymorphic VT, arousal in type II long QT syndrome.
- Binge drinking, recreational drugs abuse, and pills or supplements of uncertain ingredients.

Pharmacological therapies
- Beta-blockers suppress ventricular arrhythmias in catecholaminergic polymorphic VT and long QT syndrome, and reduce SCD in patients with MI and heart failure.
- The overall long-term benefit of amiodarone and sotalol remains controversial and should be considered as adjuncts to reduce ICD shocks or alternatives in patients reluctant or not candidates for ICD therapy.
- Other antiarrhythmic agents are probably harmful.

Non-pharmacological therapies
- Radiofrequency ablation of accessory pathway is indicated in patients with SCA due to pre-excited supraventricular tachycardia.
- Radiofrequency ablation of VT is useful to reduce ICD shocks in patients with recurrent sustained VT unresponsive to medical treatment.
- Surgical treatments including resection of arrhythmogenic focus, cardiac sympathetectomy, aneursymectomy, and cardiac transplantation may be necessary in patients with refractory VT.

ICD implantation
- ICD implantation is recommended to survivors of SCA after exclusion of completely reversible causes.
- It is dangerous to loosely attribute SCA to a reversible cause, particularly with metabolic disturbance, which is usually a triggering factor in the presence of structural or electrical heart disease rather than a causative factor itself.

Primary prevention
- Primary prevention for SCD involves the identification of at-risk population, avoidance of potential triggering factors, and implementation of general and specific preventive measures. A brief summary of drug and ICD indications is given below.

General population
- Screening and modification of risk factors for CAD
- Advise on moderate alcohol consumption (<2 drinks per day)
- Encourage regular exercise.

Patients with known or suspected ventricular arrhythmias not leading to SCA
- ICD therapy is recommended:
  - spontaneous sustained VT and structurally heart disease
  - syncope of undetermined origin and haemodynamically significant sustained VT/VF induced at electrophysiological study.
- ICD therapy is reasonable:
  - syncope in the setting of poor LVEF due to non-ischaemic cardiomyopathy
  - sustained VT/syncope despite use of beta-blockers in long QT syndrome and catecholaminergic polymorphic VT
  - sustained VT/syncope in Brugada syndrome.

Patients with CAD
- Beta-blockers, angiotensin-converting enzyme inhibitors, statins and omega-3 fatty acids (in form of fish or dietary supplement) reduce SCD in patients with CAD. Those with heart failure also benefit from angiotensin II receptor blockers and aldosterone antagonists.
- ICD therapy is indicated in CAD patients with:
  - LVEF ≤30% at least 40days post MI, and New York Heart Association (NYHA) class I symptoms
  - LVEF ≤35% at least 40days post MI, and NYHA class II/III symptoms
  - LVEF ≤40%, non-sustained VT, and inducible sustained VT at electrophysiological study.
- Inadequate evidence to support the routine use of other non-invasive testing such as signal averaged ECG, heart rate variability, baroreflex sensitivity, or T wave alternans for further risk stratification.

Patients with non-ischaemic dilated cardiomyopathy
- Beta-blockers, angiotensin converting enzyme inhibitors, angiotensin II receptor blockers and aldosterone antagonist reduce SCD in patients with heart failure.
- ICD therapy is indicated in patients with LVEF ≤35% and NYHA class II/III symptoms, and can be considered in those with NYHA class I symptoms.
- Mortality benefit of ICD implantation is independent of the time from diagnosis.

Patients with hypertrophic cardiomyopathy
- ICD implantation is reasonable for patient with major risk factors including spontaneous non-sustained VT, syncope, myocardial thickness ≥30mm, abnormal blood pressure response to exercise, and family history of SCD.

Patients with primary electrical diseases
- Beta-blockers for patients with long QT syndrome or catecholaminergic polymorphic VT to prevent VT/VF.
- ICD implantation is reasonable in patients with syncope or symptomatic VT/VF only.

Family members of patients suffered from SCA/SCD

- Family members are at higher risk of SCD if they share the following risk factors with the patient:
  - inherited risk for CAD or CAD risk factors
  - inherited monogenic myocardial or electrical disorders
  - inherited risk for SCD unrelated to known structural and electrical heart disease.
- Inform first-degree relatives of their risk of SCD and advise against high risk behaviour.
- Screening of family members for monogenic disorders is recommended (e.g. echocardiography for dilated or hypertrophic cardiomyopathy; ECG with or without exercise testing for long QT syndrome).
- Routine genetic counselling is not performed except for research purpose.

Young athletes

- Optimal screening stratagem debatable.
- A reasonable approach would be routine evaluation of personal and family history, physical examination, and resting ECG before participation of competitive sports, and additional investigations when abnormalities detected. History and physical examination should be repeated at regular intervals and self-report of symptoms should be encouraged (Buxton *et al.* 2006).

Prognosis

Short-term survival

- Meta-analysis of 79 studies on out-of-hospital SCA has revealed that 23.8% patients survived to hospital admission, but only 7.6% were discharged from hospital admission (Thompson *et al.* 2007). Factors including witnessed arrest, CPR by bystander, VT/VF as the first recorded rhythm, and return of spontaneous circulation were predictive of survival. Despite medical advancements in the past three decades, no significant change in short-term survival rate has been detected.

Long-term survival

- Registry data over 10 years have shown that post-discharge 5-year survival rates increased from 63.2% to 76.0% due to a significant fall in the risk of cardiac death. However, fewer patients have been discharged with normal neurological function (97.5% versus 81.3%), and more of them had moderate disability (8.5% versus 15.6%) (Pell *et al.* 2006).

References

Albert CM, Ma J, Rifai N, Stampfer MJ, Ridker PM. Prospective study of C-reactive protein, homocysteine, and plasma lipid levels as predictors of sudden cardiac death. *Circulation* 2002;**105**:2595–9.

Arshad A, Mandava A, Kamath G, Musat D. Sudden cardiac death and the role of medical therapy. *Prog Cardiovasc Dis* 2008;**50**:420–38.

Borjesson M, Pelliccia A. Incidence and aetiology of sudden cardiac death in young athletes: an international perspective. *Br J Sports Med* 2009;**43**:644–8.

Buxton AE, Calkins H, Callans DJ, *et al.* ACC/AHA/HRS 2006 key data elements and definitions for electrophysiological studies and procedures: a report of the American College of Cardiology/American Heart Association Task Force on Clinical Data Standards. *J Am Coll Cardiol* 2006 Dec 5;**48**:2360–96.

Chugh SS, Reinier K, Teodorescu C, *et al.* Epidemiology of sudden cardiac death: clinical and research implications. *Prog Cardiovasc Dis* 2008;**51**:213–28.

ECC Committee, Task Forces of the American Heart A. 2005 American Heart Association Guidelines for Cardiopulmonary Resuscitation and Emergency Cardiovascular Care. *Circulation* 2005;**112**(24 Suppl):IV1–203.

Eckart RE, Scoville SL, Campbell CL, *et al.* Sudden death in young adults: a 25-year review of autopsies in military recruits. *Ann Intern Med* 2004;**141**:829–34.

Epstein AE, DiMarco JP, Ellenbogen KA, *et al.* ACC/AHA/HRS 2008 Guidelines for Device-Based Therapy of Cardiac Rhythm Abnormalities: a Report of the American College of Cardiology/American Heart Association Task Force on Practice Guidelines. *J Am Coll Cardiol* 2008;**51**:e1–62.

Jouven X, Charles MA, Desnos M, Ducimetière P. Circulating non-esterified fatty acid level as a predictive risk factor for sudden death in the population. *Circulation* 2001;**104**:756–61.

Jouven X, Desnos M, Guerot C, Ducimetière P. Predicting sudden death in the population: the Paris Prospective Study I. *Circulation* 1999;**99**:1978–83.

Kark JD, Goldman S, Epstein L. Iraqi missile attacks on Israel. The association of mortality with a life-threatening stressor. *JAMA* 1995;**273**:1208–10.

Pell JP, Corstorphine M, McConnachie A. Post-discharge survival following pre-hospital cardiopulmonary arrest due to cardiac aetiology: temporal trends and impact of changes in clinical management. *Eur Heart J* 2006;**27**:406–12.

Polderman KH. Induced hypothermia and fever control for prevention and treatment of neurological injuries. *Lancet* 2008;**371**:1955–69.

Priori SG, Aliot E, Blømstrom-Lundqvist C, *et al.* Task Force on Sudden Cardiac Death, European Society of Cardiology. *Europace* 2002;**4**:3–18.

Rea TD, Page RL. Community approaches to improve resuscitation after out-of-hospital sudden cardiac arrest. *Circulation* 2010;**121**:1134–40.

Sasson C, Rogers MA, Dahl J, Kellermann AL. Predictors of survival from out-of-hospital cardiac arrest: a systematic review and meta-analysis. *Circ Cardiovasc Qual Outcomes* 2010;**3**:63–81.

Subbiah R, Gula LJ, Klein GJ, Skanes AC, White J, Yee R, Krahn AD. Workup of the cardiac arrest survivor: for the symposium on sudden cardiac death for progress in cardiovascular diseases. *Prog Cardiovasc Dis* 2008;**51**:195–203.

Thompson PD, Franklin BA, Balady GJ, *et al.* Exercise and acute cardiovascular events placing the risks into perspective: a scientific statement from the American Heart Association Council on Nutrition, Physical Activity, and Metabolism and the Council on Clinical Cardiology. *Circulation* 2007 1;**115**:2358–68.

Turakhia M, Tseng ZH. Sudden cardiac death: epidemiology, mechanisms, and therapy. *Curr Probl Cardiol* 2007;**32**:501–46.

Zipes DP, Camm AJ, Borggrefe M, *et al.* Guidelines. ECFP. ACC/AHA/ESC 2006 Guidelines for Management of Patients With Ventricular Arrhythmias and the Prevention of Sudden Cardiac Death: a Report of the American College of Cardiology/American Heart Association Task Force and the European Society of Cardiology Committee for Practice Guidelines. *Circulation* 2006;**114**:e385–e484.

Neurogenic syncope

Psuedonyms

Neurogenic syncope, also called as reflex syncope, is caused by the triggering of a vascular reflex. This gives rise to vasodilatation and/or bradycardia. The term reflex syncope avoids the suggestion that this is a neurological condition, although convulsive reflex syncope, undoubtedly mimics epilepsy often. Some other names found in the literature for this condition are vasovagal syncope, neurocardiogenic syncope, vasodepressor, neurally mediated hypotension, bradycardia syndrome, emotional fainting, pallid breath-holding spells, pallid infantile syncope, reflex anoxic seizures, reflex asystolic syncope, and malignant vasovagal syncope.

Definition

Syncope, as defined by the European Society of Cardiology, 'is a transient, self-limited loss of consciousness, usually leading to collapse. The onset of syncope is relatively rapid, and the subsequent recovery is spontaneous, complete, and usually prompt. The underlying mechanism is transient global cerebral hypoperfusion'.

Syncope is a transient symptom and needs to be differentiated from other common causes of transient loss of consciousness (T-LOC), namely epilepsy and non-epileptic attack disorder (NEAD). Also, reflex syncope needs to be differentiated from many other causes of syncope (given below).

Causes of syncope

Reflex syncope

- Vasovagal syncope
- Carotid sinus syncope
- Situational syncope (e.g. post micturition, post exercise, postprandial, cough, swallow, visceral pain).

Orthostatic hypotension

Cardiac arrhythmias as a primary cause

- Sinus node dysfunction (including tachy-brady syndrome)
- Atrioventricular conduction disease
- Ventricular tachycardia and supraventricular tachycardia
- Arrhythmias associated with inherited syndromes, e.g. long QT syndrome, Brugada syndrome, arrhythmogenic right ventricular dysplasia (ARVD)
- Implanted device (pacemaker, implantable cardioverter defibrillator) malfunction.

Structural cardiac or cardiopulmonary disease

- Severe left ventricular dysfunction
- Obstructive valvular heart disease, e.g. aortic stenosis
- Remote or acute myocardial infarction/ischaemia
- Hypertrophic obstructive cardiomyopathy
- Acute aortic dissection
- Pericardial disease/tamponade
- Pulmonary embolism/pulmonary hypertension.

Epidemiology

Syncope is a common condition. The Framingham study estimates the prevalence of syncope to be 42% during the life of a person living 70 years. It accounts for 1.0–1.5% of emergency room visits and up to 6% of general hospital admissions. It shows a bimodal age distribution with a high incidence in young populations (median age 15 years), with a second peak in older patients ≥75 years of age. Females are more prone to syncope than men. The prognosis of syncope depends on its cause. Reflex syncope, the commonest cause of syncope, has a mortality that is near to 0%, whereas cardiac syncope is an independent predictor of mortality and sudden death.

Evaluation

Typically patients with syncope are asymptomatic at the time of their initial assessment. In all patients with syncope, including reflex syncope, the initial evaluation should consist of a careful history, physical examination, including orthostatic blood pressure measurements, and a standard 12-lead electrocardiogram (ECG). Studies have shown that based on this initial evaluation, a diagnosis of syncope can be made with certainty in between 50% and 63% of patients, thus avoiding the need for additional testing. Also, further tests tend to be costly and have a low yield.

History

A carefully history on its own may be sufficient in arriving at a diagnosis of reflex syncope. Clinical features which point towards this diagnosis are:
- Absence of cardiac disease
- Long history of syncope
- T-LOC occurring after unpleasant sight, sound, smell or pain, after prolonged standing, or in crowded, hot places
- Nausea vomiting associated with syncope
- T-LOC during or in the absorptive state after a meal
- Head rotation or pressure on the carotid sinus precipitating T-LOC
- T-LOC occurring *after* exertion.

On the other hand, syncope due to cardiac arrhythmias or secondary to cardiopulmonary disease is suggested by:
- The presence of severe structural heart disease
- T-LOC *during* exertion or when supine
- T-LOC preceded by palpitation or accompanied by chest pain
- Family history of sudden cardiac death ≤40 years of age.

The yield of history taking may be limited in the presence of cognitive impairment in elderly people, a feature which one may encounter in ~5% of 65 year olds and ~20% of 80 year olds. A good history may also help to differentiate 'convulsive syncope' from epilepsy, thereby helping to prevent a misdiagnosis of epilepsy (see below). On balance, convulsive syncope is probably more common than generalized epilepsy.

Physical examination

A thorough physical examination is an important aspect of the initial evaluation of any patient with syncope. Care should be taken to assess the rate and regularity of the pulse, lying and standing blood pressure, examination for scars of previous cardiac operations, and auscultation for heart sounds and any murmurs. Abnormalities in the physical examination can point towards a diagnosis of syncope due to orthostatic hypotension, an arrhythmia, or structural heart disease. On the other hand, in reflex syncope, the examination is likely to be normal, which is reassuring.

ECG

A resting 12-lead ECG forms another essential part of the initial evaluation of patients presenting with T-LOC. It is a cheap and reliable test and must be undertaken in every patient with T-LOC. Though the diagnostic yield of electrocardiography is low, ranging from 1% to 11%, a normal 12-lead ECG is a good prognostic indicator and can be used for risk stratification of patients presenting with T-LOC. Abnormalities on the ECG that suggest or are diagnostic of a non-reflex cause of syncope are as follows:

- Mobitz II second- or third-degree atrioventricular block
- Abnormal Q waves suggesting myocardial infarction
- Rapid ventricular or supraventricular tachycardia
- Symptomatic sinus bradycardia (<50 bpm), sinoatrial block or sinus pause(s) ≥3 seconds in the absence of negatively chronotropic medications
- Prolonged QT interval
- Pacemaker malfunction with cardiac pauses
- Pre-excited QRS complexes
- Other intraventricular conduction disturbances (QRS duration ≥0.12 seconds)
- Bifascicular block (left bundle branch block or right bundle branch block combined with left anterior or left posterior fascicular block)
- Alternating right and left bundle branch block
- Right bundle branch block pattern with ST elevation in leads V1–V3 (Brugada syndrome)
- Negative T waves in right precordial leads, epsilon waves, and ventricular late potentials suggestive of ARVD.

Other investigations

Basic laboratory tests have a limited value in the investigation of patients with syncope. However, in selected cases, they may help to elucidate the cause of loss of consciousness when the clinical picture suggests blood loss or a metabolic cause.

Tilt table testing

Tilt testing is a simple, non-invasive test with a low risk of complications. Clinicians began using this test in the late 1980s following studies showing a high rate of reflex hypotension and bradycardia in patients with syncope of previously unknown origin when compared with control subjects. Subsequently, clinical practice has seen a wide range of protocols, varying in duration and angle of tilt, the use of drug provocation and, importantly, the type of patients studied. Such factors presumably underlie the variable yield of tilt table testing, which ranges from 26% and 87%. Although currently recommended by the European Society of Cardiology and the American College of Cardiology, limitations of tilt testing include its poor reproducibility, low specificity, poor reproduction of spontaneous features and its inability to predict response to treatment, either by drugs or devices. When the diagnosis of reflex syncope can be made with confidence based on the initial evaluation, tilt table testing adds little to the overall management of the patient. When simultaneously undertaken with an electroencephalogram, it is a useful test for investigating patients with psychogenic blackouts or NEAD. Recently, there have been a few reports on the usefulness of tilt table testing in the demonstration of 'counterpressure manoeuvres' and the role of 'tilt training' in patients with reflex syncope. The true value of tilt table testing for these indications awaits further confirmation.

Loop recorder implantation

Recording of physiological variables, e.g. blood pressure, heart rate/rhythm or the electrical activity of the brain during an episode of T-LOC is critical in confirming the clinical suspicion of the mechanism and/or the cause of T-LOC. However, such opportunities are rare due to the infrequent, episodic and unexpected occurrence of symptoms of T-LOC and the limitations of the currently available investigations. Although one is able to acquire high quality ECGs for short durations of time with low-cost non-invasive recording devices like the Holter monitor, the diagnostic yield is poor because of infrequent ECG symptom correlation. The implantable loop recorder is a small metallic device that is inserted on the left side of the chest under local anaesthesia. There are currently three such devices on the market. The newer devices are also capable of being remotely monitored. The largest published literature is with the Reveal family of devices, manufactured by Medtronic. The usefulness of the loop recorder is in those patients where the cause or mechanism of syncope cannot be determined on initial evaluation, or where an arrhythmic cause for syncope is suspected. A much higher ECG symptom correlation has been demonstrated with these devices than external Holter monitoring. Limitations are their high initial costs, their lack of ability to measure any other physiological variable, and the need for an invasive procedure to implant them. However, they are more cost-effective as their diagnostic yield is far higher.

Carotid sinus massage

Pressure at the site where the common carotid artery bifurcates produces a reflex slowing in heart rate and a fall in blood pressure. A ventricular pause lasting ≥3 seconds and/or a fall in systolic blood pressure of 50 mmHg is considered abnormal. When the above haemodynamic effects are accompanied by reproduction of symptoms, it is called as carotid sinus syndrome. In the absence of symptoms, it is appropriate to use the term carotid sinus hypersensitivity. Studies have shown the latter to be more common than the former.

Differential diagnosis

Reflex syncope should be differentiated from other causes of T-LOC/blackout, namely epilepsy and psychogenic blackouts, or NEAD.

Epilepsy is the most common chronic disabling neurological condition in the UK. A 'seizure' as defined by the International League Against Epilepsy (ILAE) and the International Bureau of Epilepsy (IBE) is a 'transient occurrence of signs and/or symptoms due to an abnormal excessive or asynchronous neuronal activity in the brain' A diagnosis of 'epilepsy' is reserved for those patients who have recurrent 'seizures'. Epilepsy is much less common than syncope, with a lifetime prevalence of 0.5–1.0%. A diagnosis of epilepsy is more likely when the following clinical features are present:

- Previous history of brain injury
- History of aura, e.g. unusual or distinctive smell before the event
- Prolonged tonic-clonic movements coincident with the onset of transient loss of consciousness
- Lateral tongue biting
- Suffused or cyanosed face
- Prolonged post-T-LOC confusion
- Family history of idiopathic epilepsy

- Headache or aching muscles after T-LOC
- History of cerebral birth trauma or hypoxia, severe learning disabilities or autism
- New or evolving neurological deficit.

In 'convulsive syncope' T-LOC caused by cerebral hypoperfusion can give rise to a clinical picture similar to epilepsy. Some differentiating features are facial pallor, floppy body tone initially, followed by stiffness, abnormal movements occurring after the fall that usually take the form of asymmetrical myoclonic jerks, and quick recovery from T-LOC.

Psychogenic blackouts or NEAD are 'unintentional paroxysms of altered sensation, movement, perception, or emotion that clinically resemble epileptic seizures but are not accompanied by epileptiform neurophysiological changes'. It is estimated that the incidence of NEAD is between 3 and 5 per 100 000 population and that it co-exists with epilepsy in up to 20% of patients. Most patients are women, begin to have symptoms in their late teens or early 20s, and up to 80% have a history of previous medically unexplained symptoms. Clinical features which point towards a diagnosis of NEAD are:

- Prominent motor features that wax and wane throughout a blackout
- Long duration of blackouts (over 2 minutes)
- On recovery from a blackout, able to recall events during it
- Poor response to antiepileptic drugs
- History of previous unexplained medical symptoms
- A psychiatric history or childhood traumatic experiences, e.g. sexual abuse.

If NEAD is suspected a sensitive exploration of the social history is required, and awareness of help available from neuropsychiatrists and clinical psychologists.

Management

Only about two-thirds of patients with a syncopal episode see a doctor or visit a hospital for evaluation. Treatment of patients with syncope depends on its cause.

In all patients with reflex syncope, treatment consists of:
- Education and reassurance
- Lifestyle measures, e.g. volume expansion by salt supplements, isometric leg and arm counter-pressure manoeuvres to abort an impending attack
- Avoidance of precipitating situations in patients with situational syncope

In selected cases, the following may be useful:
- Drug therapy, e.g. midodrine

Midodrine is an alpha-1-sympathomimetic drug producing a therapeutic benefit by its ability to increase blood pressure through its peripheral vasoconstrictor effect. It is not licensed in the UK, being available only on a named patient basis. Side-effects include itching of the skin, tingling of the scalp, flushing, or supine hypertension. The dose ranges from 2.5 to 10 mg tds po. There are no safety data during pregnancy.

Other drugs which have been tried in patients with reflex syncope are fludrocortisone, paroxetine, etilefrine, and beta-blockers.

Permanent pacemaker implantation (PPM)

Though widely practised, the role of permanent pacemaker implantation in patients with reflex syncope is uncertain and awaits the results of further studies. A meta-analysis of blinded and unblinded randomized controlled trials of PPM based on the results of tilt table testing has failed to show a salutary effect on symptoms. The literature suggests pacemaker implantation based on the results of an insertable loop recorder may be a better predictor of freedom from recurrence of symptoms but awaits confirmation in a currently ongoing randomized controlled blinded study. It is a Class II indication for pacing in the current (2008) Heart Rhythm Society/American College of Cardiology/American Heart Rhythm Association and the European Society of Cardiology (2007) guidelines.

Carotid sinus syndrome is a Class I indication for PPM according to the above guidelines.

Further reading

Benditt DG, Blanc JJ, Brignole M, Sutton R (eds). *The evaluation and treatment of syncope. A handbook for clinical practice.* Boston: Blackwell Publishing, 2003

Brignole M, Sutton R, Menozzi C, et al. for the International Study on Syncope of Uncertain Etiology 2 (ISSUE 2) Group. Early application of an implantable loop recorder allows effective specific therapy in patients with recurrent suspected neurally mediated syncope. *Eur Heart J* 2006;**26**:1085–92.

Fitzpatrick AP, Cooper P. Diagnosis and management of patients with blackouts. *Heart* 2006;**92**:559–68.

Fitzpatrick AP, Lee RJ, Epstein LM, et al. Effect of patient characteristics on the yield of prolonged baseline head-up tilt testing and the additional yield of drug provocation. *Heart* 1996;**76**:406–11.

Mellers JDC. The approach to patients with 'non-epileptic seizures'. *Postgrad Med J* 2005;**81**:498–504.

Perez-Lugones A, Schweikert R, Pavia S, et al. Usefulness of midodrine in patients with severely symptomatic neurocardogenic syncope: a randomized control study. *J Cardiovasc Electrophysiol* 2001;**12**:935–38.

Petersen MEV, Williams TR, Sutton R. Psychogenic syncope diagnosed by prolonged head-up tilt testing. *Q J Med* 1995;**88**:209–13.

Stokes T, Shaw EJ, Juarez-Garcia A, et al. Clinical guidelines and evidence review for the epilepsies: Diagnosis and management in adults and children in primary and secondary care. London: Royal College of General Practitioners, 2004.

Sud S, MasselD, Klein GJ, et al. The expectation effect and cardiac pacing for refractory vasovagal syncope. *Am J Med* 2007;**120**: 54–62.

The Task Force on Syncope, European Society of Cardiology. Guidelines on management (Diagnosis and Treatment) of syncope: update 2004. *Europace* 2004;**6**:467–537.

Inappropriate sinus tachycardia

Sinus tachycardia is a form of supraventricular tachycardia originating from the sinus node. It can be secondary to various physiological or pathophysiological stresses. Inappropriate sinus tachycardia (IAST) is a disorder characterized by a persistent increase in resting heart rate or sinus rate in otherwise healthy individuals, which is unrelated to, or out of proportion with, the level of physical, emotional, pathological, or pharmacological stress (Shen 2005). It has significant overlap in clinical presentation and pathogenic mechanisms with postural orthostatic tachycardia syndrome (POTS) in which symptoms and tachycardia predominantly develop in the upright position (Brady et al. 2005).

Mechanisms

The pathological basis of IAST is not well defined. It is generally believed that the underlying mechanisms are likely to multifactorial and significant heterogeneity exists among different individuals with IAST. The proposed pathogenic mechanisms can be broadly divided into cardiac and extracardiac (Table 3.7.1). It was recently suggested that the predominant primary pathogenesis is autonomic in origin and IAST is merely a secondary manifestation.

Epidemiology

The epidemiology of this patient population has not been extensively studied. Once thought to be a relatively uncommon condition, the condition has been diagnosed with increasing frequency. The prevalence has been estimated to be 1.16% in the general population (Still et al. 2005). The majority of IAST patients are young women (15–50 years old). IAST was also recognized to be associated with health professional workers and hypertension (Brady et al. 2005).

Table 3.7.1 Proposed mechanisms of inappropriate sinus tachycardia

Cardiac	Enhanced automaticity of the sinus node
	Increased sympathetic tone
	Increased sympathetic receptor sensitivity
	Blunted parasympathetic tone
	Sympathovagal imbalance
Extracardiac	Subtle or regional autonomic neuropathy
	Beta-adrenergic receptor autoantibodies
	Beta-adrenergic receptor supersensitivity
	M2 receptor abnormalities
	Depressed efferent cardiovagal reflex
	Impaired baroreflex control

Clinical approach

IAST is a diagnosis of exclusion (Fig. 3.7.1). Examinations and investigations should aim to establish the diagnosis, exclude other supraventricular tachyarrhythmias and secondary causes of sinus tachycardia (Table 3.7.2), and assess the patient's autonomic function.

The major diagnostic criteria recommended by the ACC/AHA/ESC guidelines (Blomström-Lundqvist et al. 2003) include:

1 The presence of a persistent sinus tachycardia (heart rate >100 bpm) during the day with excessive rate increase in response to activity and nocturnal normalization of rate, as confirmed by a 24-hour Holter recording.

2 Tachycardia and symptoms are non-paroxysmal

3 P-wave morphology and endocardial activation identical to sinus rhythm.

4 Exclusion of secondary causes (e.g. hyperthyroidism, pheochromocytoma, physical deconditioning).

History: key points

- Symptoms—patients may present with large variation of degree of disability. The most common symptom is palpitation; others include lightheadedness, presyncope/syncope, orthostatic intolerance, chest pain, headache, myalgia, dyspnoea, fatigue, abdominal discomfort, anxiety, depression

- Characteristics of palpitation—gradual onset and termination, non-paroxysmal, triggered by minimal exertion

- Concomitant medical history—absent of pathologies that can give rise to secondary sinus tachycardia, e.g. anaemia, hyperthyroidism, etc.

- Drug history—use of drugs that can produce sinus tachycardia (atropine, catecholamines, thyroid medications)

- Social history—alcohol consumption, cigarette smoking, caffeine.

Examination

- Regular and increased heart rate
- No evidence of structural heart diseases.

Investigations

Blood tests

- Routine and screening
  - Complete blood count
  - Fasting blood glucose
  - Thyroid function screening
- Elective
  - Orthostatic plasma noradrenaline (norepinephrine)
  - Urinary metanephrines
  - 24-hour urinary sodium excretion.

Electrocardiography

- Tachycardia may not always be detected
- P wave: axis and morphology during tachycardia similar to sinus rhythm.

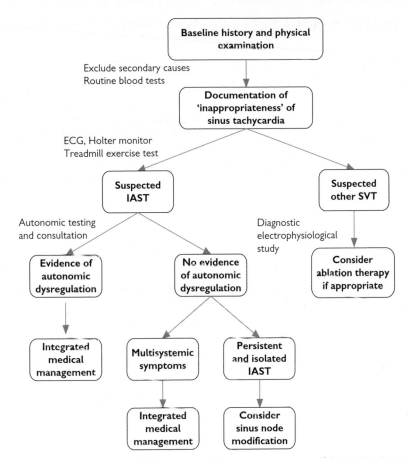

Fig. 3.7.1 Algorithm for investigation of suspected IAST. From Shen WK, *How to manage patients with inappropriate sinus tachycardia, Heart Rhythm*, copyright (2005) with permission from Elsevier.

Echocardiography
- To rule out structural heart diseases and heart failure
- Left ventricular function: mostly normal.

24-hour Holter monitoring
- Persistent elevated heart rate (>100) during the day
- Excessive increase in response to activity
- Normal or near-normal heart rate during sleep
- Mean heart rate >90
- Symptoms correlate to episodes of tachycardia.

Treadmill exercise test
- Exaggerated heart rate response to minimal exercise: increased to >130 during first 90 seconds on a standard Bruce protocol.

Diagnostic electrophysiological study (Lee and Shinbane 1997)
- Indicated when aetiology of tachycardia is uncertain or other supraventricular tachycardias are suspected
- Gradual increase and decrease of heart rate spontaneously or during initiation and termination of isoproterenol infusion
- Not influenced by atrial pacing (in contrast to re-entry or triggered atrial arrhythmias)
- Surface P wave morphology similar to that observed during sinus rhythm
- During mapping, earliest endocardial activation near the area of sinus node, with a craniocaudal direction along the crista terminalis. Site of earliest activation shifts superiorly at a higher heart rate and inferiorly at a lower rate.

Table 3.7.2 Secondary causes of sinus tachycardia

Increased demand	Exercise
	Fever
Neuropsychiatric	Anxiety
	Pain
Cardiorespiratory insufficiency	Anaemia
	Dehydration
	Pulmonary embolus
	Pulmonary oedema
	Pneumothorax
Cardiovascular disorders	Heart failure
	Pericarditis
	Cardiac rupture
	Aortic insufficiency
	Acute mitral regurgitation
	Myocardial infarction
	After ablation of SVT
Metabolic and endocrine causes	Hyperthyroidism
	Hypoglycaemia
	Diabetes
	Pheochromocytoma
Drugs and stimulants	Cocaine abuse
	Amphetamine ingestion
	Catecholamine infusion
	Anticholinergic drugs
	Tobacco
	Caffeine
	Alcohol
	Beta-blocker withdrawal

Tilt table test
- Tilt table test of short duration (up to 10 minutes) is useful to assess response to orthostatic stress
- Prolonged tilt table test usually not necessary.

Autonomic function assessment
- Routine autonomic screening tests are limited to a few selected medical centres
- May guide mechanism-based therapies.

Natural history and management

Complications

IAST is a chronic condition. During a follow-up period of 6 years, there were only minor changes in the heart rate of patients. The prognosis of IAST is benign. Tachycardia-induced cardiomyopathy was reported as a possible but uncommon complication. Majority of patients develop no clinical or echocardiographic evidence of structural heart disease.

Management strategy
- Given the benign prognosis, management of IAST is predominantly symptom driven. Pharmacological treatments are indicated when symptoms are not well controlled by non-pharmacological means. Interventional therapies should be restricted to refractory cases. A heart rate of 80–90 bpm should be aimed as the target endpoint.

Non-pharmacological approaches (Brady et al. 2005)
- Sleeping with head of the bed elevated
- Plasma volume expansion
- Compressive stockings
- Physical counter-manoeuvres
- Resistance training.

Pharmacological treatments (Blomström-Lundqvist et al. 2003)
Beta-blockers
- As the first-line medical therapy
- A non-selective beta-blocker such as propranolol (30–160 mg/day) or nadolol (40–160 mg/day) can be started at the lowest dose and titrated upwards gradually to the maximum tolerable dose
- Response can be heterogeneous. Some patients may not respond even at high dose.

Non-dihydropyridine calcium channel blockers
- Verapamil (120–480 mg/day) and diltiazem (180–360 mg/day) may be effective.

Selective If channel blocker
- Ivabradine (2.5–7.5 mg bd) may be used to specifically inhibit the pacemaker if current
- Some individual reports suggested side-effects are few but include visual disturbances (phosphenes, blurring), bradyarrhythmias, and headache.

Interventional treatments
Radiofrequency ablation (RFA) of sinus node
- Total ablation of the sinus node was reported to have a high short term success rate.
- The high risk of need of permanent pacemaker makes it less favourable.

Sinus node modification (Lee and Shinbane 1997; Olshansky 2008)
- It aims to perform RFA at the most superior aspect of the sinus node complex to eliminate symptoms of IAST while preserving sinus node function

- Indication: IAST refractory to medical treatment
- Contraindication: POTS must be excluded because ablative procedures are shown to worsen symptoms
- Prognosis: short-term success rate reaches 76–100%. However, long-term outcome is often incomplete or suboptimal. Most cardiac and extracardiac symptoms persist despite slower heart rate
- Potential adverse effects: pericarditis, phrenic nerve injury, superior vena cava syndrome, need for permanent pacing.

References

Blomström-Lundqvist C, Scheinman MM, Aliot EM. ACC/AHA/ESC Guidelines for the Management of Patients with Supraventricular Arrhythmias. *J Am Coll Cardiol* 2003;**15**:1493–531.

Brady PA, Low PA, Shen WK. Inappropriate sinus tachycardia, postural orthostatic tachycardia syndrome, and overlapping syndromes. *PACE* 2005;**28**:1112–21.

Lee RJ, Shinbane JS. Inappropriate sinus tachycardia: diagnosis and treatment. *Cardiol Clin* 1997;**15**:599–605.

Olshansky B. What's so inappropriate about sinus tachycardia? *J Cardiovasc Electrophysiol* 2008;**19**:977–8.

Shen WK. How to manage patients with inappropriate sinus tachycardia. *Heart Rhythm* 2005;**2**:1015–19.

Still AM, Raatikainen P, Ylitalo A, *et al.* Prevalence, characteristics and natural course of inappropriate sinus tachycardia. *Europace* 2005;**7**:104–12.

Antithrombotic therapy in atrial fibrillation

Atrial fibrillation (AF) is an independent predictor of mortality. AF is associated with increase in morbidity and mortality from stroke, thromboembolism, and heart failure. The risk of stroke is similar in patients either with persistent or paroxysmal AF.

The risk of stroke increases four- to fivefold across all age groups in AF patients. This accounts for 10–15% of all ischaemic stroke: 1.5% in patients <60 years old and >24% in patients >80 years old. Hence, antithrombotic therapy becomes an essential part of AF management.

The risk of stroke is not homogeneous among all AF patients. Treatment has to balance stroke risk, contraindications and co-morbidities.

Risk factors for stroke and thromboembolism are as follows:
- Previous stroke/transient ischaemic attack
- Older age
- Diabetes
- Hypertension
- Heart failure
- Vascular disease
- Moderate–severe left ventricular dysfunction on two-dimensional (2D) echocardiography
- Reduced left atrial appendage velocities, spontaneous contrast, complex aortic plaque on the descending aorta on transoesophageal echocardiography (TEE).

Standard therapy

There are numerous randomized controlled trials that have looked into thromboprophylaxis in AF. In summary:
- Adjusted warfarin with target international normalization ratio (INR) between 2.0 to 3.0
- Warfarin (adjusted dose, INR 2–3) reduces stroke risk by 64% compared with placebo
- Aspirin 75–325 mg reduces stroke risk by 22% compared with placebo
- Warfarin reduces stroke risk by 40% compared with aspirin
- In patients >75 years old, warfarin was more effective than aspirin (>50% reduction) without any excess in risk of major bleeding
- A combination of warfarin and aspirin offer no extra benefit to stroke prevention when compared with warfarin therapy alone, but increases the risk of bleeding
- In patients for whom warfarin is not suitable or contraindicated, a combination of aspirin and clopidogrel reduced the risk when compared with aspirin alone
- Warfarin remains under-prescribed, especially in high-risk patient groups (elderly people), on the basis of a presumed increased risk of haemorrhagic complications.

Stroke risk stratification

There are published risk stratification schemes to aid in the assessment of stroke and thromboembolic risk.

There are some differences among the scheme designed to stratify stroke risk in patients with AF. The proportion classified as 'high risk' varies from 11% to 77% and the proportion classified as 'low risk' varies from 9% to 49% depending on the stroke risk stratification scheme used.

Some of the commonest used schemes are:
- CHADS2
- NICE guidelines (2006) (Figure 3.8.1)
- ACC/AHA/ESC guidelines (2006).

CHADS2 is simple to be use and well validated, but it does not include echocardiographic left ventricular impairment or association with other vascular disease as high-risk factors. The CHADS2 scheme is similar in predicting stroke and vascular events when compared to the NICE risk stratification scheme (Table 3.8.1).

Annual risk of stroke:
High risk, 8–12%; moderate risk, 4%; low risk, 1%.

Bleeding risk

All patients need to be assessed individually for stroke risk and bleeding risk. The decision of whether to initiate a formal anticoagulant needs to be a joint decision between physicians and patients.

Risk factors associated with bleeding complications:
- Elderly age (>75 years)
- Uncontrolled hypertension
- Polypharmacy
- History of bleeding
- Anaemia
- Concomitant use of antiplatelet therapy.

Newer antithrombotic agents

Warfarin is very effective in the treatment of thromboembolic events and thromboprophylaxis in AF. However, its use is limited by:
- The narrow therapeutic window
- Substantial inter- and intra-individual variability
- The need for regular adjustment to keep the INR between 2.0 and 3.0
- Metabolism is influenced by genetic factors, diet and drug interactions.

These limitations have prompted the quest for new antithromotic therapy. The ideal novel anticoagulants should:

Table 3.8.1 Relationship between CHADS scores and risk of stroke

Risk factor	Individual score	Total score	Adjusted stroke rate (%)
Nil	0	0	1.9
C (CHF)	1	1	2.8
H (hypertension)	1	2	4.0
A (age)	1	3	5.0
D (DM)	1	4	8.5
S2 (previous stroke or TIA)	2	6	18.2

CHF, congestive heart failure; DM, diabetes mellitus; TIA, transient ischaemic attack

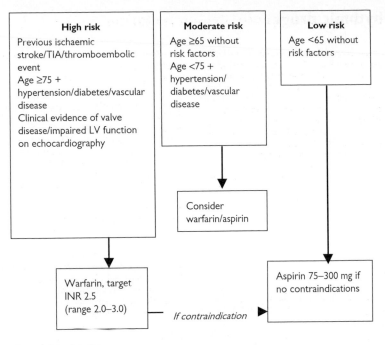

High risk	Moderate risk	Low risk
Previous ischaemic stroke/TIA/thromboembolic event	Age ≥65 without risk factors	Age <65 without risk factors
Age ≥75 + hypertension/diabetes/vascular disease	Age <75 + hypertension/diabetes/vascular disease	
Clinical evidence of valve disease/impaired LV function on echocardiography		

Consider warfarin/aspirin

Warfarin, target INR 2.5 (range 2.0–3.0)

If contraindication

Aspirin 75–300 mg if no contraindications

Annual risk of stroke:
High risk, 8–12%; moderate risk, 4%; low risk, 1%

Fig. 3.8.1 NICE guidelines for stroke risk stratification. With permission from Royal College of Physicians London.

- Have predictable pharmacokinetic and pharmacodynamic properties
- Be given in fixed doses
- Have wider therapeutic window
- Have fewer interactions with food or other drugs
- Not require regular monitoring.

Those in the most advanced clinical development stages are

- Factor Xa inhibitor (Rivaroxaban, Apixaban, Betrixaban, Edoxaban)
- Direct thrombin inhibitor (Dabigatran, AZD-0837).

Recent data from the RE-LY trial showed that dabigatran 150 mg bid was superior to warfarin for stroke prevention, with a similar rate of major bleeding; also, dabigatran 110 mg bid was not inferior to warfarin for stroke prevention with significantly less major bleeding events. Both doses of dabigatran resulted in lower intracranial haemorrhage than warfarin.

Support group: Arrhythmia Alliance, The Heart Rhythm Charity www.heartrhythmcharity.org.uk.

Further reading

Connolly SJ, Ezekowitz MD, Yusuf S, *et al*. RE-LY Steering Committee and Investigators. Dabigatran versus warfarin in patients with atrial fibrillation. *N Engl J Med* 2009 17;**361**:1139–51.

Fuster V, Ryden LE, Cannom DS, *et al*. ACC/AHA/ESC 2006 guidelines for the management of patients with atrial fibrillation: full text: a report of the American College of Cardiology/American Heart Association Task Force on practice guidelines and the European Society of Cardiology Committee for Practice Guidelines (Writing Committee to Revise the 2001 guidelines for the management of patients with atrial fibrillation) developed in collaboration with the European Heart Rhythm Association and the Heart Rhythm Society. *Europace* 2006;**8**:651–745.

Lip GY, Lim HS. Atrial fibrillation and stroke prevention. *Lancet Neurol* 2007;**6**:981–93.

National Collaborating Centre for Chronic Conditions. *Atrial Fibrillation: national clinical guideline for management in primary and secondary care*. London: Royal College of Physicians, 2006 (http://rcplondon.ac.uk/pubs/books/af/index.asp).

Stroke Risk in Atrial Fibrillation Working Group. Comparison of 12 risk stratification schemes to predict stroke in patients with nonvalvular atrial fibrillation. *Stroke* 2008;**39**:1902–10.

Antiarrhythmic drugs

Antiarrhythmic agents are used daily in clinical practice to suppress cardiac arrhythmias. Most of the antiarrhythmic agents are very potent compounds with narrow therapeutic windows. As such, they also have proarrhythmic effects. Inappropriate use of antiarrhythmic drugs either by wrong choice or wrong dosage could potentially be hazardous and life-threatening.

The safe prescribing of these agents depends on the understanding of the pharmacodynamic and pharmacokinetic properties. The choice of drug depends on numerous factors:

• Indication of usage
• Efficacy of drug
• Toxicity
• Dosing interval
• Metabolites (active and non-active)
• Bioavailability
• Drug–drug interactions
• Metabolism and clearance.

Various attempts have been made to classify antiarrhythmic agents. For example, the Sicilian gambit tried to produce a complete and accurate classification of the agents based on all mechanism of actions. However, the classification was so complex that its usage in day-to-day practice is limited. The most used classification to date is the Vaughan Williams classification.

Vaughan Williams classification

This is based on the primary mechanism of action of each agent on certain ion channels and receptors located on the myocardial cell membrane. This classification has its limitations as most antiarrhythmic agents have multiple mechanisms of action. However, it remains the clearest and most practical classification of antiarrhythmic agents. The original classification grouped antiarrhythmic agents into four major groups. This has since been revised by Harrison (Table 3.9.1).

Class I agents

These primarily block rapid inward sodium (Na) channel. Thus, they slow the rise of action potential. They are further subclassified based on electrophysiological effects:

• Ia: prolongs repolarization and refractoriness of myocardial tissue. (↑QRS and ↑QT interval). Examples include quinidine, disopyramide and procainamide. These agents are used for the treatment of supraventricular and ventricular arrhythmias. They are mainly used in ventricular arrhythmias and for the prevention of recurrent atrial fibrillation.
• Ib: shortens the action potential, limited effect on rapid inward Na channel. (minimal effect on QRS, QT, and PR intervals) Examples include lidocaine, phenytoin, mexiletine and tocainide. Traditionally, this agent was used to suppress ventricular arrhythmias.
• Ic: more potent antiarrhythmic agents that are powerful fast Na channel blockers. These agents also inhibit the His conduction system with widening QRS complexes. Besides, they markedly shortened the action potential duration of Purkinje fibres. Examples include flecainide, and propafenone. These agents are used in supraventricular and ventricular arrhythmias They are effective in paroxysmal supraventricular tachycardia and ventricular arrhythmias resistant to other agents.

Class II agents

These agents act on the beta-1-adrenergic receptor, thus decreasing sympathetic activity of the heart. They prolong AV conduction. (↑ PR interval). Examples include propanolol, esmolol, metoprolol, and atenolol. They have been shown to improve mortality, especially post myocardial infarction MI, and in systolic heart failure. These agents are also used in supraventricular and ventricular arrhythmias.

Table 3.9.1 Vaughan Williams classification of antiarrhythmic drugs

Class	Action	Effect on cardiac potential	Examples	Clinical indication
I	Block fast Na channel	Slow phase 0 rate of rise, depress phase 4 rate of rise Effect on action potential varies:		
Ia		Prolongs the action potential	Disopyramide, procainamide, quinidine	Ventricular arrhythmias, prevention of recurrent atrial fibrillation
Ib		Shortens the action potential	Lidocaine, mexiletine, phenytoin	Ventricular tachycardia, atrial fibrillation. Limited usage due to risk of asystole
Ic		No significant effect on action potential	Flecainide, propafenone	Paroxysmal atrial fibrillation, resistant tachyarrhythmias
II	Beta-adrenergic blockers	Depress phase 4 rate of rise	Propranolol, atenolol	Prevent recurrent of tachyarrhythmias
III	Potassium channel blockers that prolong repolarization	Prolong repolarization, increase action potential duration	Amiodarone, sotalol, bretylium, dofetilide, ibutilide	Ventricular tachycardia, supraventricular tachycardia (atrial fibrillation, atrial flutter)
IV	Slow calcium channel blockers	Depress phase 2 and 3	Verapamil, diltiazem	Prevent recurrence of supraventricular tachycardia, ventricular rate control in atrial fibrillation

Class III agents

These agents inhibit the outward potassium current, thus prolonging repolarization and refractories (↑QRS, QT intervals). Examples include sotalol and amiodarone. In fact, class 3 agents are often called the mixed group. Sotalol has class 2 effect and amiodarone exhibits the effects of all four classes. The prolongation of QT interval by these agents may predispose to torsades de pointes. These agents are effective in both ventricular and supraventricular arrhythmias.

Class IV agents

These are mainly calcium channel blockers that slow conduction through the AV node (↑ PR interval). They have little effect on QRS or QT interval. These agents are used in treating supraventricular arrhythmias. Examples include diltiazem and verapamil. They are effective in atrial arrhythmias by slowing the ventricular response.

Class V agents

- Digoxin inhibits the Na,K-ATPase receptor. It reduces heart rate by increasing PR interval. Its main effect is the augmentation of parasympathetic tone on the atrial and AV node. Thus, its effect is seen less during exercise.
- Adenosine is a purinergic receptor agonist. It has direct nodal inhibition effects. It reduces heart rate by increasing PR interval. It is effective in termination of supraventricular tachycardia and junctional tachycardia.

Newer antiarrhythmic agents

Numerous new antiarrhythmic agents are under investigations because of the limitations of the current available antiarrhythmic agents.

- Dronedarone is a non-iodinated amiodarone-like drug that has potent electrophysiological properties and less extracardiac toxicity than amiodarone. Numerous phase 2 and 3 clinical trials have shown the safety and efficacy of this drug. It was approved by the EU in November 2009.
- Venakalant is an intravenous antiarrhythmic agent that has proven highly effective in rapid cardioversion of recent onset (<7 days) atrial fibrillation. It has no effect on atrial flutter. Oral vernakalant is still undergoing Phase 2/3 trials.

Further reading

Kowey PR. Pharmacological effects of antiarrhythmic drugs. *Arch Intern Med* 1998;**158**:325–332.

Camm AJ, Al-Saady NM, Opie LH. Antiarrhythmic drugs. In: Opie LH, Gersh BJ, eds. *Drugs for the heart*. 5th edn. Saunders 2001: pp. 221–73.

Cardiac pacemaker

With the aging population, there has been an increasing trend in cardiac pacemaker implantation worldwide. In the United States, up to 2.25 million electronic pacemakers were implanted in the period from 1990 to 2002, and the annual implantation rate increased almost threefold. Since the first endocardial pacing lead implantation in 1958, pacemaker therapy has undergone remarkable technological advances. Nonetheless, pacemaker therapy (both implantation and long-term management) remains one of the core aspects in cardiology.

Pacemaker classification

In 2002, the North American Society of Pacing and Electrophysiology (NASPE) and British Pacing and Electrophysiology Group (BPEG) published a revised five-letter pacemaker code describing the basic function of cardiac pacemakers (Table 3.10.1) (Bernstein et al. 2002). The first and the second position of this code refer to the chamber(s) paced and the chamber(s) sensed respectively. The third position refers to the pacemaker response to the sensed event, which could be inhibited (I), triggered (T), or dual (T+I). For instance, in single-chamber, inhibited (synchronous) pacing mode (AAI and VVI), a sensed event in the chamber of interest inhibits the output and resets the timing cycle. In DDD (dual-chamber AV sequential pacing mode), a sensed atrial event inhibits the atrial output pulse but triggers an output pulse to the ventricle unless a ventricular event is sensed. The fourth position refers to the rate modulation capacity of the pacemaker, i.e. the ability to alter its pacing rate according to the patient's physiological need. The fifth position indicates the presence or absence of multisite pacing.

Indications for permanent pacemaker (Vardas et al. 2007; Epstein et al. 2008)

Pacing for bradycardia (adapted from Vardas et al. 2007; Epstein et al. 2008)

Generally speaking, patients with symptomatic bradycardia without reversible cause require pacemaker therapy.

Sino-atrial nodal dysfunction (SND)
Pacemaker therapy is indicated:
- Patients with documented symptomatic bradycardia including frequent sinus pauses,
- Patients with symptomatic chronotropic incompetence,

- Patients with documented symptomatic sinus bradycardia due to a required drug therapy for a medical condition.

Pacemaker therapy is reasonable in:
- Patients with symptomatic SND with heart rate less than 40 bpm but without a clear association between symptom and bradycardia
- In patients with unexplained syncope and electrophysiological evidences of significant SND.

Atrioventricular nodal dysfunction
- For patients with third-degree and advanced second-degree atrioventricular (AV) block at any anatomical level associated with (1) bradycardia and symptoms, (2) arrhythmia and other medical conditions requiring a drug therapy leading to symptomatic bradycardia, (3) documented asystole ≥3 seconds, escape rate <40 bpm, or escape rhythm below AV node despite the lack of symptom, (4) atrial fibrillation (AF) with pause(s) ≥5 seconds, (5) catheter AVN ablation, (6) post-cardiac surgery AV block expected not to resolve, (7) neuromuscular disease with AV block regardless of symptom, (8) exercise in the absence of myocardial ischaemia; pacemaker therapy is indicated.
- For patients with second-degree AV block with symptom regardless of the type and site of block, pacemaker therapy is indicated.
- For patients with asymptomatic third-degree AV block at any anatomic site associated with LV dysfunction or the site of block is below AVN despite the average awake ventricular rate >40 bpm, pacemaker therapy is indicated.
- For patients with alternating bundle branch block, pacemaker therapy is indicated.
- For patients with persistent asymptomatic third-degree AV block at any anatomic site with escape rate >40 bpm without cardiomegaly, pacemaker therapy is reasonable.
- For patients with asymptomatic second-degree AV block at intra- or infra-His level documented in electrophysiological study, pacemaker therapy is reasonable.
- For patients with first- or second-degree AV block with symptoms typical of haemodynamic compromise, pacemaker therapy is reasonable.
- For patients with asymptomatic second-degree AV block with narrow QRS, pacemaker therapy is reasonable.

Table 3.10.1 Revised NASPE/BPEG generic code for antibradycardia pacing

Position I	Position II	Position III	Position IV	Position V
Chamber paced	Chamber sensed	Response to sensed event	Rate modulation	Multisite pacing
O = None	O = None	O = None	O = None	O = None
A = Atrium	A = Atrium	I = Inhibited	R = Rate modulation	A = Atrium
V = Ventricle	V = Ventricle	T = Triggered		V = Ventricle
D = Dual (A+V)	D = Dual (A+V)	D = Dual (T+I)		D = Dual (A+V)

NASPE, North American Society of Pacing and Electrophysiology; BPEG, British Pacing and Electrophysiology Group. Modified from Bernstein et al. 2002

Pacing for heart failure (cardiac resynchronization therapy, CRT) (adapted from Vardas et al. 2007; Epstein et al. 2008)

- For patients with left ventricular ejection fraction (LVEF) ≤35%, QRS ≥120 ms, New York Heart Association (NYHA) functional classes III-IV while on optimal medical therapy, CRT is indicated.
- For patients with LVEF ≤35%, NYHA functional classes III-IV, and requiring frequent ventricular pacing while on optimal medical therapy, CRT is reasonable.
- The indication for milder form of heart failure (class II) to prevent remodelling is evolving.

Pacing for arrhythmia (adapted from Vardas et al. 2007; Epstein et al. 2008)

- For patients with sustained pause-dependent ventricular tachyarrhythmia with or without prolonged QT interval, pacemaker therapy is indicated.
- For patients with congenital long-QT syndrome at high risk of VT, pacemaker therapy is reasonable.

Pacing mode selection

Generally speaking, it is accepted in patients with SND, atrial-based pacing with an effort to minimize ventricular pacing should be the pacing mode of choice, which is however limited by the presence of concomitant AVD. While dual-chamber pacing can maintain AV synchrony, an alternative ventricular pacing site (RV outflow tract, or even CRT) to RV apical pacing may be needed in order to maintain ventricular synchrony due to high level of ventricular pacing.

Preoperative preparation

Prior to the operation, informed consent, standard 12-lead electrocardiogram (ECG), chest X-ray and routine blood tests including complete blood count, renal function, and clotting profile should be obtained. For pacemaker site selection, factors including the patient's hand dominance, occupation and recreational activities, previous cardiac and/or thoracic surgery, previous radiotherapy to thorax, abnormal venous drainage, and venous occlusion or thrombosis, should be taken into consideration. An intravenous catheter for drug administration, as well as for venogram if needed, should be placed over the arm of the side of the proposed pacemaker implantation site. While the use of prophylactic antibiotic remains a controversial issue, local guidelines and practice should be observed. In cases when prophylactic antibiotic is indicated, an intravenous agent with antistaphylococcal activity is generally needed. Likewise, anticoagulant and/or antiplatelet agents are commonly withheld prior to the implantation; significant variation in clinical practice and little consensus exist. The area from the angle of the jaw to the nipple line, and from both axillary lines should be shaved and washed with antiseptic agents.

Pacemaker implantation

The implantation techniques outlined here are by no means comprehensive or exhaustive, but represents some of the commonly used methods. As the left infraclavicular site is the most common site of pacemaker implantation, surface anatomical landmarks including the lateral third of the clavicle, the coracoid process, and the deltopectoral groove should be identified. A skin incision (~1 inch (2.5 cm)) is made at the level of the coracoid process, which runs perpendicular to the deltopectoral groove and somewhat parallel to the inferior border of the clavicle (Fig. 3.10.1). This incision often allows access to subclavian and axillary veins (with the puncture technique), as well as the cephalic vein (with the cutdown technique) (Table 3.10.2).

After obtaining venous access(es) with standard peel-away sheath(s) *in situ*, pacemaker lead placement could be guided by fluoroscopy. Although the right ventricular (RV) apex and right atrial appendage are generally the intended sites of pacemaker lead placement, alternative pacing sites, such as RV septum for RV pacing and interatrial septum/Bachmann bundle for atrial pacing with active fixation leads, have been gaining popularity among implanting physicians in order to provide more physiological pacing (Siu et al. 2008). After testing sensing function and pacing parameters, the leads are then attached to the generator. The generator is then placed either in a subcutaneous or submuscular pocket, and the incision is closed.

Postoperative management

Postoperatively, patients are to be monitored with continuous ECG or telemetry systems. Simple analgesic is required to minimize pain. Preoperative anticoagulant and/or antiplatelet agents can be resumed after good haemostasis is achieved. In addition, it is imperative to identify acute post-procedural complications (Table 3.10.3). Chest X-rays should be performed after the patient is transferred back to the ward in order to detect complications such as pneumothorax, haemothorax, cardiac and central venous perforation. Pacemakers should be interrogated immediately and before discharge in order to detect any lead or generator malfunction.

Follow-up

It is recommended that patients implanted with a pacemaker should be followed-up in person at 2 weeks and 3 months after implantation, and every 3–12 months thereafter (either in person or with remote monitoring). As the battery approaching elective replacement, the follow-up frequency should be increased to every 1–3 months accordingly.

During each follow-up, the devices should be interrogated for basic parameters including battery status, capture threshold, lead impedance, high rate, and automatic mode switch episodes. In addition, patients should be enquired

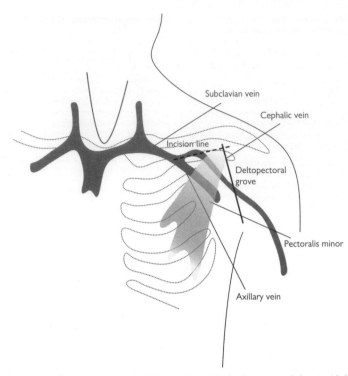

Fig. 3.10.1 Anatomy of the infraclavicular region demonstrating the relationship of axillary vein, cephalic vein, subclavian vein, and the deltopectoral grove. The dotted line represents the skin incision, which is perpendicular to the deltopectoral grove.

for symptoms for potential pacemaker syndrome. More recently, pacemakers together with home transmitters have become available from most major pacemaker manufacturers, which make remote monitoring of both the device function and patients' status possible. Information obtained from the devices either manually by patients or automatically with a wireless system can be transmitted via phone and/or GSM network. Although this may reduce the workload in outpatient clinics and provide closer monitoring of individual patients, the data generated on a day-to-day basis may overload the physicians as well as create potential medico-legal problems.

Table 3.10.2 Pros and cons for various venous accesses

	Pros	Cons
Axillary	Simple puncture technique	Small vessel size
	Minimal risk of pleural complication	
	Low risk of vascular complication	
Subclavian	Simple puncture technique	Risk of pleural complications
	Large vessel for multiple leads	Risk of vascular complications
		Subclavian crush
Cephalic	No risk of pleural complications	Surgical skill for cut-down required
	Minimal risk of vascular complications	Small vessel size

Table 3.10.3 Complications of pacemaker implantation

Acute complications
Pneumothorax
Haemothorax
Pacemaker pocket haematoma
Perforation of heart and central veins
Lead dislodgement and damage
Long-term complications
Pacemaker infection
Central venous thrombosis and obstruction
Lead fracture (e.g. subclavian crush)
Insulator break
Twiddler syndrome

References

Bernstein AD, Daubert JC, Fletcher RD, *et al.* The revised NASPE/BPEG generic code for antibradycardia, adaptive-rate, and multisite pacing. North American Society of Pacing and Electrophysiology/British Pacing and Electrophysiology Group. *Pacing Clin Electrophysiol* 2002;**25**:260–4.

Vardas PE, Auricchio A, Blanc JJ, *et al.* Guidelines for cardiac pacing and cardiac resynchronization therapy: The Task Force for Cardiac Pacing and Cardiac Resynchronization Therapy of the European Society of Cardiology. Developed in collaboration with the European Heart Rhythm Association. *Eur Heart J* 2007;**28**:2256–95.

Epstein AE, DiMarco JP, Ellenbogen KA, *et al.* ACC/AHA/HRS 2008 Guidelines for Device-Based Therapy of Cardiac Rhythm Abnormalities: a report of the American College of Cardiology/ American Heart Association Task Force on Practice Guidelines (Writing Committee to Revise the ACC/AHA/NASPE 2002 Guideline Update for Implantation of Cardiac Pacemakers and Antiarrhythmia Devices): developed in collaboration with the American Association for Thoracic Surgery and Society of Thoracic Surgeons. *Circulation* 2008;**117**:e350–408.

Siu CW, Wang M, Zhang XH, Lau CP, Tse HF. Analysis of ventricular performance as a function of pacing site and mode. *Prog Cardiovasc Dis* 2008;**51**:171–82.

Wilkoff BL, Auricchio A, Brugada J, *et al.* HRS/EHRA Expert Consensus on the Monitoring of Cardiovascular Implantable Electronic Devices (CIEDs): description of techniques, indications, personnel, frequency and ethical considerations: developed in partnership with the Heart Rhythm Society (HRS) and the European Heart Rhythm Association (EHRA); and in collaboration with the American College of Cardiology (ACC), the American Heart Association (AHA), the European Society of Cardiology (ESC), the Heart Failure Association of ESC (HFA), and the Heart Failure Society of America (HFSA). Endorsed by the Heart Rhythm Society, the European Heart Rhythm Association (a registered branch of the ESC), the American College of Cardiology, the American Heart Association. *Europace* 2008;**10**:707–25.

Implantable cardioverter-defibrillators

Despite the advances that have been made in cardiovascular therapeutics over the past two decades, mortality from cardiac disease remains high, and sudden death remains the predominant mode of death. The implantable cardioverter-defibrillator (ICD) was developed as a treatment for patients at high risk of sudden death from ventricular arrhythmias. Although initially targeted at patients who had been resuscitated from a life-threatening episode of ventricular tachycardia (VT) or ventricular fibrillation (VF), it is now being used increasingly for 'primary prevention' of sudden cardiac death in patients who are thought to be at high risk of sudden cardiac death but have not yet had a life-threatening cardiac arrhythmia.

Development of the technology

Early experiments on miniaturization of defibrillators were performed by Michel Mirowsky and colleagues in Baltimore in the 1970s, and the first human implantable defibrillator procedure was performed in 1980 (Mirowski et al. 1980). Throughout the 1980s the procedure was a prolonged and high-risk cardiac surgical procedure, requiring thoracotomy to attach the shocking and sensing electrodes to the epicardial surface of the heart. The generator (which weighed approximately 250 g) was implanted in the rectus sheath in the abdominal wall, and the leads from the epicardial electrodes were tunnelled from the chest to the abdominal generator site. The entire implant procedure could take around 4 hours (or longer if concomitant cardiac surgery was being performed), post-implant hospital stay was 7–10 days, and the implant mortality was around 5%.

Non-thoracotomy leads were developed in the early 1990s, and this simplified the procedure considerably. The lead(s) still needed to be tunnelled to the abdominal generator site, but by the mid-1990s generators had became small enough to be implanted in the pectoral position. These advances were made possible by the use of better battery technology, smaller capacitors, and the use of biphasic shocks that could defibrillate more effectively than conventional monophasic shocks.

A modern ICD weighs around 80 g, and the implant procedure often takes less than 30 minutes and is performed under local anaesthesia and sedation. A single incision approximately 5 cm in length is made inferior to the left clavicle, and a pocket is made for the generator, either subcutaneously or deep to the pectoralis major muscle. A lead is inserted via the subclavian or cephalic vein and advanced under fluoroscopy to the apex of the right ventricle. This lead is used for pacing and sensing as well as defibrillation. If necessary a right atrial pacing lead may also be implanted. Additionally, if the patient requires biventricular pacing (cardiac resynchronization therapy) for heart failure, a left ventricular lead is implanted. Once the leads are in place they are attached to the generator, which is then placed in the subcutaneous or submuscular pocket. It is then customary to test defibrillation efficacy. This is performed by inducing ventricular fibrillation (either by delivering a small shock on the T wave or a short burst of AC or DC current) and programming the device to terminate the arrhythmia. An external defibrillator is available should the implanted device fail to terminate the arrhythmia. Patients are usually discharged home the following day provided that a chest X-ray shows satisfactory lead positions and no evidence of pneumothorax.

Complications

The complications of ICD implantation are similar to those associated with pacemaker implantation, and include bleeding, infection, pneumothorax, and lead displacement. Implant-related mortality is very rare; published rates of 'operative mortality' (i.e. 30-day mortality) are around 1% and usually related to the severity of the patient's cardiac disease.

In the long term, the commonest adverse event is shocks from the device, either appropriate shocks for VT or VF or inappropriate shocks. The latter can be minimized by judicious programming and appropriate use of beta-blockers and other antiarrhythmic drugs, but occasionally inappropriate shocks can occur as a result of hardware problems such as conductor fracture or insulation break of the ventricular lead. The reason for inappropriate shocks can usually be diagnosed by interrogation of the device. Each device can store the electrograms before and after shock therapies. Lead problems often manifest with changes in lead impedance, a conductor break causing the pacing impedance to rise and an insulation break causing a fall in impedance.

Clinical trials of ICD therapy

ICDs have long been known to be effective at terminating sustained ventricular arrhythmias but until the late 1990s there was not clear evidence that they reduced all-cause mortality. Three randomized controlled trials of ICD therapy versus antiarrhythmic drugs in patients with a history of sustained VT or VF were published between 1997 and 2000, and their results are summarized in Table 3.11.1.

A meta-analysis of these three trials (Connolly et al. 2000) showed a 28% reduction in mortality in the ICD group (95% CI 60–87%; $P = 0.0006$) compared with amiodarone therapy. Patients with left ventricular ejection fraction (LVEF) of 35% or below had more to gain (34% reduction in mortality compared with amiodarone) than those with preserved ventricular function (no significant difference in mortality compared with amiodarone).

Several studies have assessed the efficacy of ICDs in the 'primary prevention' of sudden cardiac death, i.e. in patients

Table 3.11.1 Trials of ICDs in patients with VT/VF

	Number in trial	Control treatment	Mean follow-up	ICD mortality	Control mortality	p value
AVID	1016	Amiodarone or sotalol	18 months	25% at 3 years	36% at 3 years	<0.02
CIDS	659	Amiodarone	36 months	8.3% per year	10.2% per year	0.142
CASH	288	Amiodarone or metoprolol	57 months	36%	44%	0.081

who have severe structural heart disease (usually patients with severely impaired LVEF, either as a result of prior myocardial infarction or idiopathic dilated cardiomyopathy) but have not had a life-threatening arrhythmia. The earliest studies (Multicenter Automatic Defibrillator Implantation Trial (MADIT) and Multicenter Unsustained Tachycardia Trial (MUSTT)) recruited patients who had prior myocardial infarction, poor LVEF, non-sustained VT and inducible sustained VT at electrophysiological study. Both these studies showed significantly better survival with a defibrillator than without, the relative risk reduction in mortality being 54% and 60% respectively. More recently the MADIT-2 study (Moss et al. 2002) randomized 1232 patients with prior myocardial infarction and LVEF of 30% or less to receive an ICD or be treated with conventional therapy alone. After a mean follow-up of 20 months, the mortality was 14.2% in the ICD group and 19.8% in the conventionally treated group; this equates to a relative risk reduction of 31%, similar to that seen in the 'secondary prevention' trials detailed above. Subsequent analysis of the results of this trial showed that the 12-lead ECG was useful in predicting benefit from the ICD, patients most likely to gain from ICD therapy were those with a QRS complex width of 120 ms or more (relative risk reduction of 50%).

The Sudden Cardiac Death in Heart Failure trial (SCD-HeFT) (Bardy et al. 2005) is the largest ICD trial to be published. In this study, 2521 patients with symptomatic heart failure (NYHA class 2 or 3) were randomized to receive optimal medical therapy alone, medical therapy plus amiodarone, or medical therapy plus an ICD. Approximately 50% of the patients had coronary artery disease as the cause of their heart failure and 50% had non-ischaemic dilated cardiomyopathy. After a follow-up period of 5 years the mortality in the medical arm was 36.1% (7.2% per year) and amiodarone had no effect on mortality. The ICD patients had a 23% reduction in mortality compared with placebo (P = 0.007). The benefit from the ICD was most pronounced in those with an LVEF of less than 30% and in the patients with relatively mild symptoms (NYHA Class 2).

Two trials have shown a trend towards increased mortality in patients who undergo ICD implantation within a few weeks of acute myocardial infarction. The DINAMIT study (Hohnloser et al. 2004) randomized patients with significant LV dysfunction to ICD implantation or standard treatment within 6–40 days of acute myocardial infarction. The ICD reduced the risk of arrhythmic death but was associated with an increased risk of non-arrhythmic death. The total mortality was 8% higher in the ICD group than the control arm. Recently the IRIS trial has produced similar results, and published guidelines have taken account of this in recommending that primary prevention ICDs should not be implanted within 4–6 weeks of acute myocardial infarction.

Guidelines on patient selection for ICD therapy

Based on the results of these and other trials, several national and international bodies have produced guidelines for selection of appropriate patients for ICD implantation. All are agreed that ICDs should routinely be implanted for 'secondary prevention' in patients who have survived a cardiac arrest due to VT or VF, and in patients who have had sustained monomorphic VT with either severe symptoms or in the context of significant left ventricular dysfunction, unless the arrhythmia was due to a transient or reversible

cause (such as the acute phase of myocardial infarction, or as a result of electrolyte imbalance or drug toxicity).

The situation regarding 'primary prevention' ICDs is somewhat more controversial, and some national societies have produced guidelines that take into account the economic impact of increasing ICD implant numbers as well as the evidence per se. For example, the European Society of Cardiology guidelines on heart failure (Dickstein et al. 2008) recommend ICD implantation for patients with heart failure in NYHA class 2 or 3 with an ejection fraction of 35% or less, who are receiving optimal medical therapy, and have a reasonable expectation of survival with good functional status for at least 1 year.

In England and Wales, the National Institute for Health and Clinical Excellence (NICE 2006) has produced recommendations for patient selection for ICDs. These are summarized below. The NICE guidelines have taken account of new evidence, and recommended ICD therapy for patients who fulfilled the high-risk subgroup criteria in the MADIT-2 trial, i.e. LVEF <30% after myocardial infarction and QRS width of >120 ms. They did not approve MADIT-2 in its entirety, nor did they approve ICD therapy for patients who fulfil the criteria for the SCD-HeFT trial.

NICE indications for ICD implantation

Secondary prevention

For patients who present, in the absence of a treatable cause, with:

Cardiac arrest due to either VT or VF.

Spontaneous sustained VT with syncope or significant haemodynamic compromise.

Sustained VT without syncope/cardiac arrest, LVEF <35%, NYHA class 1–3.

Primary prevention

For patients with:

A history of previous myocardial infarction and all of the following:

Non-sustained VT on Holter monitoring.

Inducible VT on electrophysiological testing.

LVEF < 35%, NYHA Class 1–3.

Or

A history of previous myocardial infarction and all of the following:

LVEF <35%, NYHA Class 1–3.

QRS width > 120 ms.

A familial cardiac condition with a high risk of sudden death, including,

Long QT syndrome.

Hypertrophic cardiomyopathy.

Brugada syndrome.

Arrhythmogenic right ventricular dysplasia.

In Scotland, the Scottish Intercollegiate Guidelines Network (SIGN 2007) has produced guidelines for primary prevention ICD therapy that are somewhat at variance with the NICE guidance. SIGN has recommended that 'patients with moderate to severe LV dysfunction, in NYHA Class I–III at least 1 month after myocardial infarction should be considered for ICD therapy' and that 'patients with spontaneous non-sustained VT (especially if sustained VT is inducible), severely impaired ejection fraction (<0.25) or prolonged QRS duration (>120 ms) should be prioritized for ICD implantation'.

Lifestyle implications of ICD therapy

An ICD is not a cure. Patients are still considered to be at risk of an arrhythmia, which might cause syncope or cardiac arrest, if only for a few seconds before treatment is delivered. Inevitably many patients face significant lifestyle restrictions, and a minority of patients have severe psychological problems. Although the implant procedure is similar to pacemaker implantation, follow-up of patients with ICDs tends to be more complex. Although technical follow-up of the device may become easier with the development of systems for remote follow-up, many of the patients have coronary artery disease and poor left ventricular function and are likely to require ongoing medical therapy for their underlying cardiac condition. Some patients will have an inherited or congenital cardiac condition, and issues such as genetic counselling and screening of relatives can be complex.

Although some patients may develop an adverse psychological reaction to ICD implantation, it is important to be aware that these patients often improve with the passage of time as they become accustomed to having the device and adapt to their physical limitations. However, many patients tolerate defibrillation shocks very poorly, particularly if they experience multiple shocks (appropriate or inappropriate). For this reason, antiarrhythmic drugs may have a role in reducing the incidence of both ventricular and supraventricular arrhythmias in patients with ICDs. In one study (Pacifico et al. 1999), treatment with sotalol reduced the mean frequency of shocks (both appropriate and inappropriate) by 63% compared with placebo.

The regulations regarding fitness to drive in patients with ICDs will vary between countries, and are subject to periodic review. In the UK, the Driver and Vehicle Licensing Agency publishes its recommendations on its website (www.dvla.gov.uk). Patients who have received an ICD for 'secondary prevention' may be allowed to drive provided that the device has been implanted for at least 6 months and has not delivered shock therapy or symptomatic antitachycardia pacing therapy for 6 months (except during formal clinical testing), and if previous discharges have not been accompanied by incapacity. Patients must stop driving for 1 month if the device (lead or generator) is revised, or if any change is made in antiarrhythmic treatment. Patients who have an ICD implanted for 'primary prevention' need only refrain from driving for 1 month, unless they subsequently receive shocks from the device. Licences are subject to annual review. Patients are also advised not to use 'cruise control' in case they do suffer an arrhythmia associated with transient incapacity while driving. Patients with ICDs are permanently disqualified from driving lorries and buses. These recommendations are similar to the current North American and European guidelines on driving for patients with arrhythmias.

Modern ICDs (and pacemakers) are well protected against external sources of electromagnetic interference. However, arc welding equipment can interfere with these devices. In addition, although devices are being developed that will be safe to use in magnetic resonance imaging (MRI) scanners, at the present time ICD and pacemaker recipients are advised that they cannot undergo MRI scanning. Cellular telephones (mobile phones) can occasionally interfere with ICDs and pacemakers, but only if the telephone is within 15 cm (6″) of the generator. Patients are therefore routinely advised to use their mobile phone at the ear contralateral to the implant site, and not to carry the phone in a breast pocket overlying the device. There have been occasional reports of interference to pacemakers and ICDs caused by electronic article surveillance gates ('shoplifting detection gates'), but only if the patient is in the vicinity of the gates for several seconds. Patients can be reassured that it is safe for them to enter and exit shops via these gates as long as they 'don't lean and don't linger'. Very occasionally there are patients with these devices who work in environments where high intensity electrical or magnetic fields might interfere with the device, and such scenarios require specialist assessment which often involves collaboration among the patient's cardiologist, the engineers employed by the device manufacturer, and the occupational health physician at the place of work.

Conclusion

ICD implantation has become much more commonplace over the past decade as a result of accumulating evidence for device efficacy in different patient subgroups and the development of national and international guidelines for patient selection. The criteria for patient selection for ICDs in patients who have survived a life-threatening ventricular arrhythmia are well established. The evidence for the efficacy of ICDs in the primary prevention of sudden death is also well established in patients with poor left ventricular function, but individual clinicians should be aware of their own local or national approved guidelines when considering ICD therapy in these patients.

References

Bardy GH, Lee KL, Mark DB, et al. Amiodarone or an implantable cardioverter-defibrillator for congestive heart failure. N Engl J Med 2005;**352**:225–37.

Connolly SJ, Hallstrom AP, Cappato R, et al. Meta-analysis of the implantable cardioverter defibrillator secondary prevention trials. Eur Heart J 2000;**21**:2071–8.

Dickstein K, Cohen-Salal A, Filippatos G, et al. ESC guidelines for the diagnosis and treatment of acute and chronic heart failure 2008. Eur Heart J 2008;**29**:2388–442.

Hohnloser SH, Kuck KH, Dorian P, et al. Prophylactic use of an implantable cardioverter-defibrillator after acute myocardial infarction. N Engl J Med 2004;**351**:2481–8.

Mirowski M, Reid PR, Mower MM, et al. Termination of malignant ventricular arrhythmias with an implanted automatic defibrillator in human beings. N Engl J Med 1980;**303**:322–4.

Moss AJ, Zareba W, Hall WJ, et al. Prophylactic implantation of a defibrillator in patients with myocardial infarction and reduced ejection fraction. N Engl J Med 2002;**346**:877–83.

National Institute for Health and Clinical Excellence (NICE): Health technology appraisal 95: implantable cardiac defibrillators, January 2006. Available at http://www.nice.org.uk.

Pacifico A, Hohnloser SH, Williams JH, et al. Prevention of implantable-defibrillator shocks by treatment with sotalol. N Engl J Med 1999;**340**:1855–62.

Scottish Intercollegiate Guidelines Network (SIGN) Guideline 94: Cardiac arrhythmias in coronary heart disease, February 2007. Available at http://www.sign.ac.uk.

Electrical cardioversion

Atrial fibrillation is the most common cardiac arrhythmia observed in clinical practice. Many different therapeutic approaches are available at present but none of them can be considered the gold standard treatment. Antiarrhythmic drugs are not very effective to cardiovert persistent atrial fibrillation, and therefore the technique most frequently used to restore sinus rhythm is electrical cardioversion.

Introduction

Epidemiology and natural history of atrial fibrillation

Atrial fibrillation is a common clinical disease particularly frequent in elderly people (3–5% of the population over 60 years of age), and in patients with organic heart disease (70–80%) (Levy et al. 2002).

Atrial fibrillation may be defined as paroxysmal, persistent, and permanent according to its duration. If the episode of AF terminates by itself, it is designated paroxysmal, but if does not it is termed persistent. Permanent AF include cases of long-standing AF in which cardioversion has not been indicated or attempted (Fuster et al. 2001). Both paroxysmal and persistent forms of atrial fibrillation may evolve to permanent atrial fibrillation.

Who are the candidates for electrical cardioversion?

Several studies in recent times (RACE, AFFIRM, PIAF and STAF) have found that rate control is an acceptable alternative to rhythm control in patients with recurrent atrial fibrillation, whereas for those with severely symptomatic atrial fibrillation continued rhythm control is unavoidable. The choice between a conservative strategy (heart rate control) and a more aggressive one (rhythm control) is based on the clinical presentation of the arrhythmia and on the cultural and organizational features of different hospitals.

Electrical cardioversion is the best therapeutic approach in patients in whom the sinus rhythm could improve their quality of life and there is an important expectation for maintenance of normal rhythm after the restoration. This technique compared with pharmacological cardioversion shows some important advantages: immediate effect, high success rate, and safety in haemodynamically unstable patients.

There are three main groups of patients in whom sinus rhythm is a benefit:

- Patients with severe symptoms during the arrhythmia
- Patients with recent atrial fibrillation to prevent the long-term electrical remodelling
- Patients with structural heart disease, like hypertension and ventricular hypertrophy, who deserve haemodynamic benefit with sinus rhythm.

Prevention of embolic complications

An important concept associated with electrical cardioversion is the prevention of embolic complications. There is a high risk of atrial thrombus formation secondary to atrial stasis in patients with an atrial fibrillation longer than 48 hours. It is highly advisable to administer anticoagulant therapy to the patient before attempting cardioversion.

For this purpose there are two alternative approaches in patients with atrial fibrillation duration longer than 48 hours (Prystowsky et al. 1996). The conventional approach is outpatient systemic anticoagulation with warfarin or acecumarol to achieve an international normalized ratio (INR) of 2.0–3.0 for at least 3 weeks, followed by cardioversion. An alternative approach is a short-duration heparin treatment that showed to be sufficient if the presence of a left atrial thrombus has been ruled out with a transoesophageal echocardiogram (Klein et al. 1997); heparin can be continued with oral warfarin therapy until the INR is more than 2. In patients with atrial fibrillation duration under 48 hours, electrical cardioversion can be performed without prior anticoaugulation therapy.

After cardioversion it is necessary to continue anticoagulant treatment with warfarin for at least 4 weeks to minimize the risk for thromboembolic complications due to the atrial stunning after electrical cardioversion, especially in patients with diabetes mellitus and hypertension; these two diseases are associated with increased risk of embolization early after cardioversion (Gentile et al. 2002).

Use of antiarrhythmic drugs before or during electrical cardioversion

The success rate of electrical cardioversion is extremely high and the major causes of failure are high atrial defibrillation threshold and early reinitiation of the arrhythmia.

In patients with high atrial defibrillation threshold antiarrhythmic agents should be used before or during cardioversion. These drugs may facilitate electrical cardioversion by reducing the atrial defibrillation threshold and preventing early reinitiations of atrial fibrillation (within minutes) after successful cardioversion.

Summarizing data from literature we can conclude that both class IC and class III antiarrhythmic agents may reduce the atrial defibrillation threshold and prevent early reinitiation of atrial fibrillation; nevertheless, sometimes acute administration of these drugs during the cardioversion may lead to an increase in the defibrillation threshold, a transient bradycardia that requires temporary pacing (Timmermans et al. 1998), and is associated with a potential risk of ventricular tachycardia, especially in patients with impaired left ventricular function and in those who have been pre-treated with other oral antiarrhythmic agents.

Techniques

External transthoracic cardioversion

Electrical cardioversion of atrial fibrillation using high-voltage direct current (DC) shocks delivered between skin paddle electrodes was first described in 1962 (Lown et al. 1962) and is still standard technique for restoring sinus rhythm. The efficacy of external cardioversion increased significantly with the introduction of a biphasic waveform. Rectilinear biphasic shocks are significantly more effective than damped sine wave monophasic shocks; additionally, increased efficacy with rectilinear biphasic shocks is achieved with significantly less delivered current than with monophasic shocks (Mittal et al. 2000) (Fig. 3.12.1). Also Page et al. (2002) in an international randomized double-blind multicentre trial demonstrated the advantages of biphasic shocks over monophasic shocks in conversion of atrial fibrillation, showing how a biphasic shock waveform has greater efficacy, requires fewer shocks and lower delivered energy, and results in less dermal injury than a monophasic shock waveform.

Several steps should be followed to maximize the efficacy for external direct current cardioversion. The optimal

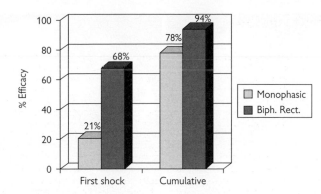

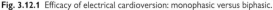

Fig. 3.12.1 Efficacy of electrical cardioversion: monophasic versus biphasic.

electrode size is 12–13 cm in diameter and self-adhesive electrode pads should be used for optimal electrode–skin contact; different electrode configurations have been used: the apex-anterior and anterorposterior positions are equally effective. Firm pressure applied to the anterior electrode during expiration to reduce impedance is useful to facilitate current delivery to the heart when non-adhesive defibrillation paddles are used (Kerber et al., 1996). Shocks should always be synchronized to the R wave to avoid the vulnerable period and the inadvertent induction of ventricular fibrillation.

Direct current external cardioversion, even using very high energy, is indeed a very safe technique without any clinical evidence of myocardial impairment or damage (Saliba et al. 1999).

The current recommendation for the initial energy for direct current external cardioversion of atrial fibrillation is 200 J using a biphasic waveform shock, considering that lower energies are associated with a higher failure rate.

Internal cardioversion

Low-energy internal cardioversion is another method, safe and effective as well, for the restoration of sinus rhythm in patients with atrial fibrillation. The spread of this technique in clinical practice has been limited by the need for an electrophysiology laboratory with fluoroscopy and of a specific technical competence for lead positioning inside the heart; furthermore, after the development of biphasic waveform defibrillators, failure of external cardioversion became a very rare event so that the need of an invasive approach to cardiovert persistent atrial fibrillation can be considered an exception as well.

Internal cardioversion may be very useful during electrophysiological procedures complicated by atrial fibrillation or during open-heart surgery. This technique is also, sometimes, indicated in obese patients and in patients with severe lung disease who have high thoracic impedance.

If we look at data we can see that the energy required for bi-atrial internal cardioversion is in the range of 2–6 J, a very low energy, which is only around 2–5% of the energy required for transthoracic cardioversion. To execute internal cardioversion three transvenous electrodes are introduced: two of them are defibrillator catheters with a large surface area (more than 6 cm) that are located in the right atrium and in the coronary sinus or in the left pulmonary artery, which are both in direct contact with the left atrium, allowing a significant reduction of the atrial defibrillation

threshold (Feinberg et al. 1995). The third catheter is collocated in the apex of the right ventricle; it is used for the synchronization with the R wave and as a temporized ventricle pacing (Fig. 3.12.2). An alternative and simplified technique to perform the internal cardioversion is the hybrid transoesophageal–endocardial cardioversion; in this configuration a catheter is positioned in the oesophagus, avoiding the lead in the coronary sinus or in the left pulmonary artery, another lead in the right atrium, and a third one placed in the right ventricular apex allows synchronization of the delivery of the shock with the QRS.

A further reduction in the overall complexity of internal cardioversion was achieved by Pandozi et al. (2003), who proposed a technique that can be performed without fluoroscopy and outside the electrophysiology laboratory, using a catheter in the oesophagus and a second lead introduced within the right atrium via the right internal jugular vein, without fluoroscopy control and avoiding the need of a third catheter in the right ventricle for shock synchronization, which was easily achievable by means of surface electrodes.

With regard to safety, low energy internal transvenous cardioversion of atrial fibrillation is very safe if synchronized to the R wave and delivered after a minimum RR interval of at least 300 ms.

Discomfort related to low-energy internal cardioversion represents an important problem of this technique. Internal cardioversion is associated with a pain perception that is not influenced by peak voltage alone and increases with the number of applied shocks so that the tolerability of the internal cardioversion may be improved using a single shock instead of a multiple shock step-up protocol (Santini et al. 1999). Despite its safety, efficacy (with an overall success rate around 90%), and tolerability under mild sedation, the spread of internal cardioversion in clinical practice is limited due to its overall complexity requiring specific skilled manoeuvres and the restricted number of indications.

Oesophageal electrical cardioversion

This type of cardioversion could obviate some limitations of external and internal cardioversion. In some patients high thoracic impedance (emphysema or a large body surface area) is a predictor of unsuccessful external cardioversion due respectively to air trapping and a weight-related increase in electrical impedance that impairs conduction of the direct current shock to the atria (Elhendy et al. 2002).

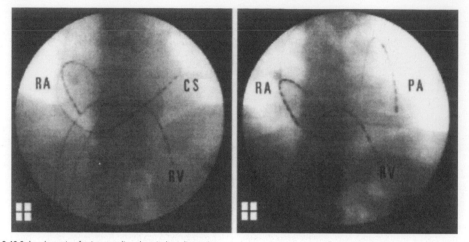

Fig. 3.12.2 Leads setting for intracardiac electrical cardioversion.

Oesophageal cardioversion provides several advantages such as:

- A lower energy requirement thanks to the proximity of the oesophagus to the left atrium, which warrants lower energy dispersion and a lower defibrillation impedance. Delivering a direct current shock using an external configuration, only around 20% of energy delivered reaches the heart, because most of the energy is dispersed in extracardiac tissues, especially in high thoracic impedance patients (Kerber *et al.* 1981).
- Avoidance of general anaesthesia or deep sedation: requiring low energies, mild sedation is sufficient to make the procedure well tolerated by most patients.
- Safety in patients with pacemaker or ICD: there is a lower risk of damage and of increasing pacing threshold, which is a shock intensity-dependent phenomenon, particularly dangerous for pacemaker-dependent patients (Li *et al.*, 1991).
- Atrial pacing back up: the oesophageal catheter may be also used to pace the atrium, should present a prolonged post-shock sinus arrest, sinus bradycardia or a pacemaker exit block.

The technique used in the most recent series about oesophageal cardioversion is oesophageal–precordial cardioversion. In this configuration, energy is applied between the electrodes of an oesophageal catheter (cathode) and one or two precordial adhesive patch electrodes (anode). Such a lead configuration provides, especially using a decapolar oesophageal catheter and two precordial leads, greater electrode surface and a larger atrial mass embraced by the leads. This configuration generates a uniform electrical field during the shock, resulting in vectors with a low atrial defibrillation threshold (Fig. 3.12.3).

In more than 40 years of oesophageal cardioversion, many studies have proven the safety of such a technique after performing histological examination of the oesophageal mucosa in animals that underwent oesophageal shocks (Cai *et al.*, 1989) or oesophageal endoscopy in patients who underwent oesophageal-intracardiac cardioversion (Santini *et al.*, 2000). McKeown *et al.* (1993) showed that no damage or dysphagia was seen in patients receiving shocks less than 100 J.

Oesophageal cardioversion is highly effective (95.3%). Furthermore, using 50 J or less 88.5% of patients can be cardioverted (Santini *et al.* 2007).

The method is quite simple and very fast, and the only criterion used to assess good positioning of the catheter is the length of catheter introduced into the oesophagus (40–45 cm from the nasal cavity), without the need for radioscopic control or oesophageal ECG. Different drugs are used for sedation, the most common is midazolam, which is effective at low dosage, safe, and easily handled. Finally, this technique is well tolerated by patients and can be performed easily in an outpatient setting.

Conclusions

Drugs don't play a significant role in cardioverting persistent atrial fibrillation; electrical cardioversion has been shown to be very safe and effective. There are different techniques to perform electrical cardioversion, each with specific indications, advantages, and limitations. The method most frequently used to restore sinus rhythm is external direct current cardioversion, which is a safe and effective technique, especially now that biphasic waveform defibrillators are widely available. Oesophageal cardioversion is an alternative method to restore sinus rhythm, warranting acute and long-term results comparable with those obtained by the conventional transthoracic technique. But external cardioversion has been recently showed to be highly effective and well tolerated, avoiding even general anaesthesia or deep sedation (Santini *et al.* 2007) so that oesophageal cardioversion shows no clear advantage; transthoracic cardioversion should remain the approach of first choice. Oesophageal cardioversion may still be the used in obese and COPD patients with high thoracic impedance. Another technique performed during the last two decades is internal cardioversion, but at the moment the advantage of this technique is limited to the small percentage of unsuccessful external cardioversions or during electrophysiological procedures.

Nowadays, we have seen how the restoration of sinus rhythm may be easily obtained by electrical cardioversion of atrial fibrillation. The real challenge for cardiologists remains preventing recurrences of atrial fibrillation. But it is also very important to correctly select candidates for

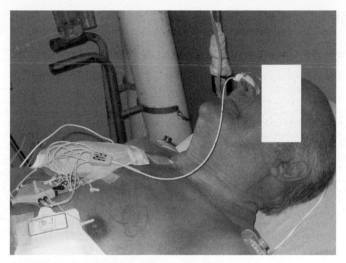

Fig. 3.12.3 Oesophageal–precordial cardioversion. See also Plate 17.

cardioversion as rhythm control is not the first treatment strategy in all patients. The choice of the best technique has to be taken basing on specific clinical conditions and on the cultural and organizational features of the different hospitals.

References

Cai YC, Fan SL, Feng DX, et al. Transesophageal low-energy cardioversion in a animal model of life-threatening tachyarrhythmias. *Circulation* 1989;**80**:1354–9.

Elhendy A, Gentile F, Khandheria BK, et al. Predictors of unsuccessful electrical cardioversion in atrial fibrillation. *Am J Cardiol* 2002;**89**:83–6.

Feinberg WM, Blackshear JL, Laupacis A, et al. Prevalence, age distribution, and gender of patients with atrial fibrillation: analysis and implications. *Arch Intern Med* 1995;**155**:469–73.

Fuster V, Ryden L, Asinger RV, et al. ACC/AHA/ESC guidelines for the management of patients with atrial fibrillation. *Eur Heart J* 2001;**22**:1852–923.

Gentile F, Elhendy A, Khandheria BK, et al. Safety of electrical cardioversion in patients with atrial fibrillation. *Mayo Clin Proc* 2002;**77**:895–6.

Kerber RE, Grayzel J, Hoyt R, et al. Transthoracic resistance in human defibrillation . Influence of body weight, chest size, serial shocks, paddle size and paddle contact pressure. *Circulation* 1981;**63**:676–82.

Kerber RE. Transthoracic cardioversion of atrial fibrillation and flutter: standard techniques and new advances. *Am J Cardiol* 1996;**78**:22–26.

Klein AL, Grimm RA, Black IW, et al. Cardioversion guided by trans-esophageal echocardiography; the ACUTE Pilot Study: a randomized, controlled trial. *Ann Intern Med* 1997;**126**:200–9.

Levy S. Epidemiology and natural history of atrial fibrillation. In: Santini M (ed.) *Non pharmacological treatment of atrial fibrillation.* Casalecchio: Arianna editrice, 2002:9–24.

Li HG, Jones DL, Yee R, Klein GJ. Defibrillation shocks increase myocardial pacing threshold: an intracellular microelectrode study. *Am J Physiol* 1991;**260**:H1973–9.

Lown B, Amarasingham R, Neuman J. New method for terminating cardiac arrhythmias: use of synchronized capacitor discharge. *JAMA* 1962;**182**:548–55.

McKeown PP, Croal S, Allen JD, et al. Transesophageal cardioversion. *Am Heart J* 1993;**125**:396–404.

Mittal S, Ayati S, Stein KM, et al. Transthoracic cardioversion of atrial fibrillation: comparison of rectilinear biphasic versus damped sine wave monophasic shocks. *Circulation* 2000;**101**:1282–7.

Page RL, Kerber RE, Russell JK, et al. Biphasic versus monophasic shock waveform for conversion of atrial fibrillation. *J Am Coll Cardiol* 2002;**39**:1956–63.

Pandozi C, Scianaro MC, Magris B, et al. Transesophageal low-energy cardioversion of atrial fibrillation without fluoroscopy outside the electrophysiology laboratori. *Ital Heart J* 2003;**4**:335–40.

Prystowsky EN, Benson DW, Fuster V, et al. Management of patients with atrial fibrillation: a statement for healthcare professionals from the subcommittee on electrocardiography and electrophysiology. American Heart Association. *Circulation* 1996;**93**:1262–77.

Saliba W, Juratli N, Chung MK, et al. Higher energy synchronized external direct current for refractory atrial fibrillation. *J Am Coll Cardiol* 1999; **34**:2031–4.

Santini L, Gallagher MM, Papavasileiou LP, et al. Transthoracic versus transesophageal cardioversion of atrial fibrillation under light sedation: a prospective randomized trial. *Pacing Clin Electrophysiol* 2007;**30**:1469–75.

Santini L, Magris B, Topa A, et al. Outpatient oesophageal-precordial electrical cardioversion of atrial fibrillation: an effective and safe technique to restore sinus rhythm. *J Cardiovasc Med (Hagerstown)* 2007;**8**:488–93.

Santini M, Pandozi C, Altamura G, et al. Single shock endocavitary low energy intracardiac cardioversion of chronic atrial fibrillation. *J Interv Card Electrophysiol* 1999;**3**:53–4.

Santini M, Pandozi C, Colivicchi F, et al. Transoesophageal low-energy cardioversion of atrial fibrillation. Results with the oesophageal-right atrial lead configuration. *Eur Heart J* 2000;**21**:848–55.

Timmermans C, Rodriguez LM, Smeets JL, et al. Immediate reinitiation of atrial fibrillation following internal atrial defibrillation. *J Cardiovasc Electrophisiol* 1998;**9**:122–8.

Catheter ablation

What is catheter ablation of cardiac arrhythmias?

The ability to deliver lesion-forming energy into myocardial tissue to prevent impulse generation or propagation by catheter ablation has revolutionized the management of patients with tachyarrhythmias. Over the past 25 years, catheter ablation, usually using radiofrequency energy—alternatively, but less often used, also cryo-energy or high-intensity focused ultrasound—has become the preferred and often first-line therapy for many supraventricular tachycardias and some ventricular tachycardias (VTs) (Table 3.13.1). In patients with structurally normal hearts, catheter ablation can often 'cure' tachyarrhythmias based on a thorough and individualized understanding of tachycardia mechanisms and identification of cardiac structures critical to the arrhythmia. In patients with structural heart disease, including patients with congenital malformations of the heart, success rates are lower, especially in atrial fibrillation (AF), multifocal atrial tachycardias, VTs, or ventricular fibrillation. In such patients, catheter ablation is limited by an incomplete understanding of arrhythmia mechanisms and by limited length and depth of ablation lesions that can be delivered using current techniques.

Table 3.13.1 Overview of indications for catheter ablation

Catheter ablation should be considered as primary, often curative therapy in patients with
AVNRT
AVRT
WPW syndrome
Isthmus-dependent atrial flutter
Idiopathic (right or left) ventricular outflow tract tachycardia (LBBB)
Idiopathic fascicular left ventricular tachycardias (RBBB/superior axis)

Catheter ablation is a reasonable second-line, often effective antiarrhythmic intervention in
Other atrial flutters
Atrial tachycardias
Atrial fibrillation (especially paroxysmal AF in patients with otherwise normal hearts)
Ventricular tachycardias in patients with structural heart disease
In these situations, catheter ablation should be part of a comprehensive patients management that includes therapy of all cardiac and extracardiac (e.g. pulmonary) conditions

Technical considerations

Access site

Catheter ablation usually requires insertion of several diagnostic catheters into the right heart and one ablation catheter into the target chamber of the heart. Most procedures use a femoral access site (femoral veins or arteries), but selected procedures may require jugular or, rarely, pericardial access sites. Many centres perform ablation procedures while the patient is lightly sedated, but this is not a requirement.

Electrophysiological study and ablation technique

Some procedures require induction of the clinical arrhythmia by programmed stimulation or drug delivery during the procedure. The ablation catheter is then placed at the critical structure that maintains the arrhythmia and radiofrequency energy is delivered.

Success rates and procedure-related risk

Many supraventricular arrhythmias can be cured with a high success rate (90–97%). The overall risk of catheter ablation is low (1–5% of severe complications, most of which can be managed without sequelae). Apart from general catheter-based complications (e.g. infection, haematoma, vessel/nerve injury) there are procedure-related risks:

- Thrombus formation and embolism (cerebrovascular event during left sided ablation)
- Valvular disruption
- Coronary occlusion
- Death (0.1%)
- Damage of cardiac and adjacent extracardiac structures, e.g. phrenic nerve, oesophagus, or pulmonary veins in ablation of AF.
- Damage of the conduction system with need for permanent pacemaker therapy (<1%, 1–2% in atrioventricular nodal re-entrant tachycardia (AVNRT))
- Pericardial effusion/tamponade with possible need for drainage/operative closure (after trans-septal puncture).

Many ablation procedures require relatively long fluoroscopy times. These can be reduced using modern catheter localization and mapping systems.

General approach to patients with tachyarrhythmias or palpitations

History of palpitations: key points

- Record frequency, duration, and symptoms of palpitations
- Is onset/offset of arrhythmia episodes sudden ('switching on/switching off', points to AVNRT or AVRT)?
- History of syncope/fainting/survived sudden death?
- Is the pulse regular or irregular during arrhythmia (irregular pulse points to AF)
- Is structural heart disease known (including congential heart disease)?

- Are the following concomitant conditions present: hypertension, cardiomyopathy, congenital heart disease, valvular heart disease, coronary artery disease, diabetes mellitus, prior myocardial infarctions, prior stroke?
- Has the heart been operated on before?
- What antiarrhythmic drugs were used (including dosage and duration of therapy), and were they effective?
- Consider beta-blockers, calcium channel antagonists, and digitalis as antiarrhythmics, although their main effect is slowing of AV nodal conduction and slowing of ventricular rate.

Examinations prior to catheter ablation: key points
- Routine ECG (rhythm, pre-excitation, signs of structural heart disease)
- ECG during arrhythmia often defines diagnosis and thereby guides therapy
- If no ECG during arrhythmia is available consider Holter/event recorders
- Echocardiography to rule out structural heart disease
- Transesophageal echo to exclude intracardiac thrombus prior to AF/flutter ablation
- Exclude pregnancy
- Antiarrhythmic medication should be stopped for more than five half-lives (mostly 48 hours), especially prior to ablation of AV nodal re-entrant tachycardia, AV re-entrant tachycardia, and idiopathic VTs
- Consent form for elective procedures (explain complications), fasting for at least 4–6 hours, inguinal shave.

Role of catheter ablation in the management of specific tachyarrhythmias
Supraventricular tachycardias
Tachycardias originating in the atria or involving the atrioventricular node are referred to as supraventricular tachycardias. Specific forms of supraventricular tachycardia are AVNRT, atrioventricular tachycardia (AVRT), atrial flutter, atrial tachycardia, and AF.

AV nodal re-entrant tachycardia and accessory pathways
- Highest incidence in second to fifth decade of life, two-thirds female patients in AVNRT, two-thirds males in AVRT
- Regular palpitations with sudden onset and end of rapid, typically lasting for about 30 minutes and occurring several times per year
- Involve the AV node in their re-entrant circuit
- Can often be terminated by vagal manoeuvres or rapid injection of adenosine
- ECG during tachycardia shows regular narrow-complex tachycardia without P waves prior to QRS complexes
  - P waves are hidden within the QRS complex or just after the end of the QRS complex in cases of AVNRT or visible in the ST segment (RP<PR) in cases of AVRT
  - Heart rate is typically around 180 bpm (wide range possible).

AVNRT
- This is a re-entrant tachycardia within the atrioventricular node that involves two functional pathways, referred to as the slow and fast pathways. In most cases the slow pathway forms the antegrade limb of the re-entrant circuit and retrograde conduction is via the fast pathway. This form is called typical (slow–fast) AVNRT.
- Treatment is driven by symptoms.
- Catheter-based modulation of the AV node targeting the slow pathway is the first treatment of choice.
- Success rates are high (> 95%), complication rates low. Rarely (1–2%), complete AV block is induced that requires implantation of a DDD pacemaker.

AVRT
- This involves an accessory atrioventricular pathway as one limb of the re-entrant circuit, the other limb is the AV node.
- Pathways that conduct antegradely during sinus rhythm can be seen by delta waves (ventricular pre-excitation) that may rarely be intermittent.
- Accessory pathways that only conduct retrogradely are called 'concealed'.
- First-line therapy is ablation of the accessory pathway.

Wolff–Parkinson–White syndrome
- Wolff–Parkinson–White (WPW) syndrome consists of ventricular pre-excitation and paroxysmal tachycardias.
- Therapy consists of catheter ablation of the accessory pathway.
- Pathways with a rapid antegrade conduction may predispose to sudden death (prognostic indication for catheter ablation).

Atrial flutter
- This often occurs in elderly people.
- It often concurs with AF.
- It is associated with a history of arterial hypertension and structural heart disease.
- The atrial rate is around 300 bpm; AV nodal conduction determines the resulting heart rate; 2:1 conduction with a resulting rate of 150 bpm is typical but slower and faster rates are possible.
- It can present as a paroxysmal arrhythmia, but typically it does not terminate spontaneously.

Isthmus-dependent atrial flutter
- This has a defined re-entrant circuit around the tricuspid valve.
- Isthmus ablation in the inferior right atrium is the treatment of choice.
- P waves usually show a saw-tooth pattern in the inferior leads ('typical') or positive in the inferior leads ('reverse type typical'). AV conduction is variable, typical is a 2:1 conduction with a resulting heart rate of 150 bpm.

Other atrial flutters
- Re-entrant circuit around a scar or patch, often including left atrial structures, occurs, e.g.
  - After open-heart surgery
  - After catheter ablation of AF
  - In grown-ups with congenital heart disease
- Ablation is technically more difficult—antiarrhythmic rug therapy is often first choice.

Atrial tachycardias
- These often occur in older patients with structural heart disease or obstructive pulmonary disease.
- Intra-atrial re-entrant circuits (similar to atrial flutters) or ectopic foci (often multifocal).
- These often occurs several times a day or per week.
- The heart rate is typically around 140–160 bpm.
- P waves precede QRS complexes. P-wave polarity allows approximation of the tachycardia origin.
- AV conduction can be variable without affecting tachycardia cycle length.
- Catheter ablation can target either ectopic foci or re-entrant circuits in the atria. Success rates are relatively low (50–70%). Especially multifocal atrial tachycardias have a tendency to recur after ablation.
- Antiarrhythmic drug therapy (sodium channel blockers in structurally normal hearts, amiodarone in others) should be considered prior to ablation or as an adjunct to therapy.

Atrial fibrillation
Unlike most other supraventricular arrhythmias, atrial fibrillation (AF) has a complex pathophysiology that involves several factors in most patients. In almost all patients, AF is a chronically progressing disease that—unlike other supraventricular arrhythmias—is associated with severe complications such as stroke and excess death. The risk for complications increases with age. Prevention of AF-related complications is the foremost therapeutic goal in AF. In the past decade, catheter-based electrical isolation of the pulmonary veins has emerged as the most effective form of therapy to prevent recurrent AF, especially in patients with paroxysmal AF and without other cardiac disease. Although systematic data to this end are lacking at present, catheter ablation is most likely only one part of a comprehensive management of atrial fibrillation that will, at least in patients at risk for stroke and death, also include antithrombotic therapy, rate control, appropriate management of concomitant conditions, and antiarrhythmic drugs.

Presentation and history: key points
- AF affects 1–2% of the population (often elderly people, increasing prevalence expected).
- Associated with a doubling of death, causes severe strokes, and markedly affects quality of life.
- Very selected patients with 'lone AF', i.e. patients without structural heart disease may carry a lower risk of these complications.
- AF is characterized by an irregular pulse and irregular RR intervals in the ECG.

Examinations: key points
- Any examination of an AF patient should search for underlying conditions that may put the patient at risk for stroke and death:
  - Hypertension
  - Cardiomyopathies
  - Vascular disease
  - Valvular disease
  - Diabetes mellitus
  - Older age, female sex
  - Prior cerebrovascular event.
- Symptoms during AF can be assessed using the EHRA score (Table 3.12.2)
- Any ECG during AF should be assessed for ventricular rate at rest and ideally during exercise (Holter ECG or exercise test).

Management of AF patients who undergo ablation: key points.
- AF management should reduce AF-related complications, treat concomitant conditions, and ameliorate symptoms.
- Lifelong antithrombotic therapy and rate control are essential parts of AF management in patients at risk for stroke. Anticoagulation is recommended for 2 months after ablation, even in patients at low risk for stroke.
- The decision for rhythm control in addition to rate control therapy should be discussed with each patient during the initial workup. A decision for rhythm control therapy is usually warranted in highly symptomatic patients.
- Catheter-based electrical isolation of the pulmonary veins is an accepted therapy in patients with 'focal' AF,

Table 3.13.2 EHRA atrial fibrillation symptoms classification. This EHRA score assesses symptoms during atrial fibrillation episodes and attempts to quantify those symptoms that are due to the arrhythmia. Modified from Kirchhof *et al*, with permission from Oxford University Press

Symptom severity	Definition
EHRA I	'No symptoms'
EHRA II	'Mild symptoms'. Normal daily activity not affected
EHRA III	'Severe symptoms'. Normal daily activity affected
EHRA IV	'Disabling symptoms'. Normal daily activity discontinued

The following items during presumed arrhythmia episodes are checked to determine the score: palpitations, fatigue, dizziness, dyspnoea, chest pain, anxiety. In addition to this score, the frequency could be classified into three groups, namely occasionally (less than once per month), intermediate (once per month—almost daily), and frequent (at least daily).

i.e. AF initiated by focal discharges that often originate from the pulmonary veins
- Catheter ablation is indicated in patients with symptomatic AF:
  - At present, AF ablation is indicated after AF recurrence on antiarrhythmic drugs
  - In selected patients with lone, highly symptomatic paroxysmal AF, catheter ablation may be first-line therapy (needs individual discussion).
- 'Extensive' ablation of AF beyond pulmonary vein isolation can increase sinus rhythm maintenance but should be performed by experienced centres only, usually as a part of controlled trial protocols.

Ventricular tachycardia

VT is a relatively organized tachyarrhythmia with discrete QRS complexes. It can be either sustained (lasting longer than 30 seconds) or non-sustained (defined as three or more beats but less than 30 seconds), and can be monomorphic or polymorphic. Polymorphic VT tends to be faster and less stable than monomorphic. The rate of VT can range from 100 bpm) to more than 300 bpm. At faster rates (usually 220 bpm or faster), VT is so rapid that it may be impossible to distinguish the QRS complex from the T wave.

Clinical approach

VT is a medical emergency that may cause sudden death. Rare exceptions are 'idiopathic' ventricular tachycardias. Whenever possible, a 12-lead ECG documentation during VT should be obtained. Most patients are at high risk of recurring ventricular arrhythmias and sudden death and usually require an implanted defibrillator. Catheter ablation can be an adjunct to implanted defibrillators in patients with frequent VT episodes.

History: key points

- In patients without structural heart disease or in patients with very slow monomorphic VT (<120 bpm), no symptoms may be noticed during VT.
- Palpitations, dyspnoea, heart failure, or chest pain. Cardiac output and blood pressure are maintained and/or when the VT is short-lived or slow (<150 bpm).
- VT is the cause of syncope in about 30% of patients with severe structural heart disease.
- History of structural heart disease:
  - Survived myocardial infarction
  - Dilated cardiomyopathy
  - Other cardiomyopathy.
- Drug-induced VT may be caused by cardiovascular drugs, non-cardiovascular drugs, and even non-prescription agents. Major causes include drugs that affect ion channels such as cardiac glycosides, QT-prolonging agents (so-called acquired QT syndrome), or sodium channel blocking drugs (e.g. flecainide or propafenone).

Physical examination: key points

- Haemodynamic distress: low blood pressure, heart failure, or cardiogenic shock.
- Polymorphic VT or rapid monomorphic VT may degenerate into ventricular fibrillation (VF).

Investigations

- Treadmill test: consider in patients with monomorphic VT after excluding acute coronary syndrome. Valuable in patients with idiopathic exercise-dependent VT (e.g. idiopathic outflow tract VT and fascicular VT) and catecholaminergic polymorphic VT (a rare ion channel disorder); may also just unmask ischaemic heart disease or even induce a polymorphic ischaemia-related VT.
- Echocardiogram: helpful to screen for structural heart disease (e.g. an old myocardial infarction, reduced left ventricular function) and congenital abnormalities (e.g. hypertrophic cardiomyopathy arrhythmogenic right ventricular cardiomyopathy (ARVCM). Search for ARVCM in patients with left bundle-branch block pattern during VT.
- Cardiac magnetic resonance imaging (MRI): MRI allows right and left ventricular function and cardiac malformations to be assessed. Delayed contrast enhancement may identify abnormalities such as myocarditis, cardiac sarcoidosis, arrhythmogenic right ventricular cardiomyopathy, or amyloidosis. Should be reserved for special circumstances.
- Angiography: useful when coronary artery disease and myocardial ischaemia are suspected. Not needed in idiopathic outflow tract VT, e.g. LBBB VT with an inferior axis and in clearly diagnosed arrhythmogenic cardiomyopathies (e.g. long QT syndrome).
- Invasive electrophysiological testing: useful when VT ablation is planned—often part of the ablation procedure. In patients with non-sustained VT and moderate left ventricular function (LVEF between 35% and 40%) and in patients with previous myocardial infarction presenting with syncope, programmed stimulation may guide the decision for implanting a defibrillator.
- In patients without structural heart disease, supraventricular tachycardias with aberrant conduction or a pre-excited tachycardia in WPW syndrome account for a substantial number of wide complex tachycardias. Be aware of atrial fibrillation with rapid ventricular rates due to AV conduction over an accessory pathway (FBI (fast, broad, irregular) tachycardia.

Management

The spectrum of therapies for VT includes drug therapy, device implantation and surgical or catheter ablation interventional techniques. The management challenge is to diagnose and treat underlying structural heart disease, to manage the VT that is the presenting symptom, and to assess the pervading risk for sudden arrhythmic death.

Acute management of VT

- In patients with sustained monomprphic VT and haemodynamic compromise a cardioversion with appropriate sedation is recommended.
- If the VT is refractory to cardioversion, amiodarone should be given.
- If the patient is haemodynamic stable, intravenous procainamide or ajmaline (only available in some European countries) can be administered. Amiodarone is only poorly effective in this situation.

- Consider therapy of underlying heart disease.
- Rarely, emergency catheter ablation can terminate 'electrical storm' not amenable to other therapy.

Catheter ablation in patients with VT

- In patients with idiopathic ventricular tachycardias (out-flow tract tachycardias, fascicular tachycardias), catheter ablation is an adequate first-line therapy. Beta-blockers or calcium channel antagonists are alternatives.
- In other VT, catheter ablation is considered palliation (at times very valuable):
  - In patients with frequent defibrillator shocks
  - In patients with long episodes of slow VT.
- Management of underlying heart disease should be optimized.
- Beta-blockers may reduce VT recurrences.
- Amiodarone is capable of reducing frequent VT episodes.
- Ongoing clinical trials evaluate whether upfront catheter ablation at the time of defibrillator implantation can prevent complications due to VT.

Further reading

Aliot EM, Stevenson WG, Almendral-Garrote JM, et al. EHRA/HRS Expert Consensus on Catheter Ablation of Ventricular Arrhythmias: developed in a partnership with the European Heart Rhythm Association (EHRA), a Registered Branch of the European Society of Cardiology (ESC), and the Heart Rhythm Society (HRS); in collaboration with the American College of Cardiology (ACC) and the American Heart Association (AHA). Europace 2009;**11**:771–817.

Calkins H, Brugada J, Packer DL, et al. HRS/EHRA/ECAS Expert Consensus Statement on Catheter and Surgical Ablation of Atrial Fibrillation: Recommendations for Personnel, Policy, Procedures and Follow-Up: A report of the Heart Rhythm Society (HRS) Task Force on Catheter and Surgical Ablation of Atrial Fibrillation Developed in partnership with the European Heart Rhythm Association (EHRA) and the European Cardiac Arrhythmia Society (ECAS); in collaboration with the American College of Cardiology (ACC), American Heart Association (AHA), and the Society of Thoracic Surgeons (STS). Endorsed and Approved by the governing bodies of the American College of Cardiology, the American Heart Association, the European Cardiac Arrhythmia Society, the European Heart Rhythm Association, the Society of Thoracic Surgeons, and the Heart Rhythm Society. Europace 2007;**9**:335–79.

Camm AJ, Luscher T, Serruys P (eds). The ESC textbook of cardiovascular medicine, 2nd edn. Oxford 2009.

Cesario DA, Mahajan A, Shivkumar K. Lesion-forming technologies for catheter ablation of atrial fibrillation. Heart Rhythm 2007; **4**(3 Suppl):S44–50.

Fuster V, Ryden LE, Cannom DS, et al. ACC/AHA/ESC 2006 guidelines for the management of patients with atrial fibrillation-executive summary: A report of the American College of Cardiology/American Heart Association Task Force on practice guidelines and the European Society of Cardiology Committee for Practice Guidelines (Writing Committee to Revise the 2001 Guidelines for the Management of Patients with Atrial Fibrillation) Developed in collaboration with the European Heart Rhythm Association and the Heart Rhythm Society. Eur Heart J 2006;**27**:1979–2030.

Goldberger JJ, Cain ME, Hohnloser SH, et al. American Heart Association/American College of Cardiology Foundation/Heart Rhythm Society scientific statement on noninvasive risk stratification techniques for identifying patients at risk for sudden cardiac death: a scientific statement from the American Heart Association Council on Clinical Cardiology Committee on Electrocardiography and Arrhythmias and Council on Epidemiology and Prevention. Circulation 2008;**118**:1497–518.

Kirchhof P, Auricchio A, Bax J, et al. Outcome parameters for trials in atrial fibrillation: executive summary: Recommendations from a consensus conference organized by the German Atrial Fibrillation Competence NETwork (AFNET) and the European Heart Rhythm Association (EHRA). Eur Heart J 2007;**28**:2803–17.

Morady F. Radio-frequency ablation as treatment for cardiac arrhythmias. N Engl J Med 1999;**340**:534–44.

Priori SG, Zipes DP. Sudden cardiac death, 1st edn. Malden: Blackwell Publishing, 2006.

Task Force and the European Society of Cardiology Committee for Practice Guidelines. Guidelines for management of patients with ventricular arrhythmias and the prevention of sudden cardiac death. Eur Heart J 2006;**27**:2099–144.

Tracy CM, Akhtar M, DiMarco JP, et al. American College of Cardiology/American Heart Association 2006 Update of the Clinical Competence Statement on Invasive Electrophysiology Studies, Catheter Ablation, and Cardioversion A Report of the American College of Cardiology/American Heart Association/American College of Physicians Task Force on Clinical Competence and Training Developed in Collaboration With the Heart Rhythm Society. J Am Coll Cardiol 2006;**48** :1503–17.

Cardiac arrhythmias: cardiac surgery

Supraventricular arrhythmias due to Wolff–Parkinson–White (WPS) syndrome, AV node re-entry, automatic atrial foci, and most forms of atrial flutter have disappeared from the realm of the surgeon because of the great success of less invasive radiofrequency catheter ablation techniques. The only supraventricular arrhythmia of significance to the cardiac surgeon is atrial fibrillation (AF).

The Cox maze procedure

Surgical procedures to prevent or to treat AF are being performed more frequently with recent advances in technologies for lesion creation. Although catheter ablation for lone AF is well established, its rationale comes from an innovative surgical procedure introduced in 1988. This is the Cox maze procedure (Cox et al. 1991), which is based on the theory that AF results from multiple macro-re-entry circuits in the atria. The operation creates a maze-like series of incisions in both atria to prevent the formation of these macro-re-entry circuits. During the procedure, the pulmonary veins are completely isolated, and both appendages are removed. This was fortuitous because the importance of the pulmonary veins in the initiation of AF has become more appreciated in recent years (Haissaguerre et al. 1998). The operation has been proved to be effective, with a high success rate and elimination of late strokes (Cox et al. 1996).

The current indications for a Cox maze III operation include drug intolerance, arrhythmia intolerance, and recurrent embolic events. There are two main groups of patients who are referred for this operation: those with symptomatic lone AF and those with AF associated with other organic cardiac disorders, especially mitral valve disease. It is likely that the underlying pathophysiology responsible for the genesis of AF in these two groups of patients is different. Therefore one can expect differences in the results of the Cox maze procedure in these two populations.

In the original operation incisions were made in both atria and then repaired by suture. To improve results Cox modified the procedure twice culminating in the Cox maze III procedure. In a recent report from Cox's group (Prasad et al. 2003), 198 patients underwent the Cox maze procedure, 112 were lone operations and 86 were concomitant procedures. The lone operation group was significantly younger (51.3 ± 1.5 years versus 58.8 ± 9.9 years) and had a higher male/female ratio (4:1 versus 2:1). There was no difference in operative mortality between groups (1.8% versus 1.2%). At a follow-up period of 5.5 ± 2.9 years, 96.6% (172/178) of all patients were free of atrial fibrillation. There was no difference between the lone operation and concomitant procedure groups (95.9% versus 97.5%).

New approaches for surgical ablation

This has been made possible by the development of ablation tools that use a variety of energy sources to facilitate rapid and safe creation of lines of conduction block under direct vision. Catheter ablation of pulmonary vein foci has proven effective at ablating paroxysmal AF (Gaita et al. 1988). Although these observations demonstrate the critical importance of the pulmonary veins in patients with paroxysmal AF, their role in persistent and permanent AF is less clear. Intraoperative left atrial mapping of patients with persistent AF has demonstrated that the left atrium acts as the electrical driving chamber (Nitta et al. 1999). In patients with persistent AF and mitral valve disease, a simple left atrial procedure successfully ablated AF in 78% of patients (Sueda et al. 1997).

Several new ablation tools have been developed. These probes and catheters rely on external energy sources to create long linear lesions that block conduction. Energy sources that have been used clinically include radiofrequency, laser, ultrasound, microwave, and cryothermy. The largest clinical experience is with radiofrequency energy that uses alternating current to heat tissue. Several different types of probe are available. Under direct vision, the probes may be placed on the epicardial or endocardial surface of the heart. Epicardial placement allows for beating heart or 'off-pump' AF ablation, although there is some concern that epicardial delivery of unipolar radiofrequency energy will not produce transmural lesions. In contrast, the bipolar radiofrequency clamp is well suited to epicardial placement; it also includes a mechanism for real time assessment of transmurality, an important advance in the surgical treatment of AF. Although there is less experience with microwave, laser, and ultrasound, these heat-based energy sources also facilitate AF ablation.

Because the surgeon has the advantage of direct vision of cardiac structures and ablation tools that allow rapid creation of transmural lesions, completion of left atrial lesion sets requires only 10–20 minutes, which contrasts with the 1 hour to perform the classic maze procedure. In addition, the risk of bleeding is virtually eliminated when alternate energy sources are used. The principle is to create transmural lesions in the atrial wall since the fibrocytes that constitute the scar will not conduct electrically. Results of AF ablation using left atrial lesion sets are complete ablation in 70–80% of patients. Most treated patients have structural heart disease and have received a mitral valve procedure in addition to AF ablation. Success is similar with different energy sources regardless of whether right atrial lesions are included.

After ablation, perioperative AF is common, occurring in approximately 60% of patients. Although 30–40% of patients leave hospital in AF, many return to sinus rhythm over the next 3 months. Factors that influence procedure success have not been identified with certainty but left atrial size (>5 cm diameter), rheumatic heart disease, and the presence of persistent AF for more than 5 years are all strongly negative predictive factors.

New developments

Surgeons are developing epicardially based, minimally invasive, and thoracoscopic approaches to offer rapid and safe AF ablation to patients with lone AF. Minimally invasive, off-pump, epicardial ablation of AF is being pursued in a number of specialized centres. Pulmonary vein isolation and excision can be performed thoracoscopically. With minor modifications in technology to ensure rapid and safe creation of transmural lines of conduction block, off-pump epicardial ablation of AF is being offered to patients in a few centres.

Ventricular arrhythmias

The success of the implantable cardioverter-defibrillator (ICD) and radiofrequency catheter ablation has led to a dramatic decrease in the number of patients referred for surgery. Nevertheless, in selected patients with coronary artery disease where the substrate for ventricular arrhythmias is ischaemia, surgery still has an important role to play. This is particularly true with the recent resurgence of interest in left ventricular surgical remodelling as a potential treatment for congestive cardiac failure. Although an ICD is effective electrical instability is only one part of a complex problem. Other sequelae of coronary artery disease include the potential for recurrent ischaemia, and in many patients progressive heart failure related to poor left ventricular function with or without mitral regurgitation. Optimal treatment in these patients would prevent further episodes of the arrhythmia, reverse ischaemia, and restore left ventricular size, shape, and geometry towards normal.

Currently, surgery would be advised in patients with coronary artery disease, poor left ventricular function, and ventricular arrhythmias, if the area of antero-apical scarring (akinesis or dyskinesis) corresponds to a region of significant thinning. At operation, the septum should be examined for scarring. All visible endocardial septal scar tissue should be excised with cryoablation at the periphery of the excision as the strategy for control of VT (Mickleborough et al. 2000). A postoperative electrophysiological study should be performed. If ventricular arrhythmias are still inducible, amiodarone should be given. Further studies are needed to confirm the effectiveness of this approach in patients with poor left ventricular function and dilated hearts. Surgery should be performed before progressive dilatation and adverse remodelling result, leaving transplantation as the only reasonable option.

Summary

Although the maze procedure is extremely effective at treating AF, new surgical procedures are far simpler and include pulmonary vein lesions, left atrial lesions, and excision of the left atrial appendage. Currently applied as an adjunct to other cardiac operations, these new approaches are being modified for thoracoscopic, minimally invasive, epicardial AF ablation.

References

Cox JL, Schuessler RB, D'Agostino HJ. The surgical treatment of atrial fibrillation lll: development of a definitive procedure. *J Thorac Cardiovasc Surg* 1991;**101**:569–83.

Haissaguerre M, Shah DC, Jais P. Spontaneous initiation of atrial fibrillation by ectopic beats originating in the pulmonary veins. *N Engl J Med* 1998;**339**:659–66.

Cox JL, Scheussler RB, Lappas DG, Boineau JP. An 8½ year clinical experience with surgery for atrial fibrillation. *Ann Surg* 1996;**224**:267–75.

Prasad SM, Maniar HS, Camillo CJ, et al. The Cox maze lll procedure for atrial fibrillation: Long-term efficacy in patients undergoing lone versus concomitant procedures. *J Thorac Cardiovasc Surg* 2003;**126**:1822–8.

Gaita F, Riccardi R, Calo L, et al. Atrial mapping and radiofrequency catheter ablation in patients with idiopathic atrial fibrillation. Electrophysiological findings and ablation results. *Circulation* 1988;**97**:2136–45.

Nitta T, Imura H, Bessho R, et al. Wavelength and conduction in homogeneity in each atrium in patients with isolated mitral valve disease and atrial fibrillation. *J Cardiovasc Electrophysiol* 1999;**10**:521–28.

Sueda T, Nagata H, Orihashi K, et al. Efficacy of a simple left atrial procedure for chronic atrial fibrillation in mitral valve operations. *Ann Thorac Surg* 1997;**63**:1070–5.

Mickleborough LL, Carson S, Tamariz M, Ivanov J. Results of revascularisation in patients with severe left ventricular dysfunction. *J Thorac Cardiovasc Surg* 2000;**119**:550–6.

Chapter 4

Hypertension

Hypertension: diagnosis and evaluation

- Hypertension occurs when the systemic arterial pressure is consistently elevated (Table 4.1.1).
- Elevated blood pressure increases the risk of stroke and myocardial infarction. It also leads to left ventricular hypertrophy and, in the long run, heart failure and renal failure.
- In the community, hypertension is often undetected and untreated. As hypertension may not cause any specific symptoms, screening in apparently healthy individuals is warranted.
- *Isolated systolic hypertension* is common in elderly people and requires treatment.
- *White coat hypertension* is present in around 20–30% of hypertensive patients whose clinic blood pressure readings are substantially higher than the blood pressure measured at home either by 24-hour ambulatory blood pressure monitoring or by an automated electronic home device (see Chapter 4.2, Ambulatory blood pressure monitoring).
- Hypertension in pregnancy may be due to pre-existing hypertension, gestational hypertension, which develops after the twentieth week, or pre-eclampsia.

Aetiology

- For the great majority of patients with hypertension, there is no single identifiable secondary cause. In the young and in severe or rapidly progressive hypertension, secondary causes should be considered. These include anatomical, endocrine, and renal causes. In the majority of patients with primary hypertension, there may be a number of predisposing factors, such as family history, obesity, high salt intake, a diet high in fat and low in fruits and vegetables, stress and excess alcohol intake.

Clinical approach

History: key points

- There are no symptoms that are characteristic of primary hypertension. Headaches, dizziness, or palpitations are often presenting symptoms that lead the blood pressure to be checked. However, the clinician should be alert to the symptoms of secondary hypertension, such as those of phaeochromocytoma. The possibility of sleep apnoea should also be considered.
- History of blood pressure readings, previous diagnosis and treatment of hypertension, complications of hypertension (e.g. stroke, myocardial infarction, heart failure, and renal disease).
- Presence of other risk factors (e.g. diabetes, hyperlipidaemia).
- Other concomitant diseases.
- Family history of hypertension, stroke, and coronary heart disease.
- Social history, including smoking, alcohol, diet, salt intake, exercise, and sexual function.

Table 4.1.1 Categories of blood pressure levels (mmHg) in the US JNC7 and the European Hypertension Society/European Society of Cardiology guidelines

Systolic		Diastolic	US JNC7	EHS/ESC
<120	and	<80	Normal	Optimal
120–129	or	80–84	Prehypertension	Normal
130–139	or	85–89	Prehypertension	High normal
140–159	or	90–99	Stage 1 hypertension	Grade 1 hypertension
160–179	or	100–109	Stage 2 hypertension	Grade 2 hypertension
≥180	and	≥110	Stage 2 hypertension	Grade 3 hypertension
≥140	and	<90	Isolated systolic hypertension	Isolated systolic hypertension

Examination: key points

The purpose is to search for secondary and reversible causes of hypertension and to detect target organ damage (e.g. left ventricular hypertrophy, albuminuria, retinopathy, and clinical manifestations of atherosclerosis) and complications of hypertension.

- General appearance on inspection: central adiposity is strongly associated with hypertension. Look for features of Cushing's syndrome and acromegaly.
- Detailed examination of the cardiovascular system, including jugular venous pressure, peripheral oedema, palpation of pulses and detection of radio-radial and radio-femoral delay, auscultation for carotid and femoral bruits, palpation of the praecordium and apex, and careful auscultation of heart sounds and any murmurs. Aortic regurgitation causes wide pulse pressure. In hypertension, the aortic second heart sound might be loud.
- The respiratory system should be examined for crackles due to heart failure, and for wheezes due to bronchial asthma, in which case beta-blockers might be contraindicated.
- Examination of the abdomen should include palpation of the liver for enlargement, the kidneys for the possibility of polycystic kidneys and the aorta for anuerysmal dilatation.
- A brief neurological examination should be performed, as hypertension is a major cause of cerebrovascular disease.
- Examination of the fundi for hypertensive retinopathy. Generalized and focal narrowing of the arterioles is common in hypertension. The presence of haemorrhages, exudates, and papilloedema indicate a more severe state and require prompt control of blood pressure.

How to take the blood pressure

- Accurate blood pressure readings are essential for diagnosis and management. As blood pressure fluctuates and can be affected by many factors, minimize variability by using recommended techniques and taking multiple readings.
- Sit the patient comfortably for at least 5 minutes. The arm should rest on a surface to ensure that the cuff is at the same level as the heart. Choose a cuff appropriate for the size of the arm. Take at least two readings, and repeat if there are large differences (e.g. >5 mmHg). Measure blood pressure in both arms and use the arm with the higher reading. Measure blood pressure in the erect position if postural hypotension is suspected.
- Hypertension is diagnosed when the systolic blood pressure is ≥140 mmHg or diastolic blood pressure is ≥90 mmHg in repeated measurements on separate occasions.

Investigations

- Ambulatory blood pressure monitoring is desirable if available and acceptable to the patient
- Full blood count
- Blood biochemistry (including sodium, potassium, urea, creatinine, and urate)
- Fasting glucose and lipids
- Urine analysis for glucose, blood and protein
- Electrocardiogram (for arrhythmia, previous myocardial infarction and left ventricular hypertrophy)
- Echocardiogram (if there is a murmur, arrhythmia, suspected malformation, left ventricular hypertrophy or heart failure)
- If available, ankle-brachial blood pressure index, pulse wave velocity and carotid ultrasound are useful in assessing the vasculature.

Elevated glucose and lipids, and albuminuria are common in hypertensive patients.

A low plasma potassium may raise the possibility of Conn's syndrome (hyperaldosteronism).

Investigation for secondary causes of hypertension (see p. 132) usually requires referral to a specialist centre. Young age (under 40), the presence of clinical features suggestive of a secondary cause, or severe blood pressure difficult to control, are good reasons to investigate for secondary causes. Renin, aldosterone, corticosteroid, and catecholamines may be measured. Imaging studies may be performed for endocrine tumours.

Assessment of overall cardiovascular risk for each patient is important as hypertension is only one of many risk factors for cardiovascular disease. This can be done using risk charts or risk scores. The level of blood pressure, the presence of other risk factors, target organ damage and overt cardiovascular disease guide the urgency and intensity of treatment.

Further reading

Chobanian AV, Bakris GL, Black HR, *et al*. The Seventh report of the Joint National Committee on Prevention, Detection, Evaluation and Treatment of High Blood Pressure: The JNC 7 Report. *JAMA* 2003;**289**:2560–72.

Mancia G, De Backer G, Dominiczak A, *et al*. Guidelines for the management of arterial hypertension: The Task Force for the Management of Arterial Hypertension of the European Society of Hypertension (ESH) and of the European Society of Cardiology (ESC). *Eur Heart J* 2007;**28**:1462–1536.

Williams B, Poulter NR, Brown MJ, *et al*. British Hypertension Society Guidelines: Guidelines for management of hypertension: report of the fourth working party of the British hypertension Society, 2004—BHS IV. *J Hum Hypertens* 2004;**18**:139–85.

Ambulatory blood pressure monitoring

Ambulatory blood pressure monitoring (ABPM) is a technique for measuring blood pressure (BP) away from the office while the patient is undertaking activities of daily living (except strenuous activity). Typically, BP measurements are made every 15–30 minutes during the day and every 30–60 minutes during the night, providing up to 70 measurements over a 24-hour period. Ambulatory blood pressure (ABP) can provide an estimate of the true, or mean, BP level, the diurnal rhythm of BP, and BP variability. Although the British Hypertension Society (BHS) and NICE do not currently recommend the use of ABPM for all patients, the BHS acknowledge that it can be helpful in specific circumstances as shown below.

Potential indications
- Possible 'white-coat hypertension' (consistently elevated office BP, normal ABPM), which can be present in 15% of the general population and one-third or more of people with hypertension
- Evaluation of drug-resistant hypertension
- Informing equivocal treatment decisions
- Unusual blood pressure variability
- Evaluation of nocturnal hypertension
- Determining the efficacy of drug treatment over 24 hours
- Diagnosis and treatment of hypertension in pregnancy
- Evaluation of symptomatic hypotension.

Contraindications
- Cardiac arrhythmias, e.g. atrial fibrillation
- Obesity where arm size is greater than the largest available cuff size.

Key points (methods)
- Use only a validated device that is serviced and calibrated regularly
- Use correct sized cuff and ensure ABP and office BP are within ±5 mmHg at set up
- Ensure that staff undertaking ABPM are trained and competent
- Perform on a typical day and encourage patients to keep a diary recording symptoms, sleep quality, and events that may influence BP during the recording
- Undertake only minimal editing of ABPM to remove gross measurement artefacts.

Clinical data analysis
- Calculate the average 24-hour, daytime, and night-time BP based on fixed times (day 07.00–22.00 and night 22.00–07.00) or activity-based timing (assess time of waking and sleeping from diary card).
- Normal values are different for office and ambulatory BP; approximate threshold values are shown in Table 4.2.1.
- The diurnal variation (change in BP during sleep) may be useful because so-called 'non-dippers' (a reduction in BP

of ≤10% overnight) is associated with increased mortality and other unwanted outcomes.

Key points (interpretation)
- ABP may be better than casual or office BP measurements in risk stratification and the prediction of absolute cardiovascular risk in untreated and treated patients.
- Emerging data suggest that ABP predicts cardiovascular events in diabetes better than office BP.
- ABP may be more accurate than clinic BP in assessing treatment response due to a higher reproducibility over time and an absent or negligible 'white coat' and placebo effect.
- On-treatment ABP has been shown to be associated with a lower rate of cardiovascular outcomes than similar achieved office BP values.
- ABP is commonly lower than clinic BP but 'masked' or 'isolated ambulatory hypertension' (ABP higher than clinic BP) occurs. The limited information available suggests that these patients have a greater prevalence of target organ damage, an increased prevalence of metabolic risk factors and some outcome studies have also suggested that masked hypertension increases cardiovascular risk.
- ABPM may be repeated but decisions as to repeat studies is largely one of clinical judgement.

Limitations
ABPM has advantages over other techniques, including self/home-measured BP but its limitations include:
- Generating only intermittent not continuous BP measurements
- Measuring BP while the individual is sedentary rather than truly 'ambulatory'
- The potential to cause a small number of patients discomfort including bruising
- Limited data from outcome trials based solely on ABPM, but there is increasing evidence suggesting that ABP is a better predictor of CVD risk
- Costs with ABPM are more expensive than conventional or home BP measurement
- Patient tolerance: some patients will not tolerate repeat recordings.

Table 4.2.1 Blood pressure thresholds (mmHg) for definition of hypertension by office and ambulatory BP (sourced from ESC and ESH guidelines, 2007)

	SBP	DBP
Office	140	90
24-hour average	125–130	80
Day	130–135	85
Night	120	70

Non-pharmacological treatment for hypertension

Non-pharmacological intervention, also commonly known as lifestyle modification, for treatment of hypertension is under-used. It produces a mild to moderate reduction in blood pressure (BP) which can be sufficed by itself in patients with less than severe hypertension. In patients with severe hypertension, non-pharmacological intervention augments the effects of antihypertensive medications and reduces the occurrence of resistant hypertension. Moreover, several novel non-pharmacological therapies are also under investigation for treatment of drug refractory hypertension.

Successful application of lifestyle interventions often requires professional support and encouragement and regular review because the long-term adherence to these strategies has been poor in many patients.

The following non-pharmacological treatments have been endorsed by the 2007 European Society of Hypertension and European Society of Cardiology Practice Guidelines for the Management of Arterial Hypertension:
- Reduction of salt intake
- Smoking cessation
- Weight reduction
- Reduction of excessive alcohol intake
- Physical exercise
- Increase in fruit and vegetable intake and decrease in saturated and total fat intake.

Reduction of dietary sodium (salt) intake
- There are evidence that the current dietary intake of salt in Western societies is an important factor in the genesis of essential hypertension and may even partly cause blood pressure-independent target organ damage, including renal damage.
- Dose–response relationship: the more sodium reduction, the greater the blood pressure decline.
- Moderate reduction of sodium intake to 1–2 g/day effectively reduces blood pressure without incurring significant side-effects.
- The absolute reduction in blood pressure with reduction of salt intake varies based on the baseline blood pressure. The higher the starting blood pressure, the greater the reduction. African-Americans and elderly patients are more responsive to sodium restriction.
- Excessive dietary sodium ingestion contributes importantly to resistance to antihypertensive treatment. In patients with resistant hypertension, reduction of salt intake is accompanied by increase in plasma renin activity and decrease in brain natriuretic peptide and creatinine clearance.

Stopping excessive alcohol consumption
- Safe level of alcohol consumption: less than two portions (one portion is 12 oz (336 mL) of beer, 4 oz (112 mL) of wine, or 1.5 oz (42 mL) of spirits) per day.
- Excessive alcohol intake is a recognized cause of hypertension.

Restriction of calorie intake
- A 4–8% body weight reduction causes an average 3 mmHg blood pressure decrease.
- The calorie-restricted group exhibited a significant reduction in BP in association with loss of body weight; their levels of low-density lipoprotein cholesterol, and triglycerides levels, and their fasting levels of glucose and insulin were also reduced compared with the calorie-non-restricted group.
- Caloric restriction improves endothelium-dependent vasodilation through an increased release of nitric oxide.

Dietary approaches to stop hypertension (DASH)
- A combination diet rich in fruits and vegetables and low-fat dairy products and low in saturated and total fat.
- A diet comprising four or five servings of fruit, four or five servings of vegetables, two or three servings of low-fat dairy per day, and <25% fat.
- A combination of a low sodium and DASH diet resulted in the most significant benefit, with decreases in blood pressure similar to those observed with antihypertensive agents.

Regular dynamic exercise
- 30–45 minutes daily, at least 4 days per week.
- Regular dynamic exercise results in a 5–10 mmHg reduction in blood pressure, accompanied by a fall in sympathetic activity.

Abstaining from smoking
- The immediate noxious effects of smoking are related to over-activation of the sympathetic nervous system, which increases myocardial oxygen consumption through a rise in heart rate, blood pressure, and myocardial contractility.
- Chronically, cigarette smoking induces arterial stiffness.
- Smoking should be avoided in any hypertensive patient because it can markedly increase the risk of secondary cardiovascular complications and enhance the progression of renal insufficiency.

Novel non-pharmacological treatment for hypertension

Vaccination against angiotensins
- Blocking the renin–angiotensin axis by targeting angiotensin I (PMD3117) or II (CYT006-AngQb) by vaccination has been proved to be an option to lower blood pressure in small trials.
- It offers the possibility for reduction of blood pressure with two to three immunizations per year, which may circumvent the need for daily medication and substantially improve patient compliance.
- No serious adverse events related to vaccination have been observed; however, the number of patients involved is small.

Renal sympathetic denervation procedure
- Renal sympathetic nerve activation enhances noradrenaline (norepinephrine) production, renin secretion, sodium resorption, and renal vasoconstriction, resulting in a decrease in renal blood flow. Therefore, renal sympathetic denervation may provide significant reduction of blood pressure.
- Catheter-based procedure using radiofrequency ablation with minimal systemic side-effects.
- Current practices and recommendations suggest that renal sympathetic denervation should be reserved for treatment-resistant patients.

Baroreceptor device
- Electric stimulation of baroreflex afferent nerves located at the carotid body could be sensed by the brain as an increase in blood pressure such that sympathetic activity and subsequently blood pressure are reduced.
- Novel implantable device produces sustained electric field stimulation of the carotid sinus wall and produced a persistent reduction of blood pressure.
- Potentially useful in treatment-resistant hypertensive patients.

Approach to the use of non-pharmacological treatment for hypertension
- Lifestyle modification is recommended in all patients, including those who require drug treatment.
- Long-term compliance with lifestyle measures is low and the blood pressure response is variable; therefore, patients should be followed up closely and commence drug treatment when needed.
- The general approach for pharmacological and non-pharmacological treatment is shown in Fig. 4.3.1.
- Future development of novel non-pharmacological treatment may provide alternative therapies to patients with treatment-resistant hypertension.

- As shown in Table 4.3.1, the degrees of reduction in BP with different non-pharmacological therapies are similar or above those achieved with any single pharmacological agent.

Table 4.3.1 Approximate reduction in systolic blood pressure by individual non-pharmacological treatment

Lifestyle modification	Approximate systolic BP reduction
Weight reduction	5–20 mmHg per 10-kg weight loss
Adopt DASH eating plan	8–14 mmHg
Dietary sodium reduction	2–8 mmHg
Physical activity	5–10 mmHg
Moderation of alcohol consumption	2–4 mmHg
Novel non-pharmacological treatment	
Vaccination against angiotensins	Up to 25 mmHg
Renal sympathetic denervation	Up to 27 mmHg
Baroreceptor device	Up to 41 mmHg

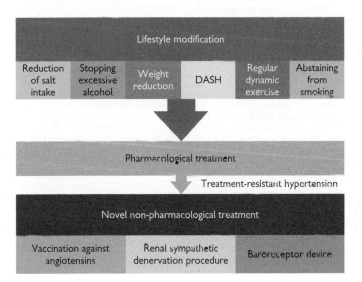

Fig. 4.3.1 General approach for pharmacological and non-pharmacological treatment for hypertension.

Further reading
Chobanian AV, Bakris GL, Black HR, *et al.* Seventh report of the Joint National Committee on Prevention, Detection, Evaluation, and Treatment of High Blood Pressure. *Hypertension* 2003;**42**:1206–52.

Doumas M, Faselis C, Papademetriou V. Renal sympathetic denervation and systemic hypertension. *Am J Cardiol* 2010;**105**:570–6.

Filippone JD, Bisognano JD. Baroreflex stimulation in the treatment of hypertension. *Curr Opin Nephrol Hypertens* 2007;**16**:403–8.

Krum H, Schlaich M, Whitbourn R, *et al.* Catheter-based renal sympathetic denervation for resistant hypertension: a multicentre safety and proof-of-principle cohort study. *Lancet* 2009;**373**:1275–81.

Mancia G, De Backer G, Dominiczak A, *et al.* 2007 ESH-ESC Practice guidelines for the management of arterial hypertension: ESH-ESC Task Force on the Management of Arterial Hypertension. *J Hypertens* 2007;**25**:1751–62.

Maurer P, Bachmann MF. Immunization against angiotensins for the treatment of hypertension. *Clin Immunol* 2010;**134**:89–95.

Tissot AC, Maurer P, Nussberger J, *et al.* Effect of immunisation against angiotensin II with CYT006-AngQb on ambulatory blood pressure: a double-blind, randomised, placebo-controlled phase IIa study. *Lancet* 2008;**371**:821–7.

Hypertension: pharmacological treatment

Blood pressure has a unimodal distribution in the general population. Therefore, any definition of high blood pressure is arbitrary. There is no apparent threshold for the graded relationship between blood pressure and cardiovascular disease morbidity and mortality. Systolic blood pressure (SBP) levels are directly and continuously related to the risk of both stroke and coronary heart disease (CHD). The incidence of both stroke and CHD continues to decline even as the lowest levels of BP are approached. Therefore, an effective BP-lowering strategy is important. It has been estimated that a decrease in population SBP by 2 mmHg would translate into a 6% reduction of stroke and a 4% reduction in CHD.

Treatment

Management of hypertension can be broadly divided into pharmacological and non-pharmacological. Non-pharmacological measures should be initiated in all patients diagnosed with hypertension and subjects with BP above 120/80. They include weight reduction, dietary sodium reduction, diet rich in fruits, vegetables, and low-fat diary products, moderation of alcohol consumption, and physical activity. These will be covered elsewhere in this book. Non-pharmacological therapy is often not enough to achieve the BP target, in which case addition of pharmacological therapy should be considered.

Initiation of pharmacological therapy

Antihypertensive treatment is evolving towards early and aggressive intervention. As recommended in the 2007 Guidelines of the European Society of Cardiology and European Society of Hypertension (ESH/ESC) guidelines, initiation of treatment should be based on the level of SBP and diastolic BP (DBP), and the level of total cardiovascular risk (Table 4.4.1). Prompt pharmacological treatment should be given in grade 3 HT and grade 1 and 2 when the total cardiovascular risk is high or very high. In patients with grade 1 and 2 hypertension with moderate total cardiovascular risk, it is justifiable to initiate pharmacological

Table 4.4.2 Target BP by ESH/ESC Guidelines

Patient characteristics	Target BP
No diabetes or renal disease	<140/90*
Diabetes or renal disease	<130/80
All high-risk hypertensives	<130/80
Proteinuria >1 g	Even lower than <130/80

*Lower values if tolerated.

treatment if BP remains uncontrolled by non-pharmacological means after several weeks. In subjects with BP in the high normal range, the presence of diabetes, established cardiovascular disease, or renal disease would necessitate pharmacological treatment.

Treatment targets

The primary objective of antihypertensive treatment is to minimize the long-term total cardiovascular risk. Different treatments targets, based on clinical studies, are adopted by various organizations. ESH/ESC and the Seventh Report of the Joint National Committee on Detection, Evaluation and Treatment of High Blood Pressure (JNC-7) recommend similar target blood pressures. BP level as low as 130/80 has been recommended by American Heart Association. Table 4.4.2 summarizes the ESH/ESC goals.

Drug classes

The drug classes that are most commonly used in clinical practice include angiotensin-converting enzyme inhibitors (ACEIs), angiotensin receptor blockers (ARBs), beta-adrenergic blockers (BBs), calcium channel blockers (CCBs), and diuretics. Their contraindications are listed in Table 4.4.3. Most of the currently available drugs lower blood pressure to similar extents, so the choice of drug may depend on co-morbidities and contraindications. Frequently, more than one drug is needed to achieve BP control. There is

Table 4.4.1 Initiation of blood pressure intervention (from Mancia et al. 2007)

Blood pressure (mm Hg)	Normal SBP 120–129 or DBP 80–84	High normal SBP 130–139 or DBP 85–89	Grade 1 HT SBP 140–159 or DBP 90–99	Grade 2 HT SBP 160–179 or DBP 100–109	Grade 3 HT SBP≥180 or DBP ≥110
No other risk factors	No BP intervention	No BP intervention	Lifestyle changes for several months then drug treatment if BP uncontrolled	Lifestyle changes for several weeks then drug treatment if BP uncontrolled	Lifestyle changes + Immediate drug treatment
1–2 risk factors	Lifestyle changes	Lifestyle changes	Lifestyle changes for several weeks then drug treatment if BP uncontrolled	Lifestyle changes for several weeks then drug treatment if BP uncontrolled	Lifestyle changes + Immediate drug treatment
≥3 risk factors, MS or OD	Lifestyle changes	Lifestyle changes and consider drug treatment	Lifestyle changes + Drug treatment	Lifestyle changes + Drug treatment	Lifestyle changes + Immediate drug treatment
Diabetes	Lifestyle changes	Lifestyle changes + Drug treatment			
Established CV or renal disease	Lifestyle changes + Immediate drug treatment	Lifestyle changes + Immediate drug treatment	Lifestyle changes +Immediate drug treatment	Lifestyle changes + Immediate drug treatment	Lifestyle changes + Immediate drug treatment

MS, metabolic syndrome; OD, hypertensive target organ damage.

some evidence that blockers of the renin–angiotensin system (ACEI, ARB) are more effective in younger people (e.g. age under 55) and are less effective in older people and in black people. For these groups, diuretics are more effective.

Alpha-adrenergic receptor blockers (alpha-blockers)
- Mechanism: selective inhibition of alpha-1-adrenergic receptors and reduction of systemic vascular resistance.
- Indications
  - Not a first-line agent
  - Benign prostatic hypertrophy.
- Side-effects
  - Postural hypotension.

Angiotensin-converting enzyme inhibitors (ACEIs)
- Mechanism: inhibition of the generation of angiotensin II from angiotensin I and degradation of vasoactive peptides.
- Indications
  - First-line for hypertension
  - Concomitant diabetes
  - Concomitant diabetic and non-diabetic nephropathy
  - Post myocardial infarction
  - Heart failure and left ventricular dysfunction.
- Side-effects
  - Usually well tolerated, up to 20% develop side-effects that necessitate termination of therapy
  - Cough most common
  - Hyperkalaemia
  - Angioedema uncommon, not dose dependent
  - Acute renal dysfunction with pre-existing renal insufficiency
  - Birth defect.

Angiotensin II receptor blockers (ARBs)
- Mechanism: selective inhibition of angiotensin II receptor type I.
- Indications
  - Same as ACEIs
- Side-effects
  - Well tolerated
  - No cough
  - Hyperkalaemia
  - Acute renal dysfunction with pre-existing renal insufficiency
  - Angioedema rare.

Beta-adrenergic receptor blockers (beta-blockers)
- Mechanism: selective inhibition of beta-adrenergic receptors and reduction of cardiac output and heart rate.
- Indications
  - No longer recommended as first-line therapy under NICE, AHA and WHO guidelines
  - Post myocardial infarction
  - Angina pectoris
  - Ventricular arrhythmias and certain atrioventricular-dependent supraventricular arrhythmias
  - Compensated congestive heart failure.
- Side-effects
  - Decrease exercise tolerance in younger patient
  - Erectile dysfunction and worsening of hyperglycaemia.

Calcium channel blockers (CCBs)
- Mechanism: inhibition of L-type voltage-gated calcium channels. Classified as dihydropyridines and non-dihydropyridines. Both can produce coronary artery dilatation but only the later slow heart rates as well.
- Indications
  - First-line for uncomplicated hypertension
  - Third-line for diabetic patients after ACEI/ARB and diuretics.
- Side-effects (dihydropyridines)
  - Headache
  - Flushing
  - Reflex tachycardia
  - Peripheral oedema exacerbated by high-salt diet and improved with ACEI/ARB.
- Side-effects (non-dihydropyridines)
  - Constipation
  - Bradycardia
  - Peripheral oedema.

Diuretics: thiazides
- Mechanism: decrease in body sodium and extracellular fluid volume, vasodilatation.
- Indications
  - First-line for uncomplicated hypertension
  - Add-on drug on top of ACEI/ARB in diabetics
  - Considered as second drug if alternative first-line agent is used.
- Side effects
  - Volume depletion and prerenal azotaemia
  - Electrolyte abnormalities, including hypokalaemia, hypomagnesaemia
  - Increased level of blood glucose
  - Hyperuricaemia
  - Erectile dysfunction: long-term use.

Table 4.4.3 Contraindications of antihypertensive agents (Cobanian *et al.* 2003; Mancia *et al.* 2007)

Drug	Contraindications
ACEIs	Pregnancy
	Angioneurotic oedema
	Hyperkalaemia
	Bilateral renal artery stenosis
ARBs	Pregnancy
	Hyperkalaemia
	Bilateral renal artery stenosis
Beta-blockers	Asthma
	AV block (grade 2 or 3)
Non-dihydropyridines	AV block (grade 2 or 3)
	Heart failure
Thiazides	Hypokalaemia

Others
- Currently approved agents for second-line therapy: clonidine, reserpine, methyldopa, moxonidine, hydralazine, minoxidil, aliskiren, spironolactone, eplerenone.
- Methyldopa and hydralazine maybe used for treatment of hypertension in pregnancy.
- Aliskiren is a newly approved renin inhibitor which is well-tolerated up to the dose of 600 mg for hypertension. Its short-term effectiveness for blood pressure control has been demonstrated by a number of clinical trials. Furthermore, it has been shown to reduce proteinuria in patients with diabetic nephropathy.
- Spironolactone is an aldosterone antagonist that may be used in Conn's syndrome and refractory hypertension. Its well-known side-effects, gynaecomastia and erectile dysfunction, are not found in the newer agent eplerenone. However, both agents can lead to hyperkalaemia, especially in patients with renal impairment.

Compelling indications

Although the aforementioned drugs have similar BP-lowering efficacy, some drugs should be preferred in the presence of compelling indications (Table 4.4.4) unless contraindicated. These considerations could help the management of co-existing conditions. For example, ACEIs were found to retard progression of renal damage in patients with renal disease. They also decrease post myocardial infarction left ventricular remodelling and left ventricular hypertrophy. These beneficial effects could not be explained solely by the BP-lowering effect. There are also situations that certain antihypertensive agents may have favourable effects on co-morbid conditions. Thiazide diuretics may reduce calcium excretion and benefit patients with osteoporosis. In men with benign prostatic hypertrophy, alpha-adrenergic receptor blockers may also relax the smooth muscle tissue in the prostate.

Table 4.4.4 Considerations for initial drug therapy (from Stergiou and Bakris 2009)

Compelling indications	Preferred drug therapy
Diabetes mellitus, type 1 and 2	ACEIs, ARBs
Diabetic and non-diabetic proteinuria	ACEIs, ARBs
Diabetes and microalbuminuria	ACEIs, ARBs
Renal insufficiency	ACEIs, ARBs
Systolic heart failure	ACEIs, ARBs, beta-blockers, aldosterone antagonists, diuretics
Myocardial infarction	Beta-blockers, ACEIs, ARBs, aldosterone antagonists
Coronary heart disease	ACEIs
Isolated systolic hypertension	Diuretics, CCBs

This table was published in *Cardiology* 3e, Crawford et al., copyright Elsevier (2010).

Suggested clinical approach

- Fig. 4.4.1 outlines a pharmacological approach in managing essential hypertension. Lifestyle modification should be advised in all patients with hypertension. Pharmacological treatment may start with a single drug, first at a low dose and slowly stepped up when BP is not well controlled.
- If the BP goal is not reached with full dose, a second drug may be added.
- The presence of compelling indications and contraindications should be considered when choosing the first antihypertensive agent.
- If there is no compelling indication, any one of the first-line agents can be used. Individual response to antihypertensive agents can be remarkably heterogeneous.

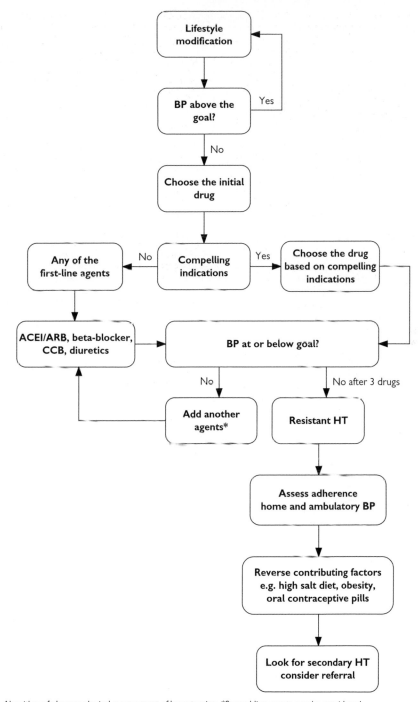

Fig. 4.4.1 Algorithm of pharmacological management of hypertension. *Second-line agents may be considered.

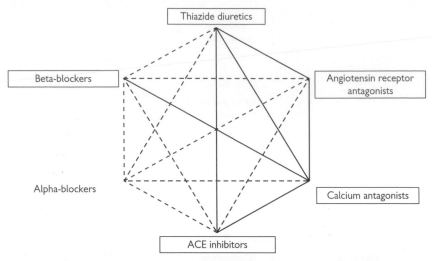

Fig. 4.4.2 Possible combinations between some classes of antihypertensive drugs. The preferred combinations in the general hypertensive population are represented as thick lines. The frames indicate classes of agents proven to be beneficial in controlled intervention trials (Mancia *et al.* 2007).

- Switching to a different class of agent is advisable if the first agent fails to decrease BP or results in significant side-effects. This approach may help identify the agent that the individual patient responds optimally. Combination therapy has been evaluated in many trials.
- The ESH/ESC guidelines recommend several drug combinations that were shown to be synergistic or more tolerable (Fig. 4.4.2).
- When initial BP is in the grade 2 or 3 range or total cardiovascular risk is high or very high, a combination of two drugs at low doses is recommended as the first treatment.

Resistant or refractory hypertension is usually defined as systolic or diastolic BP above goal when a therapeutic plan that has included attention to lifestyle measures and the prescription of at least three drugs (including a diuretic) in adequate doses. The patient adherence should be carefully assessed; 24-hour ambulatory blood pressure monitoring is often helpful to assess BP control throughout day and night, and to avoid the white coat effect on BP when it is measured in the clinic. Causes of secondary hypertension should be ruled out and referral to a specialist should be considered.

Further reading

Cobanian AV, Bakris GL, Black HR, *et al.* The Seventh report of the Joint National Committee on Prevention, Detection, Evaluation and Treatment of High Blood Pressure: The JNC 7 Report. *JAMA* 2003;**289**:2560–72.

Mancia G, De Backer G, Dominiczak A, *et al.* Guidelines for the management of arterial hypertension: The Task Force for the Management of Arterial Hypertension of the European Society of Hypertension (ESH) and of the European Society of Cardiology (ESC). *Eur Heart J* 2007;**28**:1462–536.

Messerli F, Williams B, Eberhard R. Essential hypertension. *Lancet* 2007;**370**:591–603.

Stergiou GS, Bakris GL. Pharmacological treatment. In: Crawford MH, DiMarco JP, Paulus WJ (eds) *Cardiology*. London: Mosby, 2009.

Secondary hypertension

Secondary hypertension is the presence of a specific condition linked to the kidney, the vasculature, endocrine organs, lungs, or central nervous system that is known to cause hypertension (Taler 2008). Almost all secondary causes can be cured or adequately treated medically, thus allowing for significantly better blood pressure (BP) control. Evaluation of secondary causes of hypertension depends on the history, symptoms, and laboratory abnormalities present in a given patient.

Causes associated with the kidney

Renovascular disease ranges from overt renal artery stenosis of one or both renal arteries to subtle intrarenal vascular disease detected only by kidney biopsy. Renal artery stenosis is diagnosed with a >70% narrowing of a renal artery, or >50% luminal narrowing with a post-stenotic dilatation. Not all renal stenoses are associated with hypertension. Renovascular hypertension has a physiological basis for diagnosis. Several aetiologies of renovascular hypertension exist, including fibromuscular dysplasia, atherosclerotic disease, and Takayasu's disease. Patients may present with a continuous abdominal bruit. Captopril scintigraphy remains widely available and is used to rule out high-grade renal artery disease. Magnetic resonance angiography (MRA) is the most sensitive and specific test to confirm the diagnosis. Angioplasty alone is the treatment of choice for fibromuscular dysplasia. There are three treatment options for renal artery stenosis: surgical revascularization, angioplasty with or without stenting, or medical management. Stenting is done in most cases to preserve kidney function and not to treat the hypertension.

Chronic kidney disease is probably the most common medical cause of secondary hypertension and is both a cause and a consequence of hypertension. The current BP goal for such patients is <130/80 mmHg. Angiotensin-converting enzyme (ACE) inhibitors or angiotensin receptor blockers (ARBs) are the initial agents of choice. Calcium antagonists or diuretics are usually needed to achieve this BP goal.

Renin-producing tumours arise from the juxtaglomerular cells of the kidney. Symptoms manifest as hypertension and hypokalaemia, and elevated plasma renin activity (PRA) and plasma aldosterone concentration (PAC), with the PAC/PRA ratio normal or reduced. This is a diagnosis of exclusion after eliminating other causes of renovascular hypertension. Extrarenal sites, such as adrenals, colon, lung, ovary, have been reported. Surgical excision is the therapy of choice.

Endocrine causes

Liddle syndrome is an inherited condition characterized by hypertension, metabolic alkalosis, urinary loss of potassium, and suppressed renin and aldosterone secretion. Proximal renal tubular acidosis is common and agents that inhibit sodium reabsorption in the distal tubule may be effective.

Phaeochromocytoma is a tumour of neuroectodermal origin that produces excess amounts of catecholamines (Mittendorf *et al.* 2007), explaining the rise in BP and the constellation of symptoms that accompany this disorder. The triad of headache, sweating, and palpitations is classically seen. Plasma-free metanephrines or urinary fractionated metanephrines measurements are the most sensitive and specific tests for diagnosis. Abdominal computed tomography or magnetic resonance imaging can be performed as a means of tumour localization. A mass can be further localized with ^{123}I-metaiodobenzylguanidine scanning, which has 95–100% specificity. Surgical treatment is the only effective therapeutic approach, be it benign (90%) or malignant (10%). Adequate preoperative management includes volume replacement and drug therapy that offers pure alpha-blockade. Beta-blockers are contraindicated.

Primary hyperaldosteronism is considered when hypertension and hypokalaemia co-exist. Patients may present with mild hypokalaemic alkalosis, but if hypokalaemia is severe they may present with weakness, polyuria, polydipsia, and nocturia. The diagnosis can be established with a serum potassium of <3.0 mEq/L, inappropriate urinary K^+ wasting (>30 mmol), a reduced plasma renin activity (<1.0 ng/mL/hour) and elevated 24-hour urinary aldosterone. Thin slice (2–3 mm) computed tomography is used to determine whether the cause is bilateral adrenal hyperplasia or unilateral adenoma. Adrenal vein sampling is done if imaging is negative and biochemical analyses support hyperaldosteronism. Unilateral adrenal adenomas are best treated surgically, whereas aldosterone receptor blockade is indicated in patients with bilateral hyperplasia or those at high operative risk.

Cushing syndrome results from prolonged exposure to excess glucocorticoids. The most common cause is iatrogenic as a consequence of exogenous steroid administration; the non-iatrogenic causes can be separated into ACTH-dependent and ACTH-independent causes. Diagnosis includes determination of 24-hour urinary free cortisol and the dexamethasone suppression test; 24-hour urinary cortisol should be measured as a confirmatory test. The preferred approach in Cushing's syndrome is selective excision of the pituitary adenoma by transphenoidal surgery. Adrenalectomy is done with cases of adrenal adenomas, micronodular or macronodular hyperplasia, and carcinoma. Medical management is reserved for extensive and inoperable diseases, with ketoconazole being the agent of choice. Other medical options include mitotane and mifepristone.

Hyperthyroidism is an uncommon cause of hypertension and associated with a predominant systolic component. Common symptoms include palpitations, tremor, fatigue, hyperactivity, insomnia, heat intolerance, weight loss, nocturia, diarrhoea, oligomenorrhoea, and emotional lability. Physical examination may reveal tachycardia, hypertension, hyperthermia, moist skin, lid lag, brisk reflexes, and hyperdynamic precordium. Correction of overactive thyroid activity and symptomatic management is the cornerstone of treatment. Beta-blockers are the drug of choice to control symptoms. Hypothyroidism is associated with diastolic hypertension and occurs in 20% of these patients. Elevations in TSH confirm hypothyroidism and levothyroxine is the drug of choice.

Primary hyperparathyroidism manifests as hypercalcaemia with hypophosphataemia and non-specific symptoms of weakness, lethargy, abdominal discomfort, and constipation. The pathophysiology of hypertension in hyperparathyroidism is unclear, but vasoconstriction associated with calcium levels is postulated. Surgical removal of the parathyroid gland or adenoma is the definitive treatment, and calcium antagonists may be used to help BP control.

Vascular causes

Coarctation of the aorta is a constriction that can occur anywhere in the aorta, but is most commonly found just distal to the subclavian artery (Chiong *et al.* 2008). The physical examination is typical of elevated upper extremity BP relative to the lower extremities. Patients may also present with weak femoral pulses during simultaneous palpation of the upper and lower extremity pulse. Screening tests include either transthoracic or transoesophageal echocardiography. Surgical intervention is the treatment of choice.

Neurogenic hypertension

Increase in intracranial pressure can produce substantial elevations in systemic BP. Hypertension following a closed-head injury, subarachnoid haemorrhage or acute stroke is typically transient or episodic. Treatment using nimodpine or other calcium antagonist is preferred for treatment of systemic hypertension. Brain tumours, especially in the supratentorial space or the posterior fossa, may also be associated with labile hypertension. Treatment with surgery or radiation results in normalization of BP.

Autonomic hyper-reflexia is a syndrome described in patients with cervical or high thoracic spinal cord injuries. Hypertension may develop in quadriplegic patients due to uncontrolled sympathetic output. Polyneuritis of the afferent limb of baroreflexes causes autonomic dysfunction, as seen in Guillain–Barré syndrome. Management of hypertensive episodes is difficult but best managed with short-acting parenteral agents that can be rapidly titrated and also inhibit the sympathetic system, such as beta-blockers.

Autonomic failure is characterized by orthostatic hypotension, inadequate heart rate response, and bowel, bladder, and erectile dysfunction. The most striking presentation is orthostatic hypertension. Hypertension in these types of patients is treated with drugs that decrease sympathetic tone or block alpha-adrenergic receptors.

Obstructive sleep apnoea

Obstructive sleep apnoea (OSA) is characterized by repetitive episodes of upper airway narrowing, occurring up to several hundred times per night in severe cases (Okcay *et al.* 2008). The apnoeic episodes give rise to increased sympathetic tone that results from hypoxemia and reoxygenation, leading to increases in peripheral vasoconstriction and attendant rises in BP. Continuous positive airway pressure (CPAP) is the most effective form of therapy for OSA. It has been shown to acutely attenuate sympathetic drive and nocturnal BP. As most patients with OSA are obese, weight loss is also a very effective treatment for OSA.

Illicit and therapeutic drug use

A variety of chemical substances can induce either a transient or persistent increase in BP (Grossman and Messerli 2008). Cocaine use is a common cause of hypertension. Agents containing steroids or steroid-like materials, including liquorice, carbenoxolone, ketoconazole, skin ointments, antihaemorrhoidal preparations, ophthalmic drops, nasal spray, and oral contraceptive, may activate the sympathetic nervous system. Anaesthetics and sympathomimetics also activate the sympathetic nervous system. Antiemetic drugs, such as metoclopramide, alizapride, and prochlorperazine, have also been reported. Cyclosporine A, tacrolimus, paclitaxel, cis-diamminedichloroplatinum, bevacizumab, sorafenib, sunitinib, and recombinant human erythropoietin all increases BP by either increasing endothelin or altering blood viscosity. Non-steroidal anti-inflammatory medications increase BP and interfere with antihypertensive medications, with the exception of calcium antagonists.

Obesity

Obesity is a common underlying cause of secondary hypertension. Multiple mechanisms have been suggested including elevated volume, vasoconstriction, enhanced cardiac output, and increases in aldosterone induced by the adipocyte.

Treatment for obese patients with hypertension is not well defined, but weight reduction and use of aldosterone blockers with calcium antagonists is effective. Four or more antihypertensive agents may be needed in some cases (Chiong *et al.* 2008).

Paroxysmal hypertension

Stress and emotion play a role in patients with paroxysmal hypertension. Pseudo-phaeochromocytoma is described as paroxysmal hypertension in the absence of phaeochromocytoma (Pickering and Clemow 2008). The hypertensive episodes are accompanied by tachycardia, sweating, flushing, nervousness, shaking, and other manifestations of acute sympathetic activation. Panic symptoms of autonomic origin are common in the attacks experienced by hypertensive patients. The role of hyperventilation in causing hypertension is unclear. All patients with paroxysmal hypertension should be screened for phaeochromocytoma. If the results are negative and the symptoms are consistent, evaluation for panic disorder and hyperventilation is appropriate. Treatment is focused on two areas: controlling the pressure and treating the underlying panic or anxiety state. It has been suggested that combined alpha- and beta-blockade may be beneficial in such patients.

References

Chiong JR, Aronow WS, Khan IA, *et al.* Secondary hypertension: current diagnosis and treatment. *Int J Cardiol* 2008;**124**:6–21.

Grossman E, Messerli FH. Secondary hypertension: interfering substances. *J Clin Hypertens (Greenwich)* 2008;**10**:556–66.

Mittendorf EA, Evans DB, Lee JE, Perrier ND. Pheochromocytoma: advances in genetics, diagnosis, localization, and treatment. *Hematol Oncol Clin North Am* 2007;**21**:509–25.

Okcay A, Somers VK, Caples SM. Obstructive sleep apnea and hypertension. *J Clin Hypertens (Greenwich)* 2008;**10**:549–55.

Pickering TG, Clemow L. Paroxysmal hypertension: the role of stress and psychological factors. *J Clin Hypertens (Greenwich)* 2008;**10**:575–81.

Taler SJ. Secondary causes of hypertension. *Prim Care* 2008;**35**: 489–500.

Hypertensive emergencies

Definition

A hypertensive emergency is said to be present when a severe elevation in blood pressure (BP), such as a diastolic BP above 120–130 mmHg is associated with an immediate threat to the integrity of the cardiovascular system (Table 4.6.1).

Patients with a hypertensive emergency require an immediate reduction in BP (not necessarily to normal levels) to avoid end-organ damage, generally by means of intravenous therapy in an intensive care setting.

Unlike a hypertensive emergency, patients with severe elevation in BP who have no evidence of progressive end-organ injury are classified as having 'hypertensive urgency' and require only a gradual reduction in BP over a period of 12–24 hours, often with oral therapy.

Clinical presentations

Hypertensive emergency (includes malignant phase hypertension)

Hypertensive emergency has replaced the old term malignant hypertension, by including all cases of elevated BP associated with acute target organ damage, in addition to malignant hypertension per se.

Clinical features

A proportion of patients with a hypertension emergency are asymptomatic or present at a late stage in their disease. Complications associated with hypertensive emergency can include neurological syndromes, myocardial ischaemia and infarction, acute left ventricular dysfunction, aortic dissection, acute renal failure, microangiopathic haemolytic anaemia and eclampsia.

Hypertensive encephalopathy

Hypertensive encephalopathy refers to the presence of symptoms or signs of cerebral oedema often caused by BP breaking through the autoregulatory threshold associated with hyperperfusion of the cerebral vascular bed, either from very severe hypertension or from sudden increase in BP. It is usually characterized by headache, nausea, and vomiting, followed by visual disturbances and fluctuating, diffuse neurological symptoms such as restlessness, confusion, and, if the hypertension is not treated, seizures and

coma. Papilloedema is frequently, although not universally, present. Hypertensive encephalopathy is often indistinguishable from other acute neurological complications of hypertension, i.e. cerebral infarction, subarachnoidal bleeding, or intracerebral haemorrhage. The only definite criterion to confirm diagnosis of hypertensive encephalopathy is a prompt improvement in the patient's condition in response to antihypertensive therapy. Computed tomography (CT) and magnetic resonance imaging (MRI) can help to confirm the diagnosis by excluding other neurological diseases.

Severe hypertension with acute stroke

Up to 80% of patients admitted with acute stoke will have increased BP. Usually BP will decrease spontaneously over the first week. There is no evidence of benefits or absence thereof of BP reduction in this clinical setting. Too rapid aggressive reduction of BP during acute stroke could be hazardous and should be avoided. Current national guidelines recommend lowering BP during stroke only if end-organ damage is present or if systolic/diastolic BP exceeds 220/120 or 185/110 mmHg in patients ineligible and in those eligible to receive thrombolytic drug therapy, respectively.

Severe hypertension with intracerebral haemorrhage

As a result of intracerebral haemorrhage (ICH), intracerebral pressure rises and higher intra-arterial pressure is required to perfuse the brain adequately. In this condition, hypertension may be a result of increased intracerebral pressure and may resolve spontaneously within 48 hours.

Rapid reduction in BP may indeed prevent further bleeding, but at the risk of cerebral hypoperfusion. Thus, there is no consensus with regard to the advisability of reducing BP in these patients. BP reduction should probably not exceed 20% of pre-treatment BP level. If BP is extremely elevated (diastolic pressure greater than 140 mmHg) and last more than 20 minutes, intravenous treatment is recommended.

Hypertension with heart failure or ischaemic event

Severe hypertension results in a significant increase in afterload that causes cardiac decompensation with pulmonary congestion and/or pulmonary oedema.

In patients with myocardial infarction or unstable angina an excessively high BP (>180/110 mmHg) is a definite contraindication to thrombolytic treatment. The therapeutic strategy should be focused on protecting the ischaemic myocardium. The reduction in BP should not be abrupt, and a gradual reduction over a period of 24 hours is recommended, so that further myocardial or brain ischaemia is avoided.

Hypertension with aortic dissection

Aortic dissection occurs from an intimal tear that allows the passage of blood into the media, creating a false subintimal channel within the outer medial and adventitial layers of the aorta. The dissection can extend either proximally or distally, potentially leading to cardiac tamponade, aortic regurgitation, aortic rupture, or occlusion of side branches, with end-organ ischaemia.

The majority of patients are male smokers, around the sixth decade, but pregnant women can also be affected in

Table 4.6.1 Definition of a hypertensive emergency

Moderate to severe elevation of arterial pressure associated with
1 Malignant hypertension*
2 Intracranial haemorrhage
3 Atherothrombotic cerebral infarction
4 Acute congestive heart failure
5 Acute coronary insufficiency
6 Acute renal insufficiency
7 Acute aortic dissection
8 Eclampsia

*A syndrome characterized by elevated BP accompanied by encephalopathy or nephropathy or by papilloedema and/or microangiopathic haemolytic anaemia.

labour, particularly if they have Marfan's syndrome. Typically, dissection presents with a sudden, severe, retrosternal chest pain that radiates posteriorly to the inter scapular region or the base of the neck. Signs may include new-onset aortic regurgitation, a difference in BP between the two arms, absent pulses, or evidence of haemorrhage. Aortic dissection may also present with an acute abdomen, stroke, or myocardial infarction. Most untreated patients die within 1 year, and most of the deaths occur within 2 weeks. Once diagnosis is suspected attempts should be made to decrease the shear stress to the aortic wall with suitable agents. BP should be reduced within 15–30 minutes to the lowest tolerated level that preserves adequate organ perfusion.

Renal failure in hypertensive emergency
Renal involvement in hypertensive emergency has been referred to as malignant nephrosclerosis, leading to acute renal failure, haematuria, and proteinuria. Urea and creatinine concentrations at presentation are independent predictors of survival.

Retinopathy in hypertensive emergency
Retinal flame-shaped haemorrhages, cotton-wool spots, and hard exudates, or a combination of these signs are defined as moderately severe retinopathy and corresponding to grade 3 of the Keith, Wagener, and Barker classification. When these findings co-exist with swelling of the optic disc it is defined as malignant retinopathy and the prognosis is poor. It should be noted that similar retinal appearances can be seen in patients with severe anaemia, connective tissue disease, and infective endocarditis. Benign intracranial hypertension may cause bilateral papilloedema that is usually self-limiting and minimally symptomatic. Nevertheless, severe hypertension and lone bilateral papilloedema may represent a variant of malignant hypertension, with similar clinical features and prognosis.

Severe pre-eclampsia or eclampsia
Pregnancy-induced hypertension (BP >140/90 mmHg) after the twentieth week of pregnancy that is associated with proteinuria (>300 mg/L) is often referred to as pre-eclampsia.

Clinical symptoms are common, with generalized puffiness, frontal headaches, and visual symptoms. Papilloedema may be seen. There may be epigastric pain because of hepatic oedema and brisk reflexes and ankle clonus. Urgent antihypertensive and anticonvulsant treatment is needed.

When these findings are associated with nausea, vomiting, and convulsions it is defined as eclampsia. Eclampsia is a hypertensive emergency that is associated with a high incidence of both maternal and fetal death. It is usually occurs in labour or in the puerperium. However, postpartum eclampsia has been described even 41 days after delivery. Convulsions may be preceded by auras, epigastric pain, apprehension, and hyper-reflexia, although there is little or no warning in many cases. After intense tonic–clonic seizures, the patient may become stuporous or comatose. Another complication is cortical blindness, which results in visual loss caused by petechial haemorrhages and focal oedema in the occipital cortex. Other complications include pulmonary oedema, renal failure, hepatic failure, papilloedema, retinal haemorrhages or even detachment, and cerebrovascular accidents.

Diagnostic techniques
Selection of diagnostic tests depend upon the condition and the clinical state of the patient. In severe hypertensive emergencies, such as aortic dissection, hypertensive left ventricular failure and hypertensive encephalopathy, the patient may be far too ill to undertake any 'routine' investigations for hypertension, and the strategy is to stabilize the patient, make the diagnosis and correct the problem. In contrast, many patients with hypertensive emergency present with only mild symptoms of visual disturbance, headaches, or dizziness, allowing full investigation and exclusion of secondary causes of hypertension. After stabilizations the 'work-up' of all patients with hypertensive crises should include investigations to exclude secondary hypertension, assessment of additional risk factors and co-morbidity, and evidence of target organ damage.

Evaluation of patients with hypertensive emergency
Early triage is critical in an effort to assure the most appropriate therapy for each patient. A brief but thorough history should address the duration as well as the severity of hypertension, all current medications, including prescription and non-prescription drugs, and the use of recreational drugs. Information regarding neurological, cardiovascular, and/or renal symptoms and specific manifestations, such as headache, seizures, chest pain, dyspnoea, and oedema, is important for the correct diagnosis. A history of other co-morbid conditions and prior cardiovascular or renal disease is critical for the initial evaluation.

Physical assessment should start with BP measurement in both arms. A careful cardiovascular examination including auscultation of aorta, renal arteries, palpation of femoral pulses, as well as a thorough neurological and fundoscopic examination should be conducted.

Initial laboratory evaluation should include urinalysis with sediment examination, a stat chemistry profile, blood count, electrocardiogram, and an echocardiogram. Proteinuria, red blood cells, and/or cellular casts in the urine are suggestive of renal parenchymal disease. Anaemia with fragmented red blood cells suggests microangiopathic haemolytic anaemia. Electrolyte abnormalities and evidence of renal dysfunction may suggest secondary hypertension. The electrocardiogram should identify evidence of coronary ischaemia and left ventricular hypertrophy, and differences in BP levels between arms should raise the question of aortic dissection. A CT scan or MRI of the head should be considered when encephalopathy or cerebrovascular ischaemia or haemorrhage are suspected, or in a comatose patient. The initial evaluation should help to decide whether to treat the patient with hypertensive crisis as an emergency or urgency (Fig. 4.6.1). The decision to treat as an emergency should prompt immediate admission to an intensive care unit for intravenous treatment and continuous BP monitoring.

Management
The initial goal of the antihypertensive therapy is *not* to rapidly normalize BP but rather to prevent damage to target organs by gradually decreasing BP, while minimizing the risk of hypoperfusion.

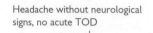

High blood pressure (e.g. >220/120 mm Hg)

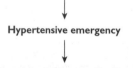

Neurological signs (hypertensive encephalopathy, haemorrhagic or ischaemic stroke).
Hypertensive retinopathy—grade 3–4.
Chest pain as a presenting symptom of ischaemic heart disease or dissecting aortic aneurysm.
Pulmonary oedema, toxaemia, catecholamine excess, acute renal failure.

Hypertensive emergency

Intravenous treatment with close monitoring in intensive care unit.
Oral treatment should be added

Headache without neurological signs, no acute TOD

Hypertensive urgency

Identify the cause

Anxiety—anti-anxiety treatment
Pain—analgesic
Unknown cause—oral antihypertensive treatment to lower blood pressure within 12–24 hours

Fig. 4.6.1 The approach to hypertensive crisis, adapted from *Comprehensive Hypertension* edited by Gregory YH Lip and John E. Hall, Fig. 1, copyright Elsevier (2007).

The urgency of interventions depends on the clinical syndrome. For example, uncomplicated malignant-phase hypertension is associated with target organ damage, which occurs over days or weeks rather than minutes, and can be referred to as a hypertensive 'urgency' rather than an emergency. By contrast, hypertensive encephalopathy, hypertensive left ventricular failure, and aortic dissection can be immediately life threatening and are more typical 'hypertensive emergencies'. Similarly, eclampsia (or severe pre-eclampsia) can result in a high maternal and fetal morbidity and mortality, if immediate and effective antihypertensive therapy is not initiated.

In hypertensive urgencies immediate and rapid reduction of BP with parenteral drugs is not indicated and aggressive treatment may place the patient at unnecessary risk. Oral antihypertensive therapy should be given. However, sublingual nifedipine should not be used in view of the negligible oral absorption, the unpredictable hypotensive effects, and an increased risk of arrhythmias, stroke, or worsening cardiac ischaemia or infarction. Clonidine loading is now a less popular choice for the treatment of hypertensive urgency.

In true emergency initial parenteral treatment should be started. Drug selection should be based on the severity of the emergency and on the specific case.

Parenteral agents

Parenteral therapy requires intensive care monitoring and should be restricted to severe hypertensive emergencies.

Several parenteral agents are available for the treatment of hypertensive emergencies. It should be noted that no outcome studies are available assessing or comparing antihypertensive therapy in hypertensive emergencies and that therefore most of the following guidelines are empirical.

Labetalol

Labetalol is a combined alpha- and beta-blocker. It is contraindicated in patients with asthma, chronic obstructive lung disease, congestive heart failure, bradycardia, and atrioventricular block. It has rapid onset of action (5 minutes or less). Labetalol can be given as an intravenous bolus or infusion. The bolus dose is 20 mg initially, followed by 20–80 mg every 10 minutes to a total dose of 300 mg. The infusion rate is 0.5–2 mg/min.

Intravenous nitrates cause venous dilatation at low doses and both arteriolar and venous dilatation at higher doses. They are of limited value in hypertensive encephalopathy because of headache, which frequently occurs with the doses required to reduce BP. Nitrates are most useful in patients with symptomatic coronary disease and in postoperative hypertension or hypertensive heart failure. The initial dose of glyceryl trinitrate is 5 μg/min, which can be increased as necessary to a maximum of 100 μg/min. The onset of action is 2–5 minutes, and the duration of action is 5–10 minutes. Headache and tachycardia are the primary side-effects.

Fenoldopam

Fenoldopam is a selective postsynaptic dopaminergic (DA1) receptor agonist with weak α_2-antagonistic properties. Fenoldopam is a natriuretic agent that has a potent vasodilator activity affecting primarily the renal vasculature.

The onset of action is within 5 minutes with the maximal response being achieved by 15 minutes. The duration of action is between 30 and 60 minutes with the pressure gradually returning to pre-treatment values without rebound upon termination of the drug. At a dose of 0.2–0.5 μg/kg/min, fenoldopam decreases BP to desired levels within 5–40 minutes. Side-effects include headache, flushing, tachycardia, and dizziness. A dose-related increase in intraocular pressure has been observed. It seems that fenoldopam can be the drug of choice in severely hypertensive patients with impaired renal function.

Nicardipine

Nicardipine is a dihydropyridine calcium antagonist with high vascular selectivity that can be administered intravenously. Its onset of action is between 5 and 10 minutes, with duration of action of 15–90 minutes. The drug may preserve tissue perfusion, and therefore may be advantageous in patients with ischaemic disorders, such as coronary, cerebrovascular, and peripheral vascular disease. The drug is given as a continuous infusion at a starting dose of 5 mg/hour followed by increments of 2.5 mg/hour every 5 minutes until either reaching a maximal dose of 30 mg/hour or achieving the desired reduction in BP. Side-effects include headache, hypotension, and nausea. Patients receiving intravenous nicardipine can then be easily switched to oral medication.

Sodium nitroprusside

Sodium nitroprusside is a direct vasodilator that acts on both arteriolar and venous vessels. It is a potentially dangerous drug, and should be administered only in the intensive care unit, where constant BP monitoring is available. Nitroprusside is metabolized to thiocyanate, potentially leading to the development of cyanide or, rarely, thiocyanate toxicity, which may be fatal. This problem, which is manifested by clinical deterioration, altered mental status and lactic acidosis, can be minimized by treatment for as short a time as possible using the lowest dose possible and by careful monitoring of the patient. Thiocyanate concentration should be measured after 48 hours of infusion. If blood levels exceed 1.7 mmol/L the infusion should be stopped. Nitroprusside should not be given to pregnant women. The drug has a rapid onset (1–2 minutes) and short duration of action (1–5 minutes). The drug is administered as a titrated continuous infusion with a starting dose of 0.25–0.5 µg/kg/min, which can be increased as necessary to a maximum dose of 8–10 µg/kg/min, although use of these higher doses should generally be avoided or limited to a maximum duration of 10 minutes. It is inactivated by light and should therefore be protected during the infusion.

Considering the potential toxicity, this drug should only be used when other intravenous antihypertensive agents are not available and then, only in specific clinical circumstances in patients with normal renal and hepatic functions.

Esmolol

Esmolol is an ultra-short-acting β1-selective adrenergic blocker. The onset of action is within 60–120 seconds and the duration of action is about 10–30 minutes. Esmolol can be easily titrated to the desired effect. The drug can be administered either as a bolus injection or as a continuous intravenous infusion. The recommended loading dose is a bolus of 250–500 µg/kg/min followed by an infusion of 50–100 µg/kg/min. Esmolol is frequently combined with direct vasodilators to provide a more desirable haemodynamic profile.

Urapidil

Urapidil is a selective postsynaptic α1-adrenoreceptor antagonist with strong vasodilating properties. Urapidil has a rapid onset of action and a high rate of response. It is given as an intravenous bolus at a dose of 12.5–25 mg followed by a continuous infusion at a rate of 5–40 mg/hour. It has no effect on coronary sinus blood flow, myocardial oxygen consumption, and myocardial lactate extraction, and it does not increase intracranial pressure. Adverse effects occur in 2% of all patients and include hypotension, headache, and dizziness. Urapidil is currently not approved by the FDA in the United States, but it is available in Europe.

Enalaprilat

Enalaprilat is the only available angiotensin-converting enzyme inhibitor that can be administered intravenously. Enalaprilat lowers BP within 15–30 minutes, but the BP response is unpredictable. The initial recommended dose is 0.625–1.25 mg administered over 5 minutes. The maximal single dose should not exceed 5 mg for patients receiving diuretics and 1.25 mg for patients with renal impairment. The initial dose can be repeated after 1 hour if clinical response is inadequate. The total daily dose should not exceed 20 mg. In patients with severe renal insufficiency the dose should be decreased because the compound is excreted primarily by the kidney. Enalaprilat may induce a dramatic fall in BP in patients who are volume depleted. It is contraindicated in patients with bilateral renal artery stenosis or unilateral stenosis of a single kidney. Enalaprilat is particularly useful in hypertensive emergencies associated with congestive heart failure or high renin levels, and can be easily replaced by oral enalapril for long-term maintenance therapy.

Arterial vasodilators

Use of diazoxide or hydralazine is rarely indicated. A beta-blocker such as propranolol or labetalol is usually given concurrently to block reflex tachycardia. It is recommended that these agents should not be used in patients with angina pectoris, myocardial infarction, pulmonary oedema, or a dissecting aortic aneurysm. Diazoxide can also cause marked fluid retention, and a loop diuretic may need to be added if oedema or otherwise unexplained weight gain is noted. Diazoxide is also longer acting and, in the currently recommended doses, requires less monitoring than nitroprusside, because the peak effect is seen within 15 minutes and lasts for 4–24 hours.

Hydralazine is currently used in pregnant women in the management of severe pre-eclampsia. The initial dose is 5–10 mg intravenously, with the maximum dose being 20 mg. The decrease in BP begins within 10–30 minutes and lasts 2–4 hours.

Phentolamine

Phentolamine is a parenteral non-specific α-adrenergic blocker with rapid onset and short-lasting hypotensive effect. It is given intravenously in boluses of 5–10 mg as necessary. Adverse effects include tachycardia, vomiting, and headache. In patients with coronary artery disease phentolamine may induce angina pectoris or myocardial infarction. It is specifically useful in treatment of catecholamine-mediated hypertensive crises. However, it is

Table 4.6.2 Preferred agents for specific hypertensive emergency

Emergency condition	Preferred agent	Comments
Hypertensive encephalopathy	Labetalol, fenoldopam, nicardipine, clevidipine sodium nitroprusside, or urapidil	Avoid methyldopa and diazoxide
Cerebrovascular accident	Sodium nitroprusside, labetalol, urapidil, esmolol, clevidine, nicardipine, nimodipine	Benefit from acute lowering of BP is uncertain
Acute left ventricular failure	Fenoldopam, or sodium nitroprusside with nitroglycerin, enalaprilat, urapidil, furosemide, morphine	Avoid labetalol, esmolol, diazoxide, hydralazine
Coronary insufficiency	Nitroglycerin, labetalol, esmolol, clevidipine, nicardipine	BP should be reduced gradually. Avoid hydralazine, diazoxide
Dissecting aortic aneurysm	Labetalol, or combination of clevidipine or nicardipine or fenoldopam or sodium nitroprusside with a beta-blocker or trimethaphan	Titrate BP to the lowest possible level. Avoid hydralazine, diazoxide
Perioperative hypertension	Clevidipine, sodium nitroprusside, nitroglycerin, labetalol, urapidil, esmolol, nicardipine	Nitroglycerine is preferred in managing post-coronary bypass hypertension
Eclampsia	Hydralazine, labetalol, urapidil, calcium antagonists	Avoid diuretics, trimethaphan, sodium nitroprusside, ACE inhibitor
Catecholamine excess	Phentolamine, labetalol	Avoid diuretics, sodium nitroprusside
Renal insufficiency	Fenoldopam, clevidipine, nicardipine, labetalol	Avoid beta-blockers, sodium nitroprusside

not consistently effective in other types of hypertensive emergencies.

Clevidipine

Clevidipine, a third-generation, intravenous, ultra-short-acting dihydropyridine calcium channel antagonist, has been approved in the United States for the management of perioperative hypertension and other hypertensive crises. Clevidipine is a potent arterial vasodilator with very little or no effect of the myocardial contractility and venous capacitance. Its short half-life allows easy titration and the drug is rapidly metabolized by tissue and plasma esterases. Clevidipine can protect against organ reperfusion injury and can augment endothelial nitric oxide bioavailability via antioxidative actions. Because of its user-friendly characteristics it promises to become the drug of choice for many if not most hypertensive emergencies.

Treatment of specific hypertensive emergencies

There is a multiplicity of disorders or diseases accompanying elevated BP that constitute a hypertensive emergency; and there is a broad spectrum of pharmacological agents that may be selected for treatment of these cases. Some agents that are useful for one hypertensive emergency may

actually be contraindicated for another. The recommended therapeutic approach for specific conditions is summarized in Table 4.6.2.

Further reading

Aggarwal M, Khan IA. Hypertensive crisis: hypertensive emergencies and urgencies. *Cardiol Clin* 2006;**24**:135–46.

Grossman E, Messerli FH, Grodzicki T, Kowey P. Should a moratorium be placed on sublingual nifedipine capsules given for hypertensive emergencies and pseudoemergencies?. *JAMA* 1996;**276**:1328–31.

Grossman E, Ironi AN, Messerli FH. Comparative tolerability profile of hypertensive crisis treatments. *Drug Saf* 1998;**19**:99–122.

Lip GY, Beevers M, Beevers G. The failure of malignant hypertension to decline: a survey of 24 years' experience in a multiracial population in England. *J Hypertens* 1994;**12**:1297–305.

Lip GY, Beevers M, Potter JF, Beevers DG. Malignant hypertension in the elderly. *QJM* 1995;**88**:641–7.

Ram CV. Immediate management of severe hypertension. *Cardiol Clin* 1995;**13**:579–91.

Varon J, Marik PE. Clinical review: the management of hypertensive crises. *Crit Care* 2003;**7**:374–84.

Varon J. Treatment of acute severe hypertension: current and newer agents. *Drugs* 2008;**68**:283–97.

Vidt DG. Emergency room management of hypertensive urgencies and emergencies. *J Clin Hypertens (Greenwich)* 2001;**3**:158–64.

Chapter 5

Ischaemic heart disease

Risk factors for ischaemic heart disease

A number of risk factors have been identified that predispose to ischaemic heart disease (IHD). Risk factors are conveniently classified as reversible and irreversible.

Prevention of IHD

In healthy populations, lifestyle modification and drugs to lower blood pressure and cholesterol can delay or prevent disease development in high-risk individuals. This is called 'primary prevention' and must be distinguished from 'secondary prevention' in which similar measures are applied in patients with established IHD to prevent myocardial infarction and coronary death.

Risk scores

Risk assessment tools quantify cumulative effects of multiple risk factors on the 10-year risk of developing IHD in asymptomatic individuals. These tools are used to guide the need for primary prevention in those with a 10-year risk of IHD that exceeds 20%. The Framingham score (Anderson et al. 1991) has been widely used, which calculates risk from an individual's age, gender, total and high-density lipoprotein (HDL) cholesterol, smoking habit, and systolic blood pressure. Because the score is based on the Framingham cohort in Massachusetts, its relevance has been questioned for the UK, where there is now increasing interest in Q-Risk, which uses a risk algorithm based on UK primary care data (Hippisley-Cox et al. 2007). Also widely used are colour-coded charts that predict risk without the need for an electronic device to enter data (British Cardiac Society 1998).

Reversible risk factors

These are important clinically because their avoidance or correction may protect against the development or progression of IHD. In INTERHEART, a case–control study conducted in 52 countries, just nine 'potentially modifiable' risk factors were found to account for >90% of the population attributable risk of myocardial infarction in all regions of the world (Yusuf et al. 2004). This implies that the risk of myocardial infarction, and other manifestations of IHD, could be substantially reduced on a global scale by avoidance or modification of these risk factors.

Smoking

The risk of IHD rises in proportion to the number of cigarettes smoked. In INTERHEART, current smokers had nearly three times the risk of heart attack than non-smokers. Smokers also put at risk those exposed to their second-hand smoke, a fact that has driven the introduction of smoke-free legislation in many countries (Jamrozik 2005). Smoke-free legislation has already produced substantial reductions in rates of myocardial infarction (Pell and Haw 2009), consistent with earlier observations that quitting smoking can decrease IHD risk to levels similar to people who have never smoked (Rosenberg et al. 1985). Smoking cessation is a key strategy in the prevention of IHD.

Hypertension

The IHD risk attributable to hypertension increases with both systolic and diastolic measurements. In INTERHEART, hypertension was associated with a twofold increased risk of myocardial infarction. A persistently raised blood pressure ≥160/100 mmHg (≥140/90 mmHg in diabetes) that

has not responded to lifestyle modification provides indication for treatment. The benefits of antihypertensive treatment for reducing risk of stroke have never been questioned, and it is now clear that parallel benefits exist for reducing IHD risk, there being no 'normal level' below which further reductions in blood pressure are not potentially beneficial. Current targets for treatment are <140/85 mmHg (<130/80 mmHg in diabetes).

Dyslipidaemia

The coronary risk attributable to hypercholesterolaemia increases almost linearly with blood cholesterol levels, the low-density lipoprotein (LDL) component being particularly damaging while the HDL component is protective. The total cholesterol/HDL ratio has been widely used as a measure of coronary risk, and is a central component of the Framingham risk score algorithm. Other lipid fractions may be yet more sensitive in risk assessment, and in INTERHEART the ratio of ApoB to ApoA1 showed a stepwise association with myocardial infarction, with a more than threefold risk for the highest quintile group. About 1:500 individuals have familial hypercholesterolaemia (FH), an inherited disorder with a high risk of premature IHD. FH requires treatment with dietary modification and statins, which should also be offered to individuals whose 10-year IHD risk is >20%.

Diabetes

In the Framingham study, diabetes increased the risk of IHD by 66% in men and >200% in women (Kannel and McGee 1997). In INTERHEART, diabetes was associated with a more than twofold risk of myocardial infarction. Subclinical glucose intolerance also increases risk (Fuller et al. 1983). Strict glycaemic control continues to be recommended in patients with diabetes to protect against microvascular complications, particularly retinal and glomerular damage, but there is little evidence that this affects the risk of IHD. Probably more important is aggressive management of lifestyle and other risk factors, particularly hypertension and dyslipidaemia.

Obesity

The obesity epidemic in Western societies is driving a parallel epidemic of diabetes, dyslipidaemia, and hypertension, all of which contribute to its association with IHD. However, obesity is itself a potent inflammatory stimulus showing independent association with IHD and because it often develops in childhood is emerging as a major risk factor for the development of premature disease in young adults. In INTERHEART, the highest tertile of abdominal obesity was associated with a 62% increased risk of myocardial infarction. Treatment of obesity is difficult, but there are likely to be direct benefits for IHD prevention as well as indirect benefits through diabetic, blood pressure and lipid control.

Psychosocial factors

The association with IHD is best documented for depression, a study of medical students followed up for 40 years showing that those who reported clinical depression had a more than twofold greater risk for subsequent IHD (Ford et al. 1998). Stress at work may also increase risk (Marmot et al. 1997), and when a package of psychosocial exposures were referenced against non-exposure in INTERHEART there was a nearly threefold greater risk for myocardial infarction. Whether treatment of depression reduces coronary risk is unknown.

Sedentary lifestyle

Ever since the demonstration of increased cardiovascular risk for London bus drivers compared with conductors, there has emerged a substantial literature confirming that a sedentary lifestyle increases the risk of IHD. Even relatively low levels of exercise taken regularly are beneficial, a study of >70 000 middle-aged women showing that brisk walking was as effective as vigorous exercise (Manson et al. 1999). In INTERHEART, exercise was associated with a 14% reduction in the risk of myocardial infarction.

Diet

The high-fat diet of Western societies has contributed importantly to the epidemic of IHD, but there is now evidence for reduced coronary risk associated with the 'Mediterranean' diet in which bread, fruit, vegetables, and fish predominate over meat, and butter and cheese products are largely replaced by vegetable and plant oils (Mente et al. 2009). In INTERHEART, a diet rich in fruit and vegetables was associated with a 30% reduction in the risk of myocardial infarction.

Alcohol

Multiple studies have reported an inverse association between alcohol consumption and IHD. Although 'abstainer error' related to sick individuals who quit drinking is a potential bias, studies that have included a sufficient number of never-drinkers suggest the observation is robust (Arriola et al. 2009). In INTERHEART, the effect of alcohol consumption was modest, being associated with a 9% lower risk of myocardial infarction. It is appropriate, therefore, to permit alcohol consumption within safe limits in individuals at increased risk of IHD.

Irreversible risk factors

These, by definition, are not amenable to modification and clinical relevance therefore is confined to risk prediction and not to treatment.

Age and gender

Incidence and mortality rates for IHD increase with age at an accelerating rate, delayed by about 10 years in women. After the age of 60, rates in women become comparable with men.

Family history

A history of premature IHD among parents doubles an individual's risk, independently of shared risk factors such as smoking, dyslipidaemia, and hypertension. The risk increases further if both a parent and sibling have a history of IHD (Nasir et al. 2007). The genetic basis for IHD is complex and has not yet been defined.

Further reading

Anderson KM, Odell PM, Wilson PW, Kannel WB. Cardiovascular disease risk profiles. Am Heart J 1991;**121**:293–8.

Arriola L, Martinez-Camblor P, Larrañaga N, et al. Alcohol intake and the Risk of coronary heart disease in the Spanish EPIC cohort study. Heart 2010;**96**:124–30.

British Cardiac Society Working Party; British Hyperlipidaemia Association and British Hypertension Society. Joint British recommendations on prevention of coronary heart disease in clinical practice. Heart 1998;**80**(Suppl 2):S1–29.

Ford DE, Mead LA, Chang PP, Cooper-Patrick L, Wang NY, Klag MJ. Depression is a risk factor for coronary artery disease in men: The Precursors Study. Arch Intern Med 1998;**158**:1422–26.

Fuller JH, Shipley MJ, Rose G, Jarrett RJ, Keen H. Mortality from CHD and stroke in relation to degree of glycaemia: the Whitehall study. BMJ 1983;**287**:867–70.

Hippisley-Cox J, Coupland C, Vinogradova Y, Robson J, May M, Brindle P. Derivation and validation of QRISK, a new cardiovascular disease risk score for the United Kingdom: prospective open cohort study. BMJ 2007;**335**:136.

Jamrozik K. Estimate of deaths attributable to passive smoking among UK adults: database analysis. BMJ 2005;**330**:812.

Kannel WB, McGee DL. Diabetes and cardiovascular risk factors: the Framingham Study. Circulation 1979;**59**:8–13.

Manson JE, Hu FB, Rich-Edwards JW, et al. A prospective study of walking as compared with vigorous exercise in the prevention of coronary heart disease in women. N Engl J Med 1999;**341**:650–8.

Marmot MG, Bosma H, Hemingway H, Brunner E, Stansfeld S. Contribution of job control and other risk factors to social variations in coronary heart disease incidence. Lancet 1997;**350**:235–9.

Mente A, de Koning L, Shannon HS, Anand SS. A systematic review of the evidence supporting a causal link between dietary factors and coronary heart disease. Arch Intern Med 2009;**169**:659–69.

Nasir K, Budoff MJ, Wong ND, et al. Family history of premature coronary heart disease and coronary artery calcification: Multi Ethnic Study of Atherosclerosis (MESA). Circulation 2007;**116**:619–26.

Pell JP, Haw S. The triumph of national smoke-free legislation. Heart 2009;**95**:1377–9.

Rosenberg L, Kaufman DW, Helmrich SP, Shapiro S. The risk of myocardial infarction after quitting smoking in men under 55 years of age. NEJM 1985;**313**:1511–14.

Yusuf S, Hawken S, Ounpuu S, et al. Effect of potentially modifiable risk factors associated with myocardial infarction in 52 countries (The INTERHEART study). Lancet 2004;**364**:937–52.

Diets and ischaemic heart disease

Adverse lifestyle choices, including the consumption of cheap, calorie-dense foods, promote the development of ischaemic heart disease (IHD), whereas a balanced healthy diet can prevent delay of onset. A 'balanced diet' meets the requirements of essential nutrients, but data describing what constitutes a healthy diet remain incomplete and often conflicting, although various recommendations exist.

Humans can turn to three sources of energy, each of which comes in a specific form: fats, proteins, or carbohydrates. Assuming a 2000-kcal diet, guidelines recommend that 60% of daily calories come from carbohydrates, ~10% from protein, and <30% from fat, including saturated fat. Newer guidelines, such as the US 'MyPyramid' recognize both the importance of a balanced diet and the amount consumed within a more active healthy lifestyle.

Quality of existing dietary advice

The quality of dietary advice depends on the quality of the studies from which they are derived, yet given the complexity of our diets there are limitations to conducting appropriate studies, particularly when interventional in nature. These studies are fraught with potential residual confounding, and lack of compliance, a major limitation in behavioural modification studies, which limit data interpretation. Many of the statements in this review are referenced in Thomas et al. (2007).

Global dietary intake

Carbohydrate is the major source of dietary energy in most populations, forming 50–80% of dietary energy in developing countries and 40–50% in developed populations. Carbohydrates are made up of starches, non-starch polysaccharides, which are the major component of dietary fibre, and sugars. In contrast, fat is the most energy-dense dietary constituent (9 kcal/g compared to 4 kcal/g for carbohydrates and protein), and are of plant and animal origin, the latter being the predominant source of saturated fat. Protein intake generally varies between 10% and 18% of total energy intake in populations.

Effects of urbanization and modernization

As a result of modernization the proportion of carbohydrate consumption is falling, although the proportion of refined carbohydrates has risen. Likewise, the proportion of fat, and in particular saturated animal fat also increases with urbanization and modernization from <15–30% in developing countries to 30–40% and more in developed countries. Only modest increases in protein consumption most protein is of plant origin which is then replaced by those of animal origin. These changes in consumption are thought to determine the observed increases in vascular risk factors and IHD.

Dietary food groups and metabolism

Fats and oils

Evidence suggests that consumption of saturated fats carries little more risk of IHD than refined carbohydrates. A Cochrane meta-analysis of fat reduction found a non-significant 9% reduction in IHD mortality, although there was a significant 16% reduction in events, with a 16–28% reduction in trials lasting more than 2 years, which also reduced all-cause mortality (Hooper et al. 2002). There are significant flaws in that analysis, including the inclusion of underpowered, limited-duration studies conducted in low-risk subjects and only assessed total fat reductions, which consistently has shown no effect on cholesterol or IHD events. Replacement of saturated fat with carbohydrate proportionally lowers both LDL and HDL cholesterol leaving the ratio unchanged with each 5% relative change being associated with a non-significant 17% increase in the risk of IHD. Replacement of saturated with unsaturated fat preferentially reduces LDL cholesterol levels and reduces risk of IHD by 42%. A high polyunsaturated to saturated fat ratio is desirable. Trans-fatty acids have particularly adverse effects raising LDL and lowering HDL cholesterol, resulting in the ratio of total to HDL cholesterol being twice that of those consuming saturated fat, and increasing mortality.

Low-carbohydrate diets, e.g. the Atkins diet

These diets reduce body weight compared with low-fat diets over 6 months, but not over longer periods (Astrup et al. 2004). Weight loss appears more associated with the duration and level of calorie restriction rather than the dietary recommendations per se. There have been reports of life-threatening complications, but up to 6 months the diet appears relatively safe, although longer term evidence is required (Astrup et al. 2004).

Fat may actually be less satiating than either protein or fibre-rich carbohydrates, particularly among those already overweight. A high dietary fat-to-carbohydrate ratio promotes passive overconsumption which in conjunction with less faecal energy loss and lower thermogenicity can result in a positive energy balance and weight gain. Additionally, fat is more readily absorbed.

Carbohydrates, dietary fibre, and glycaemic index

Epidemiological results have consistently demonstrated inverse associations between unrefined carbohydrate, especially cereal fibre and whole grain foods, and the development of diabetes and IHD. This effect is mediated by small but significant improvements in total and LDL cholesterol levels. Low glycaemic index, high-fibre foods, such as lentils, beans, and oats have been shown to significantly reduce glycaemic load, promote weight loss and protect against carbohydrate-induced hypertriglyceridaemia. However, there is insufficient evidence to show benefit on IHD events.

Fish (oils and meat)

Studies suggest that fish intake can significantly reduce both IHD and stroke even in those consuming fish once per week. The effect may be the result of differences in omega-3 fatty acid (eicosapentaenoic acid and docosahexaenoic acid) levels. Intervention studies in high-risk populations appear to benefit from increased fatty fish consumption, with 40–60 g of fish per day being optimal and associated with a risk reduction of 40–60%. Cochrane systematic reviews found that diets enriched with n-3 polyunsaturated fatty acids significantly reduced IHD mortality by 26% and sudden death by 29% (Bucher et al. 2002). This study included low-risk populations that do not appear to benefit from the intervention. No benefit or harm was found for n-3 fatty acid supplementation.

A note of caution, fish, in particular older, larger, predatory fish may contain high levels of environmental contaminants, and thus intake should be limited in pregnant or nursing women and children, but benefits may outweigh the risk for middle-aged men and postmenopausal women.

Fruit and vegetables

Cohort studies have clearly shown a beneficial effect of consuming fruit and vegetables in reducing the IHD events. A meta-analysis found a reduction in the risk of IHD and both ischaemic and haemorrhagic stroke by 4%, and 5% per portion per day of fruit and vegetable consumed, respectively, thus having clear beneficial effects on reducing IHD mortality (Willett 2006).

Electrolytes

Epidemiological studies have shown a positive correlation between sodium intake and blood pressure. Modest salt intake reductions of 78 mmol/day (4.6 g) reduced systolic and diastolic blood pressures by 5.0 and 2.7 mmHg in hypertensive subjects (He and MacGregor 2004). However, 75% of dietary sodium is found in processed food for which restriction is difficult. Supplementing dietary intake with potassium, and possibly calcium, may reduce blood pressure but the evidence is limited.

Vitamins

For vitamins and minerals, the minimum requirements are fairly straightforward, but the evidence describing their role in health and disease at higher concentrations is generally insufficient. Epidemiological studies have proposed antioxidants to be effective in the prevention of atherosclerotic vascular disease. However, despite theoretical and biological evidence of benefit, randomized, controlled trials with vitamins C, E and β-carotene have demonstrated no benefit. These vitamins may also reduce the benefit of cholesterol-lowering drugs.

Whole diet studies

Food is not consumed as isolated food groups or nutrients, for which changes may have both beneficial and detrimental effects. Therefore manipulation of whole diets is likely to be most realistic. Epidemiological studies have shown that healthy diets high in fruit, vegetable and soya, and fish are associated with reduced mortality and may offset the consumption of less healthy foods. Mediterranean-style or plant-rich and vegetarian diets with fruit, vegetables, whole grains, and a high polyunsaturated-to-unsaturated fat ratio appear to reduce IHD by about 24–46% (Willett 2006).

Dietary recommendation

Based on the evidence from well-conducted trials, a diet similar to the Dietary Approaches to Stop Hypertension (DASH) diet including 500 g/day of whole grains (wheat, corn, rice, legumes) and another 500 g/day of fruit, vegetables, and nuts (walnuts and almonds), as well as 30 g/day of canola or mustard or soy bean oil or 40–60 g/day of oily fish, with minimal sodium intake is the closest to an optimal evidence-based healthy diet to reduce IHD (Willett 2006). Vitamin supplementation appears to have no benefit.

Dietary advice

A systematic review describing dietary advice for the primary prevention of IHD found no significant effect on mortality (Ebrahim and Smith 1997). This review did not include interventions in populations with existing IHD, despite suggestions that dietary interventions may be more effective in such populations. The study also did not differentiate between the dietary targets. The study found small benefits but suggested that the interventions failed to modify lifestyle, rather than an absence of an effect from dietary modification per se. The authors therefore suggested that financial and legislative measures may be more effective for improving health (Ebrahim and Smith 1997), which have certainly proved useful in lifestyle modifications, such as promoting smoking cessation.

Integrated perspective

It is important to remember that dietary factors also modify the pathogenesis of other chronic diseases, particularly cancers, and some food items present with contrasting findings. For example, moderate alcohol consumption appears beneficial for vascular health, but is harmful at any level of intake for certain cancers (Key et al. 2004). Thus dietary recommendations should not be given in isolation, but should take account of the effects on overall health. Similarly, excessive quantities of even healthy foods will result in excess calories being stored as fat; therefore, moderate calorie intake is essential. A balanced diet is only one component of a healthy lifestyle, which also requires regular physical activity and avoidance of smoking to minimize the development of cardiovascular and other chronic diseases.

References

Astrup A, Meinert Larsen T, Harper A,. Atkins and other low-carbohydrate diets: hoax or an effective tool for weight loss? *Lancet Neurol* 2004;**364**:897–9.

Bucher HC, Hengstler P, Schindler C, et al. N-3 polyunsaturated fatty acids in coronary heart disease: a meta-analysis of randomized controlled trials. *Am J Med* 2002;**112**:298–304.

Ebrahim S, Smith GD. Systematic review of randomised controlled trials of multiple risk factor interventions for preventing coronary heart disease. *BMJ* 1997;**314**:1666–74.

He FJ, MacGregor GA. Effect of longer-term modest salt reduction on blood pressure. *Cochrane Database Syst Rev.* 2004;(3):CD004937.

Hooper L, Summerbell CD, Higgins JP, et al. Reduced or modified dietary fat for preventing cardiovascular disease. *Cochrane Database Syst Rev* 2001;(3):CD002137.

Key TJ, Schatzkin A, Willett WC, et al. Diet, nutrition and the prevention of cancer. *Public Health Nutr* 2004;**7**:187–200.

Thomas GN, Cheung BMY, Ho S, et al. Overview of dietary influences on atherosclerotic vascular disease: Epidemiology and prevention. *Cardiovasc Haematol Disorders-Drug Targets* 2007;**7**:87–97.

Willett WC. The Mediterranean diet: science and practice. *Public Health Nutr* 2006;**9**:105–10.

Exercise and ischaemic heart disease

Exercise is a core element of the contemporary management and rehabilitation of patients with stable angina and following myocardial infarction (MI) and revascularization (Wenger 2008).

Current European and US guidelines for secondary prevention of ischaemic heart disease (IHD) recommend that programmes should not only be restricted to exercise alone but also include risk factor education, psychological input, and drug therapy—so-called 'comprehensive' cardiac rehabilitation (Giannuzzi et al. 2003; Leon et al. 2005; NICE 2008; SIGN 2002). The following section summarizes the evidence base for exercise in patients with IHD and considers the practical issues in the use of exercise in this population, including pre-exercise screening and guidelines for exercise prescription, follow-up, and maintenance.

The evidence base for exercise training

In the absence of definitive randomized controlled trials (RCTs), meta-analyses of smaller RCTs have been used to assess the role of exercise training, alone or as part of a comprehensive cardiac rehabilitation programme (Clark et al. 2006; Jolliffe et al. 2001; O'Connor et al. 1989; Oldridge et al. 1988; Taylor et al. 2004). The most comprehensive meta-analysis to date includes 48 trials of ≥6 months' duration with a total of 8940 patients assessing the impact of trials of exercise alone or exercise plus other interventions (comprehensive programme) compared with usual medical care (Taylor et al. 2004). The majority of patients were young (median age 55 years), low-risk males (80% of cohort) following MI or revascularization.

Many of the trials of exercise in IHD date back to the 1970s and 1980s.

Few data were provided in these studies on the use of acute thrombolytic therapy and adjunctive cardioprotective drugs.

As shown in Fig. 5.3.1, exercise-based cardiac rehabilitation was associated with lower total and cardiac mortality rates than usual medical care. Subgroup analyses showed that mortality rates did not differ between post MI and vascularization patients or programmes limited to exercise and those providing more comprehensive secondary interventions. Favourable trends were also noted for a lower incidence of non-fatal MI and revascularization procedures in cardiac patients who received exercise-based rehabilitation, but these trends did not achieve statistical significance. Furthermore, data from a limited number of studies included in this meta-analysis showed more favourable changes in some modifiable cardiovascular risk factors (blood pressure, lipid levels, and smoking) among patients who received exercise therapy. Quality of life was assessed in only 25% of the clinical trials, via a variety of measures, and similar improvement was noted in both the exercise-based rehabilitation and control groups.

Major advances in the management of patients with IHD during the 1990s—use of antiplatelet and anticoagulant drugs, prompt coronary revascularization by thrombolysis or percutaneous interventions, and use of adjunctive cardioprotective drugs (e.g. statins)—raise a question about the independent effects of the exercise component of contemporary cardiac rehabilitation programmes. However, subgroup analysis showed that mortality effects of exercise did not differ between pre- and post-1995 studies (Taylor et al. 2004), supporting the benefits of exercise-based cardiac rehabilitation within the context of today's cardiovascular service provision.

Two UK trials have recently compared the more traditional model of supervised hospital-based cardiac rehabilitation to a rehabilitation programme delivered in the home setting in post MI and revascularization patients (Dalal et al. 2007; Jolly et al. 2008). Both hospital and home-based programmes included exercise training. Similar improvements were seen in clinical event rates and IHD risk factor outcomes in each of these two settings. Thus, patients have the choice of participating in a more traditional supervised centre-based or home-based programme according to their preference. The increased availability of home-based exercise programmes may lead to an improvement in the uptake of cardiac rehabilitation and an also improvement in long-term individual compliance (Jolliffe et al. 2001).

Pre-exercise screening

Exercise has both risks and benefits. Although the risks of complications with exercise are increased in patients with IHD compared with healthy individuals, major adverse events are nevertheless rare. Recent data indicate an occurrence of major cardiovascular events range from 1 in 60 000 to 1 in 120 000 patient hours of exercise, with only two fatalities reported per 1.5 million patient-hours of exercise (see Leon et al. 2005).

The three most important factors affecting the risk of exercise are age, presence of heart disease, and intensity of exercise (Fletcher et al. 2001). Before initiating an exercise programme, all patients should have their risk of exercise assessed on history, examination and resting ECG combined with an exercise test.

High-risk patients may be defined as those who have (SIGN 2005):

- Experienced a MI complicated by heart failure, cardiogenic shock, and/or complex ventricular arrhythmias
- Angina or breathlessness occurring at a low level of exercise
- ST segment depression ≥1 mm on resting ECG
- Undergone exercise testing with marked ST depression ≥2 mm or angina at <5 METS.

Exercise under medical supervision and monitoring (ECG and BP) is recommended for such high-risk individuals (Fletcher et al. 2001).

Exercise prescription

Trials included in meta-analyses of exercise for IHD span a wide range of exercise prescriptions. Subgroup analysis showed that the overall amount of exercise in a programme was not predictive of benefit. However, consensus-based guidelines do provide recommendation of the level of exercise that should be undertaken by patients with IHD (Table 5.3.1).

Patients are recommended to undertake aerobic (dynamic exercise in large muscle groups alternatively contracting and relaxing) exercise such as walking, jogging, cycling, or swimming exercise at a moderate intensity (40–60% maximum aerobic capacity (VO_{2max}) or 50–70% of age adjusted maximum heart rate), four or five times per week for 20–60 minutes (Fletcher et al. 2001). Each exercise session should be preceded by a warm up period and followed by a cool down period of low-intensity physical activity. Resistance (or strength) training, particularly in older individuals, can be used to improve the strength of thigh and shoulder girdle muscles and reduce the risk of falls (Fletcher et al. 2001).

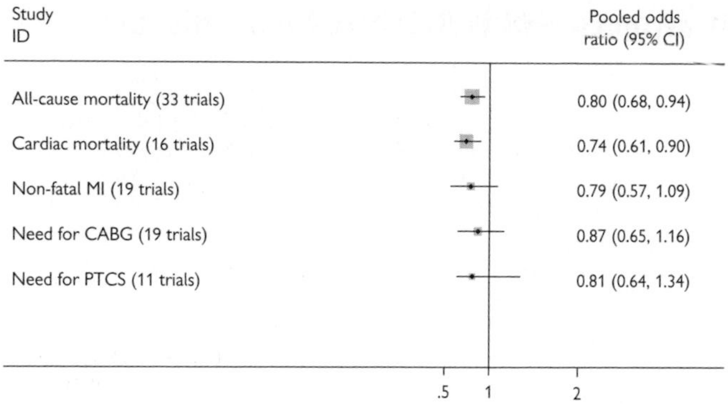

Study ID		Pooled odds ratio (95% CI)
All-cause mortality (33 trials)		0.80 (0.68, 0.94)
Cardiac mortality (16 trials)		0.74 (0.61, 0.90)
Non-fatal MI (19 trials)		0.79 (0.57, 1.09)
Need for CABG (19 trials)		0.87 (0.65, 1.16)
Need for PTCS (11 trials)		0.81 (0.64, 1.34)

.5 1 2

Fig. 5.3.1 Risk of mortality following cardiac rehabilitation (adapted from Taylor *et al.* 2004). The relative risk of mortality and morbidity following exercise based cardiac rehabilitation. A relative risk <1.00 indicates a result in favour of cardiac rehabilitation and relative risk of >1.00 indicates a result in favour of control.

Table 5.3.1 Exercise prescription recommendations for cardiac rehabilitation (Adapted from Fletcher *et al.* 2001). Shows the levels of aerobic and resistance (strength) training that cardiac patients should be asked to undertake as part of their rehabilitation

Frequency	Intensity	Duration	Modality
Aerobic exercise 3–5 days/ week	50–70% max HR 40–80% VO_{2max} or HRR	20–60 min	Walking, swimming, jogging, etc.
Resistance exercise 2–3 days/ week	1–3 sets of 8–15 RM for each muscle group		Lower or upper extremity

max HR, maximum heart rate; HRR, heart rate reserve; VO_{2max}, maximum aerobic capacity; RM, repetition maximum.

Follow-up and maintenance

The continuing benefits of exercise depend on long-term maintenance of exercise behaviour. Studies have shown that less than 50% of people who participate in cardiac rehabilitation programmes maintain an exercise regimen for as long as 6 months after completion (Daly *et al.* 2002). Some patients may devise their own exercise programme, or return to sports, or join a self-help group or a sport centre, or use walking-based home exercise programmes. Others may prefer class-based exercise programmes. In the absence of evidence that one of these options is better than another, all options should be made available, and choice should be determined by patient preference (Davies *et al.* 2009).

References

Clark AM, Hartling L, Vandermeer B, McAlister FA. Meta-analysis: secondary prevention programs for patients with coronary heart disease. *Ann Intern Med* 2005;**143**:659–72.

Dalal HM, Watt A, Evans PH, *et al.* Home-based cardiac rehabilitation versus hospital-based rehabilitation: a randomized controlled trial. *Int J Cardiol* 2007;**119**:202–11.

Daly J, Sindone AP, Thompson DR, *et al.* Barriers to participation in and adherence to cardiac rehabilitation programs: a critical literature review. *Prog Cardiovasc Nursing* 2002;**17**:8–17.

Davies P, Taylor F, Beswick A, *et al.* Promoting patient uptake and adherence in cardiac rehabilitation. *Cochrane Database Syst Rev* 2010;(7):CD007131.

Fletcher GF, Balady GJ, Amsterdam FA, *et al.* Exercise standards for testing and training: a statement for healthcare professionals from the American Heart Association. *Circulation* 2001;**104**: 1694–1740.

Giannuzzi P, Saner H, Björnstad H, *et al.* Secondary prevention through cardiac rehabilitation: position paper of the Working Group on Cardiac Rehabilitation and Exercise Physiology of the European Society of Cardiology. *Eur Heart J.* 2003;**24**:1273–8.

Joliffe JA, Rees K, Taylor RS, *et al.* Exercise-based rehabilitation for coronary heart disease. Cochrane Database of Systematic Reviews, Cochrane Library Issue 3 2004. Chichester: John Wiley & Sons Ltd; 2003.

Jolly K, Taylor RS, Lip GYH, *et al.* The Birmingham Rehabilitation Uptake Maximization study (BRUM): a randomized controlled trial comparing home-based with centre-based cardiac rehabilitation. *Heart* 2009;**95**:36–42.

Leon AS, Franklin BA, Costa F, *et al.* Cardiac rehabilitation and secondary prevention of coronary heart disease: an American Heart Association scientific statement from the Council on Clinical Cardiology (Subcommittee on Exercise, Cardiac Rehabilitation, and Prevention) and the Council on Nutrition, Physical Activity, and Metabolism (Subcommittee on Physical Activity), in collaboration with the American association of Cardiovascular and Pulmonary Rehabilitation. *Circulation* 2005;**111**:369–76.

Moore SM, Charvat JM, Gordon NH, *et al.* Effects of a CHANGE intervention to increase exercise maintenance following cardiac events. *Ann Behavioral Med* 2006;**31**:53–62.

National Institute for Health and Clinical Excellence (NICE). Post Myocardial Infarction Secondary prevention in primary and secondary care for patients following a myocardial infarction, May 2007. Available at: http://www.nice.org.uk/nicemedia/pdf/CG48NICEGuidance.pdf (accessed May 2009).

Oldridge NB, Guyatt GH, Fischer ME, Rimm AA. Cardiac rehabilitation after myocardial infarction. Combined experience of randomized clinical trials. *JAMA* 1988;**260**:945–950.

O'Connor GT, Buring JE, Yusuf S, *et al.* An overview of randomized trials of rehabilitation with exercise after myocardial infarction. *Circulation.* 1989;**80**:234–244.

Scottish Intercollegiate Guidelines Network (SIGN) Cardiac Rehabilitation. Publication No. 57. Edinburgh, United Kingdom: Scottish Intercollegiate Guidelines Network; 2002. Available at: http://www.sign.ac.uk/pdf/sign57.pdf (accessed May 2009).

Skidmore B, Stone J, Thompson DR. Exercise based rehabilitation for patients with coronary heart disease: Systematic review & meta-analysis of randomized controlled trials. *Am J Med* 2004; **116**:682–92.

Taylor RS, Brown A, Ebrahim S, *et al.* Exercise based rehabilitation for patients with coronary heart disease: Systematic review & meta-analysis of randomized controlled trials. *Am J Med* 2004;**116**:682–92.

Wenger NK. Current status of cardiac rehabilitation. *J Am Coll Cardiol* 2008;**51**:1619–31.

Psychosocial aspects and ischaemic heart disease

Introduction

All of our interventions for ischaemic heart disease (IHD) are directed towards the two aims of making people:
- Live longer = reduced mortality
- Feel better = improved quality of life (QoL).

Interventions that do not improve life expectancy sometimes improve other clinical end-points, such as symptom reduction, improved functional capacity, reduction in hospital readmissions, prevention of further acute coronary events or coronary revascularization reduction. Apart from some potential cost savings, the only benefit to the patient of reducing these non-fatal clinical end-points is improved QoL. In addition, apart from the medical illness, there are obviously a number of unrelated (or only partly related) psychological and social factors that contribute to the QoL of the patient.

Epidemiology

Many psychosocial factors have been prospectively demonstrated to be associated with:
- Increased incidence of IHD
- Worse outcome for those with existing IHD.

These factors include:
- Lower education
- Lower socioeconomic status and income
- Social isolation/low social support
- Depression.

The three most important factors contributing to presentation with acute coronary syndromes, compared with the profile of matched controls, would appear to be primarily:
- Comprehensive lipid profile using ApoB/ApoA ratios
- Smoking
- Psychosocial factors (Yusuf 2004).

Depression prevalence
- General population 5–10%
- IHD patients 30% (15% major depression)
- IHD and unipolar depression:
  - Currently the two most important causes of disability in high-income countries
  - By 2030 this will be true for all country groups (WHO 2008)
  - Just from their high prevalence, IHD and depression will commonly co-exist.

Causal relationship?
- Because of the higher prevalence of depression in IHD patients, it is likely that IHD causes an increase in depression.
- It is also possible that depression might contribute to the development of IHD and its outcome.
  - There are a few long-term population studies that have demonstrated that IHD is more likely to develop in those with depression at baseline.
  - Tightly controlled studies have demonstrated that depression is a strong, independent predictor of subsequent mortality.

- However, randomized controlled trials of treating depression in patients with IHD have so far not demonstrated any reduction in cardiac events.
- Whether or not there is a causal relationship, depression is the single most important determinant of QoL of patients and as such is important to detect and treat.

Psychosocial effects
Quality of life
- QoL is a general term.
- It covers a number of perspectives, including the psychological, functional, and social.
- For any one patient, one aspect can be more important than another.
- Probably the most commonly used generic measure is the SF-36 with its different domains.
- Being depressed is a major component of QoL and can possibly be regarded as the 'bottom line' of QoL.

Psychological
Anxiety
- Related to fear (both rational and irrational) of anticipated loss (either real or perceived).
- Anticipated losses include life, health, independence, occupation, financial security, sexual activity, social role, and previously assumed invincibility.
- Generally based on false, socially determined ideas about the consequences of coronary disease.
- The implications of their cardiac condition, and their generally good prognosis, are often unclear to them.
- Anxiety starts immediately at the onset of an acute coronary syndrome (ACS).
- Within days, anxieties and their social consequences become more difficult to reverse.
- Accurate, informed knowledge about the future needs to be imparted to the patient and their 'significant others' (close friends and family) from the very first day.

  - The earlier that this is done, the more successful the outcome in preventing or reversing these negative thought patterns;
  - Information, explanation, advice, and reassurance need to be given by someone who clearly understands the medical condition and prognosis;
  - The importance of these simple measures cannot be underestimated.

Denial
- Patients sometimes exhibit language and behavior that deny the full meaning of what has happened to them
- Can be conscious (suppression) or unconscious (repression)
- Can result in poor adherence to advice and medications
- Includes expressions of bravado, invincibility, projection of fears onto others (e.g. 'My wife is worried about me'), displacement of fears onto other situations (e.g. 'How will they cope at work without me')
- Quickly allaying the underlying fears is essential. This includes answering questions that the patient has not actually asked (e.g. You will be able to resume sexual

activity in 2 weeks and return to your usual job in 4 weeks time). Obviously this information varies a little from patient to patient.

Depression
- Depressed mood is an understandable response to illness or other life stressors
- Degrees of depressed mood are experienced over a continuous range
- We also cluster certain features as 'diagnoses' that have diagnostic utility
- Often the term 'depression' is limited to the diagnosis of 'major depression'
- Cardiac patients often have only 'minor depression'
- Depression can also be a spontaneously resolving reaction to a specific event, such as an acute coronary syndrome ('adjustment disorder with depressed mood')
- Prior to the introduction of group rehabilitation programmes, persistent depression over 1 year was found in 30% of patients after ACSs. With better supportive patient management, it is now not uncommon to see milder forms of depression undergo some improvement over time without specific depressant treatments
- Some depression can be prevented by optimal medical management, early reassurance, social support and physical activity (especially in a group setting)
- Persistent depression, especially as 'major depression', is not a healthy response, and should be identified as a disabling and treatable condition
- Pharmacological treatments
  - Patients with previous episodes of depression and/or more severe depression have been demonstrated (in three separate RCTs) to respond to SSRI antidepressant medications
  - SSRIs are safe even in patients with impaired LV function
  - The use of tricyclic antidepressants requires careful assessment
- Non-pharmacological treatments
  - Group exercise programmes
  - Cognitive behavioral therapy
  - Structured discussion
  - Dysfunctional ideas and thinking are addressed
  - Therapists in this specific setting require a detailed knowledge of cardiac patients and their true prognosis
  - Specific interpersonal psychotherapy has been demonstrated not to be generally beneficial.
- Depression is not always easy to recognize in cardiac patients
- Screening for depression is therefore essential
  - Need high sensitivity without sacrificing too much specificity
  - Should screen for all depression as well as 'major depression'
  - Many generic tools have been validated for 'major depression' screening: include BDI, HADS, PHQ9, PHQ2, CES-D; variable sensitivity and specificity; choose one
  - The CDS was derived and developed specifically in cardiac patient. It assesses depression over the full range found in cardiac patients. Unlike most measures

in cardiac patients, the CDS has a normal distribution without skewness; Therefore it is suitable for parametric statistics on the raw scores
- Its short form derivative takes <1 minute to complete with over 90% sensitivity and over 70% specificity for all depression forms (>80% for major depression).

Social
Spouse/partner/family
- Over-protectiveness is very common amongst family and friends
- Cardiac disease can result in depression in the partner as well as the patient
- The anxieties and depression in the partner can increase social friction and also depression in the patient
- Wherever possible partners should be included in discussions and programmes
- Not including partners can result in arguments caused by different perceptions of recovery
- Dispelling unsubstantiated fears:
  - Watching the patient breathe at night and, when there is a normal pause in respiration, attempting to elicit a sign of life from the patient. This occurs with the majority of couples and ceases after these respiratory pauses are explained as being entirely normal
  - Fears of the patient undertaking physical activity, such as sweeping or cutting grass. These resolve when the patient is seen to be physically active in a rehabilitation programme or undertaking a symptom limited stress test (with or without wall motion or perfusion imaging), especially when that level of activity is generalized to other daily tasks.

Employment
- Issues such as 'sick leave' or social security entitlements need to be addressed from day one
- A plan for return to work should be formulated early
- The patient should generally contact their employer at an early stage
- Many patients can return to work within two weeks. Others require longer
- For example, patient with an LVEF < 40% might need 12 weeks and a exercise stress test before returning to a job with high physical demands
- Patients with unskilled, physical employment should never be given a certificate for 'light duties'
  - In general 'light duties' do not exist for these patients
  - If any temporary restriction is required, it should be specifically stated
  - The assistance of an Occupational Therapist is extremely helpful in these situations.

Sexual activity
- In general, patients are told that they can resume sexual activity at a time when they are able to walk briskly up two flights of stairs
  - This advice can vary a little from patient to patient
  - The same information should be given to both partners, preferably together: in general, a female partner will not believe advice relayed on by a male patient on this issue and will unrealistically fear the consequences.

Leisure activities
- Vary enormously
- With the exception of very demanding activities such as rock climbing or scuba diving, most patients can return to all their previous activities without any limitation
- If the patient has particularly poor LV function and/or functional capacity, additional assessment will be required.

Physical activity
- Patients are generally told that they can exercise to a level at which they are breathing more deeply but would still be able to talk short sentences without problems.

Improving adherence to life-style change and medications
- Better patient education
  - Consistency of information
  - Understandable information, such as culture, language, educational level.
- Better education of health professionals
  - Recognise own frustrations
  - Identifying patient characteristics, such as personality, depressed mood, denial.
- More active role for patients
- Increased partner/family involvement
- More structured programme
  - Structured programmes have been shown to improve smoking cessation; improve functional capacity; reduce LDL cholesterol levels
  - Improved programme access and interest
  - Reduce waiting times.

- Increased personal contact
  - Personal re-contact for non-attendance
  - Continuity of personal contact.

Conclusion

Psychosocial aspects of ischaemic heart disease are crucial to patient management. In particular, depressed mood must be prevented and managed.

Further information on the psychosocial management of ischaemic heart disease has been published in a number of countries (Bethell 2009) and by a number of professional groups including the American Heart Association (Balady 2007). Various performance measures have also been discussed by a number of different groups and organizations (Thomas 2007).

References

Balady G, Williams MA, Bittner V, *et al.* Core components of cardiac rehabilitation/secondary prevention programs: 2007 update. *Circulation* 2007;**115**:2675–82.

Bethell H, Lewin R, Dalal H. Cardiac rehabilitation in the United Kingdom. *Heart* 2009;**95**:271–5.

Thomas RJ, King M, Lui K, *et al.* AACVPR/ACC/AHA 2007 performance measures on cardiac rehabilitation for referral to and delivery of cardiac rehabilitation/secondary prevention services. *J Am Coll Cardiol* 2007;**50**:1400–33. (http://content.onlinejacc.org/cgi/content/full/j.jacc.2007.04.033v1)

WHO. *The global burden of disease.* 2004 Update. World Health Organisation 2008; WHO Press, Geneva, Switzerland.

Yusuf S, Hawken S, Ounpuu S, *et al.* Effect of potentially modifiable risk factors associated with myocardial infarction in 52 countries (the INTERHEART study): case-control study. *Lancet* 2004;**364**:937–52.

Tobacco and ischaemic heart disease

Active smoking
UK prevalence and trends
- In the UK 9.4 million adults smoke (22% of men, 20% of women)
- Two-thirds of smokers commence smoking before 18 years of age
- Smoking prevalence is highest in:
  - 20–24 year olds (32% of men, 30% of women)
  - deprived communities (29% of manual workers versus 14% of non-manual workers)
  - Scotland (24% overall prevalence)
  - Some ethnic minority groups (especially Bangladeshi).
- Overall, smoking prevalence has declined in the past 50 years—the decline has been steeper in men than women—in 1950, smoking prevalence in men was double that in women—the prevalence in women is now equivalent to that in men
- The decline has also been steeper in older age groups.

Risk
- Smoking cigarettes predisposes to thrombosis (raised fibrinogen and platelet aggregation), endothelial dysfunction, inflammation, and dyslipidaemia.
- It increases the risk of atherosclerotic plaque formation.
- It also increases the risk of plaque instability and rupture.
- Therefore, it is a risk factor for chronic ischaemic heart disease (IHD) such as angina pectoris but an even stronger risk factor for acute events such as myocardial infarction and sudden cardiac death.
- 75% of sudden cardiac deaths due to thrombosis occur in smokers.
- The relative risk associated with smoking is higher in younger age groups.
- Smoking is a risk factor for IHD in both sexes but the relative risk in women is around double that in men—the sex difference in relative risk is greater <45 years of age.
- Smoking exhibits a dose response whereby the risk of IHD increases with the amount smoked and the duration of smoking —the dose response in relation to the amount smoked is steeper in women than men.
- On average, life expectancy is 10 years shorter in smokers than non-smokers.
- Half of all regular smokers will be killed by a smoking-related condition.
- Every year >100 000 smokers in the UK die from smoking-related conditions.
- Smoking causes 17% of IHD deaths.

Smoking cessation
UK prevalence and trends
- 28% of men and 21% of women are ex-smokers.
- 70% of current smokers want to quit.
- The most common reason for wanting to quit is health concerns.
- Half of all smokers attempt to quit each year.
- Only 2–3% of these succeed long term.

- Most smokers make repeated attempts to quit—just over half of all smokers manage to quit before they die, but many succeed too late to improve their life expectancy.
- For every year that quitting is postponed beyond 40 years of age, life expectancy is reduced by 3 months.
- The main reason that most quit attempts fail within a week is nicotine dependence.
- Half of all quit attempts are made without any form of support (pharmaceutical or psychological interventions).

Risk
- The risk of IHD gradually falls after quitting.
- Overall, the excess IHD risk among smokers is halved 1 year after quitting, and falls to normal by 3–5 years (Dobson 1991).
- However, the extent to which life expectancy reverts to that of never smokers varies depending on the life-time duration of smoking (Doll 2004).
- Smokers who quit at 30 years of age have normal life expectancy.
- Smokers who quit at 50 years of age live 6 years longer than those who continue to smoke, but 4 years shorter than life-long non-smokers.
- Patients who quit smoking following myocardial infarction have a better prognosis with regard to their risk of all-cause death, cardiovascular death, and non-fatal cardiovascular events.

Second-hand smoke exposure
- Exposure to second-hand smoke rapidly induces platelet aggregation, thrombosis, endothelial dysfunction, and inflammation.
- It is associated with an increased risk of IHD.
- >11 000 deaths per annum in the UK are attributed to second-hand smoke exposure.
- Side-stream smoke contains higher concentrations of toxins and small, respirable particles than mainstream smoke; therefore, second-hand smoke exposure carries a disproportionately high risk compared with active smoking.
- Compared with active smoking, exposure to second-hand smoke equates to around 1% of the exposure to nicotine but 50% of excess IHD risk.
- Animal experiments suggest that, in those who suffer myocardial infarction, second-hand smoke exposure results in a larger area of infarction and greater risk of ventricular hypertrophy.
- Preliminary data on humans suggest that second-hand smoke exposure may be associated with a worse early prognosis (Panagiotakos 2007).

Population interventions
Taxation
- Tobacco consumption is very price sensitive.

UK legislation
- It is prohibited to sell tobacco to anyone <18 years.
- Advertising and promoting cigarettes is prohibited, apart from limited point of sale advertising.

- Smoking in enclosed public places is prohibited.
- Cigarette packaging carries mandatory health warnings.
- Upper limits have been imposed on the tar, nicotine, and carbon monoxide content of cigarettes.

Framework Convention on Tobacco Control

(www.fctc.org)
- Produced by the WHO—this is the first global health treaty and sets internationally agreed minimum standards on tobacco control.

Individual interventions

- Healthcare workers managing patients who smoke should be supportive but not judgemental (Lancaster 2004).
- They should follow the five 'As'
  - **a**sk about smoking
  - **a**dvise patients to stop
  - **a**ssess motivation to stop
  - **a**ssist—provide prescription or refer to psychological support programme
  - **a**rrange follow-up.

Nicotine replacement therapy

- This is available in several forms (chewing gum, skin patch, lozenge, nasal spray, or inhalator).
- It is available by prescription or over the counter.
- A meta-analysis of >100 randomized control trials (RCTs) shows that all forms of nicotine replacement therapy (NRT) are roughly equally effective with regard to long-term cessation (OR 1.77, 95% CI 1.66–1.88).
- However, they can be used in combination—for example, patches can be used to provide background replacement with gum for breakthrough urges.
- Combining a patch with an acute form of NRT increases success of long-term cessation (OR 1.42, 95% CI 1.14–1.76) (Ayeyard 2007; Cochrane 2001).

Antidepressants

- Withdrawal from cigarette smoking can lead to depression.
- Bupropion is the only antidepressant licensed for use as a smoking cessation aid.
- Meta-analysis suggests that bupropion can double cessation rates (OR 1.94, 95% CI 1.72–2.19).
- There is a 0.1% risk of seizures.
- It is not clear whether the effect is additive to NRT.
- Nortriptyline has also been shown to be effective in meta-analyses.
- There is no evidence that SSRIs are effective at improving long-term smoking cessation (Ayeyard 2007; DTB 2000).

Varenicline

- This is a licensed partial agonist acting on the $\alpha_4\beta_2$ nicotine receptor.

- It is associated with a threefold increase in success compared with unassisted quit attempts (Cahill *et al.* 2008).
- Studies suggest it may be more effective than both bupropion and NRT.

Psychological support

- Support is available in a number of forms, including groups, face-to-face sessions, and telephone helplines.
- All forms have been shown to be successful at improving long-term cessation.
- Meta-analyses suggest that group support (OR 2.04, 95% CI 1.60–2.60) may be more successful than individual support (OR 1.56, 95% CI 1.32–1.84) (Stead 2005).
- Support can even be successful if provided by phone (meta-analysis OR 1.64, 95% CI 1.41–1.92) (Stead 2006).
- Psychological support can be used in isolation or as an adjunct to pharmacological interventions.
- Multiple sessions are usually required.
- Psychological support is not effective if delivered by healthcare workers who are not trained in these techniques.
- Most recently, web-based support packages have been developed, and early evidence suggests that they may be effective.
- There is no RCT evidence that acupuncture and hypnotherapy are beneficial.

Further reading

Anonymous. Bupropion to aid smoking cessation. *Drug Therapeutics Bull* 2000;**38**.73–5.

Anonymous. Nicotine replacement therapy for smoking cessation. *The Cochrane Library*, Issue 3, May 2001.

Aveyard P, West P.. Managing smoking cessation. *BMJ* 2007;**335**:37–41.

Cahill K, Stead LF, Lancaster T. Nicotine receptor partial agonists for smoking cessation. *Cochrane Database Syst Rev* 2008;(3):CD006103.

Dobson AJ, Alexander HM, Heller RF, Lloyd DM. How soon after quitting smoking does risk of heart attack decline?. *J Clin Epidemiol* 1991;**44**:1247–53.

Doll R, Peto R, Boreham J, Sutherland I. Mortality in relation to smoking: 50 years' observations on male British doctors. *BMJ* 2004;**328**.1519.

Lancaster T, Stead LF. Physician advice for smoking cessation. *Cochrane Database Syst Rev* 2004;(4): CD000165.

Panagiotakos DB, Pitsavos C, Stefanadis C. Chronic exposure to second hand smoke and 30-day prognosis of patients hopsitalised with acute coronary syndromes. *Heart* 2007;**93**:309–12.

Stead L, Lancaster T. Group behaviour therapy programmes for smoking cessation. *Cochrane Database Syst Rev* 2005;(2):CD001007.

Stead L, Perera R, Lancaster T. Telephone counselling for smoking cessation. *Cochrane Database Syst Rev* 2006;(3):CD002850.

Chronic stable angina

Introduction

Chronic stable angina is not an uncommon disabling disorder. Angina pectoris is defined as chest pain or discomfort that occurs due to myocardial ischaemia as a result of impaired coronary blood flow. Although commonly associated with atherosclerotic coronary artery disease, it can also occur as a result of severe aortic stenosis and hypertrophic cardiomyopathy. It commonly occurs during exertion and is relieved by rest or sublingual nitrates. It is often described as a heaviness or pressure in the chest that radiates to the jaw and left arm. Chronic stable angina refers to angina pectoris that is longstanding in duration, often predictable, where the intensity, frequency, and the duration of symptoms remain fairly unchanged with time, although some variability may be seen during different times of the year (seasonal or weather related).

Pathophysiology

The main pathophysiological cause of angina is an imbalance between the requirement and the supply of oxygen to the myocardium. The commonest cause is narrowing of the arterial lumen due to atherosclerosis, although other causes mentioned above can also cause angina. Typically, therefore, the blood flow reaching the myocardium at rest is sufficient for its metabolic needs. During exercise, the oxygen requirement increases, but supply is restricted due to the restricted lumen and this causes angina. Other factors such as endothelial function, the presence of collateral circulation, platelet aggregation, vascular tone, etc., can also affect the myocardial oxygen demand. Rarely, myocardial bridging can cause angina. Similarly, in the presence of a low degree of narrowing, the presence of anaemia can cause angina.

Clinical features

The diagnosis of angina can often be made on a good history. In the majority of cases (especially in the presence of coronary risk factors), it is possible to make a definite diagnosis on history alone. However, often further investigations are required to confirm the diagnosis. The pain caused by myocardial ischaemia typically comes on exertion, is localized to the substernal area and is relieved by rest. The pain or discomfort may radiate to the jaw, neck, or the left arm. Occasionally, the pain is only present in the arm or jaw and not in the chest. History should also include a history of risk factors such as presence of diabetes, hypertension, hypercholesterolaemia, and a family history of premature cardiovascular events.

In some patients, angina pectoris presents as breathlessness rather than chest discomfort and this should be suspected in patients with multiple cardiovascular risk factors especially diabetes. This is called angina equivalence.

According to the European Society of Cardiology, definite angina fulfils three criteria: (1) definite substernal discomfort of characteristic quality and duration, (2) provoked by exertion or emotional stress, and (3) relieved by rest or sublingual glyceryl trinitrate (GTN). Probable angina meets two of these criteria, and non-cardiac chest pain meets one or none of these criteria. In order to classify the severity of the symptoms, a classification such as the Canadian Cardiovascular Society Score can be used (Table 5.6.1).

There are no specific signs on clinical examination in patients with chronic stable angina. However, a full physical examination should include the blood pressure and a search for signs of diabetes, such as fundus examination, and the presence of xanthalesma as a clue for hypercholesterolaemia, etc.

Investigations

Routine laboratory blood tests do not directly aid in the diagnosis of angina pectoris. However, it is very important to check the haemoglobin to rule out anaemia as a cause of angina, as mentioned above. Renal functions, blood glucose, and blood cholesterol levels are important in the management of these patients.

All patients with a suspected diagnosis of angina should receive an electrocardiogram (ECG) as in some cases this could show ischaemic changes or changes suggestive of an old infarct. This would also help the choice of the next non-invasive test for the diagnosis of angina. For example, patients with a left bundle block pattern on resting ECG would not be suitable for an exercise ECG.

Non-invasive tests are the next step in the diagnosis. Exercise ECG (either on a treadmill or exercise bicycle), stress echocardiography, or myocardial perfusion scan help to make the diagnosis and the last two also help to localize the territory of myocardial ischaemia. Table 5.6.2 lists the sensitivity and specificity of the different tests in the diagnosis of angina. In addition to aiding the diagnosis, these tests also help in risk stratification of these patients.

Multislice coronary computed tomography (MCCT) may be indicated in patients in whom a lower probability of angina is suspected, as this would help reduce the need for an invasive test.

Invasive coronary angiography remains the gold standard in the diagnosis of coronary heart disease. This should be considered in all patients with a diagnosis of angina and those in whom any of the non-invasive tests are either strongly positive or are inconclusive.

Management

The treatment of a patient with chronic stable angina can be divided into either medical management or invasive management (revascularization).

Medical management includes non-pharmacological and pharmacological means. The non-pharmacological treatment of angina includes weight reduction, regular physical exercise, cessation of smoking, and dietary changes such as lower fatty diets, and increased fruits and vegetables. Treatment of concomitant risk factors such as

Table 5.6.1 Classification of the severity of angina according to the Canadian Cardiovascular Society Score

Class 1: Ordinary exertion does not cause angina, only comes with severe or prolonged unaccustomed exertion

Class 2: Slight limitation of ordinary activity. Angina on climbing or walking rapidly, in cold weather, or immediately after meals or in the first few hours after awakening

Class 3: Marked limitation of ordinary physical activity. Angina on walking 100–200 m on level ground or on climbing one flight of stairs

Class 4: Inability to carry out any physical activity or angina at rest

Table 5.6.2 Sensitivity and specificity of the different non-invasive tests for the diagnosis of angina

	Sensitivity (%)	Specificity (%)
Exercise ECG	68	77
Exercise echo	8–5	8–6
Exercise myocardial perfusion	8–0	7–5
Dobutamine stress echo	4–00	6–00
Vasodilator stress echo	5–2	8–00
Vasodilator stress myocardial perfusion	8–4	6–0

diabetes, hypertension, and hypercholesterolaemia is also important.

Pharmacological treatment
The goal of pharmacological therapy is to improve the quality of life (reduce symptoms, reduce need for hospitalization and invasive procedures) and to improve the overall prognosis of the patient, i.e. to prevent cardiovascular-related morbidity and mortality. The different drugs that are used are briefly reviewed below.

Antiplatelet agents
Low-dose aspirin is the cornerstone of the treatment of angina. Many trials and meta-analyses have confirmed the use of aspirin in lowering cardiovascular end-points in patients with ischaemic heart disease. It acts via irreversible inhibition of platelet COX-1 and thus thromboxane production. This effect is maximal at a low dose of 75 mg a day. At increased doses, no further platelet inhibition is seen, but there is increased risk of side-effects, including gastrointestinal bleeding.

Clopidogrel is another antiplatelet agent that can be used in angina. Clopidogrel and ticlopidine are thienopyridines, which act as non-competitive ADP receptor antagonists. Ticlopidine has gone out of favour because of a higher incidence of symptomatic side-effects and a high rate of thrombocytopenia and neutropenia. As clopidogrel is much more expensive than aspirin, in general practice, its use is often limited to patients with acute coronary syndromes and unstable angina in combination with aspirin. The CAPRIE study demonstrated its efficacy in stable angina. Clopidogrel is also often used in patients who are intolerant of aspirin. Often clopidogrel is used in patients who have had a gastrointestinal bleed with aspirin. Although clopidogrel does not have any effect on the gastric mucosa as aspirin does, any antiplatelet agent can theoretically cause gastrointestinal bleeds.

Lipid-lowering agents
Statin treatment has been shown to significantly reduce the risk of atherosclerotic cardiovascular complications in both primary and secondary prevention. Although there are no trials specifically looking at patients with stable angina, these patients often formed a large proportion of various large studies such as the Heart Protection Study and the ASCOT LLA. It is now considered that statins have effects that are over and above their lipid-lowering effect, although the nature of this effect is not completely understood. Other lipid-lowering agents such as ezetemibe, fibrates, nicotinic acid, etc., may also be used in patients

intolerant of statins, or in combination with statins, to help patients reach target levels of cholesterol. The second Joint British Societies (JBS-2) guidelines for cholesterol levels are a low-density lipoprotein (LDL) of less than 2 mmol/L and total cholesterol of less than 4 mmol/L or a reduction of 30% from baseline.

Angiotensin-converting enzyme inhibitors
These drugs are well established in the treatment of hypertension and heart failure. Studies such as EUROPA and HOPE have demonstrated a benefit with perindopril and ramipril in secondary prevention as well. Although debatable, it is thought that angiotensin-converting enzyme inhibitors (ACEIs) exert an effect over and above that due to blood pressure lowering. It is therefore advisable to add an ACEI in hypertensive and diabetic patients with stable angina who may also have impaired left ventricular function.

Beta-blockers
This group of drugs reduces the incidence of myocardial infarctions by around 30% in patients who have had a previous myocardial infarction. There is conflicting data on their use in stable angina, with studies demonstrating improvement in angina symptoms but no improvement in prognosis.

Calcium channel blockers
There is at present no data to support the use of these drugs for prognostic reasons in uncomplicated stable angina. However, in patients who are intolerant of beta-blockers, rate-lowering calcium channel blockers may be used post myocardial infarction in patients without heart failure. These agents are also the drug of choice in patients with vasospastic coronary artery disease.

Symptomatic relief
Drugs such as nitrates (short-acting sublingual or long-acting oral preparations), potassium channel blockers (nicorandil), sinus node inhibitors (ivabradine) may also be used purely for symptomatic relief with no prognostic benefit. Newer agents such as ranolazine and trimetazidine may also be used, although clinical trial data are still awaited on these agents.

Coronary revascularization
Coronary revascularization or physical relief of the atherosclerotic narrowing can be performed in two ways—either by percutaneous coronary intervention (PCI) or by coronary artery bypass grafting (CABG).

There has been considerable debate regarding the role of revascularization especially PCI in chronic stable angina. The recent COURAGE study and meta-analyses, both preceding it and following it, demonstrate that PCI is better than optimal medical therapy in improving symptoms but does not offer a survival benefit. It is therefore recommended that PCI is considered when optimal intensive medical therapy fails.

CABG on the other hand can be carried out for both symptomatic and prognostic benefit. The subgroup of patients who have been shown to have a prognostic benefit include
1 significant stenosis of the left main stem
2 significant proximal stenosis of the three main epicardial arteries
3 significant stenosis of two major coronary arteries including high grade stenosis of the proximal left anterior descending artery.

A significant stenosis angiographically has been defined as a stenosis greater than 70% for major coronary arteries and greater than 50% for the left main stem.

CABG can be offered to patients on symptomatic grounds when their coronary anatomy does not fit the above criteria, but have disease that is not suitable for PCI (multi vessel disease, diffuse calcific disease).

The recent SYNTAX study compared PCI and CABG in multivessel disease and left main stem disease. The patients in the PCI arm had more revascularization events but similar mortality and mortality to the patients in the CABG arm. CABG is therefore recommended for these patients.

The European Society of Cardiology recommend revascularization for the following patients:

1 medical therapy is unsuccessful in controlling symptoms
2 non-invasive tests reveal a substantial area of myocardium at risk
3 there is a high likelihood of success and acceptable risk of morbidity and mortality
4 the patient prefers an interventional route and is fully aware of the risks of this route.

Refractory angina

Chronic stable refractory angina can be defined as a clinical diagnosis based on the presence of symptoms of stable angina thought to be caused by ischaemia due to advanced coronary disease and which are not controllable by a combination of maximal medical therapy, bypass surgery and PCI. Some of the modalities that have been tried include:

- Neuromodulation techniques (spinal cord stimulation)
- Thoracic epidural anaesthesia
- Thoracic sympathectomy
- Stellate ganglion blockade
- Transmyocardial or percutaneous laser
- Angiogenesis
- External counter pulsation
- Heart transplantation.

Further reading

Antithrombotic Trialists' Collaboration. Collaborative meta-analysis of randomised trials of antiplatelet therapy for prevention of death, myocardial infarction, and stroke in high risk patients. *BMJ* 2002;**324**:71–86.

Boden WE, O'Rourke RA, Teo KK, et al. COURAGE Trial Research Group. Optimal medical therapy with or without PCI for stable coronary disease. *N Engl J Med* 2007;**356**:1503–16.

Brugts JJ, Ninomiya T, Boersma E, et al. The consistency of the treatment effect of an ACE-inhibitor based treatment regimen in patients with vascular disease or high risk of vascular disease: a combined analysis of individual data of ADVANCE, EUROPA, and PROGRESS trials. *Eur Heart J* 2009;**30**:1385–94.

CAPRIE Steering Committee. A randomised, blinded, trial of clopidogrel versus aspirin in patients at risk of ischaemic events (CAPRIE). *Lancet* 1996;**348**:1329–39.

Fox KM, Garcia MA, Ardissino D, et al., Task Force on the Management of Stable Angina Pectoris of the European Society of Cardiology; ESC Committee for Practice Guidelines (CPG). Guidelines on the management of stable angina pectoris: executive summary. *Eur Heart J* 2006;**27**:1341–81.

Fox KM, EURopean trial On reduction of cardiac events with Perindopril in stable coronary Artery disease Investigators. Efficacy of perindopril in reduction of cardiovascular events among patients with stable coronary artery disease: randomised, double-blind, placebo-controlled, multicentre trial (the EUROPA study). *Lancet* 2003;**362**:782–8.

Serruys PW, Morice MC, Kappetein AP, et al., SYNTAX Investigators. Percutaneous coronary intervention versus coronary-artery bypass grafting for severe coronary artery disease. *N Engl J Med* 2009;**360**:961–72.

Sever PS, Dahlöf B, Poulter NR, et al., ASCOT investigators. Prevention of coronary and stroke events with atorvastatin in hypertensive patients who have average or lower-than-average cholesterol concentrations, in the Anglo-Scandinavian Cardiac Outcomes Trial—Lipid Lowering Arm (ASCOT-LLA): a multicentre randomised controlled trial. *Lancet* 2003;**361**:1149–58.

Yusuf S, Sleight P, Pogue J, et al. Effects of an angiotensin-converting-enzyme inhibitor, ramipril, on cardiovascular events in high-risk patients. The Heart Outcomes Prevention Evaluation Study Investigators. *N Engl J Med* 2000;**342**:145–53.

Acute coronary syndromes

'Acute coronary syndromes' (ACS) are the acute clinical manifestations of coronary artery disease, when disruption or erosion of a coronary atheromatous plaque results in sufficient coronary obstruction to produce clinical and/or electrocardiographic features of ischaemia accompanied by a variable extent of myocyte necrosis. The condition may present, unheralded, as cardiac arrest or sudden death when abrupt ischaemia induces a malignant ventricular arrhythmia, predominantly ventricular fibrillation. ACS is not an inevitable consequence of plaque disruption: there may be no clinical features and no detectable ischaemia in the absence of obstruction to coronary flow ('silent' plaque disruption and atherogenesis).

There are three principal forms of ACS:

1 Unstable angina (symptoms plus ECG changes of ischaemia: ST depression or T wave inversion. *No* detectable biomarker release).

2 Non-ST elevation myocardial infarction (MI) (symptoms plus ECG changes of ischaemia: ST depression or T wave inversion, *plus* detectable biomarker release, e.g. troponin).

3 ST elevation MI (symptoms plus ECG changes of infarction: ST elevation and reciprocal ST depression, *plus* detectable biomarker release, e.g. troponin).

- Symptoms: all three forms involve symptoms of ischaemia, principally chest pain or tightness (>10-minute duration), and the discomfort may radiate to the jaw and to the arms or shoulders and uncommonly to the back. In contrast to exertional angina the symptoms come on at rest or on minimal exertion. In unstable angina a relapsing pattern of repeated episodes of pain is seen and these may progressively worsen, the 'crescendo angina' pattern. Unstable angina may develop in a patient with previously stable angina, or it may arise *de novo* or following infarction. In non-ST elevation and ST elevation MI the symptoms are typically more severe and more persistent and usually accompanied by autonomic disturbance. Oppressive chest discomfort may be described as 'breathlessness' in some patients. In the elderly people and in diabetic subjects the symptoms may be atypical or even absent.

- Clinical signs: these are of limited value in making the diagnosis of ACS. In the absence of haemodynamic and/or autonomic disturbance, there may be no abnormal signs. With ST elevation MI, pallor and sweating are commonly seen and with extensive infarction the patient may have signs of reduced cardiac output, arrhythmias, heart failure, and cardiogenic shock (see Chapter 5.8).

Electrocardiogram

ST elevation MI

Typically, horizontal ST elevation infarction is seen in adjacent leads, reflecting the distribution of the occluded artery. Reciprocal ST depression may be present. For details see Chapter 5.8.

During the early phase of ST elevation MI the earliest signs may be peaked T waves, then upsloping ST segments, then more characteristic horizontal ST elevation. The ECG is very seldom entirely normal in the early stages of infarction. Late or 'missed' ST elevation infarction may be evident as loss of R waves and the development of Q waves.

Non-ST elevation MI and unstable angina

The key features are horizontal ST depression (>1 mm (0.1 mV)) and t wave inversion. Minor ST depression (0.5 mm (0.05 mV)) is less specific but still conveys a worse prognosis than ACS without ST depression. Some patients may only have peaked t waves. The signs of ischaemia are usually more extensive in non-ST elevation MI than unstable angina.

Various other conditions may produce abnormalities of t waves and ST changes (see Chapter 5.9).

Biomarkers of necrosis

Troponin, creatine kinase MB fraction. Troponin is the reference standard and increasingly sensitive assays allow the accurate detection of very small volumes of myocyte necrosis. Hence a greater proportion of 'unstable angina' has measurable myocyte necrosis and is reclassified as non-ST elevation MI. Even very modest troponin elevations (e.g. >0.05 ng/mL) have important prognostic impact (on subsequent risk of death and MI). A Global Task Force has provided guidance on diagnostic criteria for infarction (Thygesen 2007).

Importantly, detectable troponin release only occurs 2–4 hours after onset of ischaemia so a working ACS diagnosis needs to be made and initial management based upon this.

Any cause of myocyte cell death will cause troponin release (including arrhythmias and heart failure) even in the absence of detectable coronary disease. Thus troponin release signifies myocyte cell death, *not specifically ACS*.

Imaging in ACS

Although imaging is not usually required to make the diagnosis, imaging can be valuable, especially when the clinical features are equivocal. For example, entirely normal contractile function would exclude the diagnosis of acute infarction in a patient with undefined chest pain.

- *Echocardiography* is used to assess contractile function and the presence or absence of complications like mitral regurgitation, and ventricular thrombus following infarction. It is used to assess co-existing valve disease, for example aortic stenosis, that may contribute to the extent of ischaemia.

- *Magnetic resonance* imaging provides a very accurate method of providing structural information and MR angiography is especially useful to define shunts, abnormal vascular connections, and disorders of the great vessels. Gadolinium and related contrast agents can provide an accurate assessment of the extent and distribution of infarction.

- *Computed tomography (CT)*: multislice CT can now provide a very rapid method of detecting coronary disease, but its role in screening or 'rule out' of ACS in those with chest pain is still being evaluated. CT angiography is the key investigation if pulmonary emboli are suspected.

Differential diagnoses include

- *Cardiovascular:* aortic dissection, pericarditis, myocarditis aortic stenosis, variant angina, hypertrophic cardiomyopathy, other cardiomyopathy, Tako–Tsubo syndrome.

- *Respiratory:* pulmonary embolism or infarction, pneumonia, pneumothorax, acute asthma.

- *Gastrointestinal:* oesophagitis, oesophageal spasm, hiatus hernia, peptic ulcer disease, pancreatitis, biliary colic.
- *Other:* musculoskeletal pain, cervical spondylosis, costchondritis, rib fracture, psychogenic pain.

Early management and risk stratification

ST elevation infarction is a high-risk condition requiring emergency management. Acute risk stratification is not required to guide early management. For immediate management, reperfusion therapy and later management see Chapter 5.8.

Non-ST elevation infarction and unstable angina: the conditions cannot be distinguished until sufficient time has elapsed to measure biomarkers of necrosis with sufficient diagnostic accuracy (troponin levels become diagnostic at approximately 4–6 hours). Hence a working diagnosis of non ST elevation ACS should form the basis of initial management.

Initial evaluation (Fig. 5.7.1)

The aim of the initial evaluation—usually performed in the emergency department—is to establish a working diagnosis based on clinical evaluation of the patient, the ECG, and any other relevant information including risks of ACS. It is critically important that patients with evolving ST elevation infarction are identified without delay and transferred for primary percutaneous coronary intervention (pPCI), or if unavailable within 90 minutes of first medical contact; the patient should receive thrombolysis (ideally in the pre-hospital or paramedic ambulance setting after telemetry of the ECG.

Having excluded ST elevation infarction and having established a working diagnosis of non-ST elevation ACS, the aims of treatment are:
- To reduce ischaemia
- To reduce thrombotic complications
- To risk stratify patients for acute and non-acute revascularization
- To identify patients with continuing ischaemia or ischaemic complications or evolving ST elevation MI.

Repeat clinical and ECG evaluation (ideally continuous ST monitoring) is required to identify evolving infarction.

Anti-ischaemic therapy

Nitrates: the main therapeutic benefit is related to the venodilator effects that lead to a decrease in myocardial preload and LV end-diastolic volume, and a decrease in myocardial oxygen consumption. There is evidence for their effectiveness in relieving ischaemia but no evidence that they alter outcome (death or MI). Intravenous nitrates can be titrated upwards until symptoms (angina and/or dyspnoea) are relieved within the limits of side-effects (hypotension, headache). Tolerance may occur with continuous administration. Alternatives include nitrate-like drugs such as sydnonimines or potassium channel activators (nicorandil). When symptoms are controlled intravenous nitrates may be replaced with non-parenteral alternatives, incorporating nitrate-free intervals.

Beta-blockers

The principal effects are on beta-1 receptors, resulting in a decrease in myocardial oxygen consumption. A meta-analysis

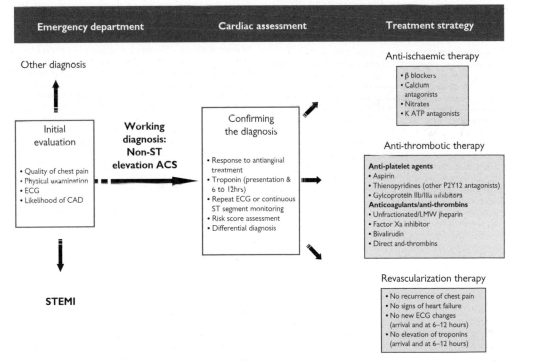

Fig. 5.7.1 Triage and early management of non-ST elevation ACS.

of smaller trials suggests that they reduce the rate of progression of unstable angina to MI; analogous studies in ST elevation MI suggest that they reduce mortality. Betablockers are recommended in NSTE-ACS in the absence of contraindications and are usually well tolerated. Most benefit may be seen in those with hypertension and tachycardia (in the absence of acute heart failure). The target heart rate is between 50 and 60 bpm. Patients with significantly impaired atrioventricular conduction, those in acute heart failure or acute LV dysfunction, or those with severe asthma should not receive beta-blockers.

Ivabradine is not a beta-blocker and it produces a reduction in heart rate without an effect on myocardial contractility. It selectively inhibits the primary pacemaker current in the sinus node and may be used in patients with beta-blocker contraindications.

Calcium channel blockers

They are vasodilator drugs and some have direct effects on heart rate and atrioventricular conduction (non dihydropyridines). They provide symptom relief in patients already receiving nitrates and beta-blockers, and are useful in patients with contraindications to beta-blockers. Their efficacy in relieving symptoms appears similar to beta-blockers. Short-acting dihydropyridines are not recommended in isolation (in the absence of beta blockade), in order to avoid the oxygen demand associated with sinus tachycardia. In vasospastic angina dihydropiridines are first-line therapy.

Antiplatelet therapy

Aspirin: aspirin (160–325 mg) is indicated (ESC Guidelines IA recommendation, NICE) in all patients once a working diagnosis of ACS is made, and is indicated for lifelong secondary prevention (75–100 mg) (IA), provided the patient does not have a true allergy or bleeding contraindication.

ADP receptor antagonists

Clopidogrel is indicated as an alternative to aspirin, where aspirin is contraindicated (IB). Dual antiplatelet therapy (aspirin plus clopidogrel) is superior to aspirin alone in ST elevation MI and non-ST elevation ACS and is indicated for 9–12 months. Dual therapy (aspirin plus thienopyridine) is indicated for at least 12 months in patients with drug-eluting stents.

Prasugrel is a more potent antiplatelet thienopyridine and has been shown to have superior efficacy but more bleeding than clopidogrel. Most benefit was seen in diabetic patients, in ST elevation MI, and in limiting stent thrombosis. Prasugrel should be avoided in those with higher bleeding risk and especially those with prior stroke or transient ischaemic attack.

Ticagrelor is a direct-acting ADP antagonist (non-thienopyridine) and results in fewer deaths/MIs/strokes than clopidogrel, and fewer deaths, and fewer stent thromboses. There was no overall excess of bleeding, but more non-coronary artery bypass graft (CABG) bleeding. It is not yet approved for administration.

Glycoprotein IIb/IIIa inhibitors (GPI)

These are potent parenteral inhibitors of platelet-to-platelet binding and they are indicated in high-risk patients, particularly those undergoing PCI in the context of an ACS. Most of the studies on GPIs pre-dated the use of dual antiplatelet therapy and their benefits on top of dual antiplatelet therapy are less certain. They increase risks of bleeding. Nevertheless, evidence supports their use,

especially in primary PCI (in view of rapid onset of action, extent of platelet inhibition, and intravenous administration). They are also indicated in high-risk non-ST elevation ACS patients undergoing PCI (for example those with ongoing ischaemia or angiographically visible thrombus). Whether they confer additional benefits or hazards in patients already treated with aspirin plus higher dose clopidogrel, or prasugrel, or ticagrelor remains uncertain.

Abciximab is indicated in high-risk ACS patients, not pretreated with a GPI, who undergo PCI (ESC Guideline 1A recommendation).

Tirofiban and eptifibatide are small molecule GPIs that are administered by intravenous infusion and they can be used in acutely ischaemic patients; for example, those with recurrent or persistent ST depression and symptoms of ischaemia despite anti-anginal therapy. They can be administered in patients while in transit to an interventional centre.

Anticoagulant therapy

Unfractionated heparin (UFH) consists of a mixture of polysaccharide molecules, with a molecular weight ranging from 2000 to 30 000 daltons. Heparin bridges thrombin and antithrombin and so inhibits factor IIa. It is administered as an intravenous infusion, but its therapeutic window is narrow, requiring frequent monitoring of the activated partial thromboplastin time (aPTT). It is used in patients undergoing PCI but care should be taken to avoid over-anticoagulation if patients were previously on low-molecular-weight heparin (LMWH). It is preferable to maintain the LMWH during PCI in order to reduce bleeding risk (as demonstrated in ExTRACT and other studies).

LMWH consist of shorter fragments of heparin (2000–10 000 daltons). They link to antithrombin through the pentasaccharide sequence and this is the basis of their anti-Xa activity. Their anti-IIa activity is lower than with UFH. The extent of anti-Xa versus anti-IIa activity varies with different LMWHs. The key advantages of LMWH over UFH is the near complete absorption after subcutaneous administration without the need for monitoring. There is less protein binding, less platelet activation, and a more predictable dose–effect relationship. Most clinical trial experience is with enoxaparin, in both non-ST elevation ACS and ST elevation MI, and it has been shown to be superior to UFH.

Factor Xa inhibitors: both direct and indirect Factor Xa inhibitors are in development and fondaparinux, a selective indirect inhibitor of Xa, is the only agent currently approved. It was shown to be superior to LMWH in DVT prevention and treatment and in non-ST elevation ACS (OASIS 5) and in fibrinolytic-treated ST elevation MI (OASIS 6). In non-ST elevation ACS it results in approximately 50% of the rate of major bleeding compared with enoxaparin and lower mortality (OASIS 5). It is the preferred anticoagulant in patients with non-ST elevation ACS, provided they are not scheduled for early revascularization (ESC Guideline 1A recommendation). In patients undergoing PCI additional UFH is required to avoid a small excess rate of sent thrombosis.

Direct thrombin inhibitors (DTI) bind directly to thrombin (factor-IIa) and so inhibit the thrombin-induced conversion of fibrinogen to fibrin. They inactivate fibrin-bound, as well as fluid-phase thrombin. DTIs in development include inhibitors of thrombin on the platelet surface receptor. The only agents currently approved are lepuridin (for patients with heparin-induced thrombocytopenia (HIT) and in ACS, bivalirudin. Bivalirudin has been tested against heparins in a large randomized open study (ACUITY) and was shown to produce less bleeding than heparin/LMWH plus glycoprotein IIb/IIIa inhibitor.

Vitamin K antagonists (warfarin, coumadin) are used for long-term anticoagulation following ACS, for example in those with prosthetic heart valves or those with atrial fibrillation.

Selecting patients for revascularization in non-ST elevation ACS

Selection for revascularization (PCI or surgical) should be based on a combination of clinical history, symptoms, ECG, biomarkers, and risk score results (ESC Guideline recommendation I-B).

Combined evidence from large randomized trials of systematic versus selective revascularization, on top of optimal medical therapy, suggests an overall benefit resulting in reduced rates of cardiovascular death/MI (FRISC II, RITA 3, TIMI 38-TACTICS, ICTUS, ESC Guideline). The main benefit is in reduced rates of MI. Pooled analyses suggest most benefit is seen in highest risk patients and no or little benefit in lowest risk patients—hence the need for robust risk stratification. Decisions based on troponin positivity, alone, are not a reliable guide to risk status (ESC Guideline).

Key points

- Evaluation of risk is a dynamic process and should be updated as the clinical situation evolves.
- A 12-lead ECG should be obtained within 10 minutes of first medical contact and interpreted immediately or sent by telemetry to a cardiac centre with appropriate expertise.
- The ECG should be repeated for persistent or recurrent symptoms (or continuous ST analysis).
- Troponin (cTnT or cTnI) should be measured promptly and should be repeated after 6–12 hours if the initial test is negative.
- Established risk scores (such as GRACE) should be used for initial and subsequent risk assessment (ESC Guideline I-B).

- In patients without recurrent pain, and normal ECG findings, and negative troponins tests, a non-invasive stress test for inducible ischaemia is recommended before discharge.

Evidence to support the timing of revascularization comes from the modest sized ISAR COOL study and the large TIMACS study. Overall, there is not robust evidence to support systematic early revascularization (within approx 6–12 hours) in all patients. However, most benefit was seen for early revascularization in high-risk patients (TIMACS). It must be recognized that highest risk patients were excluded from these comparisons.

Acute revascularization (within 6–12 hours of presentation)

In patients with continuing or recurrent ischaemia (dymamic or persistent ST depression) urgent angiography is indicated, then PCI or CABG depending on the clinical and angiographic findings. Similarly, acute ischaemia complicated by recurrent arrhythmia, or heart failure, may require urgent revascularization if the patient has failed to respond to medical therapy.

Importantly, some patients who initially present with non-ST elevation ACS *evolve ST elevation MI* during the first hours after presentation and some evolve ST elevation MI after developing recurrent ischaemia at later time intervals. Such patients with acute ST elevation MI must be detected promptly and undergo emergency reperfusion (preferably primary PCI, or if unavailable within approximately 90 minutes, then intravenous thrombolysis). See Chapter 5.18.

Early revascularization (12–72 hours of presentation)

In patients without highest risk features early revascularization is indicated in those with high-risk baseline characteristics using a formal risk score.

The risk score system recommended by the SIGN, ESC and NICE Guidelines is the GRACE risk score (Fig. 5.7.2). The recommendation is based on comparison of the performance of different risk scores in unselected

Mortality in hospital and at 6 months in low-, intermediate-, and high-risk categories of patients (GRACE risk score)

Risk category (tertiles)	GRACE risk score	In-hospital deaths (%)
Low	≤108	<1
Intermediate	109–140	1–3
High	>140	>3
Risk category (tertiles)	**GRACE risk score**	**Post discharge to 6 months deaths (%)**
Low	≤88	<3
Intermediate	89–118	3–8
High	>118	>8

For calculations, see http://www.outcomes.org/grace

Fig. 5.7.2 Risk categories in ACS derived from Fox et al., 2006.

independent populations (NICE Guideline). This risk score can be downloaded (www.outcome.org/grace) and used on a computer or handheld device.

Secondary prevention

- Lifestyle measures: all patients require secondary prevention lifestyle measures, especially smoking cessation and dietary and exercise measures.
- Antiplatelet therapy: lifelong oral aspirin 75–100 mg, or if aspirin is contraindicated then a thienopyridine (clopidogrel 75 mg) is currently recommended.
- Dual antiplatelet therapy (aspirin plus thienopyridine) is indicated after non-ST elevation ACS for 9–12 months, (clopidogrel, CURE study, or prasugrel TRITON study) and also indicated for at least 12 months in patients following drug eluting stent implantation.
- ACE inhibitors/angiotensin receptor blockers are indicated for secondary prevention.
- Lipid-lowering therapy: in addition to dietary advice lipid-lowering secondary prevention is indicated, lifelong, in patients following ACS (unless angiography demonstrates no evidence of atheromatous coronary disease).
- Additional treatment may be required for related conditions including hypertension and diabetes.

Further reading

Bassand J-P, Hamm CW, Ardissino D, *et al.* Guidelines for the Diagnosis and Treatment of Non-ST-Segment Elevation Acute Coronary Syndromes. *Eur Heart J* 2007;**28**:1598–60.

Fox KAA, Dabbous OH, Goldberg RJ, *et al.*, for the GRACE Investigators: Prediction of risk of death and myocardial infarction in the six months after presentation with ACS: a prospective, multinational, observational study (GRACE). *BMJ* 2006;**333**:1091–4.

Fox KAA, Poole-Wilson P, Clayton TC, *et al.* Long term impact of an interventional strategy in non st elevation acute coronary syndrome: 5 Year Outcome of the BHF RITA 3 Study. *Lancet* 2005;**366**:914–20.

Mehta S, Granger C, Boden W, *et al.*, for the TIMACS Investigators. Early versus delayed invasive intervention in acute coronary syndromes. *N Engl J Med* 2009;**360**:2165–75.

Thygesen K, Alpert JS, White HD, on behalf of the joint ESC/ACCF/AHA/WHF Task Force for the Redefinition of Myocardial Infarction. Universal definition of myocardial infarction. *Eur Heart J* 2007;**28**:2525–38.

Yusuf S, Mehta SR, Chrolavicius S, *et al.*, for the Fifth Organisation to Assess Strategies in Acute Ischemic Syndromes (OASIS-5) investigators. Comparison of fondaparinux and enoxaparin in acute coronary syndromes. *N Engl J Med* 2006;**354**:1464–76.

Yusuf S, Mehta SR, Chrolavicius S, *et al.*, for the OASIS-6 Randomised Trial. Effects of fondaparinux on mortality and reinfarction in patients with acute ST segment elevation myocardial infarction. *JAMA* 2006;**295**:1519–30.

Websites

http://www.sign.ac.uk
http://www.nice.org.uk

Acute ST segment elevation myocardial infarction

Worldwide, more than 3 million people each year are estimated to have an acute ST elevation myocardial infarction (STEMI). Myocardial infarction (MI) is now becoming increasingly more common in developing countries, where progressive urbanization has led to increasing rates of obesity and diabetes. Partial or complete epicardial coronary artery occlusion from plaque rupture or erosion is the commonest cause.

Diagnosis

MI is defined as myocardial cell death due to prolonged myocardial ischaemia and the clinical diagnosis is based on a combination of symptoms (chest discomfort, shortness of breath, sweating) plus electrocardiogram (ECG) changes of ST elevation ≥2 mm in men, ≥1.5 mm in women (White and Chew 2008) in V1–V3 and ≥1 mm in two adjacent level leads or left bundle branch block LBBB (not known to be old).

Right ventricular infarction should be assessed by right precordial leads. There are a number of conditions that may be confused with the ECG changes of STEMI; the most common are repolarization abnormalities and pericarditis.

Cardiac biomarkers increase later and infarction may be 'aborted' by reperfusion therapy (White and Chew 2008). Troponins are the preferred markers. There is no need to use CKMB. Troponins rise by 3 hours, with high sensitivity troponins increasing earlier. Although troponins may stay elevated for 7–14 days, reinfarction can be detected (in the presence of ischaemic symptoms or ECG changes) by a rise and/or fall of 20% (Thygesen et al. 2007).

Criteria for diagnosis of acute myocardial infarction.

The term MI should be used when there is evidence of myocardial necrosis in a clinical setting consistent with myocardial ischaemia. Under these conditions any one of the following criteria meets the diagnosis for MI.

- Detection of rise and/or fall of cardiac biomarkers (preferably troponin) with at least one value above the 99th percentile of the upper reference limit together with evidence of myocardial ischaemia with at least one of the following:
- Symptoms of ischaemia.
- ECG changes indicative of new ischaemia (new ST-T changes or new LBBB).
- Development of pathological Q waves in the ECG.
- Imaging evidence of new loss of viable myocardium or new regional wall motion abnormality.

There are five types of myocardial infarction. The prognosis and treatment differs for each.

Clinical classification of myocardial infarction

- *Type 1:* spontaneous MI related to ischaemia due to a primary coronary event such as plaque fissuring, erosion or rupture, or dissection.
- *Type 2:* MI secondary to ischaemia due to either increased oxygen demand or decreased supplies e.g. coronary artery spasm, coronary embolism (thrombus, vegetations, or atrial myxoma), anaemia, arrhythmias, hypertension, or hypotension.
- *Type 3:* sudden unexpected cardiac death with symptoms suggestive of myocardial ischaemia, accompanied by new ST elevation, or new LBBB, but dying before

blood samples could be obtained, or in the lag phase of cardiac biomarkers in the blood.

- *Type 4:* MI associated with percutaneous coronary intervention (PCI).
- *Type 4b:* Stent thrombosis.
- *Type 5:* MI associated with coronary artery bypass grafting (CABG).

Treatment

Immediate reperfusion therapy must be started within 30 minutes for fibrinolysis and 90 minutes for door to balloon time for primary PCI.

- Pain should be relieved with morphine 2.5–10 mg IV. Nausea and vomiting should be treated with metoclopramide (10 mg IV) or a phenothiazine.
- Oxygen should be administered at 2–5 L/min for 3 hours.
- Nitrates should be used to relieve pain but have no effect on mortality.
- Low potassium levels should be corrected.
- Patients should be risk stratified. The best risk score for prediction of death and MI is the Global Registry for Acute Coronary Events (GRACE) score.
- The preferred reperfusion strategy is primary PCI. If this cannot be performed in a timely manner, fibrinolytic therapy should be administered if there are no contraindications.

Fibrinolytic therapy: requirements

- Systems to ensure shortened door to needle time of <30 minutes, e.g. transmission of ECG or read in the community.

Contraindications to fibrinolysis

- Trauma and/or surgery <2 weeks
- Severe uncontrolled hypertension (BP >180/110)
- Ischaemic stroke <1 year ago
- Haemorrhagic stroke ever
- Known bleeding diathesis or current use of anticoagulation outside therapeutic range
- Significant liver or renal dysfunction
- Prior exposure to streptokinase
- Pregnancy or postpartum
- Lumbar puncture within previous month
- Non-compressible vascular punctures (e.g. subclavian central venous lines).

Fibrinolytic agents

Streptokinase
- Give as 1.5 million units over 30 minutes to 1 hour. Do not readminister because of ineffectiveness or allergy due to antibodies.
- If cost is an issue, streptokinase is a good alternative.

Recombinant tissue-type plasminogen activator (rtPA, alteplase)
- Give 15-mg bolus IV then 0.75 mg/kg over 30 minutes (not to exceed 50 mg), then 0.5 mg/kg over 60 minutes (not to exceed 35 mg).

Reteplase
- Give two IV bolus doses of 10 units 10 minutes apart.

Tenecteplase
- Give as injection over 10 seconds at 30–50 mg according to body weight (500–600 μg/kg).
- The maximum dose is 50 mg.
- It is associated with less systemic bleeding.

APSAC (anistreplase)
- Give as an IV bolus of 30 mg over 2–5 minutes.

Antiplatelet therapy
- Aspirin 150–300 mg (chewed if enteric coated) and continued indefinitely 75–150 mg od.
- Clopidogrel 300–600 mg if ≤75 years, followed by 75 mg/kg loading and daily dose if >75 years. Although the trials are for a shorter period, clopidogrel should be given for 6–12 months.
- IIb/IIIa antagonists are not recommended with fibrinolytic therapy.
- Antithrombotic therapy with fibrinolytic therapy.
- Enoxaparin is the preferred antithrombotic therapy in patients <75 years; an IV bolus of 30 mg followed by 1.0 mg/kg sc 12 hourly should be given for at least 48 hours and is recommended to be given through angiography if performed, or until hospital discharge. (Table 5.8.1).
- In patients ≥75 years the bolus should be omitted and 0.75 mg/kg given sc 12 hourly. For patients with creatinine clearance ≤30 mL/min the dose should be reduced to 1.0 mg/kg once a day.

The use of adjunctive unfractionated heparin (UFH) with streptokinase has been controversial, although a meta-analysis has shown a reduction in mortality compared with placebo. Adjunctive enoxaparin or UFH is recommended to be administered immediately with streptokinase. Although a recommendation, some hospitals prefer not to use heparin particularly if patients are older and/or have a small inferior MI.

Fondaparinux, a synthetic factor Xa inhibitor reduces 30-day death or MI in patients receiving fibrinolysis and in those not receiving fibrinolysis compared with unfractionated heparin or placebo (Table 5.8.1). In patients undergoing PCI there was no benefit with fondaparinux and there was an excess of catheter thrombosis noted.

Following fibrinolysis PCI can be performed in a variety of clinical settings
- Rescue PCI for continuing ischaemia, haemodynamic instability, or failure of 50% ST resolution 90 minutes after beginning fibrinolysis (Antman *et al.* 2008).
- Facilitated PCI following fibrinolysis to ensure there is a patent infarct-related artery (Keeley *et al.* 2006). Facilitated PCI with PCI performed within 3 hours of fibrinolysis is currently not recommended because of adverse ischaemic events seen in several trials and meta-analysis (Keeley *et al.* 2006) where mortality, reinfarction, urgent target vessel revascularization, stroke, and bleeding were all increased by this approach (Keeley *et al.* 2003).
- Early elective PCI performed within 24 hours to decrease risk of reocclusion and ischaemic events. Fibrinolysis restores flow in the infarct-related artery in 50–60% of patients. Early angiography and PCI as appropriate 3–24 hours after administration of fibrinolysis has shown

equivalent or better outcomes (death, MI, revascularization) than fibrinolysis alone or primary PCI (White 2008) and shorter duration of hospitalization than fibrinolysis alone.
- PCI for reinfarction after fibrinolysis is better than readministration of fibrinolysis.
- Late elective PCI, performed after 24 hours because of recurrent ischaemia, positive stress test or to define anatomy.
- PCI of a totally occluded artery >24 hours after STEMI is not recommended in patients without continuing ischaemia, ventricular arrhythmias or haemodynamic instability (Hochman *et al.* 2006).

Table 5.8.1 Usage and dosage of antiplatelet and anticoagulant agents for patients treated with fibrinolytic agents or PCI

Antiplatelet agent	Fibrinolysis	PCI
Aspirin	150–300 mg	150–300 mg
Clopidogrel	600 mg loading for 7 days if ≤75 years, followed by 75 mg/kg od if >75 years no loading and 75 mg od	600 mg loading followed by 150 mg for 7 days and then 75 mg for 1 month with bare metal stent and 12 months with drug eluting stent
Prasugrel	Not recommended	60 mg followed by 10 mg instead of clopidogrel for 15 months
IIb/IIIa antagonists	Not recommended	Abciximab IV bolus of 0.25 μg/kg followed by 0.125 μg/kg/hour infusion for 12 hour
Antithrombotic agents		
UFH	60 U/kg bolus followed by 12 U/kg, maximum of 1000 U/hour adjusted to APTT 50–70 seconds for 24–48 hours	IV bolus of 100 U/kg (60 U/kg if GP IIb/IIIa antagonists used)
Fondaparinux	2.5 mg IV followed by 2.5 mg sc daily up to 8 days or hospital discharge	Bivalirudin: IV bolus of 0.75 mg/kg followed by 1.75 mg/kg/hour terminated at end of procedure
Enoxaparin	30 mg IV and 1.0 mg/kg 12 sc hourly if <75 years. If ≥75 years give 0.75 mg/kg sc 12 hourly. In patients with creatinine clearance ≤30 mL/min give 1.0 mg/kg od	Not recommended

The ESC Guidelines (Silber *et al.* 2005) support routine angiography after fibrinolysis in most patients. The ACC/AHA Guidelines (Antman *et al.* 2008) recommend angiography in patients with recent MI (readministration of fibrinolysis is not recommended), moderate to severe ischaemia, or stress testing. PCI of a haemodynamically significant stenosis is thought to be reversible.

Beta-blockade
- Beta-blockers have been shown to be harmful with an increase in the incidence of cardiogenic shock (Chen *et al.* 2005) in patients with a Killip class III or IV but are recommended in other patients without contraindications (heart rate <60 per minute, systolic blood pressure <100 mmHg, advanced AV block), because of a reduction in recurrent MI and ventricular fibrillation.
- Short-acting agents are recommended, e.g. metoprolol 5 mg at 5-minute intervals to a maximum of 20 mg.
- Long-acting agents (carvedilol, bisoprolol, and metoprolol succinate) are recommended for patients with heart failure.

Angiotensin-converting enzyme inhibitors
- All patients without contraindications (BP <100 mmHg) should receive an angiotensin-converting enzyme (ACE) inhibitor to reduce left ventricular remodelling (in small initial doses, e.g. ramipril 1.25 mg od, captopril 6.25 mg tds). Patients with anterior MIs and patients with impaired left ventricular function benefit most.
- If a patient is hypotensive and cannot tolerate a beta-blocker and an ACE inhibitor, the ACE inhibitor should be given first due to the beneficial effects on left ventricular remodelling.

Angiotensin receptor blockers
- Angiotensin II receptor blockers (ARBs) have a role when ACE inhibitors are not tolerated.

Statin therapy
- Initiation of statin therapy should be begun in hospital (e.g. simvastatin 40 mg or atorvastatin 80 mg) with an aim to reduce low-density lipoprotein (LDL) to <2.0 mmol/L.

Implantable defibrillators
- Robust evidence supports the use of implantable cardioverter-defibrillators in patients with life-threatening ventricular arrhythmias especially in the presence of reduced ejection fraction at least 40 days after MI.

Other therapies
- Smoking cessation advice with nicotine patches should begin in the coronary care unit; spironolactone or eplerenone should be given to patients with heart failure or decreased ejection fraction; all patients should be referred for rehabilitation.
- STEMI: an invasive strategy is generally preferred if:
  - skilled PCI laboratory is available with or without surgical back-up
  - medical contact-to-balloon or door-to-balloon time is <90 minutes
  - high risk
  - Killip class ≥3

- cardiogenic shock
- contraindications to fibrinolysis, including increased risk of bleeding and ICH
- symptom onset >3 hours ago.

STEMI: time to treatment
Time to treatment is the most important factor determining outcome. If the difference between door-balloon-door to needle time is >114 minutes, the advantage of primary PCI is lost.

Strategies to reduce door to balloon times
- ECGs performed in the community
- ECGs may be transmitted to be read or read by ambulance personnel
- Catheterization laboratory may be activated bypassing emergency department (ED)
- ED activates the catheterization laboratory while the patient still en route
- ED physicians activate the catheterization laboratory
- Single call to a central operator activates catheterization laboratory
- Catheterization laboratory staff to arrive within 20 minutes
- Having staff receive real-time feedback.

Primary PCI: requirements
Systems to ensure shortened door-to-balloon time
- Transmission of ECG; one call to activate team, bypassing ED, straight to catheterization laboratory: door-to-balloon time <90 minutes.

Antiplatelet agents
- Aspirin 150–300 mg chewed if enteric coated.
- Clopidogrel 600 mg and 150 mg for 7 days followed by 75 mg od. About 30% of patients are resistant, due to polymorphisms and other causes, with decreased impairment of platelet function following clopidogrel. Given for 1 month with bare metal stents and 12 months with drug-eluting stents.
- Prasugrel 60 mg loading followed by 10 mg od for 15 months can be used as an alternative to clopidogrel. It is not associated with platelet resistance and works earlier than clopidogrel. Decreases cardiovascular death, MI, and stroke by about 20% compared with clopidogrel (Wiviott *et al.* 2007). Groups that benefit most are diabetics, patients receiving stents and patients undergoing primary or rescue PCI. Bleeding occurs more frequently than with clopidogrel in elderly people, and low-weight females. Patients with prior stroke or TIA or patients in whom there is a possibility of coronary artery bypass surgery because of the unacceptable bleeding rates should not be prescribed prasugrel.
- The IIb//IIIa antagonist abciximab reduces mortality without increasing bleeding (Table 5.8.1).

Antithrombotic agents
- Bivalirudin or UFH
- Bivalirudin is the antithrombotic agent of choice as it is associated with decreased mortality at 30 days and one year and decreased bleeding compared with UFH (Stone *et al.* 2008).

PCI equipment
- Extraction catheters
- Stents, either bare metal or drug eluting
- *Other therapies:*
  - ACE inhibitors, ARBs, beta-blockers, statins, smoking cessation advice with nicotine patches begun in coronary care unit, spironolactone or eplerenone in patients with heart failure or decreased ejection fraction, and rehabilitation should be as with fibrinolytic therapy.
  - The success of PCI and fibrinolysis for STEMI has meant that the need for urgent surgical reperfusion is limited to a few selected patients.

Complications of myocardial infarction

Mortality from myocardial infarction has been decreasing

Most deaths in hospitalized patients with MI are due to heart failure and mechanical complications including myocardial rupture, mitral regurgitation due to papillary muscle dysfunction or chordal rupture, and ventricular septal rupture. Despite contemporary therapies including reperfusion, emergent revascularization, and intra-aortic balloon pumping, half of patients with cardiogenic shock will die. Compared with the pre-reperfusion era, fatal ventricular tachyarrhythmias are now less common, although sudden cardiac death remains a substantial cause of late mortality in those with severe impairment of left ventricular function (ejection fraction <35%).

Cardiogenic shock

An early invasive approach is the treatment of choice for patients with cardiogenic shock (Hochman et al. 1999). Patients admitted to hospitals without PCI facilities should be immediately transferred. Fibrinolytic therapy can be given (if indicated), inotropes begun and an intra-aortic balloon pump inserted (if available) if the tertiary centre is distant.

An evidence-based approach to management is needed

- Need for hub and spoke primary PCI centres with audit of door-to-balloon times <90 minutes
- For patients where this cannot be achieved, fibrinolysis should be administered within 30 minutes with close monitoring for failed reperfusion
- Close relationships with PCI centres need to be maintained, and enhanced if necessary to ensure rapid transfer

of patients with failed fibrinolysis, continuing symptoms, or haemodynamic compromise.

References

Antman EM, Hand M, Armstrong PW, et al. 2007 Focused Update of the ACC/AHA 2004 Guidelines for the Management of Patients With ST-Elevation Myocardial Infarction: a report of the American College of Cardiology/American Heart Association Task Force on Practice Guidelines: developed in collaboration With the Canadian Cardiovascular Society endorsed by the American Academy of Family Physicians: 2007 Writing Group to Review New Evidence and Update the ACC/AHA 2004 Guidelines for the Management of Patients With ST-Elevation Myocardial Infarction, Writing on Behalf of the 2004 Writing Committee. *Circulation* 2008;**117**:296–329.

Chen ZM, Pan HC, Chen YP, et al. Early intravenous then oral metoprolol in 45,852 patients with acute myocardial infarction: randomised placebo-controlled trial. *Lancet* 2005;**366**:1622–32.

Hochman JS, Lamas GA, Buller CE, et al. Coronary intervention for persistent occlusion after myocardial infarction. *N Engl J Med* 2006;**355**:2395–407.

Hochman JS, Sleeper LA, Webb JG, et al. Early revascularization in acute myocardial infarction complicated by cardiogenic shock. SHOCK Investigators. Should We Emergently Revascularize Occluded Coronaries for Cardiogenic Shock. *N Engl J Med* 1999;**341**:625–34.

Keeley EC, Boura JA, Grines CL. Comparison of primary and facilitated percutaneous coronary interventions for ST-elevation myocardial infarction: quantitative review of randomised trials. *Lancet* 2006;**367**:579–88.

Keeley EC, Boura JA, Grines CL. Primary angioplasty versus intravenous thrombolytic therapy for acute myocardial infarction: a quantitative review of 23 randomised trials. *Lancet* 2003;**361**:13–20.

Silber S, Albertsson P, Aviles FF, et al. Guidelines for percutaneous coronary interventions. The Task Force for Percutaneous Coronary Interventions of the European Society of Cardiology. *Eur Heart J* 2005;**26**:804–47.

Stone GW, Witzenbichler B, Guagliumi G, et al. Bivalirudin during primary PCI in acute myocardial infarction. *N Engl J Med* 2008;**358**:2218–30.

Thygesen K, Alpert JS, White HD. Universal definition of myocardial infarction. *J Am Coll Cardiol* 2007;**50**:2173–95.

White HD, Chew DP. Acute myocardial infarction. *Lancet* 2008;**372**:570–84.

White HD. Systems of care: need for hub-and-spoke systems for both primary and systematic percutaneous coronary intervention after fibrinolysis. *Circulation* 2008;**118**:219–22.

Wiviott SD, Braunwald E, McCabe CH, et al. Prasugrel versus clopidogrel in patients with acute coronary syndromes. *N Engl J Med* 2007;**357**:2001–15.

Non-ST-segment elevation acute coronary syndromes

Introduction
Unstable angina (UA) and non-ST-segment elevation myocardial infarction (NSTEMI) are an integral part of the spectrum of acute coronary syndromes. The usual pathophysiology is characterized by coronary thrombosis following a ruptured atherosclerotic plaque with compromise of coronary blood flow and resulting myocardial ischaemia. Whereas ST-segment elevation myocardial infarction (STEMI) is generally caused by total occlusion of the coronary artery, UA/NSTEMI usually relates to suboc-clusive coronary events, often accompanied by distal embolization.

At least one-third of patients thought initially to present with UA are now appreciated to sustain myocardial necrosis and receive the diagnosis of NSTEMI: this relates to the enhanced sensitivity for its detection by cardiac tro-ponins as opposed to conventional creatine kinase (CK) measures.

Classification
A recent consensus document has proposed a clinical classi-fication of myocardial infarction (MI) (Thygesen *et al.* 2007).
- *Type 1*: MI due to a pathological process in the coronary arterial wall (plaque erosion/rupture, fissuring, dissection).
- *Type 2*: MI due to increased oxygen demand or decreased supply (e.g. coronary spasm, embolism, anaemia, arrhyth-mias, hypotension, hypertension).
- *Type 3*: sudden unexpected cardiac death before cardiac biomarkers could be obtained or appear in the blood.
- *Type 4a*: MI associated with percutaneous coronary intervention (PCI).
- *Type 4b*: MI associated with stent thrombosis.
- *Type 5*: MI associated with coronary artery bypass surgery (CABG).

Pathophysiology
The five major pathophysiological processes that can result in UA/NSTEMI are discussed below (Braunwald 1998).

Non-occlusive thrombus
The most common mechanism of UA/NSTEMI is rupture or fissuring of an atherosclerotic plaque with superim-posed thrombus formation resulting in severe or subtotal obstruction of the coronary artery. Patients often possess more than one ulcerated plaque: plaque erosion especially among females is also a pathogenetic factor.

Progressive mechanical obstruction
Progressive luminal narrowing resulting in UA/NSTEMI is often seen in patients with restenosis following PCI but can also be seen with accelerated atherosclerosis.

Dynamic obstruction
Vasoconstriction may occur in both atheromatous and angiographically normal epicardial coronary arteries as well as in the coronary microvasculature. Triggers include local vasoconstrictor substances (serotonin, thromboxane A_2), endothelial dysfunction, adrenergic stimuli, cold expo-sure, and cocaine. Prinzmetal's angina is characterized by spontaneous episodes of angina in association with ST elevation as a result of focal spasm of an epicardial coronary artery.

Inflammation
Activated macrophages and T-lymphocytes are involved in processes leading to plaque instability, rupture, and throm-bosis. Increased levels of C-reactive protein (CRP) and interleukin 6 (IL-6) are found in patients with UA/NSTEMI and are associated with worse clinical outcomes.

Secondary unstable angina
UA/NSTEMI can result from a mismatch between myocar-dial oxygen supply and demand due to conditions unrelat-ed to coronary artery disease. Reduced oxygen supply may be due to anaemia, hypoxaemia, and hypotension (volume depletion or sepsis). Increased oxygen demand may be due to tachyarrhythmias, fever, thyrotoxicosis, hyperadrener-gic states, and high afterload states (hypertension, aortic stenosis).

Epidemiology
Observational studies have documented a consistent inci-dence of MI across a variety of time periods; however, there has been an increase in the proportion of patients with NSTEMI relative to STEMI. In the GUSTO-IIb trial, patients with NSTEMI had comparable 30-day mortality (5.7% versus 6.1%) but higher 1-year mortality (11.1% ver-sus 9.6%) than those with STEMI (Armstrong 1998). This likely relates to the higher risk profile of patients with NSTEMI than with STEMI, i.e. older, more co-morbidities (diabetes, renal failure), more extensive coronary artery disease, and prior MI.

Clinical approach
History: key points
- The three principal presentations of UA are (Anderson *et al.* 2007):
  - *Rest angina*: prolonged (>20 minutes) angina at rest
  - *New-onset angina*: new-onset severe angina of at least Canadian Cardiovascular Society (CCS) Class III severity
  - *Progressive angina*: previously diagnosed angina that becomes more frequent or severe, lasts longer, or occurs at a lower threshold.
- Rest angina is a more frequent presentation (80%) than new-onset or crescendo angina (20%).
- Atypical symptoms including indigestion, dyspnoea, syn-cope, or non-anginal pain are more frequently observed in elderly people, in women, and in diabetic patients.
- Approximately 80% of patients with UA/NSTEMI will have a history of cardiovascular disease and/or risk factors.
- Conditions that may result in myocardial oxygen supply–demand mismatch should be identified, e.g. anaemia, infec-tions, thyrotoxicosis, hypertension, tachyarrhythmias.
- Important differential diagnoses to consider include pul-monary embolism (PE) and aortic dissection.

Physical examination: key points
- The physical examination is often normal but may become abnormal during pain as evident by an S4 gallop, paradoxical S2, or mitral insufficiency.
- Signs of heart failure (jugular venous distension, S3, rales), poor perfusion (pale cool skin), and haemody-namic instability (tachycardia, hypotension) suggest a large myocardial territory at risk.

- The physical examination may be particularly useful in excluding other diagnoses such as costochondritis, pericarditis, aortic dissection, and pulmonary disorders.

Investigations

ECG

- ECG abnormalities occur in up to 50% patients with UA/NSTEMI, are more frequent during pain/symptoms, and include ST depression, transient (<20 minutes) ST elevation, and T-wave inversion.
- ST depression and its extent is an independent predictor of death or MI with ST depression ≥2 mm carrying the greatest risk (Westerhout et al. 2006). Transient ST elevation occurs in 10% of patients and portends the worst outcomes.
- Whereas the prognostic significance of isolated T-wave inversion is unclear, deep symmetrical T-wave inversions in the precordial leads, i.e. Wellen's sign, often signifies critical proximal left anterior descending (LAD) artery stenosis.
- Approximately 20% of patients with NSTEMI will have no ECG changes. Ischaemia in the territory of the left circumflex artery is recognized as often being silent on ECG.
- *Continuous ECG monitoring* allows for identification of arrhythmias and dynamic ST-segment changes, mainly ST depression, that occurs in 15–30% of patients. Silent myocardial ischaemia is common and prognostically relevant.

Biochemical markers

- Markers of myocardial injury
  - Evidence of myocardial necrosis is a cornerstone in the diagnosis of MI and distinguishes NSTEMI from UA.
  - Troponins (I or T) are preferred as they are more sensitive and specific than creatine kinase (CK) or its isoenzyme MB (CKMB). Up to one third of patients with NSTEMI are CK or CKMB negative yet troponin positive. An independent and linear relationship exists between level of troponin and mortality in patients with NSTEMI (Antman et al. 1996).
  - A rise in troponin occurs after 3–4 hours of MI and can remain elevated for up to 2 weeks.
  - Troponin elevation also occurs in the setting of non-ischaemic myocardial injury (e.g. myopericarditis, aortic dissection, PE, congestive heart failure (CHF) exacerbation) and renal failure and should never be used as the sole criteria for diagnosing NSTEMI.
- Other markers
  - Other prognostically relevant biochemical markers include elevated serum glucose, reduced creatinine clearance (CrCl), elevated C-reactive protein (CRP), and white blood cell count (markers of inflammation), and elevated B-type natriuretic peptide (BNP, marker of neurohormonal activation and LV dysfunction). BNP, in particular, has been demonstrated to have a strong and independent impact on prognosis.

Echocardiography

- LV systolic function is a strong prognostic variable.
- Transient wall motion abnormalities at rest or during stress echocardiography may be helpful in patients with atypical symptoms and a non-diagnostic ECG.

- Certain differential diagnoses may be identified, e.g. PE, aortic dissection, aortic stenosis, hypertrophic cardiomyopathy.

Stress testing

Exercise or pharmacological stress testing (with or without echocardiographic, scintigraphic, or magnetic resonance imaging) should be considered in the following situations:

- Patients with presumed ischaemia or low-risk UA identified with normal or minor ECG changes and negative serial biomarkers. Stress testing in a chest pain unit or as an outpatient within 72 hours is useful in such individuals and detects those who can be managed as outpatients.
- Hospitalized patients with UA/NSTEMI initially managed conservatively should undergo stress testing to evaluate the extent of residual ischaemia and guide further therapy including coronary angiography with or without revascularization.
- Patients with established multivessel CAD may undergo stress testing with imaging to identify the relative physiological significance of coronary lesions.

Coronary angiography

- Coronary angiography allows evaluation of the extent of coronary artery disease, identification of potential culprit lesion(s) and suitability for revascularization.
- In the TIMI-IIIB, FRISC-2, and TACTICS-TIMI 18 trials, 13–19% of patients had no significant (>50–60%) coronary stenosis, 26–38% of patients had single vessel disease, 44–62% had multivessel involvement, and 4–9% had left main disease.

Early risk stratification

- Risk stratification begins upon presentation and is a dynamic process that requires updating as the clinical situation evolves. It allows identification of high-risk patients who are likely to derive greater benefit from more aggressive therapies. Several risk scores that combine clinical, ECG, and laboratory data have been developed from clinical trials (TIMI, PURSUIT, GUSTO IV-ACS risk scores) and large registries (GRACE risk score).
- The seven-point TIMI risk score (Antman et al. 2000) is endorsed by the ACC/AHA guidelines (Anderson et al. 2007). The TIMI risk score is simple to use and useful in determining which patients will benefit from certain therapies, e.g. early invasive versus conservative approach, GP IIb/IIIa inhibitors. However it is less accurate than other well-validated risk scores in predicting long-term events.
- The PURSUIT risk score is more complex than the TIMI risk score but its strengths lie in a higher discriminatory power and the inclusion of heart failure as a prognostic factor.
- The GUSTO-IV ACS risk score includes among other factors the degree of ST-depression, creatinine clearance, and multiple biomarkers (troponin, BNP, CRP) in a model with excellent discriminatory power (c-statistic >0.80 for 30-day and 1-year death) (Westerhout et al. 2006). ST depression had the highest prognostic value in this model.
- The GRACE risk score (Fig. 5.9.1) offers excellent in-hospital and 1-year prognostic capability (Eagle et al. 2004). The ESC guideline endorses the GRACE risk score for use on admission and at discharge in routine clinical practice (Bassand et al. 2007).

Risk calculator for 6-month post-discharge mortality after hospitalization for acute coronary syndrome

Record the points for each variable at the bottom left and sum the points to calculate the total risk score. Find the total score on the x-axis of the nomogram plot. The corresponding probability on the y-axis is the estimated probability of all-cause mortality from hospital discharge to 6 months.

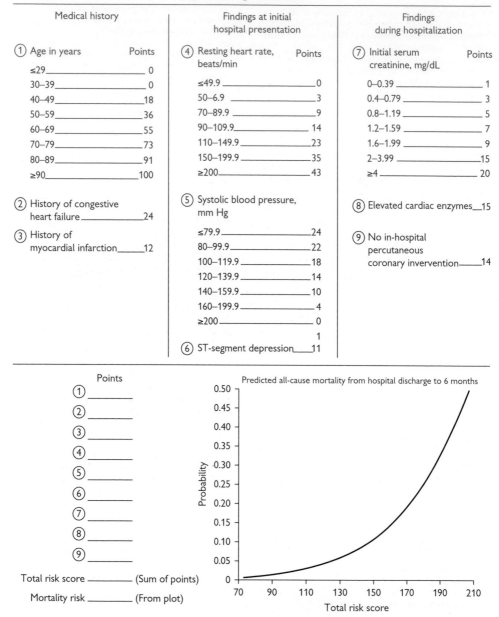

Medical history	Findings at initial hospital presentation	Findings during hospitalization
① Age in years Points	**④ Resting heart rate, beats/min** Points	**⑦ Initial serum creatinine, mg/dL** Points
≤29 ———— 0	≤49.9 ———— 0	0–0.39 ———— 1
30–39 ———— 0	50–6.9 ———— 3	0.4–0.79 ———— 3
40–49 ———— 18	70–89.9 ———— 9	0.8–1.19 ———— 5
50–59 ———— 36	90–109.9 ———— 14	1.2–1.59 ———— 7
60–69 ———— 55	110–149.9 ———— 23	1.6–1.99 ———— 9
70–79 ———— 73	150–199.9 ———— 35	2–3.99 ———— 15
80–89 ———— 91	≥200 ———— 43	≥4 ———— 20
≥90 ———— 100		
② History of congestive heart failure ———— 24	**⑤ Systolic blood pressure, mm Hg**	**⑧ Elevated cardiac enzymes** ___ 15
③ History of myocardial infarction ___ 12	≤79.9 ———— 24	**⑨ No in-hospital percutaneous coronary invervention** ———— 14
	80–99.9 ———— 22	
	100–119.9 ———— 18	
	120–139.9 ———— 14	
	140–159.9 ———— 10	
	160–199.9 ———— 4	
	≥200 ———— 0	
	1	
	⑥ ST-segment depression ___ 11	

Points

① ____
② ____
③ ____
④ ____
⑤ ____
⑥ ____
⑦ ____
⑧ ____
⑨ ____

Total risk score ———— (Sum of points)

Mortality risk ———— (From plot)

Predicted all-cause mortality from hospital discharge to 6 months

Probability (y-axis: 0, 0.05, 0.10, 0.15, 0.20, 0.25, 0.30, 0.35, 0.40, 0.45, 0.50)

Total risk score (x-axis: 70, 90, 110, 130, 150, 170, 190, 210)

Fig. 5.9.1 GRACE nomogram for all-cause mortality from discharge to 6 months. Reprinted with permission from Eagle KA, Lim MJ, Dabbous OH, *et al.* A validated prediction model for all forms of acute coronary syndrome: estimating the risk of 6-month post-discharge death in an international registry. *JAMA* 2004;291:2727–33. © 2004 American Medical Association. All rights reserved.

Management

Fig. 5.9.2 presents a simplified algorithm for the management of UA/NSTEMI. The class of recommendations shown in this section is in accordance with the ACC/AHA guidelines (Anderson *et al.* 2007).

Goals

- Relief of pain with anti-ischaemic and analgesic therapy
- Prompt and dynamic risk stratification

- Rapid initiation of antiplatelet and anticoagulant therapy
- Appropriate and timely triage into an early invasive strategy versus an initial conservative approach
- Institution of secondary prevention measures.

General measures

- High-risk patients should be admitted to a coronary care unit (CCU). A telemetry-capable unit may suffice for those at low to intermediate risk.

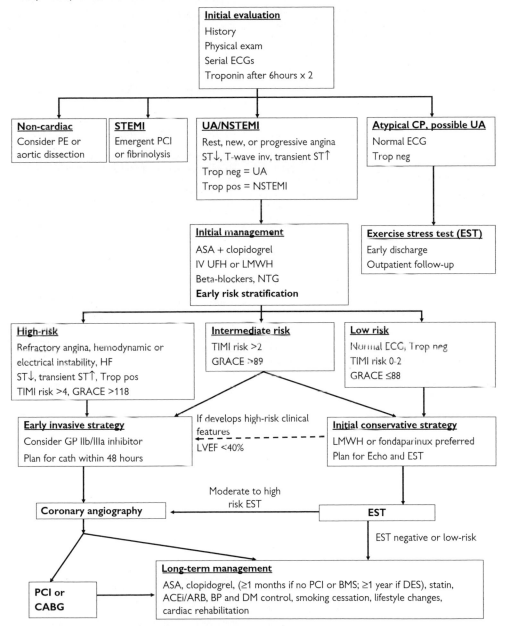

Fig. 5.9.2 Algorithm for management of UA/NSTEMI. Adapted from Anderson *et al.*, 2007. ACEi, angiotensin-converting enzyme inhibitor; ARB, angiotensin receptor blocker; ASA, atrial septal aneurysm; BMS, bare metal stent; BP, blood pressure; CABG, coronary artery bypass graft; CP, chest pain; DM, diabetes mellitus; ECG, electrocardiogram; GP, glycoprotein; LMWH, low molecular weight heparin; LVEF, left ventricular ejection fraction; NSTEMI, non-ST elevation myocardial infarction; NTG, nitroglycerin; PCI, percutaneous coronary intervention; PE, pulmonary embolism; Trop, troponin; UA, unstable angina; UFH, unfractionated heparin.

- Initial bed rest is recommended in the early hospital phase.
- Supplemental oxygen is required for patients with respiratory compromise or an arterial saturation <90%.
- Morphine (1–5 mg IV q5–30 minutes) is effective in relieving pain and anxiety.

Anti-ischaemic therapy

Nitrates

- Nitrates improve the myocardial oxygen supply–demand profile via coronary vasodilation and preload reduction.
- Sublingual nitroglycerin (NTG) 0.4 mg is given q5 minutes for three doses (Class I). IV NTG can be used for persistent ischaemia, heart failure, or hypertension.
- Main contraindications include significant hypotension and use of phosphodiesterase inhibitors e.g. sildenafil (Viagra®) in the previous 24–48 hours.

Beta-blockers

- The salutary effect of beta-blockers derive from inhibition of beta-1 adrenergic receptors with a resultant decrease in cardiac work and myocardial oxygen demand.
- Evidence for benefit of beta-blockers in UA/NSTEMI is limited and largely extrapolated from studies in stable angina and STEMI.
- Low to moderate dose oral beta-blockade should be initiated within 24 hours in the absence of AV block, bronchospasm, persistent hypotension, and acute heart failure (Class I). Long-term beta-blockade is recommended in patients with LV dysfunction and reasonable for all UA/NSTEMI patients.

Calcium channel blockers

- Calcium channel blockers (CCBs) are vasodilators and some also affect AV conduction. The evidence for benefit of CCBs in UA/NSTEMI is mainly limited to symptom control.
- Non-dihydropyridine CCBs, i.e. verapamil or diltiazem, are preferred in the absence of severe LV dysfunction, particularly in patients with contraindications to beta-blockers.
- Immediate-release nifedipine should not be given without a beta-blocker because of increased adverse outcomes.

Antiplatelet agents

Aspirin

- Aspirin (ASA) blocks thromboxane A_2-induced platelet activation and decreases overall platelet aggregation.
- ASA reduces death or MI by approximately 50% versus placebo in multiple randomized trials.
- ASA is given at a loading dose of 160–325 mg followed by 75–100 mg/day indefinitely (Class I). Higher doses are associated with increased bleeding without further benefit.

Thienopyridines

- Clopidogrel and ticlopidine inhibit ADP-induced platelet activation and subsequent aggregation. Ticlopidine's haematological depression has resulted in clopidogrel being preferred.
- In the CURE trial, ASA + clopidogrel conferred a 20% reduction in CV death, MI or stroke maintained through 1 year versus ASA alone (9.3% versus 11.4%; OR 0.80, 95% CI 0.72–0.90, P<0.001) (Yusuf *et al.* 2001).

Pre-treatment with clopidogrel prior to PCI confers a 29% reduction in CV death or MI in a meta-analysis.

- Clopidogrel is given at a loading dose of 300 mg followed by 75 mg/day (Class I): 600 mg may be used to load for those undergoing immediate PCI. Patients not undergoing PCI and those receiving a bare metal stent should remain on clopidogrel for at least 1 month and ideally up to 1 year. Patients who receive a drug-eluting stent should remain on clopidogrel for at least 1 year.

Glycoprotein IIb/IIIa inhibitors

- GP IIb/IIIa inhibitors block the fibrinogen-mediated cross-linkage of platelets, the final common pathway of platelet aggregation.
- A meta-analysis showed a 9% reduction in death or MI at 30 days with the use of GP IIb/IIIa inhibitors among UA/NSTEMI patients not routinely scheduled for PCI (10.8% versus 11.8%; OR 0.91, 95% CI 0.85–0.98, P = 0.015) (Boersma *et al.* 2002). This benefit is enhanced in patients who undergo PCI and in patients with high-risk features: positive troponins, ST depression, diabetes, or TIMI risk score >3.
- In patients undergoing an early invasive strategy, GP IIb/IIIa inhibitors are recommended as either an alternative to (Class I) or in addition to (Class IIa) clopidogrel. In conservatively managed patients, a Class IIb recommendation exists for adding a GP IIB/IIIa inhibitor to clopidogrel.
- IV epitifibatide and tirofiban are the preferred GP IIb/IIIa inhibitors. Abciximab is indicated only in conjunction with coronary angiography and PCI. GP IIb/IIIa inhibitors must be combined with an anticoagulant.

Anticoagulants

Unfractionated heparin (UFH)

- A meta-analysis showed a nominally significant 33% reduction in death or MI at one week comparing UFH with placebo or control ASA therapy (7.9% versus 10.4%; OR 0.67, 95% CI 0.45–0.99, P = 0.045) (Eikelboom *et al.* 2000).
- UFH is given as a weight-adjusted dose (60 U/kg bolus and 12 U/kg/hour infusion) and titrated to achieve an aPTT of 50–70 s (Class I). UFH may be discontinued after 48 hours or post PCI.
- Adverse effects include bleeding especially when aPTT is above target and heparin-induced thrombocytopenia (HIT).

Low-molecular-weight heparin

- Compared to UFH, low-molecular-weight heparin (LMWH) has greater bioavailability, more predictable dose response, greater ability to inhibit thrombin generation, and causes less thrombocytopenia.
- A meta-analysis showed that LMWH (plus ASA) offers a 66% reduction in death or MI versus ASA alone (1.6% versus 5.2%; OR 0.34, 95% CI 0.20–0.58, P <0.0001) (Eikelboom *et al.* 2000).
- Contemporary data suggest that LMWH and UFH have comparable efficacy and the use of either is recommended. However, patients managed conservatively appear to have less CV events when treated with enoxaparin versus UFH. In patients managed with an early invasive strategy, UFH may be preferable due to the increased risk of bleeding with enoxaparin in the SYNERGY trial.

- Enoxaparin is the preferred LMWH and is given 1 mg/kg sc q12 hours for the duration of hospitalization up to 8 days and can be stopped post PCI (Class I in ACC/AHA guidelines, Class IIa in ESC guidelines). If CrCl is <30 mL/min, enoxaparin should be dosed once daily or UFH used instead.

Fondaparinux
- Fondaparinux is a synthetic pentasaccharide that is a selective antithrombin-mediated inhibitor of factor Xa.
- In the OASIS-5 trial (Yusuf et al. 2006), the rates of death, MI, or refractory ischaemia at 9 days were similar with fondaparinux and enoxaparin (5.8% versus 5.7%). However, major bleeding rates were halved with fondaparinux (2.2% versus 4.1%, P<0.001).
- Fondaparinux is given 2.5 mg sc once daily for the duration of hospitalization up to 8 days and can be stopped post PCI. It is contraindicated in patients with CrCl <30 mL/min. Enoxaparin or fondaparinux is preferred over UFH for patients managed conservatively (Class IIa).

Direct thrombin inhibitors
- Unlike UFH and LMWH, direct thrombin inhibitors (DTIs) inhibit both fibrin-bound and fluid-phase thrombin and provide stable levels of anticoagulation without risk of thrombocytopenia.
- Bivalirudin is the only DTI approved for use in UA/NSTEMI but only with an early invasive strategy (Class I). The ACUITY trial showed that bivalirudin was similar to enoxaparin or UFH combined with a GP IIb/IIIa inhibitor (but with less bleeding) in reducing death, MI, or unplanned revascularization among patients undergoing an early invasive strategy.

Early invasive versus initial conservative strategies
- Urgent coronary angiography followed by revascularization with PCI or CABG should be performed in patients with refractory angina, and haemodynamic or electrical instability.
- Patients initially stabilized should be triaged into an early invasive strategy, i.e. routine coronary angiography and revascularization within 48–72 hours or an initial conservative approach, i.e. medical therapy with selective coronary angiography in those who destabilize, have an LVEF <40%, or have significant residual ischaemia on stress testing.
- A meta-analysis of contemporary randomized trials found lower mortality at 2 years from an invasive versus conservative approach (4.9% versus 6.5%, RR 0.75, 95% CI 0.63–0.90) (Bavry et al. 2006). The benefit of an early invasive strategy appears limited to patients with intermediate to high-risk clinical features (Cannon et al. 2001).

Coronary revascularization
- Once the coronary anatomy is defined, the selection criteria for revascularization and choice of modality (PCI versus CABG) in patients with UA/NSTEMI are similar to those for patients with stable coronary disease (see Chapters 5.18 and 5.20).
- *PCI:* stenting and contemporary antithrombotic strategies have markedly improved outcomes of PCI. Compared to bare-metal stents (BMS), drug-eluting stents (DES) reduce the rate of in-stent restenosis at the expense of more frequent late stent thrombosis especially when clopidogrel is stopped. Thus BMS is preferred in those anticipated to require surgery necessitating clopidogrel interruption <1 year after PCI, when long-term compliance is problematic or high risk of bleeding on dual antiplatelet therapy is likely. In patients with multivessel disease, staged PCI may be considered with PCI of the culprit lesion followed by non-invasive stress imaging to assess the need for subsequent intervention.
- *CABG:* CABG is preferred in patients with left main stenosis >50%, three-vessel disease, especially with LV dysfunction or diabetes, or two-vessel disease involving the proximal LAD and either LV dysfunction or ischaemia on stress testing. Whereas PCI has lower short-term morbidity and mortality than CABG, it has higher need for repeat revascularization.

Secondary prevention
Lipid lowering with statins
- The PROVE-IT TIMI 22 trial (Cannon et al. 2004) showed that when compared with moderate lipid-lowering therapy with pravastatin 40 mg/day, intensive therapy with atorvastatin 80 mg/day resulted in a 16% reduction in the primary end-point (death, MI, UA, revascularization, or stroke) at 2 years (22.4% versus 26.3%, P=0.005) already apparent at 30 days.
- A fasting lipid profile should be obtained within 24 hours of hospitalization. Statin therapy should be titrated to achieve target LDL <100 mg/dL (<2.6 mmol/L). Further titration to achieve LDL <70 mg/dL (<1.8 mmol/L) is reasonable.

Angiotensin-converting enzyme (ACE) inhibitors
- ACE inhibitors are recommended for patients recovering from UA/NSTEMI who have heart failure and LVEF <40%, hypertension, or diabetes. The HOPE and EUROPA trials suggest their use may be reasonable for all patients with UA/NSTEMI. Angiotensin receptor blockers (ARBs) should be used in patients who are intolerant of ACE inhibitors and/or who have heart failure and LVEF <40%.

Blood pressure control
- Targets of <140/90 mmHg in non-diabetics and <130/80 mmHg in diabetics and those with chronic kidney disease. BP control should be achieved with lifestyle interventions including physical activity, weight loss, and dietary modifications. Initial pharmacotherapy should include beta-blockers and/or ACE inhibitors.

Diabetes management
- A fasting blood glucose level should be obtained in all patients. In diabetics, the goal is to achieve a haemoglobin A1c level <7% through lifestyle measures and pharmacotherapy.

Lifestyle changes
- Durable smoking cessation often requires a combination of counselling, referral to special programmes, and pharmacotherapy (i.e. nicotine replacement).
- In the recovery phase, regular physical activity involving 30–60 minutes of moderate aerobic activity, e.g. brisk walking at least 5 days per week is recommended.
- Targets for weight loss are a BMI <25 kg/m^2 and waist circumference <102 cm in men and <88 cm in women.

Cardiac rehabilitation programmes
- These programmes are recommended for all patients with UA/NSTEMI, particularly those with multiple modifiable risk factors and intermediate to high-risk patients who require supervised titration of an exercise prescription.

Selected complications

Bleeding

- Bleeding is the most common non-cardiac complication of therapy for patients with UA/NSTEMI and is prognostically relevant. Major bleeding in the GRACE registry occurred in 4.7% of NSTEMI patients and was associated with more frequent in-hospital death (OR 1.64; 95% CI 1.18–2.28) (Moscucci et al. 2003).
- Predictors of major bleeding in the GRACE registry include: advanced age, female sex, prior bleeding, renal insufficiency, invasive procedures (PCI, right heart catheterization), and use of GP IIb/IIIa inhibitors (Moscucci et al. 2003).
- Prevention of bleeding involves matching therapy to the risk of bleeding, appropriate drug dosing (for age, body weight, and renal function), radial instead of femoral approach for PCI, avoidance of central lines and PA catheters, and use of proton pump inhibitors in patients with peptic ulcers.
- Management of major bleeding at non-compressible sites (intracranial, GI, retroperitoneal) includes discontinuation with or without reversal of antithrombotic therapy and judicious use of blood transfusion. Haemostatic interventions at vascular access sites include firm pressure and closure devices.
- Blood transfusion was associated with higher 30-day mortality in a meta-analysis of 24 112 patients with UA/NSTEMI even after adjustment for bleeding events.

Renal dysfunction

- Renal dysfunction frequently complicates UA/NSTEMI, increases bleeding risk, necessitates dosage adjustment of many drugs, and is a strong risk factor for mortality.
- Contrast induced nephropathy following coronary angiography is not uncommon. Risk factors include older age, diabetes, underlying renal dysfunction, hypovolaemia, large contrast volume, and the use of high osmolar contrast.

Heart failure (HF)

- Overt HF, severe LV dysfunction, and cardiogenic shock identify patients at high risk for whom urgent coronary angiography and revascularization are warranted.
- In the GRACE registry, 16% of NSTEMI patients presented with Killip II or III HF. They had threefold increased mortality in-hospital (10% versus 3%) and from discharge to 6 months (11% versus 4%). HF developing after admission was associated with even higher in-hospital mortality (18%).

Specific populations

Women

- Compared to men, women with UA/NSTEMI are older and have more co-morbidities including diabetes, renal dysfunction, and HF. After adjustment for baseline characteristics, female gender is usually not associated with worse outcomes.
- Women are more likely to present with dyspnoea and atypical symptoms and less often have biomarker elevation than men. Although women have similar rates of ST depression, they more often have T-wave inversion.
- Women have less extensive CAD than men and up to 37% of women in clinical trials have non-obstructive CAD.

- Women less frequently receive evidence-based therapies than men yet derive similar benefit from most of them. GP IIb/IIIa inhibitors and/or an early invasive strategy should be reserved for women with positive troponins or a TIMI risk score >2.

Elderly people

- Elderly patients defined as either ≥65 or ≥75 years old have more co-morbidities and more likely present with atypical symptoms, HF, and a non-diagnostic ECG. In the GRACE registry, in-hospital mortality rates adjusted for baseline risk profile increased markedly with age (OR 15.7 in patients ≥85 years versus <45 years).
- The combination of polypharmacy, reduced renal function, and lower body weight puts elderly people at risk of excessive dosing of antithrombotics and adverse drug interactions which are prognostically relevant.
- Patients ≥75 years constitute over one-third of patients with UA/NSTEMI yet are underrepresented in clinical trials. In general, the elderly patients derive comparable benefit from evidence-based therapies, including an early invasive strategy at the expense of more frequent bleeding.
- Treatment aggressiveness in elderly patients should take into account patient wishes, life expectancy, general health, co-morbidities, cognitive status, and bleeding risk.

Diabetics

- Diabetics constitute ~20–30% of UA/NSTEMI patients. They more often present with atypical symptoms and silent ischaemia, and have more extensive CAD and unstable lesions. Diabetes is a strong independent predictor of death.
- Although admission glucose level is an independent predictor of mortality, the optimal management of hyperglycemia in the acute phase of UA/NSTEMI is unclear. Guidelines recommend tight control with insulin if necessary to achieve normoglycaemia in the first few days.
- GP IIb/IIIa inhibitors should be considered for all diabetics as the benefit appears enhanced in this population.
- The optimal revascularization modality for diabetics with three-vessel disease is unclear in the current era of PCI with DES although traditionally CABG is preferred.

Controversies and future directions

- Enhanced risk profiling UA/NSTEMI is the cornerstone of management and future risk scores will rely on a combination of clinical characteristics, ECG features, multiple biomarkers, and non-invasive imaging techniques.
- The potential for novel anticoagulants and antiplatelet agents to reduce ischaemic events and bleeding is a promising area of active research. The optimal choice of the many existing antithrombotic therapies and combinations continues to be debated, e.g. enoxaparin is recommended at a Class I level by the ACC/AHA but at a Class IIa level by the ESC guidelines.
- The optimal timing of an early invasive strategy is uncertain and likely depends on the risk profile with patients at higher risk benefitting more from earlier intervention.
- Although the use of multiple evidence-based therapies (i.e. antiplatelet agents, ACE inhibitors, beta-blockers, statins, etc.) improves survival these therapies

Table 5.9.1 UA/NSTEMI top 10 messages

1 The most common mechanism of UA/NSTEMI is rupture of an atherosclerotic plaque with thrombus formation resulting in subtotal obstruction of the coronary artery and myocardial ischaemia.

2 NSTEMI patients have worse long-term outcomes than STEMI patients because of older age, more co-morbidities, and more extensive CAD.

3 Troponin is the preferred biomarker in patients suspected to have UA/NSTEMI.

4 Risk stratification should begin on presentation and is a dynamic process that allows tailoring of therapy to match the risk level.

5 Patients with possible UA but normal ECG and negative serial troponins should have a stress test prior to or within 72 hours of discharge.

6 Initial therapy of patients with UA/NSTEMI includes ASA, clopidogrel, an anticoagulant, and anti-ischaemic therapy with beta-blockers and/or nitrates.

7 Patients at low risk should undergo an initial conservative strategy involving stress testing to guide the need for coronary angiography. In these patients, enoxaparin or fondaparinux are the preferred anticoagulants.

8 Patients at high risk should undergo an early invasive strategy involving coronary angiography within 48 hours and possible revascularization. In these patients, enoxaparin or UFH are the preferred anticoagulants and GP IIb/IIIa inhibitors are recommended.

9 Bleeding is the most common non-ischaemic complication of therapy for patients with UA/NSTEMI and is prognostically relevant. Prevention involves matching therapy to bleeding risk and appropriate dosing of antithrombotics.

10 Women, elderly people, and diabetics are groups with adverse outcomes that have unique presenting features and therapeutic considerations.

are underutilized. Research efforts to enhance adherence to current guidelines and patient compliance will lead to substantial improvements in survival after UA/NSTEMI (White and Willerson 2004).

• Key summary messages are noted in Table 5.9.1.

Expert advisors: Paul W. Armstrong, MD, University Professor and Michael C. Tjandrawidjaja, MD, Cardiology Resident, University of Alberta, Edmonton, Alberta, Canada.

References

Anderson JL, Adams CD, Antman EM, et al. ACC/AHA 2007 guidelines for the management of patients with unstable angina/non-ST-elevation myocardial infarction: a report of the American College of Cardiology/American Heart Association Task Force on Practice Guidelines. *Circulation* 2007;**116**:e148–e304.

Antman EM, Cohen M, Bernink PJLM, et al. The TIMI risk score for unstable angina/non-ST elevation MI: a method for prognostication and therapeutic decision making. *JAMA* 2000;**284**:835–842.

Antman EM, Tanasijevic MJ, Thompson B, et al. Cardiac-specific troponin I levels to predict the risk of mortality in patients with acute coronary syndromes. *N Engl J Med* 1996;**335**:1342–49.

Armstrong PW, Fu Y, Chang WC, et al. Acute coronary syndromes in the GUSTO-IIb trial: prognostic insights and impact of recurrent ischemia. *Circulation* 1998;**98**:1860–8.

Bassand JP, Hamm CW, Ardissino D, et al. The Task Force for the Diagnosis and Treatment of Non-ST-Segment Elevation Acute Coronary Syndromes of the European Society of Cardiology. Guidelines for the diagnosis and treatment of non-ST-segment elevation acute coronary syndromes. *Eur Heart J* 2007;**28**:1598–660.

Bavry AA, Kumbhani DJ, Rassi AN, et al. Benefit of early invasive therapy in acute coronary syndromes a meta-analysis of contemporary randomized clinical trials. *J Am Coll Cardiol* 2006;**48**:1319–25.

Boersma E, Harrington RA, Moliterno DJ, et al. Platelet glycoprotein IIb/IIIa inhibitors in acute coronary syndromes: a meta-analysis of all major randomised clinical trials. *Lancet* 2002;**359**:189–98.

Braunwald E. Unstable angina: An etiologic approach to management. *Circulation* 1998;**98**:2219–22.

Cannon CP, Braunwald E, McCabe CH, et al. Intensive versus moderate lipid lowering with statins after acute coronary syndromes. *N Engl J Med* 2004;**350**:1495–504.

Cannon CP, Weintraub WS, Demopoulos LA, et al. Comparison of early invasive and conservative strategies in patients with unstable coronary syndromes treated with the glycoprotein IIb/IIIa inhibitor tirofiban. *N Engl J Med* 2001;**344**:1879–87.

Eagle KA, Lim MJ, Dabbous OH, et al. A validated prediction model for all forms of acute coronary syndrome: estimating the risk of 6-month postdischarge death in an international registry. *JAMA* 2004;**291**:2727–33.

Eikelboom JS, Anand SS, Malmberg K, et al. Unfractionated heparin and low-molecular-weight heparin in acute coronary syndrome without ST-elevation: a meta-analysis. *Lancet* 2000;**355**:1936–42.

Moscucci M, Fox KA, Cannon CP, et al. Predictors of major bleeding in acute coronary syndromes: the Global Registry of Acute Coronary Events (GRACE). *Eur Heart J* 2003;**24**:1815–23.

Thygesen K, Alpert JS, White HD, on behalf of the Joint ESC/ACCF/AHA/WHF Task Force for the Redefinition of Myocardial Infarction. Universal definition of myocardial infarction. *J Am Coll Cardiol* 2007;**50**:2173–95.

Westerhout CM, Fu Y, Lauer MS et al. Short and long term risk stratification in acute coronary syndromes: the added value of quantitative ST-segment depression and multiple biomarkers. *J Am Coll Cardiol* 2006;**48**:939–47.

White HD, Willerson JT. We must use the knowledge that we have to treat patients with acute coronary syndromes. *Circulation* 2004;**109**:698–700.

Yusuf S, Mehta SR, Chrolavicius S, et al. Comparison of fondaparinux and enoxaparin in acute coronary syndromes. *N Engl J Med* 2006;**354**:1464–76.

Yusuf S, Zhao F, Mehta SR, et al. Effects of clopidogrel in addition to aspirin in patients with acute coronary syndromes without ST-segment elevation. *N Engl J Med* 2001;**345**:494–502.

Cardiac syndrome X

Definition

Cardiac syndrome X (CSX) should be diagnosed in presence of:

1 angina episodes exclusively or predominantly related to efforts, typical enough to suggest obstructive coronary artery disease (CAD);

2 findings compatible with myocardial ischaemia and/or coronary blood flow (CBF) abnormalities during spontaneous or provoked angina, mainly ST-segment depression on exercise stress test (Fig. 5.10.1);

3 normal or near normal (i.e. stenosis <20%) coronary arteries at angiography;

4 absence of specific forms of cardiac disease or abnormalities (e.g. variant angina, cardiomyopathy, valvular heart disease, or even left ventricular hypertrophy and/or dilatation) and/or specific systemic disease (e.g. autoimmune diseases).

Patients with CSX constitute about 20% of those who come to clinical attention because of typical effort angina and evidence of myocardial ischaemia on non-invasive tests.

Pathogenetic mechanisms

Evidence from clinical studies indicates that abnormalities in coronary microcirculation function is responsible for CSX. The pathogenetic mechanisms of CMVD in CSX patients are probably multiple and heterogeneous among patients (Fig. 5.10.2). Impairment of endothelial function, increased adrenergic activity, insulin resistance, inflammation, structural abnormalities and, in women, oestrogen deficiency have been suggested to play a role. An impairment of coronary microvascular dilation and increased coronary microvascular constriction can variably contribute to anginal episodes in individual patients.

In some patients an increased painful perception of normally innocuous stimuli of the heart is present, which can explain the severe symptoms of some patients despite the low grade of ischaemia.

Clinical approach

- In contrast with patients with obstructive CAD, those with CSX are more often women, who constitute up to 70–80% of this population; thus a diagnosis of CSX should always be considered in female patients with effort angina, in particular when they are in the age of 45–55 years and/or in a menopausal age.

- Some characteristics of chest pain suggest CSX rather than obstructive CAD; they include:

  1 persistence of a dull pain for several minutes after the interruption of an effort;

  2 incomplete or slow response to short-acting nitrates.

- Cardiovascular risk factors are similar to those of CAD patients, although, compared with the latter group, there is a lower prevalence of smoking.

- Physical examination is unremarkable in CSX patients.

Diagnostic investigation

- 99mTc-sestamibi or 201-thallium stress myocardial scintigraphy show typical reversible perfusion defects in 50% to 75% of patients.

- Strong clues to the diagnosis of CSX, compared with the presence of obstructive CAD, include:

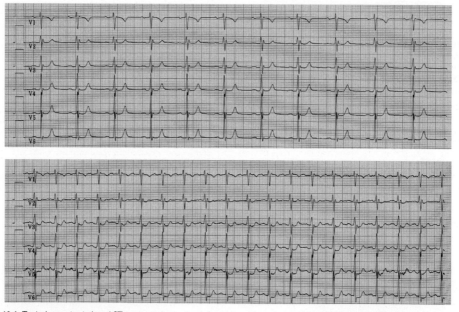

Fig. 5.10.1 Typical exercise-induced ST-segment depression in a patient with cardiac syndrome X (reproduced from Lanza GA, Cardiac syndrome X: a critical overview and future perspective. *Heart* 93:159–66, copyright (2007) with permission from BMJ Publishing Group Ltd).

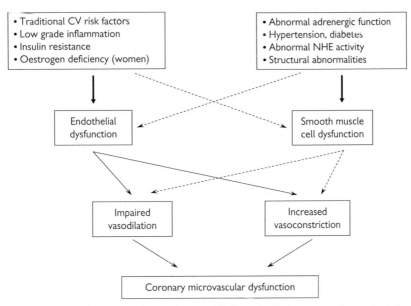

Fig. 5.10.2 Scheme of the main pathogenetic mechanisms that can variably be involved in the coronary microvascular dysfunction of patients with cardiac syndrome X. CV, cardiovascular (reproduced from Lanza GA, Cardiac syndrome X: a critical overview and future perspective. *Heart* 93:159–66, copyright (2007) with permission from BMJ Publishing Group Ltd).

• the evidence of totally normal left ventricular function at echocardiography despite the occurrence of typical angina and ST-segment depression during pharmacological stress test (either adenosine, dipyridamole or dobutamine).

• lack of improvement, or even worsening, of exercise-induced ECG abnormalities after preventive administration of short-acting nitrates.

• The confirmation of the diagnosis requires the documentation of normal coronary arteries at angiography, which, however, can be avoided when the results of echo-stress clearly show absence of regional wall motion abnormalities in the presence of angina and typical ischaemic ST segment changes.

Documentation of CMVD

• In CSX patients, transthoracic echocardiographic Doppler recording is the simplest method to conform CMVD. By this method coronary blood flow velocity can be measured in the epicardial coronary arteries (mainly the LAD), and its changes in response to vasodilator stimuli can be assessed; a ratio between diastolic blood flow velocity at peak adenosine (or dipyridamole) and blood flow velocity at rest <2.0 strongly suggests significant CMVD.

• Other non-invasive methods to assess CMVD include contrast echocardiography, cardiovascular magnetic resonance, and positron emission tomography. These methods, however, are expensive and/or complex and/or not largely available.

• The confirmation of CMVD can also be obtained by assessing the response of coronary blood flow/resistances to vasodilator stimuli (e.g. adenosine, dipyridamole, etc.) during coronary angiography, in particular by intracoronary Doppler recording. However, such tests are expensive, time-consuming and would expose patients to unhelpful (although small) additive risk.

Clinical outcome

All studies on CSX patients have consistently reported an excellent clinical outcome at long-term follow-up, with an incidence of major acute coronary events (i.e. cardiac death, acute myocardial infarction) similar to those of the healthy population.

In contrast to the excellent prognosis, however, 15–20% of CSX patients present significant impairment of quality of life, with worsening of symptoms that become more frequent, long-lasting, and also appearing at rest.

Therapeutic options (see Fig. 5.10.3)

Anti-ischaemic drugs are the first-line form of treatment. If not contraindicated, treatment with a beta-blocking agent should be preferred; in particular when evidence of increased adrenergic tone or reactivity is evident (e.g. high heart rate at rest or rapid increase in heart rate during exercise). A non-dihydropiridine calcium antagonist is an alternative choice. A dihydropiridine calcium antagonist and/or a long-acting nitrate can be added as a second-line treatment.

Alternative drugs that can variably be added to standard anti-ischaemic medications include (1) xanthine derivatives (e.g. bamiphylline or theophylline), which can cause an anti-algogenic effect through anti-adenosine effect but also favouring redistribution of coronary blood flow to ischaemic areas; (2) ACE inhibitors, which may contrast a possible involvement of the renin–angiotensin system in coronary microvascular dysfunction, in particular when hypertension is present; (3) alpha-antagonist drugs, which might decrease alpha-mediated micorvascular constriction;

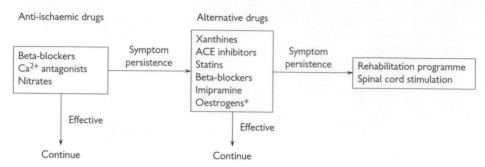

Fig. 5.10.3 Stepwise therapeutic approach to patients with cardiac syndrome X. *In menopausal women (reproduced from Lanza GA, Cardiac syndrome X: a critical overview and future perspective, *Heart* 93:159–66, copyright (2007) with permission from BMJ Publishing Group Ltd).

(4) statins, which might improve endothelium-mediated coronary vasodilation; (5) oestrogens in postmenopausal women. In severely symptomatic patients imipramine, which inhibits pain transmission from visceral tissues, can be tried. In patients with refractory angina episodes, beneficial effects have been reported with spinal cord stimulation.

Further reading

Camici PG, Crea F. Coronary microvascular dysfunction. *N Engl J Med* 2007;**356**:830–40.

Lanza GA. Cardiac syndrome X: a critical overview and future perspective. *Heart* 2007;**93**:159–66.

Maseri A, Crea F, Kaski JC, Crake T. Mechanisms of angina pectoris in syndrome X. *J Am Coll Cardiol* 1991;**17**:499–506.

Thrombolytic agents

Introduction

ST-segment myocardial infarction (STEMI) is caused by occlusion of a major coronary artery. This is generally triggered by rupture of a vulnerable plaque, with subsequent formation of an occlusive thrombus (see Chapter 5.8). Rapid restoration of coronary blood flow is essential in preventing myocardial necrosis. Early reperfusion of the infarct-related artery limits infarct size and improves outcome.

Reperfusion of the infarct-related artery can be achieved by mechanical reperfusion using primary percutaneous coronary intervention (PCI), or by pharmacological reperfusion using thrombolytic agents. Compared with thrombolysis, primary PCI achieves higher patency rates and is associated with better clinical outcomes. Current STEMI guidelines therefore recommend primary PCI as the preferred method for reperfusion. Unfortunately, only a minority of hospitals worldwide has immediate access to a catheterization facility. Moreover, hospitals with a catheterization laboratory often do not offer primary PCI during off-office hours. Even in hospital network systems where STEMI patients are transferred from a non-PCI centre to a PCI centre, transfer times can still be deplorably long. As a consequence, only a minority of primary PCI patients are actually treated within the recommended 90–120 minutes after first medical contact. Thrombolysis, in contrast, is universally available and does not require advanced logistics. Lytic therapy therefore is a valuable alternative, and is still used for the treatment of acute myocardial infarction in many centres worldwide.

The agents

Thrombolytic agents convert plasminogen to plasmin, which then degrades fibrin (Fig. 5.11.1). They are generally divided in fibrin-specific agents and non-fibrin-specific agents. Fibrin-specific drugs, such as alteplase, tenecteplase, or reteplase, are more efficient in dissolving thrombi and do not deplete systemic coagulation factors, in contrast with non-fibrin-specific agents such as streptokinase. The characteristics and dosing regimens of the current lytic agents are given in Table 5.11.1.

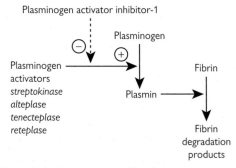

Fig. 5.11.1 Mechanism of action of thrombolytic agents.

Streptokinase

Streptokinase is a non-fibrin-specific fibrinolytic agent that indirectly activates plasminogen. Because of its lack of fibrin specificity, streptokinase depletes systemic coagulation factors, inducing a lytic state. Pre-existing anti-streptokinase antibodies may impede reperfusion after treatment with streptokinase. In addition, administration of streptokinase also invariably induces anti-streptokinase antibodies, precluding safe readministration.

Alteplase

Recombinant tissue-type plasminogen activator (rt-PA or alteplase) is a single-chain tissue-type plasminogen activator molecule. It has considerably greater fibrin specificity than streptokinase, but induces nevertheless mild systemic fibrinogen depletion. Because of its short half-life, alteplase requires a continuous infusion.

Reteplase

Reteplase, a second-generation fibrinolytic agent, was a first attempt to improve on the shortcomings of alteplase. It is a mutant of alteplase in which the finger, the kringle-1 domain, and epidermal growth factor domains are removed. This causes decreased plasma clearance, allowing double-bolus administration. The removal of the finger domain somewhat diminishes fibrin specificity.

Tenecteplase

Tenecteplase (TNK-t-PA) is also derived from alteplase, after mutations at three places. These changes enhance fibrin binding and specificity, plasma half-life, and resistance to PAI-1. Its slower clearance allows convenient single-bolus administration. Tenecteplase leads to faster recanalization than alteplase, and also has higher fibrinolytic potency on platelet-rich clots than its parent molecule. Non-cerebral bleeding complications occurred less frequently with tenecteplase than with alteplase.

Indications and contraindications for thrombolytic therapy

Indications

In the absence of contraindications and if primary PCI cannot be performed within 90–120 minutes after the first medical contact, thrombolytic therapy should be started as soon as possible. Pre-hospital initiation of therapy is recommended to save time.

Contraindications

Absolute and relative contraindications to thrombolysis are in essence precautions to avoid excessive haemorrhage in patients with co-morbidities that increase the risk of bleeding complications (Table 5.11.2). In these patients, especially those with a previous history of stroke or recent major surgery, primary PCI should be considered. Since arterial hypertension increases the risk for intracranial haemorrhage, patients presenting with persisting high blood pressure at presentation are usually also not eligible for lytic therapy, although a history of systemic hypertension in itself does not predispose to intracranial haemorrhage with lytic therapy. It is less clear whether fibrinolytic

Table 5.11.1 Characteristics and dosing regimens of thrombolytic agents

	Streptokinase	Alteplase	Reteplase	Tenecteplase
Fibrin specificity	No	++	+	+++
Half-life (min)	18–23	3–4	18	20
Antigenicity	+++	No	No	No
Administration	1-hour infusion	Bolus & 90-min infusion	Double bolus	Single bolus
Dose	1.5 MU	15-mg bolus 0.75 mg/kg IV (max 50) over 30 min 0.5 mg/kg over 60 min	10 U + 10 U 30 min apart	Weight adjusted: <60 kg: 30 mg 60–69.9 kg: 35 mg 70–79.9 kg: 40 mg 80–89.9 kg: 45 mg ≥90 kg: 50 mg

agents can be safely administered after successful treatment of high blood pressure at initial presentation. Nevertheless, because there is a substantial mortality benefit with fibrinolytic agents in patients even presenting with hypertension, fibrinolysis should still be considered in patients with high blood pressure on admission after successful initiation of antihypertensive treatment, when primary PCI is not available.

Adjunctive antithrombotic therapy with lytics

Antiplatelet therapy

Aspirin
Low-dose aspirin remains the cornerstone of antithrombotic therapy in patients receiving lytic therapy.

Clopidogrel
Clopidogrel given as a loading dose of 300 mg and a maintenance dose of 75 mg in patients <76 years improves patency rates by preventing reocclusion rather than through facilitating early reperfusion. It remains uncertain whether

Table 5.11.2 Contraindications for fibrinolysis

Absolute

Previous haemorrhagic stroke or stroke of unknown origin at any time
Non-haemorrhagic stroke in preceding 6 months
Known bleeding diathesis
Suspected aortic dissection
Intracranial neoplasm
Central nervous system trauma
Non-compressible punctures

Relative

Surgery or trauma within past 2–4 weeks
Uncontrolled hypertension on presentation (>180/100 mmHg)
Prolonged resuscitation
Oral anticoagulant use with INR >2.3
Recent (internal) bleeding
Active peptic ulcer
Previous use of streptokinase

dual antiplatelet therapy is safe in elderly patients treated with lytic therapy.

Glycoprotein IIb/IIIa inhibitors
Combination therapy with half dose of a lytic agent and abciximab results in a significant reduction in ischaemic complications after acute myocardial infarction, but this benefit is offset by an increased risk of bleeding complications, particularly in elderly people. These agents are not recommended together with lytic therapy.

Anticoagulant therapy

Unfractionated heparin and low-molecular-weight heparin
Unfractionated heparin (UFH) has been standard adjunctive anticoagulant therapy with thrombolytic agents since GUSTO-I, although other studies were unconvincing. Several fibrinolytic trials have studied the use of low-molecular weight heparin (LMWH), which does not require monitoring of its anticoagulant effect and can be given subcutaneously. In the EXTRACT trial an age-adjusted dose of enoxaparin did not increase the risk of intracranial haemorrhage while still reducing the risk of ischaemic complications when compared with heparin and is the recommended anticoagulant together with fibrin-specific lytic agents.

Fondaparinux
Fondaparinux, a synthetic pentasaccharide, is a selective indirect factor Xa inhibitor. Fondaparinux is recommended as adjunctive therapy to streptokinase but not to fibrin-specific agents since only a limited number of patients have been studied with the combination of fondaparinux and a fibrin-specific agent.

Dosing regimens of antithrombotic agents are given in Table 5.11.3.

Fibrinolysis and time to treatment

The advantages of thrombolytic therapy are time dependent. Although administering lytic agents up to 12 hours after the onset of symptoms may be beneficial in terms of outcome, every minute that reperfusion is postponed will unavoidably result in more extensive necrosis and worse outcome. Early in the course, the thrombus may be smaller and easier to lyse, which might in part explain the more prominent benefit of lytics in the first hours after symptom onset.

Table 5.11.3 Antithrombotic co-therapies with fibrin-specific fibrinolytics

Antiplatelet co-therapy	
Aspirin	150–325 mg orally or 250 mg IV if ingestion is not possible and continue 75–100 mg per day
Clopidogrel	Loading dose 300 mg (75 mg if age >75) and continue 75 mg per day

Anticoagulant co-therapy	
Unfractionated heparin	IV bolus of 60 U/kg (max 4000 U)
	Infusion of 12 U/kg (max 1000/hour) for 24–48 hours
	Target aPTT: 50–70 seconds; first monitoring after 3 hours
Enoxaparin	<75 years IV bolus of 30 mg sc 1 mg/kg bid (first dose 15 minutes after IV bolus) until discharge first two doses ≤100 mg
	>75 years no IV bolus SC 0.75 mg/kg bid (first dose 15 min after IV bolus) until discharge first two doses ≤75 mg
	Creatinine clearance <30 mL/min: same doses qd
Fondaparinux	IV bolus of 2.5
	SC 2.5 mg qd until discharge

Further reading

Antman EM, Morrow DA, McCabe CH, et al. Enoxaparin versus unfractionated heparin with fibrinolysis for ST-elevation myocardial infarction. N Engl J Med 2006;**354**:1477–88.

Assessment of the Safety and Efficacy of a New Thrombolytic Regimen (ASSENT)-3 Investigators. Efficacy and safety of tenecteplase in combination with enoxaparin, abciximab, or unfractionated heparin: the ASSENT-3 randomised trial in acute myocardial infarction. Lancet 2001;**358**:605–13.

GUSTO investigators. An international randomized trial comparing four thrombolytic strategies for acute myocardial infarction. The GUSTO Investigators. N Engl J Med 1993;**329**:673–82.

Sabatine MS, Cannon CP, Gibson CM, et al. Addition of clopidogrel to aspirin and fibrinolytic therapy for myocardial infarction with ST-segment elevation. N Engl J Med 2005;**352**:1179–89.

Van De Werf F, Adgey J, Ardissino D, et al. Assessment of the Safety and Efficacy of a New Thrombolytic (ASSENT-2). Single-bolus tenecteplase compared with front-loaded alteplase in acute myocardial infarction: the ASSENT-2 double-blind randomised trial. Lancet 1999;**354**:716–22.

Van de Werf F, Bax J, Betriu A, et al. Management of acute myocardial infarction in patients presenting with persistent ST-segment elevation: the Task Force on the Management of ST-Segment Elevation Acute Myocardial Infarction of the European Society of Cardiology. Eur Heart J 2008;**29**:2909–45.

Van de Werf FJ, Topol EJ, Sobel BE. The impact of fibrinolytic therapy for ST-segment-elevation acute myocardial infarction. J Thromb Haemost 2009;**7**:14–20.

Antiplatelet agents

Antiplatelet agents are used commonly for acute treatment and secondary prevention of occlusive vascular thrombotic events in general, including coronary artery disease, stroke or transient ischaemic attack (TIA), and peripheral vascular disease in particular. These drugs target various platelet receptors involved in cell adhesion, aggregation, secretion, and release of procoagulant mediators. The universal goal for these agents is to inhibit platelet activity, and protect platelets from excessive stickiness, which in turn is mandatory for thrombus formation.

Classes

1 COX inhibitors (aspirin)

2 PDE antagonists (cilostazol, dipyridamole)

3 P2Y12 receptor blockers (ticlopidine, clopidogrel, prasugrel)

4 GP IIb/IIIa inhibitors (abciximab, eptifibatide, tirofiban).

Drugs

Aspirin

Aspirin and related compounds block a variety of prostaglandins including thromboxane, a potent inductor of platelet activity. Aspirin is a cornerstone of antiplatelet therapy and is used usually in combination with other agents for all indications with the exception of stroke and TIA, in which monotherapy is preferred. Numerous trials suggest unquestionable benefits of aspirin in the reduction of second vascular events such as acute coronary syndromes, including non-fatal myocardial infarction, and strokes. Aspirin therapy is consistently associated with the trends towards mortality reduction; the ISIS-2 study shows absolute mortality benefit of moderate-dose aspirin, but the benefit is never seen for higher doses.

- Dose—oral, non-coated, indefinitely long, at least 50 mg but no more than 162 mg/day. Higher doses: short term, during the acute phase only.
- Adverse effects—bleeding, gastric discomfort, allergy.

Cilostzsol

Cilistazol is a cyclic AMP PDE Type 3 inhibitor causing increase in AMP in platelets and blood vessels, leading to inhibition of platelet activity and vasodilatation. Clinical trials strongly indicate improvement of walking distance in patients with intermittent claudification. No outcome data in atherothrombosis are available beyond the functional improvement in patients with peripheral artery disease.

- Dose—100–200 mg/daily for 12–24 weeks
- Adverse effects—headache, diarrhoea, dyspepsia, allergy.

Dipyridamole

- Dipyridamole is a cyclic AMP and cyclic GMP PDE Type 5 inhibitor causing increase in plasma adenosine and release of nitric oxide. An at least dual mechanism of action suggests that dipyridamole is not a pure antiplatelet agent, rather than an antithrombotic. Since the drug can be stored in lipophylic cell membranes, it is well suited for chronic use. Extended-release dipyridamole in combination with very-low-dose aspirin is used for second stroke/TIA prevention. Cardiovascular applications and effects on mortality are unknown.
- Dose—200–400 mg/daily for 2 years after stroke.
- Adverse effects—headache, dizziness, diarrhoea, nausea.

Ticlopidine

Ticlopidone, thienopyridine, is an irreversible platelet P2Y12 inhibitor, targeting predominantly ADP-induced aggregation. Ticlopidone is used to reduce risk of stroke, and stent thrombosis after coronary interventions. Present use is limited due to high risk of bone marrow toxicity.

- Dose—250–500 mg/day for 6 months after an acute event.
- Adverse effects—neutropenia, agranulocytosis, TTP, aplastic anaemia, bleeding.

Clopidogrel

Clopidogrel is a second-generation thienopyridine with the mechanism of action similar to ticlopidine. Clopidogrel is a prodrug, requiring two-step metabolization. However, clopidogrel exhibits much better safety profile with similar efficacy in preventing thrombosis. Many studies confirm the vascular outcome benefit of clopidogrel in atherothrombosis, including absolute mortality reduction in patients with acute myocardial infarction in the COMMIT trial.

- Dose—600 mg loading (only before coronary angioplasty) followed by 75 mg/day for 1 year or indefinitely dependent on atherosclerotic burden, concomitant diseases, type of stent, and bleeding events.
- Adverse effects—bleeding, especially gastrointestinal, allergy, skin rash.

Prasugrel

Prasugrel is a very potent third-generation thienopyridine, also an irreversible P2Y 12 inhibitor, requiring single step metabolization. The drug is approved in Europe for acute coronary syndromes indication.

- Dose—60 mg loading, followed by 10 mg maintenance for 1 year, 5 mg/day for elderly people and low-weight patients.
- Adverse effects—high bleeding risks, potential cancer risks, especially in women.

Abciximab

Abciximab is a Fab fragment of himeric human–murine monoclonal antibody 7E3. Abciximab binds to GP IIb/IIIa and vitronectin platelet receptors, completely preventing platelet aggregation. Abciximab is indicated as an adjunct to PCI, or in patients with unstable angina not responding to conventional therapy to prevent periprocedural ischaemic complications. Safety and efficacy of abciximab beyond PCI are not established.

- Dose—IV 0.35 mg/kg bolus 10–60 minutes before PCI, followed by a continuous infusion of 0.125 µg/kg/min (10 mg/min maximum) for 12 hours.
- Adverse effects—bleeding, thrombocytopenia, anaphylaxis, hypotension, bradycardia.

Eptifibatide

Eptifibatide is a cyclic heptapeptide binding to GP IIb/IIIa, and blocking platelet aggregation. Eptifibatide is indicated for treatment of acute coronary syndromes, and patients undergoing PCI. Randomized trials indicate the reduction of combined endpoint of death, new myocardial infarction, and need of urgent revascularization.

- Dose—IV 180 µg/kg bolus immediately after diagnosis, followed by a continuous infusion of 2 µg/kg/min for

72–96 hours. With creatinine clearance <50 mL/min, a half dose of 1 µg/kg/min is recommended.
- Adverse effects—bleeding, thrombocytopenia.

Tirofiban
Tirofiban is a small non-peptide molecule with the high affinity to GP IIb/IIIa, causing profound inhibition of platelet aggregation. Tirofiban is indicated in patients with acute coronary syndromes, including medically managed patients, and those undergoing coronary angioplasty or atherectomy. Tirofiban has been shown to reduce the combined incidence of deaths, new myocardial infarction or refractory ischaemia/repeat cardiac procedures.
- Dose—IV initially 0.4 µg/kg/min for 30 minutes, followed by 0.1 µg/kg/min. No dose reduction required in elderly people; a half-dose for patients with renal failure
- Adverse effects—bleeding.

Role of antiplatelet agents
Primary prevention
The role of aspirin, ticlopidine, and clopidogrel for the reduction of a first vascular occlusive event risk despite numerous trials is unclear, and with the other antiplatelet agents is unknown. Use of low-dose aspirin, but not thienopyridines in men at high risk for vascular disease may be currently justified.

Secondary prevention
Mortality
Moderate-dose aspirin and no loading regimen with clopidogrel were associated with absolute mortality reduction. More potent antiplatelet strategies including prasugrel and GP IIb/IIIa inhibitors consistently lack death benefit.

Non-fatal acute coronary syndromes
There is consistent evidence that all antiplatelet agents moderately reduce the risk of a second event. Most impressive prevention is observed for early periprocedural events, while the outcome benefit is diminishing over time, being minimal for late events. The benefit is heavily dependent on the definition of myocardial infarctions, when surrogate or 'enzymatic' ischaemic episodes may be summarized with classical clinical events.

Stroke
Many studies suggest that delicate rather than aggressive antiplatelet regimens are preferable for stroke management. Combination antiplatelet strategies should be avoided (ESO Summary).

Diabetes
Patients with diabetes consistently exhibit high baseline platelet activity, and low response to conventional antiplatelet regimens. More aggressive strategies, and/or higher doses may be recommended in diabetics.

Bleeding
Bleeding is the most common complication of antiplatelet therapy. The incidence and severity of bleeding is directly related to the potency and length of antiplatelet therapy. There is no evidence that future bleeding, especially serious, may be predicted in a particular patient. Although superficial minor haemorrhages are associated with the degree of platelet inhibition, major catastrophic episodes are usually unexpected, and may manifest hidden genetic defects.

Compliance
Several reports consistently document a high (10–35%) rate of non-compliance during antiplatelet therapy. The main causes are repeated annoying minor bleeding episodes, and lack of immediate outcome benefit.
Expert adviser: Anonymous.

Further reading
COMMIT Collaborative Group. Addition of clopidogrel to aspirin in 45852 patients with acute myocardial infarction: randomized placebo-controlled trial. *Lancet* 2005;**366**:1607–21.

European Stroke Organisation (ESO) Executive Committee; ESO Writing Committee. Guidelines for management of ischaemic stroke and transient ischaemic attack 2008. *Cerebrovasc Dis* 2008;**25**:457–507.

ISIS-2 Trial Investigators. Randomised trial of intravenous streptokinase, oral aspirin, both, or neither among 17,187 cases of suspected acute myocardial infarction: ISIS-2. ISIS-2 (Second International Study of Infarct Survival) Collaborative Group. *Lancet* 1988;**2**:349–60.

Antithrombotic agents

Formation of thrombus

The first stage in the formation of arterial thrombus involves exposure of subendothelial tissue factor and collagen to circulating blood. This is the consequence of disrupted vascular endothelium following erosion or atherosclerotic plaque rupture. Tissue factor is a member of the cytokine receptor superfamily, and it acts as a receptor and an essential cofactor for factors VII and VIIa. A tissue factor–factor VIIa complex on the cell surface leads to the activation of factor X and initiates coagulation (Fig. 5.13.1). Tissue factor is constitutively expressed in cells surrounding blood vessels, forming a haemostatic barrier, but it can also be induced in vascular cells in response to a number of inflammatory stimuli, such as adhesion molecules (e.g. P-selectin and CD40 ligand), cytokines, and oxidized low-density lipoproteins.

Superficial erosion or denudation of the endothelial cells over the surface of the plaque accounts for about 25% of all cases of fatal coronary thromboses, and plaque rupture occurs in the remainder. Coagulation factors are activated rapidly, generating thrombin (Fig. 5.13.1). As a result, fibrinogen is converted to fibrin, with fibrin degradation products (FDP$_{1+2}$) as byproducts. At the same time, platelet adhesion, activation, and aggregation occur as thrombin acts on the platelets attached to the site of injury. Activated platelet receptors promote aggregation by cross-linking, resulting in the formation of a platelet plug. Thrombin is generated by coagulation factors and also by platelets, and thrombin powerfully stimulates platelet adhesion and aggregation. The formation of fibrin helps to stabilize the platelet plug (which would otherwise fragment in blood flow). Fibrin forms polymer cross-links, creating the thrombus 'clot', which also contains tightly bound aggregates

of platelets. The thrombus attaches to disrupted vessel wall by platelet adhesion.

The typical arterial thrombus at the site of a coronary plaque disruption has a platelet-rich component ('white thrombus') and a friable clot, forming distally ('red thrombus') due to stasis beyond the lesion.

Although anticoagulant and antiplatelet therapies are considered separately, there is functional amplification of platelet aggregation by thrombin, and, similarly, platelet activation results in augmentation of thrombus formation. Thus, anticoagulant therapy needs to be seen not only in the clinical and interventional context, but also in the context of the extent of platelet inhibition (see below).

Anticoagulant therapy

Unfractionated heparin (UFH) is a natural product, usually obtained from porcine intestinal mucosa, and it consists of a mixture of mucopolysaccharide molecules, with a molecular weight ranging from 2000 to 30 000 daltons. About a third of the heparin chains have a specific pentasaccharide sequence with high affinity for antithrombin III; this fraction is responsible for most of the anticoagulant activity of heparin. Heparin bridges thrombin and antithrombin and so inhibits factor IIa. It is administered as an intravenous infusion, but its therapeutic window is narrow, requiring frequent monitoring of the activated partial thromboplastin time (aPTT). This is because several plasma proteins compete with antithrombin III for heparin binding, reducing anticoagulant activity. The levels of these heparin-binding proteins vary among patients and this contributes to the variable anticoagulant response to heparin and to heparin resistance. Heparin binds to endothelial cells and macrophages and in high concentrations

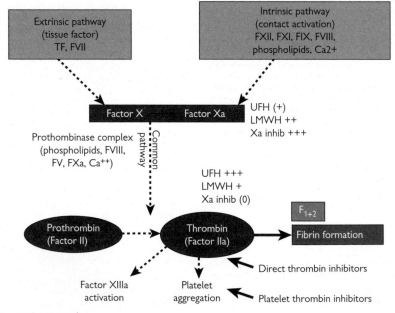

Fig. 5.13.1 The coagulation cascade.

(above clinical therapeutic) it has additional properties. UFH is used in patients undergoing PCI but care should be taken to avoid over-anticoagulation if patients were previously on low-molecular-weight heparin (LMWH). It is preferable to maintain LMWH during PCI in order to reduce bleeding risk (as demonstrated in ExTRACT and other studies). The main complication of all antithrombotics is bleeding; in addition, prolonged administration of UFH may result in heparin-induced thrombocytopenia (HIT) and osteoporosis. HIT is the result of antibodies against an epitope on platelet factor 4 (PF4), with the forming heparin/PF4 complexes.

LMWHs have replaced UFH for various indications. They consist of shorter fragments of heparin (2000–10 000 daltons) that link to antithrombin through the pentasaccharide sequence; this is the basis of their anti-Xa activity. Their anti-IIa activity is lower than with UFH. The extent of anti-Xa versus anti-IIa activity varies with different LMWHs. The key advantages of LMWH over UFH is the near-complete absorption after subcutaneous administration without the need for monitoring. There is less protein binding, less platelet activation, and a more predictable dose–effect relationship. Most clinical trial experience is with enoxaparin, in both non-ST elevation acute coronary syndrome (ACS) and in ST elevation myocardial infarction (MI), and it has been shown to be superior to UFH. Pooled analyses of trials of LMWH versus UFH show modest superiority (mainly lower rates of MI) compared with UFH (ESC Guideline: approximately 1% absolute reduction in death or MI). In ACS there is a modest increased risk of bleeding: but this is more marked in those with impaired renal function, co-administration of UFH, or potent antiplatelet agents including GP IIb/IIIa inhibitors. In ST elevation MI enoxaparin was shown to be superior to UFH in those treated with thrombolytics (ExTRACT trial). LMWHs are cleared via the kidneys; they can accumulate in patients with impaired renal function, and thus contribute to bleeding risk. LMWHs are also indicated for deep venous thrombosis prophylaxis and treatment.

Factor Xa inhibitors also do not require monitoring and they can be administered subcutaneously. Both direct and indirect factor Xa inhibitors (acting via antithrombin III) are in development and fondaparinux, a selective indirect inhibitor of Xa, is the only agent currently approved. It was shown to be superior to LMWH in DVT prevention and treatment and in non-ST elevation ACS (OASIS 5) and in fibrinolytic treated ST elevation MI (OASIS 6). In non-ST elevation ACS it results in approximately 50% of the rate of major bleeding compared with enoxaparin, and lower mortality (OASIS 5). It is the preferred anticoagulant in patients with non-ST elevation ACS, provided they are not scheduled for early revascularization (ESC Guideline 1A recommendation). In patients undergoing PCI, additional UFH is required to avoid a small excess rate of sent thrombosis.

Direct thrombin inhibitors (DTI) bind directly to thrombin (factor-IIa) and so inhibit the thrombin-induced conversion of fibrinogen to fibrin. They inactivate fibrin-bound and fluid-phase thrombin. Hirudins are polypeptides first isolated from the salivary glands of the medicinal leech. They are bivalent inhibitors that bind to the active site and to the fibrin binding site of thrombin (largely irreversible).

There is no selective antagonist of hirudin or bivalirudin, but bivalirudin is degraded by hepatic metabolism and proteolytic cleavage (half-life approximately 25 minutes). The main indications for bivalirudin are in patients undergoing percutaneous coronary intervention where they reduce the rate of major bleeding (compared with UFH or LMWH plus GP IIb/IIIa inhibitors). Bivalirudin has been tested against heparins in a large randomized open study (ACUITY) and was shown to produce less bleeding than heparin/LMWH plus glycoprotein IIb/IIIa inhibitor. In primary PCI they also reduce bleeding, with lower subsequent death rates (HORIZONS trial). DTIs in development include inhibitors of thrombin on the platelet surface receptor. The only agents currently approved are lepuridin (for patients with HIT), and in ACS, bivalirudin.

Vitamin K antagonists (warfarin, coumadin) are used for long-term anticoagulation following ACS, for example in those with prosthetic heart valves or those with atrial fibrillation. They are also indicated in patients with ventricular or apical thrombus and in heart failure patients with dilated ventricles (many develop atrial fibrillation).

Oral alternatives to warfarin: ximelagatran was the first agent developed and although it showed promise in terms of efficacy, it was removed from the market on account of hepatic side-effects. Dibigatran was tested in patients with atrial fibrillation who were either on warfarin or had an indication for warfarin in atrial fibrillation (anticoagulant naïve). Two separate doses of dibigatran were tested against warfarin (110 mg bd) (RE-LY study). The lower dose produced similar efficacy and reduced bleeding and the higher dose (150 mg bd) produced superior efficacy and similar rates of major bleeding. Dabigatran is likely to provide an oral alternative to warfarin and without the need for monitoring. Other oral anti-Xa agents are also being tested against warfarin (for example rivaroxaban) and also tested in ACS. Rivaroxaban is superior to enoxaparin for DVT prophylaxis and treatment.

Further reading

Bassand J-P, Hamm CW, Ardissino D, et al. Guidelines for the Diagnosis and Treatment of Non-ST-Segment Elevation Acute Coronary Syndromes. *Eur Heart J* 2007;**28**:1598–660.

Connolly SJ, Ezekowitz MD, Yusuf S, et al. The Randomized Evaluation of Long-Term Anticoagulation Therapy (RE-LY). *N Engl J Med* 2009;**361**:1139.

Stone GW, McLaurin BT, Cox DA, et al. Antiplatelet therapy in patients with acute coronary syndromes. Methods Study Design The Acute Catheterization and Urgent Intervention Triage Strategy (ACUITY) trial was a prospective, open-label, randomized, multicenter trial in which we compared heparin plus a glycoprotein IIb/IIIa inhibitor, bivalirudin. *N Engl J Med* 2006;**355**:2203.

Stone GW, Witzenbichler B, Guagliumi G, et al. Methods Trial. The Harmonizing Outcomes with Revascularization and Stents in Acute Myocardial Infarction (HORIZONS-AMI) study was a prospective, open-label, randomized, multicenter trial that compared bivalirudin alone with heparin plus a glycoprotein IIb/IIIa. *N Engl J Med* 2008;**358**:2218.

Yusuf S, Mehta SR, Chrolavicius S, et al., for the Fifth Organisation to Assess Strategies in Acute Ischemic Syndromes (OASIS-5) investigators. Comparison of fondaparinux and enoxaparin in acute coronary syndromes. *N Eng J Med* 2006;**354**:1464–76.

Yusuf S, Mehta SR, Chrolavicius S, et al., for the OASIS-6 Randomised Trial. Effects of fondaparinux on mortality and re-infarction in patients with acute ST segment elevation myocardial infarction. *JAMA* 2006;**295**:1519–30.

Anti-ischaemic agents

Introduction

Lifestyle advice and interventions to control cardiovascular risk factors are recommended for all patients with ischaemic heart disease (IHD), the main clinical presentation of which is angina pectoris. Comprehensive guidelines on the management of stable angina from the European Society of Cardiology (ESC) (Fox et al. 2006) and Scottish Collegiate Guidelines Network (SIGN 2007) are available. Guidance from the National Institute for Health and Clinical Excellence (NICE) is currently in preparation. Please refer to the Summary of Product Characteristics (SPC) for more detailed information for individual drugs described. In the absence of contraindications, aspirin, beta-blockers, statins, and angiotensin-converting enzyme inhibitors (ACEIs) are among the most widely currently prescribed agents which influence prognosis in IHD.

Nitrates

Nitrates are the mainstay of treatment in angina pectoris. They control symptoms and improve exercise capacity but do not influence prognosis. They have a direct relaxant effect on vascular smooth muscle cells where they are metabolically converted to nitric oxide (NO) and dilatation of coronary vessels improves myocardial oxygen supply. They also dilate peripheral veins thereby reducing preload and afterload to reduce myocardial oxygen consumption. Sublingual, buccal glyceryl trinitrate (GTN) tablets or spray should be used to prevent exertional anginal attacks and for immediate pain relief. Side-effects include headache, which may wear off but if intolerable will require alternative treatments. Occasionally postural hypotension can occur and nitrates should not be co-administered with phosphodiesterase-5 inhibitors such as sildenafil. Nitrate-tolerance can develop rapidly with continuous use and may be lessened by using preparations that provide nitrate-low or nitrate-free intervals. Molsidomine is a vasodilator that is nitrate-like with similar efficacy, but it is not available in many countries.

Nicorandil

Nicorandil is a hybrid compound that is a potassium channel opener with a nitrate moiety. Nicorandil may mimic ischaemic preconditioning, which is a powerful protection against myocardial necrosis. The Impact Of Nicorandil in Angina study (IONA 2002) showed that nicorandil 20 mg twice daily, in addition to standard antianginal therapy, improved outcomes in terms of reducing events related to acute coronary disease and the associated requirement for admission to hospital. The drug may therefore have a useful role in treatment of angina which is unresponsive to initial medical treatment.

Heart rate-lowering agents

Beta-blockers

Oral beta-blockers are recommended for long-term use in all patients without contraindications who recover from an acute myocardial infarction (MI). By extrapolation, beta-blockers may also be cardioprotective in stable angina pectoris. Agents such as bisoprolol are also firmly established in the treatment of chronic heart failure. Beta-blockers, by their heart rate and blood pressure-lowering effects, reduce the overall workload of the heart. It is conventional to adjust the dose of beta-blocker to reduce resting heart rate to 55–60 bpm. Evidence suggests that high resting heart rates carry an adverse prognosis (Borer 2008) and that heart rate lowering per se may be beneficial (Borer 2008).

Most evidence of benefit with beta-blockers is available for propranolol, timolol and metoprolol from studies conducted in the pre-thrombolysis era and without a background of aspirin and statins. Although atenolol is widely used it has been inadequately evaluated. A recent meta-analysis of placebo-controlled trials of atenolol in hypertensives (Carlberg et al. 2004) suggests no advantage of the atenolol over placebo in terms of reducing mortality (all-cause, cardiovascular or from MI). One possible explanation for this is that atenolol has a short plasma half-life (6–9 hours) and it does not provide 24-hour therapeutic levels when prescribed at a typical antianginal dose of 50 mg od. Twice a day dosing may be more appropriate, or increasing the dose increases its duration of action. Target doses for beta-blockers are atenolol 100 mg od, bisoprolol 10 mg od and metoprolol CR 200 mg od.

Beta-blocker side-effects are less likely to occur with beta-1-selective agents but these include fatigue, lethargy, cold periphery, etc. They are contraindicated in patients with asthma and bronchospastic disease. Some beta-blockers are poorly tolerated and about 20% of patients do not respond to any beta-blocker (Thadani 1991), which may require switching them to a heart rate-lowering calcium antagonist, e.g. diltiazem or the sinus node inhibitor, ivabradine.

Sinus node inhibitors

Ivabradine, the first clinically available sinus node inhibitor, is licensed for the symptomatic treatment of chronic stable angina pectoris in patients with normal sinus rhythm who have a contraindication or intolerance for beta-blockers; or in combination with beta-blockers in patients inadequately controlled with an optimal beta-blocker dose and whose heart rate is >60 bpm. Heart rate is controlled by inhibiting the If current, which plays a central role as a pacemaker in the sinoatrial node. Inhibiting this current reduces the slope of the diastolic depolarization curve and causes a dose-related decrease in heart rate. Ivabradine is a pure bradycardic agent that, at a maximum dose of 7.5 mg twice daily, decreases heart rate similarly to a beta-blocker, but has no effect on systemic blood pressure. It is not negatively inotropic but has effective anti-ischaemic and antianginal activity, which is superior to placebo and as effective as atenolol and amlodipine. The landmark, BEAUTIFUL trial (Fox et al. 2008) showed that ivabradine did not improve outcomes in all stable IHD patients with left ventricular (LV) dysfunction but could be used to reduce outcomes (admission to hospital for fatal and non-fatal MI and coronary revascularization) in a subgroup of patients with heart rates >70 bpm. The SHIFT trial showed that in patients with high testing heart rate, ivabradine did improve outcomes in patients with heart failure.

Ivabradine is generally well tolerated but generally transient, and mild visual disturbances, described as 'luminous phenomena (phosphenes)' may occur generally during the early phase of dosing. Other side-effects include bradycardia, heart block, and ventricular extrasystoles. It is important therefore to avoid use of ivabradine in patients with resting heart rates below 60 bpm or in those with heart block or arrhythmias.

Non-dihydropyridine calcium antagonists
Although calcium antagonists share the common property of inhibition of calcium into the cell, resulting in vasodilatation of vascular smooth muscle and relaxation of myocardial muscle, they have quite distinctive pharmacological and haemodynamic properties (Purcell et al. 1989). Diltiazem and verapamil reduce heart rate and blood pressure and are negatively inotropic (thus contraindicated in heart failure and in heart block). Calcium antagonists may retard the atherosclerotic process, but more complete clinical data are required to establish if they have any role other than symptom control in angina. Diltiazem and verapamil are generally as effective as beta-blockers in monotherapy or they may have additive anti-ischaemic effects if combined. Care is needed not to reduce the heart rate excessively. Adverse effects include flushing, dizziness, constipation, and fluid retention.

Dihydropyridine calcium antagonists
These include nifedipine and amlodipine, which have minimal effects on heart rate or cardiac contractility. Short-acting preparations of nifedipine are inappropriate to use as they cause reflex tachycardia. Long-acting once a day formulations are available and amlodipine 5–10 mg od is a widely used and it can also be used to treat, angina in patients with compensated heart failure.

Late sodium current inhibitors
Ranolazine is a metabolically active agent that selectively inhibits the late sodium current which is activated during ischaemia and leads to calcium overload and other effects (Nash and Nash 2008). Ranolazine reduces these ionic imbalances, and the reduction in calcium overload is expected to improve myocardial relaxation and thereby decrease LV diastolic stiffness and improve anginal symptoms. It does not affect blood pressure or heart rate. Ranolazine at a maximal dose of 750 mg twice daily is indicated as add-on therapy for angina patients who are inadequately controlled or intolerant to first-line antianginals such as beta-blockers or calcium antagonists. Three randomized trials have shown efficacy for ranolazine in increasing exercise capacity and reducing anginal episodes and GTN consumption. Side-effects include dizziness, nausea, constipation, and the potential to prolong the QT interval, but no increase in significant arrhythmias has been observed and the compound appears to provide a safe addition (being mindful to avoid certain co-administrations, e.g. CYP 3A4 such as ketoconazole) to traditional antianginal agents.

Trimetazidine, another metabolically acting drug, is available in many European countries but not the UK. It preserves energy balance during myocardial ischaemia and stimulates glucose oxidation and acts as a partial fatty acid oxidation inhibitor.

Antianginals have varying haemodynamic effects (Table 5.14.1). Patients who are hypotensive, for example, may benefit more from an agent that does not affect blood pressure. Similarly, a beta-blocker or ivabradine may be inappropriate in patients with bradycardia.

Rational prescribing
Antianginal treatment should be tailored to the individual patient. It is important to improve prognosis as well as minimize or abolish symptoms. No one antianginal has shown consistently greater efficacy in relieving chest pain or reducing exercise-induced ischaemia (Purcell and Kaddoura 2001). The dosing of one drug should be

Table 5.14.1 Effects of antianginal drug therapy on haemodynamic parameters

	Reduces heart rate	Reduces blood pressure	Vasodilatory effect
Beta-blocker	Yes	Yes	No
Dihydropyridine calcium antagonist	No	Yes	Yes
Non-dihydropyridine calcium antagonist	Yes	Yes	Yes
Long-acting nitrate	No	No	Yes
Nicorandil	No	Yes	Yes
Ivabradine	Yes	No	No
Ranolazine	No	No	No

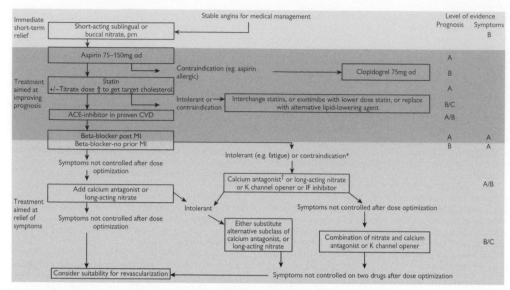

Fig. 5.14.1 Algorithm for medical management of stable angina. From Fox *et al.*, Guidelines on the management of stable angina pectoris, in *Eur Heart J* 2006;27:1341–81, copyright 2006.

optimized before adding another. Combinations of drugs may be additive and logical combinations are shown in the ESC angina treatment algorithm (Fig. 5.14.1) (Fox *et al.* 2006). Since this was published, ivabradine can now be prescribed with a beta-blocker if symptoms are uncontrolled and heart rate is >60 bpm. The evidence for combining three drugs is limited and patients whose symptoms are not controlled on maximum doses of two agents should be referred for cardiological assessment with a possible view to revascularization.

Further reading

Borer JS. Heart rate: from risk marker to risk factor. *Eur Heart J* 2008;**10**(Suppl F):F2–F6.

Carlberg B, Samuelsson O, Lindholm LH. Atenolol in hypertension: is it a wise choice? *Lancet*. 2004;**364**:1684–9.

Fox K, Ford I, Steg PG, Tendera M, Ferrari R, on behalf of the BEAUTIFUL Investigators. Ivabradine for patients with stable coronary artery disease and left-ventricular systolic dysfunction (BEAUTIFUL): a randomized, double-blind, placebo-controlled trial. *Lancet* 2008;**37**:807–16.

Fox K, Garcia MAA, Ardissino D, *et al.* Guidelines on the management of stable angina pectoris. *Eur Heart J* 2006;**27**:1341–81.

Nash DT, Nash SD. Ranolazine for chronic stable angina. *Lancet* 2008;**372**:1335–41.

Purcell H, Kaddoura S (eds). *Angina. A systematic guide to investigation and treatment.* London: Mosby, 2001.

Purcell H, Waller DG, Fox K. Calcium antagonists in cardiovascular disease. *Br J Clin Prac* 1989;**43**:369–79.

Scottish Intercollegiate Guidelines Network (SIGN). 96. Management of stable angina. A national clinical guideline. February 2007. (www.SIGN.ac.uk).

Thadani U. Medical therapy of stable angina pectoris. In: Abrams J (ed.), *Cardiology clinics: angina pectoris.* London: WB Saunders, 1991;9:73–87.

The IONA Study Group. Effect of nicorandil on coronary events in patients with stable angina: the Impact of Nicorandil in Angina (IONA) randomised trial. *Lancet* 2002;**359**:1269–15.

Lipid-lowering agents

The introduction of effective lipid-lowering therapies has had a very considerable, if sometimes controversial, impact on the prevention and management of cardiovascular disease. The great majority of this effect is due to the HMG-CoA reductase inhibitors, usually called statins. Despite their undoubted efficacy they have shortcomings and leave some unmet therapeutic needs, as discussed below. Nevertheless, the data available on these drugs far outweigh that on all other lipid-lowering agents combined and represents one of the largest accumulations of information of any class of drugs in any therapeutic field.

Statins

These agents are inhibitors of the first and probably rate limiting enzyme in the synthesis of cholesterol. The key target is the hepatocyte, where inhibition of cholesterol synthesis leads to upregulation of cell membrane low-density lipoprotein cholesterol (LDL-C) scavenger receptors, which then promote the uptake of circulating LDL particles and therefore reduce serum levels of LDL. At present there are six statins commercially available:

- Lovastatin (in the USA, not generally in Europe)
- Pravastatin
- Simvastatin
- Fluvastatin
- Atorvastatin
- Rosuvastatin.

They are listed in the chronological order in which they were introduced. Analysis of the data from over 70 studies suggests the following equivalences:

Daily doses of:
- Pravastatin 20–40 mg
- Lovastatin 10–20 mg
- Simvastatin 10 mg
- Fluvastatin 40 mg: reduce LDL-C by 20–30%
- Lovastatin 20–40 mg
- Simvastatin 30 mg
- Fluvastatin 80 mg
- Atorvastatin 10 mg: reduce LDL-C by 30–40%.

Atorvastatin and rosuvastatin at doses of 20 mg daily and above can reduce LDL-C by up to 60%. The statins have an unusual dose–response relationship: doubling the dose of any statin decreases LDL-C by 6%, the 'rule of sixes'. This means that adverse effects can increase more rapidly with dosage than does efficacy.

Primary and secondary prevention

Although most of the pivotal clinical trials in cardiovascular, and specifically coronary, disease prevention were secondary (in patients with known atheromatous disease), there is a remarkable degree of similarity in terms of relative risk reduction across all classes of patients based on data from over 150 000 individuals. A recent analysis suggests that for every 25 mg/dL (0.65 mmol/L) reduction in LDL-C there is:

- 11% reduction in cardiovascular mortality
- 14% reduction in major cardiovascular events
- 16% reduction in coronary events
- 10% reduction in stroke.

Other estimates over the last 5 years have produced similar figures. Note that the reduction in stroke is due wholly to fewer non-haemorrhagic events. There is strong correlation between LDL-C reduction and reduced risk, and it is safe to assume that this is the main factor responsible for the improvement. It is well known that statins have so-called pleiotropic effects, that is actions not directly related to lipid lowering, but the role of these (notably an anti-inflammatory effect) is not established in chronic therapy.

In a different perspective the clinical trials have produced an approximately 30% reduction in relative risk across many trials. Therefore the cost-effectiveness of statin therapy is crucially dependent on the initial level of absolute risk.

Percutaneous coronary interventions

There is strong evidence that high-dose statins, given periprocedurally reduce the short- to medium-term occurrence of myocardial infarction and other cardiac events. This action is too rapid to be due to LDL-C reduction and the anti-inflammatory properties of statins may be relevant.

LDL-C targets

The current guidelines in the USA, with general agreement elsewhere, recommend an LDL goal of approximately 3 mmol/L in general primary prevention and 2.5 mmol/L or less in high-risk patients. Even lower targets have been proposed (<2 mmol/L) but this may be at the expense of increased adverse effects.

Adverse effects and toxicity

The most serious toxicity associated with statins is skeletal muscle damage, that is to say myopathy. In its mildest form this is myalgia, at its most severe rhabdomyolysis, which is potentially fatal. Overall the incidence of myopathy is less than 1% and for rhabdomyolysis approximately 0.1%, although these figure are up to fourfold higher for simvastatin 80 mg daily. Financial pressures to use this dose of simvastatin should be resisted. The incidence of liver damage, as indicated by raised serum transaminases, is estimated at 0.5–1%, However, the clinical significance of this is controversial. Statin toxicity is enhanced (for simvastatin, atorvastatin, and lovastatin) by inhibitors of cytochrome P450 such as macrolide antibiotics and cimetidine, since these reduce drug clearance. Outside clinical trials there is a high discontinuation rate for statins, with median persistence of 5–6 months. The reasons for this are not clear but numerous 'minor' adverse effects have been reported such as disturbed sleep, memory disturbance, and erectile dysfunction. These may be more minor for the prescriber than the patients.

Fibrates

The fibric acid derivates (bezafibrate, ciprofibrate, fenofibrate, and gemfibrozil) act through the nuclear receptor peroxisome proliferator activator (PPAR)-α. The predominant effect is to reduce triglyceride (TG) synthesis, with usually only a modest effect on LDL-C, and in the case of gemfibrozil virtually none. They are therefore useful in patients with diabetes or severe insulin resistance where TG levels may be high, in extreme cases increasing the risk of acute pancreatitis. But fenofibrate has been reported in some studies to reduce LDL-C by as much as 40% and having virtually no effect in others. Importantly, the fibrates have a greater effect in raising high-density lipoprotein cholesterol (HDL-C) by up to 20%, more than the statins. Low HDL-C is a significant cardiovascular risk factor, especially in diabetic patients and individuals of South Asian origin, many of whom become diabetic later.

There is much less clinical trial data on fibrates than statins, and some of it is of worse quality. Overall the conclusion is that fibrates lower the risk of non-fatal myocardial infarction but not of coronary or cardiovascular mortality. One trial has demonstrated that mortality is reduced if the focus is on patients with low HDL-C levels but unfortunately subsequent trials have not properly taken this into account.

The fibrates can also cause myopathy, though very rarely a severe one, especially if renal function is impaired. They can also themselves cause some deterioration in renal function.

Niacin

Niacin, or nicotinic acid, has a complex mode of action in the liver and adipose tissue. It has in many ways the ideal profile for a lipid-modulating drug:
- reduces LDL-C by 20–30%
- reduces TG by 20–30%
- increases HDL-C 20–40%.

It therefore has a far more positive effect on HDL-C than any currently available agent. It also has the unique property of reducing serum levels of lipoprotein (a), an LDL-related lipoprotein with pro-atherogenic and prothrombotic properties. Unfortunately, trials with niacin have generally involved small numbers. One study has shown an 11% reduction in total mortality but others have shown reductions only in non-fatal myocardial infarction.

The main obstacle to the wider use of niacin has been the frequency of adverse effects: flushing and hepatotoxicity. These have been to some extent minimized by an extended-release formulation of the drug, and more recently by combining this with laropiprant, which is an antagonist of the prostaglandin D2 receptor thought to be responsible for the flushing.

Ezetimibe

Ezetimibe is a potent inhibitor of cholesterol absorption from the small intestine, whether the cholesterol is endogenous or dietary. Alone it can reduce LDL-C by 15–20%, although this is very variable. It may be an alternative to statins in patients who cannot tolerate them. However, outcome data will not be available for several years, although trials have shown no improvement in carotid intima-media thickness, a surrogate marker for atherosclerosis. Again myalgia and very rarely muscle damage may occur.

Bile acid sequestrants

These were the first drugs shown to reduce LDL-C. They do this by inhibiting the reabsorption of bile acids from the gut, so promoting the conversion of more cholesterol to bile acids, which are excreted. They can reduce LDL-C by 15–20% but are poorly tolerated because of gastrointestinal side-effects. Their only significant use is as part of multiple drug therapies in patients with familial hypercholesterolaemia.

Combination therapies

This is much more controversial than in hypertension. Briefly:
- Statins + fibrates: possibly increased risk of myopathy, but almost certainly exaggerated except with gemfibrozil, which should always be avoided.
- Statins + niacin: small studies suggest enhance LDL-C reduction and improved outcomes.
- Statins + ezetimibe: enhanced LDL-C reduction, equivalent to two- to fourfold increase in statin dosage, but no evidence of equivalent effect on outcomes.

New therapies

The two major challenges are patients who do not tolerate or do not respond to statins; and patients with low levels of HDL-C. One solution to the latter is inhibition of cholesterol transfer protein (CETP), so preventing the conversion of HDL-C to LDL-C. The first drug to do this, torceprapib, reached late clinical trials but was withdrawn due to increased mortality. This was due to an unexpected increase in blood pressure because of an 'off target' effect, that is one unrelated to the primary mechanism of action of the drug. Similar drugs without blood pressure effects are in development, e.g. dalcetrapib.

Further reading

Brugts JJ, Yetgin T, Hoeks SE, et al. The benefits of statins in people without established cardiovascular disease but with cardiovascular risk factors: meta-analysis of randomised controlled trials. BMJ 2009;**338**:b2376.

Chapman MJ, Redfern JS, McGovern ME, Giral P. Niacin and fibrates in atherogenic dyslipidemia: pharmacotherapy to reduce cardiovascular risk. Pharmacol Ther 2010;**16**:314–45.

Davidson MH, Robinson JG. Safety of aggressive lipid management. J Am Coll Cardiol 2007;**49**:1753–62.

Delahoy PJ, Magliano DJ, Webb K, et al. The relationship between reduction in low-density lipoprotein cholesterol by statins and reduction in risk of cardiovascular outcomes: an updated meta-analysis. Clin Ther 2009;**31**:236–44.

Karalis D. Intensive lowering of low-density lipoprotein cholesterol levels for primary prevention of coronary artery disease. Mayo Clin Proc 2009;**84**:345–52.

Mega S, Patti G, Cannon CP, di Sciascio G. Preprocedural statin therapy to prevent myocardial damage in percutaneous coronary intervention. A review of randomized trials. Crit Pathways in Cardiol 2010;**9**:19–22.

Preiss D, Sattar N. Lipids, lipid modifying agents and cardiovascular risk: a review of the evidence. Clin Endocrinol 2009;**70**:815–28.

Rozman D, Monostory K. Perspectives of the non-stain hypolipidemic agents. Pharmacol Ther 2010;**127**:19–40.

Weng T-C, Kao Yang Y-H, Lin S-J, Tai S-H. A systematic review and meta-analysis on the therapeutic equivalence of statins. J Clin Pharmacy Ther 2010;**35**:139–51.

Diabetes and ischaemic heart disease

Ischaemic coronary heart disease (CHD) is common in diabetes and 60–80% of mortality is due to macrovascular disease in both type 1 and type 2 diabetes. The risk of cardiovascular disease (CVD) events in patients with type 2 diabetes presenting in middle age is increased two- to threefold in men and three- to fivefold in women. After 10 years of diabetes the risks of CHD events in patients with diabetes are considered equivalent to nor-moglycaemic patients with established CHD. This concept is termed 'cardiovascular risk equivalence' and is used as the basis of all treatment guidelines. Epidemiological studies in type 1 diabetes show that risk is increased 10- to 30-fold compared with normoglycaemic control subjects. Cardiovascular risk in maturity-onset diabetes of the young or that associated with teenage onset of type 2 diabetes for other reasons is unclear but is assumed to be high over a lifetime, thus prompting the need to consider treatment in these age groups.

Cardiovascular risk in patients with dysglycaemia (either impaired fasting glucose or impaired glucose tolerance) is a continuous exponential risk variable even before patients cross the arbitrary threshold used to define diabetes. These patients have elevated levels of CVD risk even before they formally are diagnosed with diabetes. Many epidemiological studies have identified that both plasma glucose or HbA$_{1c}$ levels can be used to identify the additional risk due to dysglycaemia. Patients with dysglycaemia and unidentified type 2 diabetes have similar rates of CHD events to patients with diagnosed diabetes (Fig. 5.16.1).

Often dysglycaemia accompanies other features of the metabolic syndrome: visceral adiposity, hypertriglyceridae-mia, low HDL-C, and raised blood pressure. The presence of the metabolic syndrome is also associated with eleva-tion in markers of inflammation, e.g. C-reactive protein, fibrinogen, serum amyloid A, adhesion molecules, and markers of thrombotic risk, including PAI-1 and abnormal purine metabolism–uric acid. A number of definitions of the metabolic syndrome exist and all identify subtly different features of disease associated with dysglycaemia. The modified US NCEP (2001) definition used for the metabolic syndrome is based on the presence of three out five qualifying characteristics:

- visceral adiposity (40 inches or 102 cm for Caucasian men; 35 inches or 95 cm for women)
- different (lower cut-offs) apply to other ethnic groups e.g. Indian Asians or Chinese
- triglycerides >150 mg/dL (1.7 mmol/L)
- HDL-C <40 mg/dL (1.09 mmol/L) men or <45 mg/dL (1.20 mmol/L) women
- systolic blood pressure >130 mmHg
- fasting plasma glucose >100 mg/dL (5.6 mmol/L).

In contrast, the IDF specified that visceral adiposity was paramount and that two out of the remaining four were necessary factors to diagnose metabolic syndrome. The World Health Organization definition added centiles of insulin resistance and the presence of microalbuminuria as key features.

The significance of the metabolic syndrome is that it not only identifies patients more likely to develop type 2 dia-betes or have accelerated progression of type 1 diabetes but also highlights factors that contribute to cardiovascular risk in diabetes. The NCEP definition seems to identify patients with CVD risk more efficiently, and the IDF defini-tion is better for the identification of diabetes and possibly microvascular complications. All patients with diabetes should be considered to be high risk for cardiovascular dis-ease. The risk profiles of cardiovascular disease differ between type 1 and type 2 diabetes.

Clinical approach

History: Key points

- Symptoms of IHD including central chest pain and classi-cal angina, shortness of breath, tiredness; however, the incidence of silent ischaemia approaches 25% in patients with diabetes
- Symptoms of vascular disease: transient ischaemic attacks or claudication
- Family history of IHD, stroke, peripheral arterial disease
- Duration and type of diabetes

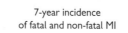

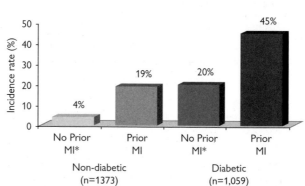

7-year incidence
of fatal and non-fatal MI

Fig. 5.16.1 Comparison of event rates in patients with established coronary disease and with diabetes. Haffner SM, *et al. N Eng J Med*;339:229–34, Copyright © 1998, Massachusetts Medical Society. All rights reserved.

Table 5.16.1 Risk factors for CHD in diabetes

Type 1	Type 2
Duration of DM	Duration of DM
Blood pressure	LDL-C
Microalbuminuria	HDL-C
Glycaemia	Blood pressure
TC: HDL-C ratio	Glycaemia

- Concomitant complications of diabetes including presence of hypertension, nephropathy (albuminuria), retinopathy, or erectile dysfunction
- Other environmental risk factors: history of previous or current smoking; obesity.

Examination: key points
- Central obesity—record waist and hip circumferences and diagnose using appropriate ethnic specific cut-offs
- Measurement of blood pressure using appropriate cuff size
- Measurement of ankle–brachial blood pressure index (ABI) if symptomatic of claudication. A value <0.7 is considered significant.
- Signs of target organ damage:
  - left ventricular hypertrophy, atrial fibrillation on ECG
  - nephropathy (dipstick test for proteinuria or micro-albuminuria)
  - retinopathy (fundoscopy/retinal eye screening)
  - erectile dysfunction as assessed by Sexual Health in Men (SHIM) score.

Biochemical investigations
- Hyperlipidaemia/dyslipidaemia.
- Measurement of a full lipid profile including total cholesterol, triglycerides; HDL-C, LDL-C.
  - Many lipid profiles are performed non-fasting in diabetes and the commonly used calculated LDL-C will underestimate actual levels due to post-prandial hypertriglyceridaemia. Calculated LDL-C is not reliable in patients with fasting TG >400 mg/dL (4.5 mmol/L). Measurement of direct LDL-C is preferable in diabetes.
  - Triglycerides mark added risk in type 2 diabetes due to the presence of small dense LDL particles and triglyceride-rich remnants. A value >150 mg/dL (1.7 mmol/L) (at HDL-C 1 mmol/L) indicates a potential added risk. Significant extra risk has been seen with levels >200 mg/dL (2.3 mmol/L).
  - In type 1 diabetes with good control lipid levels may appear normal. However apolipoprotein glycation and oxidation (advanced glycosylation end-products) means that these lipoproteins may not be handled normally and thus pose an increased CVD risk.
  - Apolipoproteins. In non-fasting samples levels of apolipoprotein B more accurately measure risk of CHD in diabetes due to particle numbers and atherogenic small dense LDL-C.
  - Particle size and number. These can be measured and may add to risk prediction over and above lipids and apolipoprotein concentrations though this is controversial and they are not routinely offered.

- Renal function
  - Estimation of creatinine clearance: this should be performed with a weight independent method: MDRD as hyperfiltration leads to artefactually normal estimated glomerular filtration rate (eGFR) in early nephropathy.
  - Albuminuria: albuminuria is an exponential risk factor in diabetes irrespective of concentration. Levels <0.7 for albumin: creatinine ratios are considered low risk though cut-offs >2.5 and >10 are taken as indicative of micro- and macro-albuminuria.
  - Uric acid. Urate is related to the metabolic syndrome and a CVD risk factor.
- Glycaemia: both current blood glucose and markers of glycaemic control (HbA$_{1c}$) levels should be measured. In type I diabetes especially hyperglycaemia associated with poor control is associated with hypertriglyceridaemia and may confound accurate determination of lipids.
- Inflammation; measurement of C-reactive protein levels in diabetes may be confounded by the high rates of intercurrent infection associated with poor glycaemic control and may not accurately reflect CVD risk. Other markers of inflammation such as LpPLA2 also correlate with risk in diabetes.

Calculation of CVD risk is not recommended in diabetes. All patients should be considered high risk. However demonstration of potential risk of CVD may be useful in counselling patients. The Framingham algorithm underestimates risk and shows significant discrepancies with the risk calculated from the UKPDS calculator which aligns better with actual event rates.

Radiological investigations
- Ultrasonic angiology: this may lead to a diagnosis of established atherosclerosis and is most useful in patients with symptoms of claudication or previous possible transient ischaemic attacks. Vasculopathy affecting one bed has a high likelihood of affecting others and thus combined carotid and femoral scanning may be useful in potential arteriopaths.
- Carotid intima-media thickness: this is strongly associated with risk of future CVD events and can be a useful risk discriminator. Values >1 mm in the common carotid artery denote patients at high risk.
- Coronary calcium scanning. This investigation adds to risk definition over and above classical risk factors. However in patients with diabetes and especially those with nephropathy adventitial calcification (Monkeberg's sclerosis) can confound the intimal calcification score used as the basis of this investigation.

Natural history and management

All patients with diabetes are high-risk for CHD events and 60–80% will develop cardiovascular complications as a result of macrovascular disease. Microvascular disease contributes an additional risk of macrovascular complications. The most substantial evidence base relates to the management of CVD risk in type 2 diabetes. The evidence base in type 1 diabetes is far more limited and based on extrapolation from epidemiological studies and from type 2 diabetes. Similarly guidelines for treatment of paediatric and young adult diabetes rely on epidemiological studies and the concept of greatly magnified relative as opposed to absolute CVD risk.

Management strategy

The management strategy of diabetes relies on aggressive management of all cardiovascular risk factors.

- Smoking cessation. Patients with diabetes should be managed aggressively using all cessation strategies. Quit rates are higher with the use of varenicline than bupropion or nicotine replacement therapies.
- Weight loss. In modern societies most patients with diabetes are overweight or obese. Obesity contributes markedly to the prevalence and progression of both type 2 and type 1 diabetes. All forms of calorie reduction diets will result in weight loss provided that long term adherence is maintained. There may be additional benefits to changes in diet composition to decrease saturated fat and salt intakes and increase intakes of fruits, nuts and vegetables. Most evidence in this area relates to the DASH diet, which has shown benefits on many CVD risk factors though it has not been assessed in end-point trials. A weight reduction of 7 kg as achieved in the DPP trial leads to two-thirds reduction in progression to type 2 diabetes. Similarly use of orlistat and a consequent 7-kg weight loss in the XENDOS study led to a 48% reduction in new type 2 diabetes. Data from the STORM study with sibutramine and the (prematurely terminated) CRESCENDO study with rimonabant, which both included subgroups of patients with diabetes, may give an indication of the likely effects of weight loss on CHD events. In the STRADIVARIUS trial with rimonabant the reduction in rate of progression of IVUS-assessed coronary atherosclerosis was not significant at 2 years but did correlate with the change in lipids associated with drug therapy.
- Exercise. Exercise should be encouraged as this can promote weight loss and consequent improvement in glycaemic control and in established atherosclerosis aid collateral circulation growth in patients with peripheral arterial disease or CHD.

Drug therapy

Drug therapy for CHD in diabetes relates to interlinked control of thrombosis, hyperlipidaemia, hypertension, and glycaemia. The focus is slightly different for type 1 and type 2 diabetes, with more emphasis on glycaemia and blood pressure control in type 1 diabetes and control of hyperlipidaemia in type 2 diabetes based on current evidence.

Thrombosis

Antithrombotic therapy is well established in atherosclerosis.

Aspirin

- The antiplatelet trialists' collaboration showed a 20–25% reduction in CVD events with the use of aspirin 75–600 mg. The lowest dose of 75 mg is commonly used. However, in the diabetes subgroup this analysis showed no benefit to aspirin therapy. Diabetes is known to be associated with hypercoagulability and it may be that the actual necessary dose is higher. One underpowered trial specifically in diabetes has shown no benefit with aspirin 81 mg. The ASCEND study of aspirin in diabetes may resolve the issue.

Dipyridamole

- Meta-analyses of dipyridamole have shown no benefit of monotherapy or aspirin–dipyridamole on CHD events except possibly in patients with stroke (ESPRIT-2).

Clopidogrel

- Comparison of aspirin and clopidogrel in the CAPRIE showed similar results with both agents with a marginal benefit with clopidogrel (9%; P = 0.04). Clopidogrel showed extra benefit (24%; P = 0.003) in patients with peripheral arterial disease and an analysis in the diabetes subgroup suggested a 21% extra benefit. In acute coronary syndromes in the CURE trial clopidogrel added to aspirin showed a 24% added benefit in all patients and in the subgroup undergoing PCI with equal benefits in all subgroups including diabetes. In chronic CHD in the CHARISMA trial the combination of aspirin and clopidogrel showed no extra benefits on CVD events and an increased rate of bleeds even in patients with diabetes. More recently in the TRITON (TIMI-38) study prasugrel added to aspirin showed a 25% extra benefit over aspirin–clopidogrel with clear superiority in patients with diabetes. Currently aspirin treatment is recommended for all patients with diabetes but there is no agreed dose.

Antihypertensives

Three classes of antihypertensives delivered equivalent CHD event reductions in the ALLHAT trial including the subgroup with diabetes with ACEIs, CCBs, or thiazide diuretics. The doxazosin arm was stopped early. There has been a debate whether any class of antihypertensive was superior to others. Thiazides and beta-blockers are known to increase risks of developing new diabetes by 1.5-fold, CCBs are neutral whereas ACEIs reduce risk by 15%, although in the DREAM study only a non-significant 11% benefit was shown with ramipril. Given the known benefit of high dose ACEIs or ARBs on microvascular end-points and progression to renal disease in both type 1 (DCCT) and type 2 (RENAAL, IDNT, PRIME) these drugs are used as first-line therapy in diabetes and show small non-significant benefits on CHD events in these trials.

Previously in patients with type 2 diabetes the UKPDS had shown that improved blood pressure control (140/85 mmHg) gave added reductions in CVD events compared with usual therapy (155/90 mmHg) which translated into mortality benefits after 10 years. More recently the ADVANCE study showed no added macrovascular disease benefit but improved microvascular benefits with improved blood pressure control to 130/80 mmHg. The results of the similarly designed ACCORD study are due in 2009. Guidelines recommend controlling blood pressure to <130/80 mmHg.

Lipid-lowering drugs

Patients with diabetes were initially excluded from lipid-lowering trials but specific trials have been performed with newer drugs and some post hoc analyses have been conducted over older drugs (Fig. 5.16.2).

Statins

- Statins were specifically investigated in type 2 diabetes in the CARDS, HPS, and ASPEN trials (Fig. 5.16.3). Meta-analysis confirmed similar benefits to non-diabetes with a 9% reduction in mortality and 22% reduction in CHD events per 1 mmol/L reduction in LDL-C. They are established first-line therapy for diabetes with guidelines recommending targets of LDL-C <70–80 mg/dL (<2 mmol/L).

Fibrates

- Patients with diabetes were excluded from early fibrate trials. Post hoc analyses of patients with metabolic

Lipid trials in diabetes

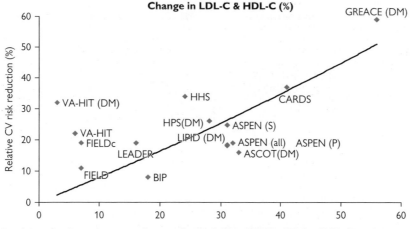

Fig. 5.16.2 Correlation of cardiovascular events reduction with sum of relative changes in LDL-C and HDL-C in trials in patients with type 2 diabetes. Reprinted from Wierzbicki, *Diab Vasc Dis Res* 3(3):166–71, copyright © 2006. Reprinted by permission of SAGE.

syndrome or diabetes suggested a 56% reduction in CHD events. In patients with low HDL-C (32 mg/dL; 0.85 mmol/L) gemfibrozil reduced CHD events by 24% in the VA-I IIT trial. In the DAIS trial in type 2 diabetes fenofibrate reduced angiographic coronary heart disease progression. However in the FIELD study fenofibrate therapy though confounded by statin drop-in showed an 11% reduction in CVD events but a non-significant 11% reduction in CHD events. There were additional benefits on progression of albuminuria grade and retinopathy. Meta-analysis suggests that fibrates reduce non-fatal myocardial infarcts and PCI but not CHD or stroke mortality.

Niacin
- Niacin improves lipids by increasing HDL-C and reducing TGs, LDL-C and lipoprotein(a). However, in patients with diabetes it can increase HbA$_{1c}$ by 0.3% if hypoglycaemic therapy titration is allowed. Some patients (5%) may show a rise in HbA$_{1c}$ of 1%. In a *post hoc* analysis of the CDP trial niacin reduced CHD events by 28% in patients with glucose >120 mg/dL (7 mmol/L). It is suggested that

the CHD event benefit of niacin exceeds the excess risk due to hyperglycaemia but not all guidelines agree on this.

Bile acid sequestrants and ezetimibe
- There is little data on the specific benefits of these drugs in diabetes. Meta-analyses suggest that any form of LDL-C reduction will result in benefits on CHD.

Omega-3 fatty acids
- Omega-3 fatty acids at high doses reduce triglycerides by 25%. At lower doses (1 g EPA or 0.5 g DHA/0.5 g EPA) they reduced CHD events in patients with CHD in GISSI-Prevenzione, JELIS, and in the GISSI heart failure trials. These trials included few patients with diabetes. The ASCEND study is investigating the efficacy of omega-3 fatty acids on CHD events in type 2 diabetes.

Combination therapy
- Trials currently underway are exploring the benefits of adding fibrates or niacin to optimal statin therapy in patients with type 2 diabetes in the ACCORD trial due in 2009 and in the HPS-2/THRIVE trial due in 2012.

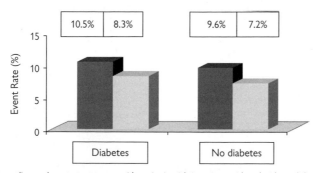

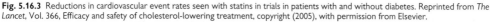

Fig. 5.16.3 Reductions in cardiovascular event rates seen with statins in trials in patients with and without diabetes. Reprinted from *The Lancet*, Vol. 366, Efficacy and safety of cholesterol-lowering treatment, copyright (2005), with permission from Elsevier.

STENO-2: Composite end-point of death from CV causes, nonfatal MI, CABG, PCI, nonfatal stroke, amputation, or surgery for PAD:

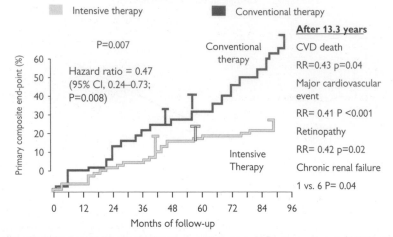

Intensive therapy   Conventional therapy

After 13.3 years

P=0.007   Conventional   CVD death
                 therapy
                                     RR=0.43 p=0.04
Hazard ratio = 0.47
(95% CI, 0.24–0.73;   Major cardiovascular
P=0.008)   event

                                     RR= 0.41 P <0.001

                                     Retinopathy

                 Intensive   RR= 0.42 p=0.02
                 Therapy
                                     Chronic renal failure

                                     1 vs. 6 P= 0.04

Months of follow-up

Fig. 5.16.4 Benefits of intensive control of glucose, blood pressure and lipids on cardiovascular event rate sin the Steno-2 trial. Gæde P, et al., *N Engl J Med*;348:383–93. Copyright © 2003, Massachusetts Medical Society. All rights reserved.

Glycaemic control

The benefits of improved glycaemic control on microvascular events were shown in type I diabetes in the DCCT study. In the 17-year follow-up of intensive glycaemic control in DCCT also reduced macrovascular CVD events by 57%. In type 2 diabetes the UKPDS showed that improved glycaemic control (HbA$_{1c}$ 7.0% versus 7.9%) was associated with microvascular benefits and a 15% reduction in CHD events. After 10 years therapy metformin in obese patients was associated with 35% reduction in CHD events while sulphonylurea (glimepride) therapy was associated with a 20% non-significant reduction in CHD events. Further improved glycaemic control (HbA$_{1c}$<6.5%) showed a non-significant 6% and 10% reductions in CHD events in the ACCORD and ADVANCE studies but was associated with additional microvascular benefits.

Polypharmacy

The efficacy of polytherapy or hypertension, lipids and glycaemia was investigated in the Steno-2 trial (Fig. 5.16.4).

After 7 years a 50% reduction in CHD events was found which translated into a 50% reduction in mortality after 13 years. The problems of polypharmacy, which can reduce adherence, may be ameliorated by single tablet 'poly-pill' therapies of which the Polycap has been the first to demonstrate good efficacy and tolerability. Based on the results of the Steno-2 study, tight control of lipids, blood pressure, and glycaemia are recommended in diabetes.

Expert advisors: Anthony S Wierzbicki DMDPhil FRCPath FAHA, Consultant in Metabolic Medicine/Chemical Pathology, Guy's & St Thomas' Hospitals, London UK. Adie Viljoen MBChB, MMed, FRCPath, MBA, Consultant in Metabolic Medicine/Chemical Pathology, Lister Hospital, Stevenage, UK.

Further reading

Alberti KG, Zimmet P, Shaw J. The metabolic syndrome—a new worldwide definition. *Lancet*, 2005;**366**(9491):1059–62.

American Diabetes Association. Standards of medical care in diabetes—2009. *Diabetes Care* 2009;**32**(Suppl 1):S13–S61.

Anti-Platelet Trialists' Collaboration. Collaborative meta-analysis of randomised trials of antiplatelet therapy for prevention of death, myocardial infarction, and stroke in high risk patients. *BMJ* 2002;**324**:71–86.

Buse JB, Ginsberg HN, Bakris GL, et al. Primary prevention of cardiovascular diseases in people with diabetes mellitus: a scientific statement from the American Heart Association and the American Diabetes Association. *Circulation* 2007;**115**:114–26.

Expert Panel on Detection Evaluation and Treatment of High Blood Cholesterol In Adults (Adult Treatment Panel III) 2001. Executive Summary of The Third Report of The National Cholesterol Education Program (NCEP). *JAMA* **285**:2486–97.

Haffner SM, Lehto S, Ronnemaa T, et al. Mortality from coronary heart disease in subjects with type 2 diabetes and in nondiabetic subjects with and without prior myocardial infarction. *N Engl J Med* 1998;**339**:229–234.

Hartweg J, Farmer AJ, Perera R, et al. Meta-analysis of the effects of n-3 polyunsaturated fatty acids on lipoproteins and other emerging lipid cardiovascular risk markers in patients with type 2 diabetes. *Diabetologia* 2007;**50**:1593–602.

Holman RR, Paul SK, Bethel MA, et al. 10-year follow-up of intensive glucose control in type 2 diabetes. *N Engl J Med* 2008a;**359**:1577–89.

Holman RR, Paul SK, Bethel MA, et al. Long-term follow-up after tight control of blood pressure in type 2 diabetes. *N Engl J Med* 2008b;**359**:1565–76.

Howard BV, Best LG, Galloway JM, et al. Coronary heart disease risk equivalence in diabetes depends on concomitant risk factors. *Diabetes Care* 2006; **29**:391–7.

Kavey RE, Allada V, Daniels SR, et al. Cardiovascular risk reduction in high-risk pediatric patients: a scientific statement from the

American Heart Association Expert Panel on Population and Prevention Science; the Councils on Cardiovascular Disease in the Young, Epidemiology and Prevention, Nutrition, Physical Activity and Metabolism, High Blood Pressure Research, Cardiovascular Nursing, and the Kidney in Heart Disease; and the Interdisciplinary Working Group on Quality of Care and Outcomes Research: endorsed by the American Academy of Pediatrics. *Circulation* 2006;**114**:2710–38.

Kearney PM, Blackwell L, Collins R, *et al.* Efficacy of cholesterol-lowering therapy in 18,686 people with diabetes in 14 randomised trials of statins: a meta-analysis. *Lancet* 2008;**371**:117–25.

Laing SP, Swerdlow AJ, Slater SD, *et al.* Mortality from heart disease in a cohort of 23,000 patients with insulin-treated diabetes. *Diabetologia* 2003;**46**:760–5.

Lewington S, Whitlock G, Clarke R, *et al.* Blood cholesterol and vascular mortality by age, sex, and blood pressure: a meta-analysis of individual data from 61 prospective studies with 55,000 vascular deaths. *Lancet* 2007;**370**:1829–39.

Nathan DM, Lachin J, Cleary P, *et al.* Intensive diabetes therapy and carotid intima-media thickness in type 1 diabetes mellitus. *N Engl J Med* 2003;**348**:2294–303.

Saha SA, Kizhakepunnur LG, Bahekar A, Arora RR. The role of fibrates in the prevention of cardiovascular disease—a pooled meta-analysis of long-term randomized placebo-controlled clinical trials. *Am Heart J* 2007;**154**:943–53.

Thomas DE, Elliott EJ, Naughton GA. Exercise for type 2 diabetes mellitus. *Cochrane Database Syst Rev* 2006;(3):CD002968.

Abbreviations

ACCORD, Action to Control Cardiovascular Risk in Diabetes; ADVANCE, Action in Diabetes and Vascular Disease; ALLHAT, Anti-hypertensive and Lipid-Lowering Treatment to Prevent Heart Attack Trial; ASCEND, A Study of Cardiovascular Events iN Diabetes; ASPEN, Atorvastatin Study for Prevention of Coronary Heart Disease Endpoints in Non-Insulin-Dependent Diabetes Mellitus; CAPRIE, Clopidogrel vs. Aspirin in Patients at Risk of Ischemic Events, CARDS, Collaborative Atorvastatin Diabetes Study; CDP, Coronary Drug Project; CHARISMA, Clopidogrel for High Atherothrombotic Risk and Ischemic Stabilization, Management and Avoidance; CRESCENDO, Comprehensive Rimonabant Evaluation Study of Cardiovascular ENDpoints and Outcomes; CURE, Clopidogrel in Unstable angina to prevent Recurrent Ischaemic Events; DAIS, Diabetes Atherosclerosis Intervention Study; DASH, Dietary Action on Sodium & Health; DCCT, Diabetes Care & Control Trial; DHA, Docosahexaenoic acid; DPP, Diabetes Prevention Program; DREAM, Diabetes reduction approaches with ramipril and rosiglitazone Medications; EPA, Eicosapentaenoic acid; ESPRIT-2, European/Australasian Stroke Prevention in Reversible Ischaemia Trial; FIELD, Fenofibrate Intervention on Endpoint Lowering in Diabetes; GISSI, Gruppo Italiano per lo Studio della Sopravvivenza nell'Infarto Miocardico; HPS, Heart Protection Study; HPS-2/THRIVE, Heart Protection Study 2-Treatment of High density lipoprotein to Reduce the Incidence of Vascular Events; IDF, International Diabetes Federation; IDNT, Irbesartan in Diabetic Nephropathy Trial; JELIS, Japan EPA Lipid Intervention Study; LpPLA2, Lipoprotein-associated phospholipase A2; MDRD, Modified Diet in Renal Disease; MODY, Maturity Onset Diabetes of the Young; NCEP, National Cholesterol Education Program; PAI-1, Plaminogen activator inhibitor-1; PCI, Percutaneous coronary intervention; PRIME, Program for Irbesartan Mortality and Morbidity Evaluation; RENAAL, Reduction of Endpoints in NIDDM with the Angiotensin II Antagonist Losartan; STORM, Sibutramine Trial on Obesity Reduction and Maintenance; STRADIVARIUS, Strategy to Reduce Atherosclerosis Development Involving Administration of Rimonabant - The Intravascular Ultrasound Study; TRITON, Trial to Assess Improvement in Therapeutic Outcomes by Optimizing Platelet Inhibition with Prasugrel; UKPDS, UK Prospective Diabetes Study; VA-HIT, Veteran's Affairs-HDL Intervention Trial; XENDOS, Xenical in the Prevention of Diabetes in Obese Subjects.

Post myocardial infarction: medical therapy

In the UK the yearly incidence of acute myocardial infarction for men and women between the ages of 30 and 69 years is 600 and 200 per 100 000 respectively. Approximately 25% of victims die out of hospital, up to 15% in hospital, <1–10% in the first year after discharge; thereafter the rate is ≤5% per year. Prognosis is influenced by age, the extent of coronary disease and residual left ventricular function, the occurrence of ventricular tachyarrhythmias, and co-morbidities such as diabetes, hypertension, smoking, sloth, and socioeconomic deprivation. For many patients the infarct occurs unheralded with no prior cardiovascular events or record of risk factors. For such patients the psychological impact of the infarct can impair attempts at rehabilitation.

For all survivors, irrespective of ST segment elevation myocardial infarction (STEMI) or non-STEMI (NSTEMI), treatment is aimed at symptom control, risk reduction with the ever-increasing range of medical and interventional secondary prophylactic treatments, and appropriate lifestyle changes. Ideally many treatments will have been started in hospital and arrangements made to attend rehabilitation classes and a post-infarct clinic, where access to and compliance with therapies can be ascertained. Some medical treatments, such as beta-blockers and angiotensin-converting enzyme inhibitors, have both symptomatic and prognostic benefits.

The recommendations made here largely conform to the NICE clinical guideline 48, MI: Secondary prevention, issued May 2007.

Drugs for secondary prophylaxis

Antiplatelets and anticoagulants
- Aspirin 300 mg oral loading dose then 75 mg od indefinitely
  plus
- Clopidogrel 300 mg oral loading dose then 75 mg od for a minimum of 12 months.

Vitamin K antagonists
- Warfarin INR 2–3 IF neither aspirin nor clopidogrel are tolerated
- Warfarin INR 2–2.5 **plus** aspirin 75 mg old if clopidogrel not tolerated
- **note** Warfarin plus clopidogrel is not yet a tested combination
- more convenient alternatives to warfarin, such as antifactor Xa and antithrombins, are currently in clinical trials.

Beta-adrenoceptor blockers
A range of beta-blockers have been assessed when given very early in acute MI (AMI), initially in patients without left ventricular (LV) dysfunction, then in such patients whether symptomatic or not:
- Without LV dysfunction
  - Intravenous then oral atenolol or metoprolol, oral acebutalol, metoprolol, propranolol or timolol.
- With LV dysfunction
  - Oral bisoprolol, carvedilol or long-acting metoprolol. These are best started once fluid retention has been treated, the starting doses must be low and increments made gradually to the ceiling doses studied in clinical trials (see *British National Formulary* for details).

Calcium-channel blockers
Drugs in this class have markedly different effects on myocardial contractility, the cardiac conduction system, and vascular smooth muscle.

Verapamil more than diltiazem depresses myocardial contractility but both can cause sinus bradycardia or atrio-ventricular block. In acute myocardial infarction they can be given cautiously in place of beta-blockers provided there is no significant LV impairment.

Of the dihydropyridine calcium channel blockers none has a proven positive role in acute myocardial infarction, but amlodipine, felodipine, nicardipine, and nifedipine can be used as additional antianginal therapies. Flushing, headache, and ankle oedema may limit their use.

Renin–angiotensin–aldosterone inhibitors
Angiotensin-converting enzyme inhibitors
These can be started early after myocardial infarction, irrespective of LV function, at low dose, with gradual increments to trial targets. Hypotension may reduce the rate of dose increase, so review the dose/need for concomitant drugs such as diuretics and antianginals. Renal function should be monitored regularly but the level at which risk exceeds benefit is not established, for most trials imposed an upper creatinine level of 220 µmol/L. They should be avoided in patients with known renovascular disease. Treatment is long term. Major side-effects are dry cough, rash, hyperkalaemia, and angioedema.

Angiotensin II receptor antagonists
These should be considered as *alternatives* to ACE inhibitors when the latter are not tolerated, e.g. for dry cough. Fewer have been tested in acute myocardial infarction, especially in patients with preserved LV function, and trials have shown comparability with an ACE inhibitor. There is no indication for dual therapy for prophylaxis, although in severe worsening heart failure combination therapy is sometimes given. As well as monitoring renal function and serum potassium, they should be used cautiously in patients with aortic or mitral valve stenosis or hypertrophic cardiomyopathy.

Aldosterone antagonists
The selective aldosterone blocker eplerenone can be started ≥3–14 days post myocardial infarction to patients with LV ejection fraction <40% and clinical/radiological evidence of pulmonary oedema (not required for diabetic patients) and already receiving ACE inhibitors with or without beta-blockers, provided serum creatinine <200 µmol/L and K+ <5.0 mmols/L. Dose 25 mg od 4 weeks, then 50 mg od. If K+ >5.5 mmol/L reduce to the lower dose. In patients developing severe heart failure after 14 days post infarction (the upper limit of the eplerenone trial), spironolactone 25 mg od can be given instead with the same biochemical cautions.

Hypolipidaemic drugs
Statins
- Statins inhibit 3-hydroxy-3-methylglutaryl co-enzyme A therapy, reducing cholesterol synthesis. The aim is to achieve a total cholesterol <4 mmol/L or low-density lipoprotein (LDL) <2 mmol/L. They can be started early in high dose, e.g. atorvastatin 80 mg od, simvastatin 40 mg od and continued indefinitely.

- Myalgia may necessitate a reduction in dose, but rhabdomyolysis occurs rarely (1/100 000 treatment years).
- Liver transaminases may increase ×3 but should not in themselves lead to discontinuation of therapy.

Ezetimibe, fibrates, niacin
- Little evidence in the acute infarct period.
- Bezafibrate or gemfibrazil can be offered to patients intolerant of statins or if hypertriglyceridaemia persists. Combination treatment increases the risk of muscle toxicity, especially with gemfibrazil, which should not be coadministered with a statin.
- Ezetimibe 10 mg old reduces the intestinal absorption of cholesterol and can be used as an adjunct to statin treatment.
- Nicotinic acid derivatives should be *avoided* in the acute infarct period but can be added to, or given as, an alternative to a statin. Side-effects are common and likely to limit their use.

Omega-3-acid ethylesters and omega-3-marine triglycerides
These are not indicated acutely, but can be added to a statin when significant hypertriglyceridaemia persists. Their benefit for secondary cardiovascular prophylaxis is controversial.

Lifestyle modifications
All patients should be enrolled in a post-discharge rehabilitation programme where adherence to secondary prophylactic medication and lifestyle advice can be assessed. In addition, patient-specific issues can be raised and specialist referral arranged. Gentle exercise not only improves confidence and morale but may encourage some patients to include it as part of their usual routine thereafter. Rehabilitation also forges new friendships and increases membership of patient support groups.

Although the prophylactic value of some aspects of rehabilitation and lifestyle changes remain uncertain, they have laudable goals that may have benefits outwith cardiovascular protection.

Smoking cessation
Not only reduces the risk of further heart attacks and worsening angina, but also benefits peripheral and cerebrovascular circulations. There is also a reduced risk of several cancers. Sustained cessation, however, is achieved in a minority of patients.
- Advice regarding locally available behavioural support groups.
- Nicotine replacement therapy is available as patches, gums, lozenges, sublingual and nasal sprays, and as an inhalation. It should be offered only to those who agree to quit smoking, the dose and duration of therapy depending on the prior level of smoking and the likelihood of a relapse. Nicotine replacement therapy should not start in the acute phase of myocardial infarction.
- Bupropion hydrochloride: possibly works via central neurotransmitters. It is contraindicated in patients having seizures, eating disorders, a CNS tumour, or having symptoms of alcohol or benzodiazepine withdrawal. Usually started 1–2 weeks before an agreed quit date, then up to 7–9 weeks afterwards.
- Varenicline: is a selective nicotine receptor partial agonist but may induce depression and suicidal thoughts. Begin 1–2 weeks before agreed quit date, then up to 12 weeks thereafter.

Exercise
Three or more *aerobic* exercise sessions per week lasting 20–30 minutes and sufficient to keep heart rate within age-predicted limits (brisk walking, swimming, aquarobics, rowing simulators, cycling, jogging).

Diet
- The inclusion of more wholemeal bread, fruit, vegetables, and oily fish in the diet, with a reduction in meat, butter, and cheese.
- Extra vitamins are *not* required.
- Alcohol: although 'moderate' levels of alcohol may be cardioprotective, levels in excess of current guidelines (14 units/week for women and 21 for men) start to increase the risk of hepatotoxicity and some cancers. The units should be consumed evenly throughout the week and not in a few binge sessions.

Obesity
- Dietary alterations and participation in regular exercise groups should encourage weight loss, especially if combined with a reduced calorie diet. Weight loss might also reduce the incidence of diabetes or improve its control, increase mobility, and self-esteem.
- Anti-obesity drugs: Should only be considered for patients with a body mass index ≥ 30 kg/m^2 and as part of an agreed dietary plan. Choice is limited.
  - Orlistat is a lipase inhibitor that reduces the absorption of dietary fat. It may also reduce the absorption of fat-soluble vitamins.
  - Sibutramine hydrochloride inhibits the reuptake of noradrenaline and serotonin in the central nervous system. It is contraindicated in patients with coronary artery disease.
  - Rimonabant has been withdrawn because of serious psychiatric adverse reactions.

Other risk factors
- Vigorous attention to control hypertension and diabetes.
- Consider further investigations if angina persists despite medical treatment.
- Consider dual chamber pacing (cardiac resynchronization therapy) for patients with left ventricular ejection fraction (LVEF) $\leq 35\%$ and either a QRS duration or ≥ 150 ms or 120–149 ms with ventricular dissymmetry on echocardiography, and are in NYHA class III–IV.
- Consider implantable cardioverter-defibrillator (ICD) to detect and cardiovert potentially lethal ventricular arrhythmias when
  - Myocardial infarction >4 weeks
  and either
  - LVEF $\leq 35\%$ and non-sustained VT
  - On a 24-hour ECG
  or
  - LVEF <30% and QRS duration ≥ 120 ms.

Summary
The treatment of the post-infarct patient is complex and formidable, with the potential for drug interactions or proven therapies being overlooked. Benefit is measured in single figures to several tens per 1000 patients treated, sometimes with a reduction in mortality or new non-fatal cardiovascular events. Patients require clear explanations of the different therapies being recommended and encouragement for compliance.

Percutaneous coronary intervention

Indications
The indications for percutaneous coronary intervention (PCI) are covered in the chapters on stable angina, acute coronary syndromes (ACS), and ST and non-ST elevation myocardial infarction (NSTEMI).

Preparation pre-procedure
Medication
- Regular medication should be taken on the day of the PCI, apart from anticoagulants and oral hypoglycaemics.
- Warfarin must be stopped for 3–5 days pre-PCI; international normalization ratio (INR) level should be <1.5 before arterial puncture. Patients with prosthetic valves should be admitted for IV heparin cover pre- and post procedure, maintaining an activated partial thromboplastin time (aPTT) of 1.5–2.5. Heparin should be discontinued 4 hours pre-procedure. Careful consideration must be made to the type of stent used, and the duration of dual antiplatelet therapy (DAPT) in those on warfarin.
- Metformin should be stopped for 48 hours pre- and post PCI. Diabetics should be preferentially done at the beginning of the list to minimize chances of hypoglycaemia.
- Aspirin and clopidogrel are covered in the chapter adjunctive therapies in PCI.

Contrast induced nephropathy
Contrast-induced nephropathy (CIN) is defined as either >25% increase in serum creatinine (SCr) or an absolute increase in SCr of 0.5 mg/dL post procedure. The risk of CIN varies from 2% to 30% in patients undergoing PCI, and it is associated with a significant increase in morbidity and mortality. Patients with (1) pre-existing renal impairment (eGFR<60 mL/min); (2) pre-existing diabetes; and (3) reduced intravascular volume are at high risk of CIN.

The incidence can be reduced through recognition of high-risk patients by routine use of eGFR coupled with appropriate periprocedural management. Some patients with raised SCr benefit from prophylactic haemodialysis.

Periprocedural management:
- Low-risk (eGFR >60 mL/1.73 m^2): Optimize hydration
- High risk (eGFR<60 mL/1.73 m^2):
  - Manage medication: withhold, if clinically appropriate, potentially nephrotoxic drugs, and administer N-acetylcysteine 600 mg orally bd for 2 days, starting the day before the PCI and continuing the day after.
  - Manage intravascular volume: avoid dehydration by administering 1 mL/kg/hour of isotonic (normal) saline 12 hours pre- and 12 hours post procedure or sodium bicarbonate 154 mEq/L at 3 mL/kg/hour starting 1 hour pre-procedure, and 1 mL/kg/hour for 6 hours post procedure.
  - Use minimal volumes of low or iso-osmolar contrast.
  - Post PCI obtain SCr after 48 hours, and consider withholding medication such as metformin and non-steroidal anti-inflammatory drugs (NSAIDs) until renal function returns to normal.
- Multislice CT scan.

Multislice computed tomography (MSCT) has a role in the assessment of a patient having PCI, particularly in those with complex lesions. In patients with bifurcations and left main stem lesions (LMS) it can identify the exact morphology and plaque burden within the lesion, helping with choice of equipment and stenting technique.

In chronic total occlusions (CTO) MSCT can identify those angiographic characteristics, such as a tapered stump without a side branch, that confer a high chance of procedural success with PCI. In addition, it can provide information on the 'missing segment' not seen on angiography, such as tortuosity, and calcification.

MSCT can readily identify calcified lesions, which are associated with an increased risk of procedural failure, and adverse clinical events. This prior knowledge is helpful when selecting equipment, and leads to a lower threshold for the use of adjunctive therapies such as rotational atherectomy (RA).

Access site
Usually dependent on operator preference, although certain patient factors such as bleeding risk, and peripheral vascular disease (PVD) may be decisive. Radial access is associated with significantly fewer bleeding complications than femoral access; however, there is an initial learning curve when longer procedural times have been noted. Catheter choice may be limited for complex cases, as only large radial arteries will accommodate 7F sheaths. However, sheathless guide catheters (GC) are available; a 7.5F sheathless GC has a smaller diameter than a standard 6F introducer sheath.

Equipment
The correct choice of equipment can be the difference between a successful procedure and a disastrous failure.

Sheath
- Size: must be compatible with guide catheter.
- Length: In patients with PVD, or tortuous peripheral vessels longer length sheaths are advisable if the radial route is not an option or not preferred. These improve guide catheter torque, facilitate delivery of equipment, and minimize complications such as peripheral vascula-ture dissections, or 'knotting' of the guide catheter.

Guiding catheter
A large variety is available, and choice should only be made after reviewing the diagnostic angiograms. The guide catheter must provide a suitable level of support to enable delivery of PCI equipment, and be appropriate for the patient's anatomy. Factors to consider are:
- Size:
  - 5F can be used subject to the availability of compatible coronary stents. Some complain of problems with visualization, but groin complications and ambulatory times are reduced.
  - 6F is the commonest used sheath, and enables delivery of the majority of PCI equipment.
  - 7F provides greater support and is preferable to enable adequate visualization when using RA or when dealing with lesions that may require kissing balloon dilatation, such as bifurcations. 7F is mandatory for kissing stent techniques.
- Catheter choice: dependent on operator preference and patient anatomy. Judkins and XB catheters are suitable for the majority of left coronary arteries.

Judkins, 3DRC or Amplatz catheters are suitable for most right coronary arteries (RCAs). The ART catheter is suited for the 'shepherd's crook' RCA.

- Side holes can be used in cases of ostial lesions, or where catheter engagement causes pressure damping and contrast hold up, which can exacerbate ischaemia. They cannot be used in conjunction with pressure wires, and may increase overall contrast load. Importantly, when using side-hole catheters careful attention must be paid to ECG changes, because the early pressure changes normally seen with ischaemia will be lost.

Improving guide catheter support

Several techniques can be employed to improve GC support to aid the deployment of stents:

- A large rigid GC well seated into the ostium of the target vessel, e.g. Amplatz catheter; however, this is associated with an increased risk of dissection.
- The use of an anchor balloon, which involves leaving a small inflated balloon in a side branch.
- Deeply intubating the GC into the target vessel which can be achieved by gently rotating and advancing the GC over the guidewire into the target vessel to a point just proximal to the lesion or past the area of tortuosity. An alternative is to use a specialized mother-child catheter where a 5F soft tipped catheter is inserted through a 6F GC to a point proximal to the lesion.

Choice of balloon

- Compliant balloons will experience an increasing diameter with increasing inflation pressure. They are routinely used for pre-dilatation, but can also be used to help provide support for guidewires. They are available in mono-rail or as over the wire (OTW) balloons.

Mono-rail balloons have a greater choice of size, and enable rapid exchange, resulting in lower radiation times.

OTW balloons are limited in size, but provide greater guidewire support. They have two ports, one for balloon inflation, and one central port which not only allow contrast to be injected into the coronary artery but also facilitate guidewire exchange, without the loss of distal wire position which is useful when dealing with a CTO.

- Non-compliant balloons maintain a constant diameter despite increasing pressure, and are primarily used for post dilatation. They can be used pre-stenting in lesions that will not dilate adequately with compliant balloons, i.e. calcified lesions.
- Cutting balloons score the plaque in a longitudinally fashion causing controlled plaque disruption resulting in reduced vessel injury. They are indicated for in-stent restenosis (ISR), bifurcation lesions, ostial lesions, small vessels, and resistant lesions. Low inflation pressures are required (4–8 atm) for lesion dilatation, leading to a decreased risk of ISR, although this has not been shown in treatment of simple lesions. The device size should approximate a 1.1:1 ratio of the diameter of the vessel proximal and distal to the stenosis.
- Drug eluting balloons consists of a conventional coronary angioplasty balloon, coated with an antiproliferative drug, usually paclitaxel, that is immediately released on balloon inflation. Studies in patients with ISR have shown these balloons have lower rates of repeat target lesion revascularization (TLR) than paclitaxel eluting stents (Unverdorben 2008).

Choice of stent

The benefits of reduced restenosis rates with drug eluting stents (DES) offset their increased risk of very late (>1 year) stent thrombosis compared with bare metal stents (BMS). Ultimately the overall net clinical benefit favours the use of DES, but some important factors to consider when choosing a stent are:

- Patient's ability to take DAPT. The early cessation of DAPT has consistently been shown to be the greatest risk factor for stent thrombosis. Consider BMS in those with planned surgery, or with a history of bleeding problems or poor compliance.
- Use of warfarin and indication. The use of warfarin and DAPT exposes patients to a higher risk of bleeding. In some cases warfarin can be temporarily stopped if it is a low-risk indication, such as those in atrial fibrillation and a low $CHADS_2$ score allowing 12 months of DAPT. If warfarin is compulsory a balanced decision must be taken following discussion with the patient.
- Lesion length and vessel diameter. The NICE guidelines state that DES are only currently indicated for those lesions >15 mm in length, or vessels <3 mm in diameter (provided the cost difference between DES and BMS <£300) (NICE 2008).
- Indication for PCI. Evidence is continuously emerging demonstrating the safety of DES in patients having PCI for a variety of indications such as ACS, STEMI, and saphenous vein graft (SVG) interventions. Indication is no longer a deciding factor on its own.
- Covered stent: see Major complications, p. 204.

Guidewire selection

Guidewires are made of different physical components, and this variation facilitates their use in different situations. Most operators will use their 'work-horse' wire for the majority for their cases; however, in the remaining, lesion, and vessel characteristics influence the choice. Factors to consider are:

- Length: standard ~175–200 cm; exchange wires of 300 cm are available to aid removal of OTW balloons or microcatheters. A docking wire can extend a standard wire to enable it to be used as an exchange wire; be aware that the 'dock' is an area where the wires are easily kinked.
- Tip load represents the force needed to bend the wire when exerted on a straight guidewire tip, 1 cm from the tip. The greater the load the greater the ability of the wire to penetrate through hard substances such as the calcified proximal cap of a CTO; however, the stiffer tip also increases the chances of perforation.
- Degree of support is an important property of the wire which is a measure of steerability and trackability. Steerability is the ability to deliver the tip of the guidewire to the desired position in the vessel. Trackability is the ability of the wire to follow the tip without kinking.
- Supportive wires (e.g. Mailman) are able to straighten out vessels, which may improve the ability to deliver stents in tortuous vessels, but in turn they can cause pleating artefacts on angiography. It is not uncommon however for supportive wires to straighten vessels out *too* much, making deployment more arduous, and in these situations a soft or medium support wire (e.g. Choice floppy, balance middle weight) may be useful on

its own. Soft and medium-support wires are typical used as workhorse wires, providing suitable support to deploy stents in the all but the most tortuous vessels. In challenging anatomy a supportive wire can be passed alongside the less supportive wire, to act as a 'buddy,' aiding the deployment of balloons and stents.

- Coating: wires with a hydrophilic coating attract water. When they are dry, they are non-slippery; however, once wet they mimic a gel. This reduces friction and improves trackability and crossibility. Importantly tactile feedback decreases as the lubricity of the wire tip increases; hence risk of perforation is greatest with hydrophilic wires.

Adjunctive devices

Rotational atherectomy (RA) relies on the principle of differential cutting selectively ablating hard lesions, especially those that are calcified, with little destruction of the surrounding soft tissue. RA improves rates of successful balloon dilatation, stent delivery, and facilitates complete stent expansion. At present there is no evidence that RA has any benefit in terms of reduced mortality, TLR, and restenosis in either native or restenotic lesions.

- Indications: severely calcified lesions, instent restenosis.
- Contraindications: occlusions in which the wire cannot cross the lesion, presence of thrombus, severe left ventricular (LV) dysfunction and PCI in the last remaining vessel.
- Prophylactic temporary pacing wire insertion is essential during RA of dominant RCA or circumflex artery lesions as heart block is common.
- Burrs come in seven sizes from 1.25 mm (needs ≥6F GC) to 2.5 mm (needs ≥9F GC) and size should not exceed a burr–artery diameter ratio of 0.70.
- Wire: 0.09" stainless steel rota wire is not easy to torque; consider using a floppy wire first and then exchanging for a rota wire using an OTW balloon. The distal wire tip should be left free in a large branch to reduce risk of distal vessel trauma.
- Complications include intimal dissection, spasm, perforation, no-reflow, acute vessel closure, and NSTEMI.

Fractional flow reserve

Fractional flow reserve (FFR) is defined as the ratio of maximum flow in the presence of a stenosis to normal maximum flow. It is a well-validated method of assessing the significance of a coronary lesion. An FFR <0.75 (before balloon angioplasty), <0.90 (after balloon angioplasty), and <0.96 (after stenting) is indicative of haemodynamic significance.

The FAME (Tonino et al. 2009) study showed 35% of angiographic lesions (>50% stenosis) were haemodynamically insignificant, and an FFR-guided PCI was associated with reduced major adverse cardiovascular events (MACE), contrast use, and cost compared to angiographic guided PCI.

Equipment: the GC should not have side holes or be too large for the vessel.

Adenosine is the usual agent for inducing maximum hyperaemia. It is safe and well tolerated, particularly if patients are warned of side-effects beforehand. It is preferably administered IV through a femoral sheath, however in those where there is a concern regarding asthma it can be used intracoronary (IC).

- IV dose 140 μg/kg/min; peak effect <1 minute.
  - Effects wear off 1 minute after stopping infusion.
  - Suitable for pullbacks and ostial lesions.
  - Infusion should be continued for 2 minutes unless not tolerated, or FFR reaches <0.75.
- IC initially give IC glyceryl trinitrate (GTN) to reduce spasm.
  - Bolus dose: 40 μg RCA, 60 μg left system.
  - Peak effect <10 s; duration of action <20 s.

Symptoms or a 10–20% fall in blood pressure (BP) or heart rate indicate that adenosine has been delivered.

Thrombectomy

Numerous different devices are available ranging from mechanical devices (e.g. Angiojet, Possis) to manual devices (e.g. Export catheter, Medtronic). Numerous underpowered studies have shown improvement in the surrogate markers of reperfusion, such as ST segment change and myocardial blush grade; but this has not resulted in improvements in MACE. A recent meta-analysis, which included the TAPAS trial, has shown that the use of manual thrombectomy devices in primary PCI reduces mortality (Bavry et al. 2008).

Embolic protection device

Several different embolic protection devices (EPDs) are available: the proximal occlusion device (e.g. Proxis, St. Jude Medical); the distal occlusive device (e.g. GuardWire, Medtronic) and the distal filter device (e.g. FilterWire Ex™, Boston Scientific). Evidence demonstrates the effectiveness of EPDs on the reduction of MACE in the management of SVG lesions, while a neutral effect has been shown from their use in primary PCI (Bavry et al. 2008).

Major complications

No reflow

No reflow is defined as the reduction of antegrade flow, despite a patent artery, and occurs because of obstruction to the coronary microvasculature due to distal embolization of atheromatous and thrombotic debris caused by balloon inflation or stent implantation. It is common, occurring in 1–5% of all PCIs, and 10–15% of primary PCIs. Among reperfused patients, those experiencing no-reflow are in a higher risk group. At follow-up they have reduced LV function and LV remodelling; and higher morbidity, and mortality. Major predictors of no-reflow on initial coronary angiography are higher plaque burden and thrombus, and TIMI grade 0 flow.

- Prevention: it is no longer sufficient to just open the infarct-related artery—attention must be paid to prevention of no-reflow. The reduction of embolic material by the use of antiplatelet agents; and the removal of thrombus and an extensive plaque burden by appropriate use of thrombectomy can be useful in prevention.
- There is no definitive treatment. A variety of agents can be tried, BP allowing: IC GTN, i.c. nitroprusside, IV adenosine, IV verapamil. Anticoagulation must be checked to ensure the ACT >200 s, and glycoprotein IIb/IIIa inhibitors (G2b/3a) should be given. Repeated contrast injections should be avoided as this exacerbates

ischaemia. An intra-aortic balloon pump can be helpful if no-reflow is poorly tolerated.

Dissection

Coronary dissections are usually the result of PCI, through either baro-trauma or GC dissection; however, they can also result from an aortic dissection extending into the coronary artery, or rarely they can occur spontaneously. The beneficial effects of angioplasty are the result of plaque fracture, intimal splitting, and controlled localized medial dissection. However, large uncontrolled dissection tears within the media or those extending through the adventia (resulting in vessel perforation) are associated with morbidity and mortality.

The use of coronary stents has dramatically reduced the incidence of acute vessel closure following coronary artery dissection. The risk of dissection is higher in lesions that are complex, calcified, long, eccentric, and in tortuous vessels.

Although Amplatz GC provide good support, they tend to deep seat in the ostium during engagement and this predisposes them to an increased risk of dissection, which can be either antegrade, and/or retrograde into the ascending aorta.

The principle in management is to seal the dissection flap with coronary stents. Initial care must be taken to ensure the guidewire is in the true lumen, and once this has been established prompt stenting is required. Antegrade flow within the vessel can propagate dissection tears distally, and therefore to prevent distal extension of the dissection, stenting should be distal to proximal.

Dissection in small vessels (<2 mm) may be managed medically with analgesia and antianginals. Cases where there is inability to re-enter the true lumen, and/or stent the vessel, and those involving an aortic dissection should be referred for emergency cardiac surgery.

Perforation and tamponade

Extension of a controlled or uncontrolled dissection through the adventia results in perforation, and it follows that the causes of perforations are similar to those of dissection. Notably the risk is increased with a balloon to artery ratio of >1.1:1; with devices that ablate or remove tissue; and with the high-pressure jets created by a pinhole balloon rupture. Major perforations at the site of angioplasty are clinically and angiographic obvious; however, care must be taken to avoid missing small distal vessel perforations due to guidewires.

- Initial management is prolonged balloon inflation (>10 min) at the site of the perforation; if balloon occlusion is not tolerated, a perfusion balloon should be used. This is usually sufficient to seal small perforations. If the above measures fail proximal and mid vessel perforations can be treated using polytetrafluoethylene or pericardial

covered stents. Distal vessel perforations which are not amenable to balloon tamponade or covered stents can be treated with micro-coils or gelofoam which obliterate the vascular lumen. Emergency coronary artery bypass graft (CABG) is indicated in cases where perforations cannot be sealed percutaneously.

- To minimize the risk of vessel thrombosis, the reversal of heparin using protamine sulphate should only be performed in cases of major perforation. G2b/3a should be discontinued immediately. Platelets are required to reverse abciximab, whilst the discontinuation of tirofiban and eptifibatide is sufficient due to their short half-life.
- Urgent echocardiography is required with immediate pericardiocentesis if tamponade is clinically evident. Echocardiography and close surveillance is mandatory for 12–24 hours post PCI in case a frank perforation develops from one that was previously sealed.

Vascular closure devices (VCD)

Vascular complications post PCI are associated with significant morbidity. To minimize these, numerous vascular closure devices (VCDs) are available all of which have demonstrated improved haemostasis, and decreased time to ambulation compared to manual compression. Suture-based devices (e.g. Starclose™ Abbott) that rely on primary closure of the puncture have the greatest learning curve and greatest risk of device or operator failure. Collagen-based devices (e.g. Angio-seal™, St. Jude) are technically easier to use and rely on secondary healing of the puncture site where the collagen plug initiates coagulation by activating platelets. Complications comprise device failure, infection, and thrombotic and thromboembolic events.

FAQs—Driving and flying

- When can I fly? Uncomplicated PCI <5 days. Individual discretion is required particularly if there has been a vascular access problem.
- When can I drive? No driving for a week post PCI (DVLA regulation).

References

Bavry AA, Kumbhani DJ, Bhatt DL. Role of adjunctive thrombectomy and embolic protection devices in acute myocardial infarction: a comprehensive meta-analysis of randomized trials. *Eur Heart J* 2008;**29**:2989–3001.

National Institute for Health and Clinical Excellence. Drug eluting stents for the treatment of coronary artery disease. (http://www.nice.org.uk/nicemedia/pdf/TA152Guidance.pdf 2008).

Tonino PA, De Bruyne B, Pijls NH, *et al.* Fractional flow reserve versus angiography for guiding percutaneous coronary intervention. *N Engl J Med* 2009;**360**:213–24.

Unverdorben M. *Paclitaxel-eluting PTCA-balloon catheter in coronary artery disease: II ISR trial.* 2007, TCT, Washington DC, USA.

Adjunctive medical therapy in percutaneous coronary interventions

Introduction

In essence, the purpose of adjunctive medical therapy in percutaneous coronary intervention (PCI) is prevention of thrombotic complications. Both antiplatelet agents and anticoagulant therapy should be given in the acute phase of the intervention (Table 5.19.1).

Nitroglycerine

Pretreatment with an intracoronary bolus of nitroglycerine (100 μg) is useful to unmask vasospasm, to assess the true vessel size, and to reduce the risk of vasospastic complications during the procedure.

Aspirin

Aspirin plays an important role for reducing ischaemic complications related to PCIs. If patients are not on aspirin or when there is doubt about medication compliance, a loading dose of 160–325 mg orally should be given more than 3 h prior to the intervention or 250–500 mg intravenously directly prior to the procedure.

Ticlopidine and clopidogrel

There is compelling evidence that for a reduction in the risk of acute and subacute stent thrombosis following PCI with stent implantation, the combination therapy of a

thienopyridine plus aspirin is superior to aspirin alone or aspirin plus an oral anticoagulant. Clopidogrel is at least as effective as ticlopidine. Compared with ticlopidine, clopidogrel has fewer side-effects and is better tolerated.

To ensure sufficient platelet inhibition, clopidogrel should be initiated at least 6 hours prior to the procedure with a loading dose of 300 mg, ideally administered the day before a planned PCI; 600 mg should be given if more rapid onset of action is required (ST segment elevation myocardial infarction (STEMI) undergoing primary PCI, non-ST-segment elevation acute coronary syndrome (NSTE-ACS) requiring urgent PCI). In STEMI patients ≤75 years and treated with thrombolytic agents, 300 mg should be given together with aspirin and an anticoagulant. In STEMI patients >75 years treated with thrombolysis, 75 mg of clopidogrel should be given (no loading dose).

After stenting, clopidrogrel should be continued for 4 weeks in case of a bare metal stent or for 6–12 months when a drug-eluting stent has been placed. In NSTE-ACS and STEMI patients a maintenance dose of 75 mg of clopidogrel for 1 year after PCI is recommended, irrespective of whether or not stenting of the culprit lesion was performed.

Glycoprotein IIb/IIIa inhibitors

Glycoprotein (GP) IIb/IIIa inhibitors are the most potent antiplatelet drugs that block the fibrinogen receptor. Two small molecules (eptifibatide and tirofiban) and one monoclonal antibody (abciximab) are available.

Whenever there is a higher than average risk of complications in stable coronary artery disease, GP IIb/IIIa inhibitors are beneficial as bail-out medication (e.g. acute vessel closure, visible thrombus, or no/slow-reflow phenomenon).

In high-risk NSTE-ACS patients (positive troponins, ST deviations, diabetes) early (upfront) treatment with eptifibatide or tirofiban (together with unfractionate heparin (UFH), a loading dose of clopidogrel and aspirin) has a small beneficial effect. The same treatment should be maintained during PCI. In high-risk NSTE-ACS not pretreated with a GP IIb/IIIa inhibitor and in STEMI patients undergoing primary PCI abciximab should be given during the procedure on top of UFH, aspirin, and a loading dose of clopidogrel.

Unfractionated heparin

UFH has been used as the standard anticoagulant for many years. UFH is given as an IV bolus either under activated clotting time (ACT) guidance (ACT in the range of 250–350 seconds or 200–250 seconds, if a GP IIb/IIIa receptor inhibitor is given) or in a weight-adjusted manner (usually 100 IU/kg or 50–60 IU/kg, if GP IIb/IIIa receptor inhibitor is given). Because of marked variability in UFH bioavailability, ACT-guided dosing is recommended. UFH should be stopped at the completion of the procedure.

Low-molecular-weight heparins

Switching from UFH to LMWH and vice versa should be avoided. In most cardiovascular studies the LMWH enoxaparin has been used. If enoxaparin has been administered prior to PCI (e.g. in NSTE-ACS patients), an additional intravenous dose of enoxaparin should be given if the last

Table 5.19.1 Doses of different antithrombotic agents in PCI

Oral antiplatelet therapy
Aspirin initial dose: 160–325 mg non-enteric formulation, followed by 75–100 mg daily
Clopidogrel 75 mg/day after a loading dose of 300 mg (600 mg when rapid onset of action is wanted)

Anticoagulants
UFH intravenous bolus 60–70 U/kg (maximum 5000 IU) followed by infusion of 12–15 IU/kg/hour (maximum 1000 U/hour) titrated to aPTT 1.5–2.5 times control
Enoxaparin 1 mg/kg subcutaneously every 12 hours. An additional intravenous dose of 0.3 mg/kg if last subcutaneous dose was >8 hours before. In patients >75 years: 0.75 mg/kg and in case of renal failure (creatinine clearance < 30 mL/min): 1 mg/kg every 24 hours
Bivalirudin intravenous bolus of 0.1 mg/kg and infusion of 0.25 mg/kg/hour. Additional intravenous bolus of 0.5 mg/kg and infusion increased to 1.75 mg/kg/hour before PCI

GP IIb/IIIa inhibition
Abciximab 0.25 mg/kg intravenous bolus followed by infusion of 0.125 μg/min (maximum 10 μg/min) for 12–24 hours
Eptifibatide 180 μg/kg intravenous bolus (second bolus after 10 min for PCI) followed by infusion of 2.0 μg/kg/min for 72–96 hours. If renal failure (creatinine clearance <50 mL/min): infusion at 1.0 μg/kg/min
Tirofiban 0.4 μg/kg/min intravenously for 30 min followed by infusion of 0.10 μg/kg/min for 48–96 hours. A high-dose regimen (bolus 25 μg/kg + 0.15 μg/kg/min infusion for 18 hours) was proven to be effective and save in acute coronary syndrome patients

subcutaneous dose was given more than 8 hours before the PCI procedure. There are no data currently available on the use of LMWH for primary PCI.

Bivalirudin

Bivalirudin is an intravenous, reversible, direct thrombin inhibitor. Both in NSTE-ACS and in STEMI patients bivalirudin (with provisional GP IIb/IIIa antagonists) was associated with fewer bleeding complications than UFH and GP IIb/IIIa antagonists. Also in stable patients, bivalirudin was associated with less bleeding.

Further reading

Bassand JP, Hamm CW, Ardissino D, et al. Task Force for Diagnosis and Treatment of Non-ST-Segment Elevation Acute Coronary Syndromes of European Society of Cardiology. Guidelines for the diagnosis and treatment of non-ST-segment elevation acute coronary syndromes. *Eur Heart J* 2007;**28**:1598–660.

De Luca G, Suryapranata H, Stone GW, et al. Abciximab as adjunctive therapy to reperfusion in acute ST-segment elevation myocardial infarction: a meta-analysis of randomized trials. *JAMA* 2005;**293**:1759–65.

Ferguson JJ, Califf RM, Antman EM, et al. Enoxaparin vs unfractionated heparin in high-risk patients with non-ST-segment elevation acute coronary syndromes managed with an intended early invasive strategy: primary results of the SYNERGY randomized trial. *JAMA* 2004;**292**:45–54.

Giugliano RP, White JA, Bode C, et al. Early versus delayed, provisional eptifibatide in acute coronary syndromes. *N Engl J Med* 2009;**360**:2176–90.

Lincoff AM, Bittl JA, Harrington RA, et al. Bivalirudin and provisional glycoprotein IIb/IIIa blockade compared with heparin and planned glycoprotein IIb/IIIa blockade during percutaneous coronary intervention: REPLACE–2 randomized trial. *JAMA* 2003;**289**:853–63.

Silber S, Albertsson P, Avilés FF, et al. Guidelines for percutaneous coronary interventions. The Task Force for Percutaneous Coronary Interventions of the European Society of Cardiology. *Eur Heart J* 2005;**26**:804–47.

Stone GW, McLaurin BT, Cox DA, et al. Bivalirudin for patients with acute coronary syndromes. *N Engl J Med* 2006; **355**:2203–16.

Stone GW, Witzenbichler B, Guagliumi G et al. Bivalirudin during primary PCI in acute myocardial infarction. *N Engl J Med* 2008;**358**:2218–30.

Van de Werf F, Bax J, Betriu A et al. Management of acute myocardial infarction in patients presenting with persistent ST-segment elevation: the Task Force on the Management of ST-Segment Elevation Acute Myocardial Infarction of the European Society of Cardiology. *Eur Heart J* 2008;**29**:2909–45.

Van't Hof AW, Ten Berg J, Heestermans T, et al. Prehospital initiation of tirofiban in patients with ST-elevation myocardial infarction undergoing primary angioplasty (On-TIME 2): a multicentre, double-blind, randomised controlled trial. *Lancet* 2008;**372**:537–46.

Coronary artery bypass surgery

The principle of coronary artery bypass graft (CABG) surgery is to simply restore myocardial blood supply through bypassing stenosed or occluded sections of coronary arteries using biological conduit. Conventionally, surgery is performed through a midline sternal incision. Cardiopulmonary bypass is used to support the circulation during surgery, during which the heart is temporarily arrested using hyperkalaemic cardioplegia.

Principal features of CABG

- CABG is the most intensively studied surgical procedure ever, with over 20 years of follow-up data
- CABG is highly effective in relieving the symptoms of coronary heart disease
- CABG improves life expectancy in certain anatomical subsets, and this benefit is increased in the presence of impaired left ventricular (LV) function
- Despite an ageing surgical population with increasing co-morbidity, CABG is a safe procedure with hospital mortality of 1–2%
- CABG has been demonstrated to be extremely cost effective in the long term.

The evidence base for coronary artery surgery

CABG is carried out either to relieve symptoms or improve prognosis. It has been compared with medical therapy in three large randomized trials; the Coronary Artery Surgery Study (CASS), the Veterans Administration Study, and the European Coronary Surgery Study.

The studies and their registries have undergone a process of continuing meta-analysis, and have defined the indications for coronary surgery for over 20 years. According to ACC/AHA (2004) guidelines, Class I evidence for prognostic and symptomatic effectiveness of CABG exists as follows;

A. Elective surgery

- Significant left main stenosis (LMS)
- 2VD (vessel damage) with significant proximal left anterior descending (LAD) and circumflex stenoses
- 3VD with impaired LV function.

B. Urgent surgery

- Unstable angina/NSTEMI (non-ST segment elevation myocardial infarction) and patient falls into Group A above
- Failed PTCA (percutaneous transluminal coronary angioplasty) with ongoing ischaemia
- Life-threatening ventricular arrhythmia

In addition there are situations in which CABG would not normally be recommended.

C. Contraindications to surgery

- Asymptomatic patients, unless there is threatening anatomy with a high risk of myocardial infarction (MI) or death.

- Chronic stable angina in patients with 1VD or 2VD not involving the LAD and controlled by medical therapy, as there is no proven prognostic benefit for surgery.
- Unstable angina in patients not in Group A should be treated non-surgically at first.
- Acute MI. There is a high operative risk in the early phase after MI, and no prognostic benefit in the long term.
- Poor LV. CABG should not be used to treat poor LV function without evidence of reversible ischaemia and viable myocardium.
- Elderly patients. Surgery for relief of symptoms and quality of life should always be considered, but extrapolation of the study survival data to elderly patients is difficult.
- Poor-quality target vessels. This involves a subjective judgement, and as such is a surgical decision. Often, subcomplete revascularization will bring some improvement in symptoms, which properly consented patients will appreciate.

The situation has more recently been confused by changes in the conduct of CABG as well as the controversy surrounding the relative merits of CABG and PCI.

Choice of conduit for coronary artery surgery

Although the long saphenous vein has long been the mainstay conduit for CABG, it is susceptible to endothelial damage and does present problems with long-term graft patency. In 1986 a landmark paper from the Cleveland Clinic emphasized the importance of the internal mammary artery graft on patency and patient survival. Almost immediately left internal mammary artery (LIMA) to LAD became the standard for CABG, with vein being used for the remaining grafts. Before long, however, enthusiasts extrapolated the Cleveland Clinic data to other arterial conduits on the basis that 'if one arterial graft is good than two (or more) must be better'.

- The long saphenous vein is the mainstay conduit for CABG, but is susceptible to endothelial damage and occlusion.
- Reported vein graft failure rates of 50% at 10 years pre-date the routine usage of aspirin and statins and patency rates in the current era are much higher.
- Higher patency rates for the LIMA graft are well established and LIMA graft to the LAD is the gold standard for surgical revascularization.
- Total arterial revascularization (using a wide range of alternative arterial conduits) has been shown in some studies to produce additional long-term benefit, but is not widespread practice.
- Patency of all grafts including arterial grafts is dependent on the grafted vessel and the degree of competitive flow.
- A combination of LIMA and vein grafts remains a conventional choice for many surgeons.

- The saphenous vein remains a key conduit and determination of its availability is an essential part of preoperative assessment.

Off-pump and minimally invasive coronary artery surgery

In an effort to eliminate the harmful effects of bypass, some surgeons have adopted off-pump, beating heart surgery (OPCAB). Progress in this venture was greatly aided by improvements in heart stabilization devices, allowing construction of coronary anastamoses in a relatively still and bloodless field. Despite these technical aids, beating heart surgery is, above all, a matter of personal preference.

- Cardiopulmonary bypass (CPB) and hypothermic cardioplegic arrest provide a still bloodless operating field, ideal for fine anastamotic work.
- CPB has deleterious systemic effects, and the current aged surgical population are increasingly susceptible to these.
- CABG may be performed by experienced surgeons on a beating heart without CPB (so-called off pump or OPCAB surgery) with equivalent outcomes to conventional surgery.
- Randomized trials and meta-analyses have been unable to detect any significant improvement in mortality, post operative MI, stroke, or other major morbidity for off-pump surgery. However, there are some groups of patients for whom OPCAB may be preferable.
- Minimal access, OPCAB, and robotic surgery are all dependent on, and driven by advances in technology.

Surgery or PCI?

CABG has been the gold standard for the treatment of patients with severe multivessel or left main stem coronary artery disease whereas PCI has generally been used to treat patients with one- or two-vessel disease. Restenosis following PCI has long been a problem, but drug-eluting stents claim to reduce the occurrence of this complication and there has been a massive growth in PCI, including in patients with more severe forms of the disease. PCI is now performed at least three times as frequently as CABG.

The expansion in PCI rates raises three questions:

1 Is the expansion in activity evidence based?

2 Is PCI cost-effective compared with CABG?

3 Are patients given the opportunity to make informed decisions about the options for treatment?

This is a controversial area but the following is known:

- In appropriately chosen patients PCI is an extremely valuable and effective treatment.
- Trials comparing PCI with surgery were flawed in design, inaccurately reported and led to inappropriate management of patients with severe coronary artery disease.
- PCI continues to have high reintervention rates, is poor value, and according to some reports is associated with an increased risk of death.

- Latest data from the SYNTAX study comparing PCI with CABG in severe CAD shows rates of major adverse cardiac or cerebrovascular events at 12 months were 17.8% in the PCI group and 12.4% in the CABG group. Death rates were similar in both groups.
- 1 year after treatment for severe coronary artery disease, quality of life is significantly better in patients having CABG compared than in PCI.
- It is recommended that all patients with multivessel or left main stem coronary artery disease be discussed at a multidisciplinary team meeting and be given the opportunity to arrive at a fully informed decision about treatment.

Carotid disease

- The risk of stroke during CABG is 1–2%, and increases with age rising to 5–10% in patients over 80.
- The single most important intervention to reduce the risk of intraoperative stroke is the detection and management of carotid disease.
- Asymptomatic patients with mild disease do not benefit from carotid surgery.
- Symptomatic patients with severe disease should undergo carotid endarterectomy, either as a staged procedure or combined with CABG.
- Asymptomatic patients with severe disease should be considered for prophylactic carotid surgery, although this may be controversial.

Risk stratification models and analysis of surgical outcomes

Coronary artery bypass surgery has been just about the most intensively studied interventional therapy ever. High volumes and easily definable outcomes make an ideal substrate for outcome measurement, but crude mortality data do not paint the whole picture and adjustments need to be made for case mix. Risk stratification systems have been developed to account for relevant risk factors and provide a numeric score that can be used to predict the risk of death. The two best known are the Parsonnet and the Euroscore, which are both simple additive systems. The additive Euroscore was derived from a large pan-European database, is seen as an improvement on Parsonnet, and gives a score that fairly accurately equals the predicted risk, especially in low- to medium-risk patients. The additive Euroscore is shown in Table 5.20.1, and can be seen to be easy to use. It is claimed that a computer modelled Logistic Euroscore provides marginally greater accuracy, but in doing so it loses much of the appealing simplicity of the additive model. The mortality data are now used to monitor an individual surgeons' performance, using either a Cumulative Summation (CUSUM) plot or a Variable Life Adjusted Display (VLAD).

- The Euroscore is a simple, additive, and accurate risk stratification model, providing patients and carers with a reasonable estimate of the operative risk

Table 5.20.1 The additive Euroscore

Factor		Definition	Score
Patient related factors	Age	Per 5 years or part thereof over 60	1
	Gender	Female	1
	COPD	Long term use of bronchodilators or steroids for lung disease	1
	Extracardiac arteriopathy	Any one or more of claudication, carotid occlusion or >50% stenosis, previous or planned surgery on the abdominal aorta, limb arteries or carotid	2
	Neurological dysfunction	Disease severely affecting ambulation or day to day living	2
	Previous cardiac surgery	Previous surgery requiring opening of the pericardium	3
	Serum creatinine	>200 μmol/L pre-op	2
	Endocarditis	Still under antibiotic therapy foe endocarditis at the time of surgery	3
	Critical preoperative state	Ventilation before arrival in anaesthetic room, preoperative inotropic support, intraortic balloon counterpulsation or preoperative acute renal failure with oliguria <10 mL/hour	3
Cardiac factors	Unstable angina	Angina requiring IV nitrates until arrival in the operating room	2
	LV dysfunction	Moderate (EF 30–50%)	1
		Poor <30%	3
	Recent MI	<90 days	2
	Pulmonary hypertension	Systolic PA pressure >60 mmHg	2
Operative factors	Emergency	Carried out on referral before the beginning of the next working day	2
	Other than isolated CABG	Major cardiac operation other than or in addition to CABG	2
	Surgery on the thoracic aorta	Ascending or descending aorta	3
	Post infarct VSD		4

- CUSUM and VLAD plots can be used to track unit or individual surgeon outcomes over time, and are useful performance indicators
- Monitoring of performance, as part of an integrated package of quality improvement, leads to improved surgical outcomes
- Individual surgeons profile and outcomes are publicly available, enhancing the patient's ability to make informed treatment decisions.

Further reading

Barnett HJM. Carotid endarterectomy. *Lancet*, 2004;**363**:1486.

Chambers BR, Donnan GA. Carotid endarterectomy for asymptomatic carotid stenosis. *Cochrane Database Syst Rev* 2005;(4):CD001923.

Chikwe J, Beddow E, Glenville B. *Cardiothoracic surgery* Oxford University Press, 2006.

Eagle KA, Guyton RA, Davidoff, *et al.* ACC/AHA guidelines update for coronary artery bypass surgery. *Circulation* 2005 Apr **19**;111:2014.

Hill R, Bagust A, Bakhai A, *et al.* Coronary stents: a rapid systematic review and economic evaluation. *Health Technol Assess* 2003;**8**:35.

Keogh BE, Kinsman R (on behalf of the Society of Cardiothoracic Surgeons of Great Britain and Ireland). The fifth national adult cardiac surgical database report: improving outcomes for patients. (The Blue Book) 2003 SCSGBI.

Kouchoukos NT, Blackstone EH, *et al. Cardiac surgery*, 3rd edn Churchill Livingstone. 2003.

Loop FD, Lytle BW, Cosgrove DM, *et al.* Influence of the internal mammary artery on 10 year survival and other cardiac events. *N Engl J Med* 1986; **314**:1.

Serruys *et al.* on behalf of the SYNTAX investigators. Percutaneous Coronary Intervention versus Coranary artery bypass grafting for severe coronary artery disease. *N Engl J Med* 2009;**360**:961–72.

Straja S, Widimsky P, Jirasek K, *et al.* Off-pump versus on-pump coronary surgery. Final results from a prospective randomized study PRAGUE-4. *Ann Thorac Surg* 2004;**77**:789.

Taggart DP. Thomas B. Ferguson Lecture. Coronary artery bypass grafting is still the best treatment for multivessel and left main disease, but patients need to know. *Ann Thorac Surg* 2006;**82**:1966.

Treasure T, Hunt J, Keogh B, Pagano D. *The evidence base for cardiothoracic surgery*. tfm Publishing, 2005.

Yusuf S, Zucker D, Peduzzi P, *et al.* effect of coronary artery bypass graft surgery on survival: overview of 10-year results from randomized trials by the Coronary Artery Bypass Graft Surgery Trialists Collaboration. *Lancet* 1994;**344**:563.

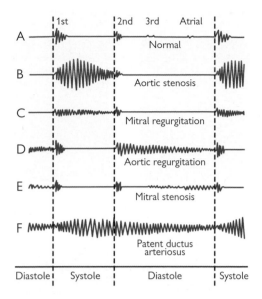

Plate 1 Murmurs. See also Fig. 1.1.1, p. 3.

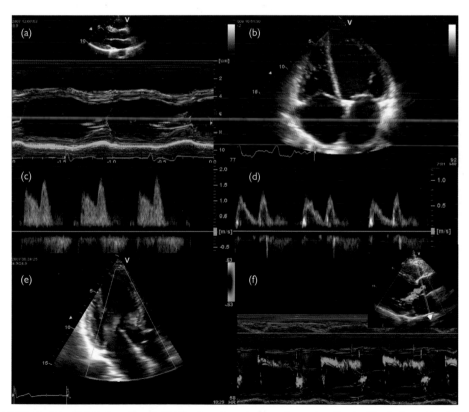

Plate 2 Echocardiographic techniques. M-mode (a), 2D echocardiography (b), continuous wave Doppler (c), pulsed wave Doppler (d), colour Doppler imaging (e) and colour Doppler M-mode (f). See also Fig. 1.4.1, p. 13.

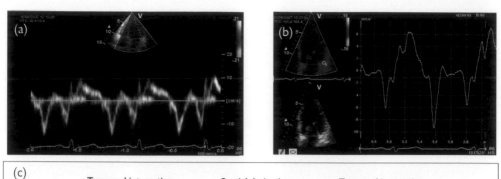

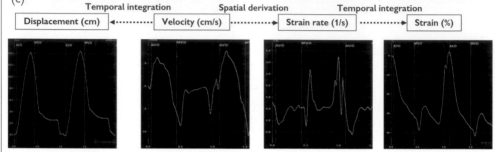

Plate 3 Tissue Doppler imaging (TDI). Pulsed wave tissue Doppler (a) and colour-coded TDI (b). (c) From colour-coded TDI, several parameters of left ventricular mechanics can be measured: velocity, displacement, strain rate and strain. See also Fig. 1.4.2, p. 14.

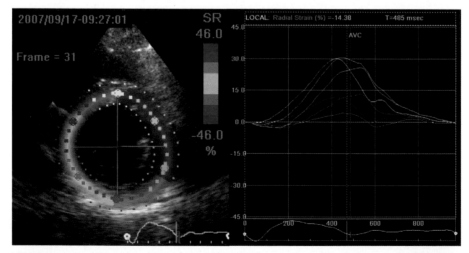

Plate 4 Two-dimensional speckle tracking imaging. By applying this echocardiographic technique to mid-ventricular parasternal short-axis view of the left ventricle, myocardial strain can be measured. The example illustrates the measurement of radial strain (myocardial thickening). See also Fig. 1.4.3, p. 15.

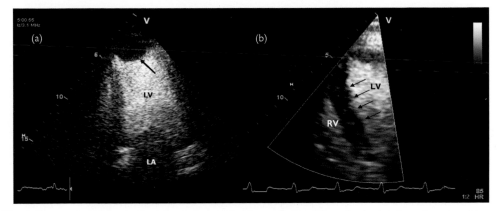

Plate 5 Contrast echocardiography. Current contrast agents allow for opacification of the cardiac chambers, improving endocardial border detection and identification of intracardiac mass (a, apical thrombus). By increasing the mechanical index, myocardial perfusion can be assessed (b, example of a patient with septal myocardial infarction; the arrows indicate the large perfusion defect). LA, left atrium; LV, left ventricle; RV, right ventricle. See also Fig. 1.4.4, p. 15.

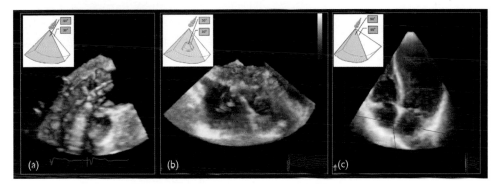

Plate 6 Real-time three-dimensional echocardiography acquisition modes: (a) real-time mode or narrow-angle mode, that displays the cardiac structures in real-time within a narrow sector (50° × 30°), (b) zoom mode, that displays a smaller, magnified pyramidal dataset (30° × 30°) with a high resolution; wide-angle mode (c) includes a large cardiac volume in a pyramidal data set of 90° × 90°. (Adapted with permission from Hung J et al. J Am Soc Echocardiogr 2007). See also Fig. 1.4.5, p. 16.

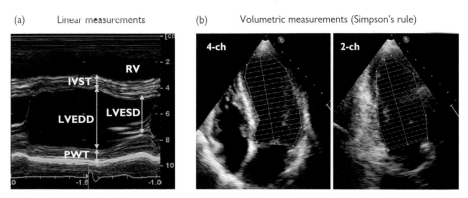

Plate 7 Left ventricular dimensions. Linear measurements of the left ventricle are usually obtained from long-axis parasternal M-mode recordings (a). Biplane Simpson's rule is the preferred method to measure left ventricular volumes and ejection fraction (b): the endocardial border of the left ventricle is traced on the apical four- and two-chamber views at the end diastolic and end-systolic frames. IVST, interventricular septum thickness; LVEDD, left ventricular end-diastolic diameter; LVESD, left ventricular end-systolic diameter; PWT, posterior wall thickness; RV, right ventricle. See also Fig. 1.4.6, p. 16.

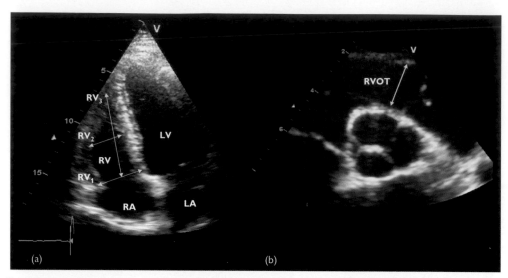

Plate 8 Right ventricular dimensions. Linear dimensions of the right ventricle are measured at the apical four-chamber view (a), including the basal (RV1), mid-ventricular (RV2), and longitudinal (RV3) diameters. From parasternal short-axis view at the level of the aortic valve, the diameter of the right ventricular outflow tract can be measured (b). LA, left atrium; LV, left ventricle; RA, right atrium; RV, right ventricle; RVOT, right ventricular outflow tract. See also Fig. 1.4.7, p. 18.

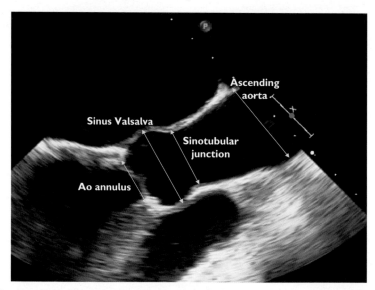

Plate 9 Aortic dimensions. Linear dimensions of the aortic root includes the diameters of the aortic annulus, sinus of Valsalva, sinotubular junction, and ascending aorta. See also Fig. 1.4.8, p. 19.

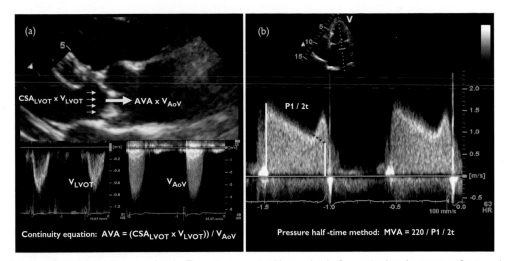

Plate 10 Estimation of the effective valvular area. The continuity equation (a) states that the flow passing through a stenotic orifice is equal to the flow proximal to the stenosis. Flow is equal to the product of velocity and cross-sectional area (CSA). Therefore, at a known CSA of the LV outflow tract (LVOT) and flow velocity at that location (by pulsed wave Doppler) and velocity through the aortic valve (continuous wave Doppler), aortic valve area can be obtained. To evaluate mitral stenosis, pressure half-time method (b) yields accurate estimations of the mitral valve area (MVA). The formula expresses the time needed to reduce by 30% the peak stenotic velocity. See also Fig. 1.4.9, p. 19.

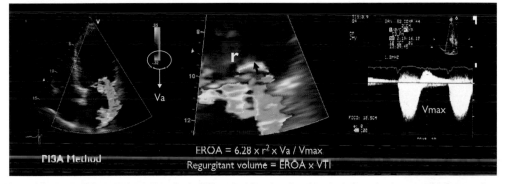

Plate 11 Estimation of the regurgitant volume by the PISA method. By colour Doppler echocardiography, the regurgitant flow is evaluated. The Nyquist limit is adjusted to clearly visualize the different velocity hemispheric surfaces that the flow forms when converges towards the regurgitant orifice. The effective regurgitant orifice area (EROA) is calculated by the product of the area of the hemisphere and the aliasing velocity (Va), given by the Nyquist limit, and divided by the maximal velocity of the regurgitant flow (Vmax). The regurgitant volume can be then calculated as the product of the EROA and the velocity time integral of the regurgitant flow. See also Fig. 1.4.10, p. 20.

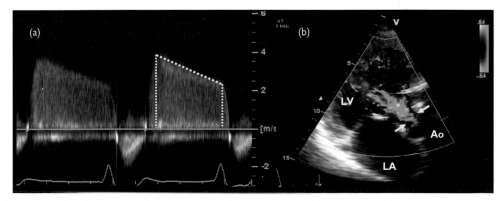

Plate 12 Evaluation of aortic regurgitation severity. The severity of the aortic regurgitation can be evaluated by measuring the pressure half-time of the continuous wave Doppler recordings of the regurgitant jet (a) or the measurement of the vena contracta at the level of the aortic valve on color-Doppler image (arrows, b). Ao, aorta; LA, left atrium; LV, left ventricle. See also Fig 1.4.11, p. 20.

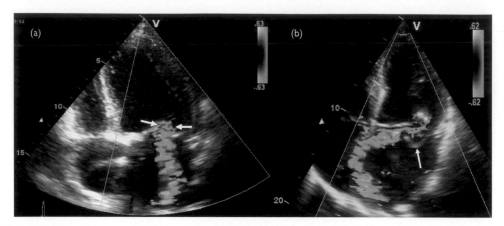

Plate 13 Evaluation of mitral valve regurgitation. Colour-Doppler imaging displays the direction of the regurgitant jet and yields clues to define the underlying mechanism of the lesion: in functional mitral valve regurgitation, left ventricular remodelling and dilatation of the mitral annulus result in tethering of the mitral leaflets and coaptation failure and a central regurgitant jet is usually observed (a). In contrast, mitral valve prolapse is characterized by anatomically abnormal mitral valve (i.e. prominent flail leaflets) showing eccentric regurgitant jets, impinging on the wall of the left atrium (coanda effect). (b) The white arrow shows the prolapse of the posterior mitral leaflet and, consequently, the regurgitant jet is directed towards the interatrial septum. See also Fig. 1.4.12, p. 21.

	Normal	Mild (Grade 1)	Moderate (Grade 2)	Severe (Grade 3)	Severe (Grade 4)
Pulsed wave mitral inflow					
E/A	0.9–1.5	<0.9	0.9–1.5	>2.0	>2.5
DT (ms)	160–240	>240	160–240	<160	<130
IVRT (ms)	70–90	>90	<90	<70	<70
Tissue Doppler imaging					
e'(cm/s)	≥10	<10	<8	<5	<5
E/e'	1–14	≥15	≥15	≥20	≥25
Mitral inflow propagation					
Vp (cm/s)	≥50	<50	<50	<50	<50
E/Vp	≤1.5	>1.5	>1.5	>1.5	>1.5
Pulmonary vein flow	S≥D	S>>D	S<D	S<<D	S<<D
Indexed LA volume (ml/m²)	22±6	>28	>28	>35	>40

E/A = the ratio of the early (E) and atrial (A) components of the mitral inflow spectral velocity recording; e', tissue Doppler early diastolic velocity; D, pulmonary vein diastolic forward flow velocity; DT, deceleration time; IVRT, isovolumetric relaxation time; LA, left atrial; S, pulmonary vein systolic forward velocity; Vp, mitral inflow propagation velocity.

Plate 14 Left ventricular diastolic function assessment by echocardiography (adapted with permission from Lester SJ *et al. J Am Coll Cardiol* 2008). See also Table 1.4.3, p. 22.

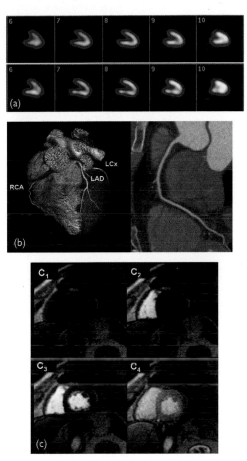

Plate 15 Examples of the different imaging modalities to detect coronary artery disease. (a) Myocardial perfusion imaging with SPECT; vertical long-axis reconstructions during adenosine stress (top) and rest (bottom) show normal myocardial perfusion. (b) Non-invasive coronary angiography with 320-slice MDCT: (left) a 3D volume-rendered reconstruction showing the left anterior descending coronary artery (LAD), left circumflex coronary artery (LCx) and right coronary artery (RCA) is provided; (right) a curved multiplanar reconstruction of the RCA showing a normal coronary artery without stenosis. (c) Myocardial perfusion imaging with magnetic resonance imaging: (1–4) consecutive images in the short-axis orientation showing the arrival of a bolus of gadolinium contrast in the myocardium. Normal homogeneous enhancement is visible in 4. See also Fig. 1.5.1, p. 25.

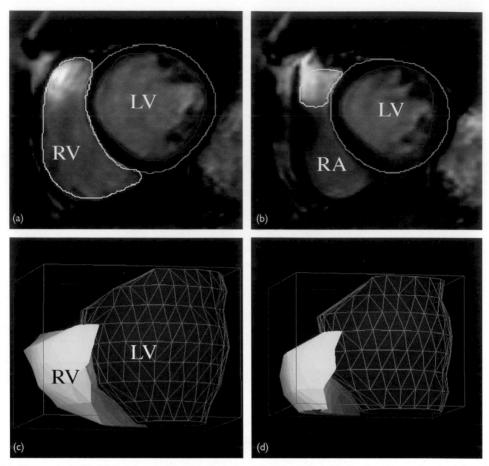

Plate 16 Example of LV function assessment with magnetic resonance imaging in a patient with dilated cardiomyopathy using dedicated software (MASS software package (Medis, Leiden, The Netherlands). (a, b) Short-axis mid-ventricular end-diastolic (ED) and end-systolic (ES) images after drawing of the epi- and endocardial LV contours. (c, d) are graphical 3D representations of the ED and ES volumes of the LV and the right ventricle (RV). See also Fig. 1.5.2, p. 26.

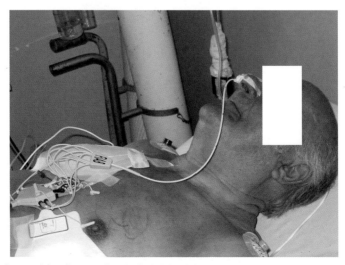

Plate 17 Oesophageal–precordial cardioversion. See also Fig. 3.12.3, p. 109.

Intra-aortic balloon pump

Indications
- Cardiogenic shock
- Haemodynamic compromise during and after cardiac catheterization and coronary intervention
- Refractory unstable angina
- High-risk percutaneous coronary intervention
- Post-coronary bypass operation to allow for weaning from cardiopulmonary bypass.

Principles
Intra-aortic balloon pump (IABP) consists of an inflatable 32- to 40-cc balloon connected to a console. It is triggered to inflate with helium immediately after aortic valve closure (i.e. early diastole) and deflate with opening or aortic valve (i.e. end of diastole). The rapid filling of the balloon during the early diastole augments the diastolic pressure and leads to an improvement in the coronary perfusion pressure, whereas deflation of the balloon at the end-diastole reduces effective aortic volume and decreases aortic systolic pressure, leading to lower left ventricular afterload (Mejia and Naidu 2008). The resultant effect is a decrease in myocardial oxygen consumption from lower systolic wall tension and an increase in the coronary flow velocity and perfusion pressure, thus improving the myocardial supply and demand balance. As a result, the cardiac output, mean pressure, cerebral perfusion, and renal perfusion will increase due to the improvement in the myocardial contractility as a result of the increased coronary blood flow and the reduced afterload. At the same time, the systemic vascular resistance will be reduced, resulting in an improvement in the peripheral perfusion.

Method
It is important to evaluate for any significant iliac or femoral arterial disease prior to insertion of IABP. It is contraindicated in patients with severe aortic insufficiency, abdominal or aortic aneurysm, and severe aorto-iliac disease. The balloon is normally inserted in the contralateral femoral artery to the interventional site. An access to the femoral artery is obtained by a Seldinger method with a long wire in a sheathless manner or via an 8- or 9-Fr sheath if there is a scar or thick layer of subcutaneous fat at the groin. Then, the balloon is de-aired with a large syringe attached to the one-way valve to ensure the lowest possible profile of the balloon during insertion. The balloon catheter is then advanced under fluoroscopy guidance over the stiff, 0.021-inch-long (0.533 mm) guidewire until the radiopaque tip of the balloon positioned just distal to left subclavian artery. The guidewire is then removed and the central lumen of the balloon catheter is flushed with normal saline and connected to the pressure transducer via its side hub at the proximal end. The end-hub of the proximal end is then connected to the console and the balloon catheter is purged with helium, and counter-pulsation can then be started. The timing and inflation/deflation or the balloon should be assessed and optimized to achieve peak haemodynamic support.

Complications
- Lower limb vascular complications including ischaemia, dissection, and thromboembolism
- Infection
- Bleeding
- Balloon leak
- Death.

At risk groups: women, peripheral vascular disease, older patients (Ferguson et al. 2001).

References
Ferguson JJ 3rd, Cohen M, Freedman RJ Jr, et al. The current practice of intra-aortic balloon counterpulsation: results from the Benchmark Registry. J Am Coll Cardiol 2001;**38**:1456–62.

Mejia VM, Naidu SS, Herrmann. Support device for high-risk percutaneous coronary intervention. In: Topol E (ed.) Textbook of interventional cardiology, 5th edn, Saunders Elsevier, 2008: pp 641–53.

Cardiac rehabilitation

Cardiac rehabilitation is the provision of comprehensive long-term services involving medical evaluation; prescriptive exercise; cardiac risk factor modification; and education, counselling, and behavioural interventions (Wenger 2008). The goal of such multifaceted and multidisciplinary services is to limit the adverse physical and psychosocial effects of cardiac illness, to reduce the risk of death or recurrence of the cardiac event, to control symptoms, and to enhance physical, psychosocial, and vocational status, thereby improving health-related quality of life. Patients with the following are likely to gain health benefits and should be referred for cardiac rehabilitation (Williams et al. 2006):

1 myocardial infarction
2 coronary artery bypass graft surgery
3 percutaneous coronary interventions
4 heart or heart/lung transplantation
5 stable angina
6 stable chronic heart failure
7 peripheral arterial disease with claudication
8 surgical procedures for heart valve repair/replacement.

Despite evidence attesting to the benefits of cardiac rehabilitation (Taylor et al. 2004; Clark et al. 2005), and guidance declaring its implementation as a key priority (NICE 2007), many patients likely to benefit are not offered it (Bethell et al. 2008).

Benefits of cardiac rehabilitation include (Taylor et al. 2004; Clark et al. 2005):

• Improvement in exercise tolerance
• Improvement in symptoms
• Improvement in lipid profile
• Improvement in psychosocial status
• Reduction in tobacco use
• Reduction in stress
• Reduction in mortality.

Cardiac rehabilitation and secondary prevention should be considered an integral part of cardiac care. Guidelines recommend that the process should start at the time of the cardiac event, continue through the hospital stay, and seamlessly to aftercare in the community (Thompson et al. 1997). The time course should be spanned by three essential elements, which are interlinked and may be overlapping:

1 the process of explanation and understanding
2 specific rehabilitation interventions including, where appropriate, secondary prevention, exercise training, and psychological support—all tailored to the needs of the individual patient and the setting of the specific medical diagnosis
3 the long-term process of readaptation and re-education.

Thus, a flexible, menu-driven approach, based on individual assessment of need is warranted, with particular attention being paid to under-represented groups such as women, elderly people, and ethnic groups (Beswick et al. 2004). Ideally, patients should be offered a choice of home- or hospital-based rehabilitation as the former does not produce inferior outcomes when compared with the latter (Dalal et al. 2007; Jolly et al. 2009).

Clinical approach

Every discharge summary after a cardiac event should confirm the diagnosis and include results of investigations, future management plans, and advice on secondary prevention (Skinner et al. 2007). An assessment of cardiovascular symptoms, the cardiovascular risk profile and the patient's perceived health status and/or health-related quality of life should be included (Wenger 2008).

All healthcare professionals caring for patients with cardiac conditions should (BACR 2007; Skinner et al. 2007):

• Offer cardiac rehabilitation to all patients
• Provide access regardless of the patient's age, sex, ethnicity, socioeconomic status, or co-morbidities
• Assess patient anxiety, depression, illness beliefs, misconceptions, and expectations
• Advise patients, where necessary, to take regular exercise, stop smoking, eat a healthy diet, consume safe amounts of alcohol, achieve and maintain a healthy weight, when to activities of daily living, including resuming sexual activity and return to work
• Take into account, where necessary, the patient's physical and psychological status, social support network and economic needs, and status as well as the nature of work and its environment
• Involve, where appropriate, partners, or carers
• Refer, where appropriate, patients who need specialist psychological (Linden et al. 2007) or psychiatric intervention
• Monitor referral to, enrolment in, and completion of cardiac rehabilitation
• Use validated outcome measures (Lewin et al. 2004)
• Maintain a database of all patients referred for cardiac rehabilitation
• Measure programme performance (AACVPR 2004).

Core components

Education

Use high-quality teaching methods and resources to enable patients (and partners/carers) to learn about their condition and management, including:

• Unhelpful beliefs and misconceptions
• Pathophysiology and symptoms
• Physical activity, smoking and diet
• Other risk factors: blood pressure, lipids, and glucose
• Psychological issues
• Vocational issues
• Sexual issues
• Pathophysiology and symptoms
• Pharmaceutical/surgical issues, including devices
• Cardiopulmonary resuscitation.

Lifestyle management

Address exercise and physical activity, healthy diet, and avoidance of obesity and smoking.

• Risk stratification and baseline assessment of physical activity status, and exercise/functional capacity.
• Venue choice: home, community centre, or hospital.
• Body mass index and waist circumference.
• Smoking status and nicotine dependence.

- Motivation for/access to smoking cessation counselling.
- Pharmacological support.

Psychosocial management

Assess psychological and social state using validated measures or interviews and, where necessary, intervene appropriately, including referral to specialist expertise for:
- Anxiety
- Depression
- Anger/hostility
- Social isolation
- Family distress
- Sexual dysfunction
- Substance abuse.

Enrolment, maintenance, and continuity

Cardiac rehabilitation is invariably concerned with the long-term management of a chronic disease and its success depends on the patient being able and willing to assume responsibility, and supported by adequate provision of services. Patient referral to, enrolment in and completion of cardiac rehabilitation has traditionally been largely confined to those with a myocardial infarction or who have undergone coronary artery bypass graft surgery. It is apparent that many who could benefit do not. For instance, factors associated with non-attendance include older age, being alone, lower income, greater deprivation, and denial of severity of illness. Barriers to participation include weak communication between healthcare service sectors, and confused roles and identities of staff. Physician endorsement and involvement enhances enrolment.

To enhance participation, attention should be given to social characteristics, individual patient needs, and preferences and location and availability of cardiac rehabilitation programmes.

Maintenance and continuity of rehabilitation are essential and individuals should be encouraged to use local community opportunities that suit their own circumstances and preferences. Partners, carers, and families can play a key role in ensuring that patients adhere to their rehabilitation programme and attain their desired goals.

Other family members

Offer support to families, especially the partner and, where feasible, include them in the rehabilitation programme as this may boost the confidence and morale of the patient as well as the partner and also allay fears, dispel myths, and correct misconceptions.

Surveillance

Ensure surveillance of patients and family members with, or at risk of developing, a cardiac condition and arrange cardiological follow-up.

Support group:

British Heart Foundation www.bhf.org.uk; Tel. 020 7554 0000.

Expert adviser: Anonymous.

References

American Association of Cardiovascular and Pulmonary Rehabilitation. *Guidelines for cardiac rehabilitation and secondary prevention*, 4th edn. Champaign, IL: Human Kinetics, 2004.

Beswick AD, Rees K, Griebsch I, *et al.* Provision, uptake and cost of cardiac rehabilitation programmes: improving services to under-represented groups. *Health Technol Asess* 2004;**8**:1–152.

Bethell HJN, Lewin RJP, Dalal HM. Cardiac rehabilitation: it works so why isn't it done?. *Br J Gen Pract* 2008;**58**:677–9.

British Association for Cardiac Rehabilitation. *Standards and core components for cardiac rehabilitation.* London: BACR, 2007.

Clark AM, Hartling L, Vandermeer B, McAlister FA. Meta-analysis: secondary prevention programs for patients with coronary artery disease. *Ann Intern Med* 2005;**143**:659–72.

Dalal HM, Evans PH, Campbell JL, *et al.* Home-based versus hospital-based rehabilitation after myocardial infarction: a randomized trial with preference arms—Cornwall Heart Attack Rehabilitation Management Study (CHARMS). *Int J Cardiol* 2007;**119**:202–11.

Jolly K, Lip GY, Greenfield S, *et al.* The Birmingham Rehabilitation Uptake Maximisation study (BRUM): a randomized controlled trial comparing home-based with centre-based cardiac rehabilitation. *Heart* 2009;**95**:36–42.

Lewin RJP, Thompson DR, Roebuck A. Development of the BACR/BHF minimum dataset for cardiac rehabilitation. *Br J Cardiol* 2004;**11**:300–1.

Linden W, Phillips MJ, LeClerc J. Psychological treatment of cardiac patients: a meta-analysis. *Eur Heart J* 2007;**28**:2972–84.

National Institute for Health and Clinical Excellence. Clinical guideline 48: MI: secondary prevention in primary and secondary care for patients following a myocardial infarction. London: NICE, 2007.

Skinner JS, Cooper A, Feder GS, on behalf of the Guideline Development Group. Secondary prevention for patients after myocardial infarction: summary of NICE guidance. *BMJ* 2007;**334**:1112–3.

Taylor RS, Brown A, Ebrahim S, *et al.* Exercise-based rehabilitation for patients with coronary heart disease: systematic review and meta-analysis of randomized controlled trials. *Am J Med* 2004;**116**:682–92.

Thompson DR, Bowman GS, de Bono DP, Hokins A. Cardiac rehabilitation: guidelines and audit standards. London: Royal College of Physicians, 1997.

Wenger NK. Current status of cardiac rehabilitation. *J Am Coll Cardiol* 2008; **51**:1619–31.

Williams MA, Ades PA, Hamm LF, *et al.* Clinical evidence for a health benefit from cardiac rehabilitation: an update. *Am Heart J* 2006;**152**:835.

Coronary restenosis and stent thrombosis

Coronary restenosis is *morphologically* (angiographically or pathologically) defined as proven significant (>50%) recurrent segmental narrowing of the coronary artery (or coronary bypass graft) lumen after previous percutaneous coronary intervention (PCI).

Pathophysiologically, restenosis is a slowly progressive (chronic) process of neointimal hyperplasia within the previously stenotic and successfully dilated coronary segment—in other words it is a hypertrophic healing reaction to the endothelial damage caused by PCI (every PCI procedure causes some degree of endothelial damage). The more extensive is endothelial (and subendothelial) damage during PCI, the more likely restenosis occurs in the coming few months. Furthermore, the likelihood of future restenosis is influenced to a large extent by the diameter of the stent implanted during the initial PCI procedure.

Stent undersizing (e.g. implantation of the 2.5-mm stent to a 3-mm coronary artery) is one of the most frequent causes of restenoses in real life clinical practice.

Clinical presentation of restenosis largely varies from entirely asymptomatic (in more than half of angiographic restenoses, usually when restenosis is in the range 50–70% luminal diameter) through slowly progressive recurrent exertional angina pectoris (most typical clinical presentation, usually in patients with restenosis involving >70% luminal diameter) to an extremely rare more dramatic manifestation (acute coronary syndrome or sudden cardiac death).

Incidence

Restenosis after PCI (with bare metal stents) occurs within approximately 6 months after intervention in rates 5–10% (clinical manifestation) or 10–20% (angiographic manifestation). It is more frequent after plain balloon angioplasty and less frequent after PCI with drug-eluting stents.

Prevention and treatment

In the past, many pharmacological agents were tested without any success: no drug used systemically is able to decrease the likelihood of restenosis. Currently the most effective approach to the prevention and treatment of restenosis are drug-eluting stents.

Coronary stent thrombosis is *morphologically* (angiographically or pathologically) defined as complete (or very rarely incomplete) thrombotic occlusion of the previously implanted coronary stent.

Pathophysiologically, stent thrombosis is an acute (or rarely subacute) thrombosis within the incompletely endothelialized and/or suboptimally deployed stent, usually in a patient with suboptimal platelet inhibition.

Stent endothelialization lasts 3–4 weeks after bare metal stent (BMS) implantation and several months or even several years after drug eluting stent (DES) implantation.

Dual antiplatelet therapy during this period is essential.

Suboptimal stent deployment means, that the stent was damaged during its deployment (struts fractures) and/or free space was left between the stent and vessel wall (incomplete stent apposition).

Clinical manifestation of stent thrombosis is usually dramatic—either as a large acute myocardial infarction (with in-hospital mortality 20–40%!) or even as sudden cardiac death. Rarely, the patient presents with angina pectoris (mostly unstable). Very rarely, stent thrombosis occurs without symptoms (e.g. when the coronary artery supplies an area with old post-infarction scarring).

The *incidence* of stent thrombosis is approximately 1–2% during the first month after stent implantation for both stent types (BMS and DES). After the first month, stent thrombosis is very rare in BMS, although in DES it occurs in approximately 0.6% per annum during the subsequent 3 (or more) years. Stent thrombosis is best *prevented* by optimal stent deployment (including the stent–artery diameter ratio approximately 1.2:1) and by uninterrupted dual antiplatelet therapy (aspirin + clopidogrel) of appropriate duration (1 month after BMS implantation, at least 12 months after DES implantation). Some patients do not respond adequately to standard doses of clopidogrel (clopidogrel non-responders) and these can significantly benefit from a new drug—prasugrel. *Treatment* of stent thrombosis is similar to treatment of any acute ST elevation myocardial infarction: aspirin, heparin, prasugrel (rather than clopidogrel), GPIIb/IIIa inhibitors, primary PCI.

Summary

Coronary restenosis is a chronic benign (mortality <1%) slowly progressive iatrogenic disease best prevented and treated by DES. Stent thrombosis is an acute deadly (mortality >20%) disease, best prevented by optimal stent deployment followed by effective dual antiplatelet therapy. DES are used to significantly decrease restenosis rates at the price of slightly increasing stent thrombosis rates.

Chapter 6

Heart failure

Diagnosis and evaluation

Heart failure is a syndrome not a diagnosis. This oft-repeated statement indicates that the disorder heart failure is a syndrome recognized by a particular pattern of symptoms, processes, and outcomes and associated with beneficial responses to a number of therapies, but it does not have a single pathological process or aetiology. This chapter will focus on the most common disorder, that of chronic heart failure due to left ventricular (LV) systolic dysfunction, but the reader is referred to the chapters on diastolic heart failure and acute heart failure for related disorders.

Presentation
Several incidence studies of heart failure have reported the mode of presentation. The majority (>80%) (Cowie et al. 1999) have been as an emergency admission to hospital, indicating that acute heart failure is a precedent to chronic heart failure in most people. This means that most cases should be diagnosed when the more sophisticated armoury of a hospital admission is available and when the presence of pulmonary oedema is more likely. Diagnosis in this setting will depend on the presence of cardiac dysfunction (usually detected by echocardiography (see Chapter 1.4)) combined with acute dyspnoea and pulmonary congestion (detected usually by chest X-ray) or less frequently peripheral oedema and a raised jugular venous pressure (JVP). Diagnostic uncertainty is therefore mainly seen in those 20% of patients who present with more insidious symptoms of exertional breathlessness or fatigue and without an episode of acute pulmonary oedema.

Definitions
The definition of heart failure has changed over time as the interest in clinical investigation has progressed, from the importance of fluid retention in its manifestations, through an interest in the damage to the muscle of the heart to the recognition of the importance of neurohormonal activation in its progression and treatment. One of the more recent (and perhaps longest) definitions (Heart Failure Society Of America 2006) tries to encapsulate all these features:

HF is a syndrome caused by cardiac dysfunction, generally resulting from myocardial muscle dysfunction or loss and characterized by left ventricular dilation or hypertrophy. Whether the dysfunction is primarily systolic or diastolic or mixed, it leads to neurohormonal and circulatory abnormalities, usually resulting in characteristic symptoms such as fluid retention, shortness of breath, and fatigue, especially on exertion. In the absence of appropriate therapeutic intervention, HF is usually progressive at the levels of cardiac function and clinical symptoms. The severity of clinical symptoms may vary substantially during the course of the disease process and may not correlate with changes in underlying cardiac function. Although HF is progressive and often fatal, patients can be stabilized and myocardial dysfunction and remodeling may improve, either spontaneously or as a consequence of therapy.

In physiologic terms, HF is a syndrome characterized by elevated cardiac filling pressure or inadequate peripheral oxygen delivery, at rest or during stress, caused by cardiac dysfunction.

These statements are unfortunately are not useful as practical guides to diagnosis of heart failure in the absence of acute pulmonary oedema. Perhaps the simplest is that of the European Society of Cardiology (Swedberg et al. 2005), which describes two or three features: symptoms of heart failure (at rest or during exercise), objective evidence (preferably by echocardiography) of cardiac dysfunction (systolic and/or diastolic) (at rest), and (in cases where the diagnosis is in doubt) a response to treatment directed towards heart failure, although it includes circular logic that make it unattractive as a definitive guide.

Diagnosing non-acute chronic heart failure
History: key points
- Insidious onset of exertional breathlessness (usually) or fatigue.
- Requires demonstration of impaired LV systolic function chronically.
- Exclusion of alternative principal cause of symptoms, e.g. lung disease, anaemia.

Examination: key points (not all need to be present)
- Cardiac dysfunction: displaced apex beat, S4 gallop rhythm
- Signs of fluid retention: raised jugular venous pressure (JVP), peripheral pitting oedema, pulsatile hepatomegaly (due to triscuspid regurgitation (TR)), ascites
- Signs of tissue congestion: enlarged liver (possibly pulsatile), pulmonary congestion.

Investigations
Full blood count
- Haemochromatosis as cause or anaemia as consequence.

Urea and electrolytes
- Coincident renal disease common
- Hypocalcaemia as rare cause.

Other blood tests
- Lipids
- Thyroid function as rare causes
- Glucose or HbA1c for diabetes.

ECG
- No characteristic changes but look for signs of old myocardial infarction (MI), ischaemia, LVH, tachyarrhythmias.

Chest X-ray
- Increased cardiothoracic ratio
- Enlarged pulmonary arteries
- Signs of the possible lung congestion.

Doppler echocardiography (see Chapter 1.4)
- Determination of LV dimensions and systolic and diastolic function
- May provide clues to cause, e.g. regional dysfunction in ischaemic heart disease, hypertrophy in hypertensive heart disease, thickening in amyloid or infiltrative cardiomyopathies, restrictive pattern in restrictive cardiomyopathy
- Flow patterns by Doppler can document severity and intracardiac pressures

- Detection of valvular disease as cause or complication of heart failure.

Cardiac magnetic resonance imaging
- Allows non-invasive assessment of right and left heart structure and function
- Can help differentiate ischaemic disease from dilated cardiomyopathy.

Exercise testing
- Useful in monitoring functional exercise capacity and for prognosis
- Reduced exercise capacity with patient having exceeded anaerobic threshold gives indication of impaired cardiac reserve if the absence of simultaneous arterial oxygen desaturation which can exclude significant lung disease as the cause of the reduced exercise capacity.

Prognostic markers in heart failure

Symptom severity, e.g. NYHA class.
LVEF.
Systolic blood pressure.
Age.
Ischemic aetiology.
Echo measures of LV performance (systolic and diastolic).
Functional measures (6-minute corridor walk test, peak oxygen consumption, anaerobic threshold, peak METS).
Ve/VCO$_2$ slope from cardiopulmonary exercise testing
Neurohormonal (plasma noradrenaline (norepine-phrine), adrenomedullin, natriuretic peptides).
Plasma sodium, creatinine, liver enzymes, bilirubin, thyroid enzymes, uric acid.
QRS duration, ventricular arrhythmias, reduced heart rate variability, previous resuscitated sudden death, persistent tachycardia, T-wave alternans.
Diabetes.
Low body mass index.
Serum troponin levels.

Cardiac catheterization
- May be necessary to exclude or to document coronary artery disease as cause of heart failure and to determine possible need for revascularization
- Rarely for biopsy, e.g. specific cardiomyopathies/acute myocarditis (see specific chapters).

Natriuretic peptides and other biomarkers
- BNP, N-terminal pro-BNP, mid-regional ANP, and mid-regional pro-adrenomedullin have all been shown to both identify heart failure and to predict mortality in established disease (Lainscak *et al.* 2009). Their role in screening and in diagnosing heart failure is unclear, and has rarely been used in routine care, although low values can effectively exclude significant (if untreated at the time of assessment) heart failure.

Prognostic markers

A variety of features have been shown to predict a higher than average risk of death in heart failure patients. These cover the measurements of haemodynamics, structural aetiological, neurohormonal, functional, electrolyte changes, and other organ dysfunction. How best to use these in routine practice to guide therapy is far from clear.

References

Cowie MR, Wood DA, Coats AJ, et al. Incidence and aetiology of heart failure; a population-based study. *Eur Heart J* 1999;**20**:421–8.

Heart Failure Society Of America. Conceptualization and working definition of heart failure. *J Card Fail* 2006;**12**:e10–1.

Lainscak M, Anker MS, von Haehling S, Anker SD. Biomarkers for chronic heart failure: diagnostic, prognostic, and therapeutic challenges [Review]. *Herz* 2009;**34**:589–93.

Swedberg K, Cleland J, Dargie H, et al., Task Force for the Diagnosis and Treatment of Chronic Heart Failure of the European Society of Cardiology. Guidelines for the diagnosis and treatment of chronic heart failure: executive summary (update 2005). *Eur Heart J* 2005;**26**:1115–40.

Pharmacological therapy of heart failure

There is an abundance of clinical trial evidence for most of the pharmacological interventions in all stages of systolic heart failure. There is, however, a paucity of evidence for pharmacological agents in patients with diastolic dysfunction/heart failure with normal ejection fraction (HFNEF). None of the current available therapies have been proven to reduce mortality in this group. The following section will address each of the classes of drugs in the management of systolic chronic heart failure (CHF).

Angiotensin-converting enzyme inhibitors

One of the first studies to demonstrate a mortality reduction was the Cooperative North Scandinavian Enalapril Survival Study (CONSENSUS) I. This study demonstrated a 40% reduction in mortality in patients on enalapril compared with standard therapy (mainly digoxin and diuretics). Since then, angiotensin-converting enzyme (ACE) inhibitors have been shown to reduce mortality in mild to moderate heart failure (Studies of Left Ventricular Dysfunction (SOLVD) trial and others). A systematic review of trials including more than 100 000 patients showed that early initiation (within 36 hours) of an ACE inhibitor post myocardial infarction (MI) resulted in a 7% proportional reduction in 30-day mortality. This was particularly evident in certain high-risk groups, such as Kilip class 2–3, heart rate ≥100 bpm at entry and in anterior MI. The incidence of non-fatal acute heart failure (AHF) post MI was also significantly reduced.

Overall, meta-analysis of the major clinical trials of ACE inhibitor use in CHF show a 23% relative risk reduction (95% CI 33–12%) and an absolute risk reduction of 6.1%. ACE inhibitor therapy also reduces hospitalization for heart failure by 35% (95% CI 26–43%). It is therefore a Grade A recommendation for all NYHA functional classes of heart failure due to left ventricular systolic dysfunction in the major published guidelines.

Owing to hypotensive effects as well as adverse renal effects, ACE inhibitors should be commenced at an appropriate starting dose and titrated upwards, every 2 weeks or so. Because of the possibility of renal impairment secondary to bilateral renovascular disease and of hyperkalaemia, patients should have their renal function and electrolytes monitored within the first 2 weeks of initiation of therapy. Other adverse effects such as cough might warrant switching to an alternative agent. Angioedema occurs in up to 0.2% of all patients treated with an ACE inhibitor (Agostoni and Cicardi 1998) and up to 17% of all hospital admissions for angioedema are due to ACE inhibitor therapy (Vleeming 1998). Any patient who suffers from angioedema should have their ACE inhibitor therapy withdrawn immediately. A recent meta-analysis suggests that the risk of angioedema with angiotensin receptor blockers (ARBs) in patients who have had angioedema on ACE inhibitors is between 2% and 17% (Haymore et al. 2008).

Other contraindications to ACE inhibitor therapy include significant aortic stenosis, known bilateral renal artery stenosis or baseline serum potassium >5.0 mmol/L. Patients should have their renal function checked at baseline and 10 days after every dose up-titration.

Although there was no significant difference, the ATLAS study showed a 15% relative risk reduction in death or heart failure hospitalization in the high-dose lisinopril group versus the low-dose group. Patients should therefore be up-titrated to the evidence-based or maximal tolerable dose of their ACE inhibitor.

Angiotensin receptor blockers

ARBs inhibit the action of the renin–angiotensin system by blocking the angiotensin type I (AT1) receptors. They therefore have similar effects to ACE inhibitors but due to the unopposed action of ACE on bradykinin breakdown (an effect of ACE inhibitor therapy may be the enhancement of the vasodilator action of bradykinin, as well as its role in producing the ACE inhibitor cough), there is a markedly reduced incidence of cough. There have been concerns that unopposed stimulation of angiotensin II type 2 receptors may have deleterious effects such as hypertrophy and fibrosis (Levy 2004).

ELITE II (Pitt et al. 1997) was the first mortality/morbidity trial to compare an ACE inhibitor with an ARB in heart failure. It showed that despite improved tolerability, losartan was not superior to the ACE inhibitor captopril. Despite criticisms about the dosing in the trial, it had the benefit of assessing ACE inhibitor-naïve patients, a feat that cannot be ethically repeated in a trial today.

The CHARM-Alternative study (Granger et al. 1997) showed that the ARB candesartan resulted in a significant 23% relative risk reduction in cardiovascular death or hospitalization in ACE inhibitor intolerant CHF patients. Data from the recent TRANSCEND trial suggests that in high CV risk patients who are intolerant of an ACE inhibitor, the ARB telmisartan failed to reduce a composite primary endpoint of cardiovascular death, myocardial infarction, stroke, or hospitalization for heart failure. However, it appears to reduce cardiovascular hospitalizations and drug discontinuation due to intolerance (Yusuf et al. 2008).

The CHARM-Preserved study in patients with HFNEF suggests that candesartan may be beneficial in reducing hospitalizations but had no effect on CV death compared with placebo (Yusuf et al. 2003). The I-Preserve study also found no benefit for irbesartan in HFNEF (Massie et al. 2008).

The addition of an ARB to an ACE inhibitor acutely in the ValHeFT trial did not reduce mortality but significantly reduced the combined endpoint of heart failure hospitalization and mortality by 13%. However, patients already on an ACE inhibitor and a beta-blocker fared worse when valsartan was added to their treatment regime (Cohn et al. 2001).

ARBs are therefore recommended for patients with heart failure who do not tolerate an ACE inhibitor. Data from the CHARM-Added study would suggest that patients who are still symptomatic on maximal therapy may benefit from the addition of an ARB to their ACE inhibitor in terms of a reduced risk of the composite endpoint of the composite of cardiovascular death or hospital admission for CHF, but the effect on total mortality was not significant.

Beta-blockers

The four beta-blockers with clinical trial evidence for the treatment of heart failure are bisoprolol (CIBIS II 1999), carvidelol (COPERNICUS) (PACKER et al. 2002), nebivolol (SENIORS) (Flather et al. 2005), and extended-release metoprolol succinate (MERIT-HF) (Hjalmarson et al. 2000). On average, there has been a 33% mortality reduction across the randomized controlled trials (RCTs). In the acute setting, beta-blockers may worsen decompensation and therefore are recommended in stable CHF patients in all NYHA classes. In the event of decompensation, the European Society of Cardiology (ESC) guidelines for the management of heart failure recommend increasing the diuretic dose and continuing the beta-blocker (if possible) at a lower dose (Dickstein et al. 2008).

Significantly, these benefits were seen in patients already treated with an ACE inhibitor or ARB. The SENIORS trial also showed that older (mean age 76 years) patients equally benefit from beta-blocker therapy (Flather et al. 2005). Chronic obstructive pulmonary disease (COPD) is NOT a contraindication to beta-blocker therapy. In a study of post-MI patients with COPD, beta-blockers reduced mortality by 40% (Gottlieb et al. 1998). However, asthma, symptomatic hypotension, second- and third-degree heart block, untreated sick sinus syndrome, and pre-existing bradycardia remain contraindications to therapy with beta-blockers.

Stable patients should be initiated on low doses and up-titrated every 4 weeks or so according to tolerability. The MOCHA study showed a dose-related improvement in LV function, mortality, and hospitalization rate with carvedilol (Bristow et al. 1996). Patients should therefore be up-titrated to the evidence-based target dose (Table 6.2.1) or maximal tolerated dose.

Aldosterone antagonists

Aldosterone antagonists should be prescribed to all NYHA III and IV patients with LVEF <40% and already on maximal ACE inhibitor (or ARB) and beta-blocker therapy.

Table 6.2.1 Dosages of commonly used drugs in heart failure (from Dickstein et al. 2007, by permission of Oxford University Press)

	Starting dose (mg)	Target (mg)
ACEi		
Captopril	6.25 tid	50–100 tid
Enalapril	2.5 bid	10–20 bid
Lisinopril	2.5–5.0 od	20–35 od
Ramipril	2.5 od	5 bid
Trandolapril	0.5 od	4 od
ARB		
Candesartan	4 or 8 od	32 od
Valsartan	40 bid	160 bid
Aldo antagonist		
Eplerenone	25 od	50 od
Spironolactone	25 od	25–50 od
Beta-blocker		
Bisoprolol	1.25 od	10 od
Carvedilol	3.125 bid	25–50 bid
Metoprolol succinate	12.5/25 od	200 od
Nebivolol	1.25 od	10 od

The two pivotal studies of aldosterone antagonists are the Eplerenone Post-Acute Myocardial Infarction Heart Failure Efficacy and Survival Study (EPHESUS) (Pitt et al. 2005) and the Randomised Aldactone Evaluation Study (RALES 1996).

EPHESUS studied patients with post-MI LVEF <40% and either signs of heart failure or diabetes. Patients were commenced on eplerenone early on (3–14 days post MI). The study found a 31% reduction in all-cause mortality, 13% reduction (P = 0.002) in CV death or hospitalization and a 21% relative risk reduction (RRR) in sudden death. Eplerenone causes less gynaecomastia than spironolactone and may be an option for patients on spironolactone (up to 10% in RALES) who develop this side-effect (George and Struthers 2007).

RALES specifically assessed 25–50 mg/day spironolactone in NYHA III and IV patients with severe LV systolic dysfunction (EF<35%) already on an ACE inhibitor (95%) and digoxin (74%). Beta-blocker use in heart failure was not widespread (11%) when this trial was conducted. The study showed a 30% reduction in all-cause mortality and a 31% reduction in cardiac mortality. Spironolactone also reduced hospitalization for heart failure by 35% (RALES 19960. An ongoing trial, EMPHASIS, is investigating the use of eplerenone in patients with mild to moderate heart failure.

Both spironolactone and eplerenone should not be commenced in patients with baseline potassium >5.0 mmol/L or serum creatinine >220 µmol/L (Dickstein et al. 2007; Network, SIG, 2007) as they are more likely to have a significant deterioration in their renal function. Monitoring of renal function is mandatory. The 2008 ESC Heart Failure guidelines suggest monitoring renal function 1 week and 4 weeks post dose increase (Dickstein et al. 2007).

Diuretics

It is not clear if diuretics improve mortality. However, diuretics are the mainstay of symptom control management in CHF. In most cases a loop diuretic such as furosemide should suffice in reducing signs of fluid retention. The risk of hypokalaemia can be offset by concurrent treatment with an ACE inhibitor (or ARB) and an aldosterone antagonist. Diuretics also upregulate the renin–angiotensin system and therefore should be used in conjunction with these agents.

The doses must be titrated according to symptoms and adjusted to the lowest dose necessary to maintain the patients 'dry body weight' (weight when there are no clinical signs of fluid retention).

The use of potassium-sparing diuretics in patients on an ACE inhibitor/ARB or aldosterone antagonist is not recommended due to the risk of hyperkalaemia. In loop diuretic resistant patients, other options include the addition of a thiazide diuretic such as metolazone or hydrochlorthiazide.

Statins

The majority of patients with heart failure will have an ischaemic aetiology. Therefore, a statin is clearly indicated in these groups. Most of the landmark statin trials excluded patients with CHF. There is currently no evidence that statins benefit patients with a non-ischaemic aetiology for their heart failure. The CORONA study showed a reduction in hospitalization with rosuvastatin in patients with systolic heart failure. The study failed to demonstrate any mortality benefit (Kjekshus et al. 2007). The GISSI-HF trial

(Gissi *et al.* 2008) showed no mortality benefit with rosuvastatin in CHF of any aetiology but a modest 8% RRR in death and hospitalization for heart failure with n-3 polyunsaturated fatty acids (n-3 PUFA) but these benefits were only seen at 2 years (Tavazzi *et al.* 2008).

Antiplatelet therapy

Most patients with CHF have an ischaemic aetiology. There have been suggestions from the WASH study that aspirin may increase hospitalization in heart failure. The subsequent WATCH study failed to show any significant differences between aspirin, clopidogrel, and warfarin for the primary endpoint of all-cause mortality, non-fatal MI, and non-fatal stroke. In the absence of any firm evidence for the withdrawal of antiplatelet agents, these should not be withdrawn in newly diagnosed HF patients. Patients on warfarin or other combinations of antiplatelet agents for anticoagulation purposes should continue on their therapy. Warfarin was more effective than antiplatelet agents in preventing thromboembolic events in patients with AF, in the WASH study.

Digoxin

Digoxin is a cardiac glycoside with inotropic activity via inhibition of the Na^+,K^+-ATPase pump. It also has effects on the AV node and therefore may be used for control of the ventricular rate in atrial fibrillation. There is only one published major study of digoxin in heart failure, the Digitalis Investigation Group (DIG) study (1997), which showed a reduction in overall and heart failure hospitalizations (absolute risk reduction 7.9%) but no effect of digoxin on mortality. However, this study was conducted before the use of beta-blockers became commonplace in the management of heart failure. Digoxin could be considered in patients who are still symptomatic despite optimum therapy.

It is important to note that digoxin itself can be arrhythmogenic in the presence of hypokalaemia as digoxin competes with the potassium ion for the same binding site on the Na^+,K^+-ATPase pump. Renal function monitoring is essential in patients on digoxin as concomitant diuretic treatment may cause hypokalaemia.

Isosorbide dinitrate (ISDN) and hydralazine

This combination is an option for patients intolerant to either an ACEi or an ARB. This combination was first tested in the 1986 Veterans Administration Study (Cohn *et al.* 1986). In patients on a combination of digoxin and a diuretic, ISDN and hydralazine (ISDN-H) produced a RRR of 34% at 2 years and a significant improvement in LVEF at 1 year compared with placebo. However, in the V-HEFT II trial, there was a trend towards increased mortality (RRI 28%) in the ISDN + hydralazine arm (Cohn *et al.* 1991). None of the patients on this trial was treated with a beta-blocker.

The A-Heft study added the combination to optimum therapy in African-American patients with NYHA III–IV. The addition of ISDN-H produced a RRR in mortality by 43% and HF hospitalization by 33%.

Hydralazine is contraindicated in those with any lupus syndrome or severe renal failure.

Further reading

Agostoni A, Cicardi M. Drug-induced angioedema without urticaria. *Drug Saf* 2001;**24**:599–606.

Bristow MR, Gilbert EM, Abraham WT, *et al.* Carvedilol produces dose-related improvements in left ventricular function and survival in subjects with chronic heart failure. MOCHA Investigators. *Circulation* 1996;**94**:2807–16.

Cardiac Insufficiency Bisoprolol Study II (CIBIS-II): a randomised trial. *Lancet* 1999;**353**:9–13.

Cohn JN, Johnson G, Ziesche S. *et al.* A comparison of enalapril with hydralazine-isosorbide dinitrate in the treatment of chronic congestive heart failure. *N Engl J Med* 1991;**325**:303–10.

Cohn JN, Archibald DG, Ziesche S, *et al.* Effect of vasodilator therapy on mortality in chronic congestive heart failure. Results of a Veterans Administration Cooperative Study. *N Engl J Med* 1986;**314**:1547–52.

Cohn JN, Tognoni G. the Valsartan Heart Failure Trial, A Randomized Trial of the Angiotensin-Receptor Blocker Valsartan in Chronic Heart Failure. *N Engl J Med* 2001;**345**(23):1667–1675.

Demers C, McMurray JJ, Swedberg K, *et al.* Impact of candesartan on nonfatal myocardial infarction and cardiovascular death in patients with heart failure. *JAMA* 2005;**294**:1794–8.

Dickstein K, Cohen-Solal A, Filippatos G, *et al.* ESC guidelines for the diagnosis and treatment of acute and chronic heart failure 2008: the Task Force for the diagnosis and treatment of acute and chronic heart failure 2008 of the European Society of Cardiology. Developed in collaboration with the Heart Failure Association of the ESC (HFA) and endorsed by the European Society of Intensive Care Medicine (ESICM). *Eur J Heart Fail* 2008;**10**:933–89.

Digitalis Investigation Group, The Effect of Digoxin on Mortality and Morbidity in Patients with Heart Failure. *N Engl J Med* 1997;**336**:525–33.

Flather MD, Shibata MC, Coats AJ, *et al.* Randomized trial to determine the effect of nebivolol on mortality and cardiovascular hospital admission in elderly patients with heart failure (SENIORS). *Eur Heart J* 2005;**26**:215–25.

George J, Struthers AD. Evaluation of the aldosterone-blocking agent eplerenone in hypertension and heart failure. *Expert Opin Pharmacother* 2007;**8**:3053–9.

Gissi-HF Investigators. Effect of rosuvastatin in patients with chronic heart failure (the GISSI-HF trial): a randomised, double-blind, placebo-controlled trial. *Lancet* 2008;**372**:1231–9.

Gottlieb SS, McCarter RJ, Vogel RA. Effect of beta-blockade on mortality among high-risk and low-risk patients after myocardial infarction. *N Engl J Med* 1998;**339**:489–97.

Granger CB, McMurray JJ, Yusuf S, *et al.* Effects of candesartan in patients with chronic heart failure and reduced left-ventricular systolic function intolerant to angiotensin-converting-enzyme inhibitors: the CHARM-Alternative trial. *Lancet* 2003;**362**:772–6.

Haymore BR, Yoon J, Mikita CP, Klote MM, DeZee KJ. Risk of angioedema with angiotensin receptor blockers in patients with prior angioedema associated with angiotensin-converting enzyme inhibitors: a meta-analysis. *Ann Allergy Asthma Immunol* 2008;**101**:495–9.

Hjalmarson A, Goldstein S, Fagerberg B, *et al.* Effects of controlled-release metoprolol on total mortality, hospitalizations, and well-being in patients with heart failure: the Metoprolol CR/XL Randomized Intervention Trial in congestive heart failure (MERIT-HF). MERIT-HF Study Group. *JAMA* 2000;**283**:1295–302.

Kjekshus J, Apetrei E, Barrios V, *et al.* Rosuvastatin in older patients with systolic heart failure. *N Engl J Med* 2007;**357**:2248–61.

Levy BI. Can angiotensin II type 2 receptors have deleterious effects in cardiovascular disease? Implications for therapeutic blockade of the renin-angiotensin system. *Circulation* 2004;**109**:8–13.

Massie BM, Carson PE, McMurray JJ, *et al.* Irbesartan in patients with heart failure and preserved ejection fraction. *N Engl J Med* 2008;**359**:2456–67.

Packer M, Fowler MB, Roecker EB, *et al.* Effect of carvedilol on the morbidity of patients with severe chronic heart failure: results of the carvedilol prospective randomized cumulative survival (COPERNICUS) study. *Circulation* 2002;**106**:2194–9.

Pitt B, White H, Nicolau J, *et al.* Eplerenone reduces mortality 30 days after randomization following acute myocardial infarction in patients with left ventricular systolic dysfunction and heart failure. *J Am Coll Cardiol* 2005;**46**:425–31.

Pitt B, Segal R, Martinez FA, et al. Randomised trial of losartan versus captopril in patients over 65 with heart failure (Evaluation of Losartan in the Elderly Study, ELITE). Lancet 1997;**349**:747–52.

Randomized Aldactone Evaluation Study (RALES). Effectiveness of spironolactone added to an angiotensin-converting enzyme inhibitor and a loop diuretic for severe chronic congestive heart failure. Am J Cardiol 1996;**78**:902–7.

Scottish Intercollegiate Guidelines Network. SIGN 95: Management of chronic heart failure. 2007. SIGN, Edinburgh.

Strauss MH, Hall AS. Angiotensin receptor blockers may increase risk of myocardial infarction: unraveling the ARB-MI paradox. Circulation 2006;**114**:838–54.

Tavazzi L, Maggioni AP, Marchioli R, et al. Effect of n-3 polyunsaturated fatty acids in patients with chronic heart failure (the GISSI-HF trial): a randomised, double-blind, placebo-controlled trial. Lancet 2008;**372**:1223–30.

Vleeming W, van Amsterdam JG, Stricker BH, de Wildt DJ. ACE inhibitor-induced angioedema. Incidence, prevention and management. Drug Saf 1998;**18**: 171.

Yusuf S, Pfeffer MA, Swedberg K, et al. Effects of candesartan in patients with chronic heart failure and preserved left-ventricular ejection fraction: the CHARM-Preserved Trial. Lancet 2003;**362**:777–81.

Yusuf S, Teo K, Anderson C, et al. Effects of the angiotensin-receptor blocker telmisartan on cardiovascular events in high-risk patients intolerant to angiotensin-converting enzyme inhibitors: a randomised controlled trial. Lancet 2008;**372**:1174–83.

Non-pharmacological treatment

Guidelines for the management of patients with chronic heart failure emphasize the need for appropriate drug therapy and drug titration to the target doses shown to be of value in clinical trials. This guidance has led in part to the development of heart failure services, but good heart failure management is more than simply dispensing medication.

Dietary intervention

A very few patients have a specific dietary deficiency as the cause of their heart failure and replacement can resolve the condition. Examples include selenium or calcium replacement in appropriate cases.

Patients with alcoholic cardiomyopathy can become deficient in thiamine (vitamin B1), and where there is a suspicion of high alcohol intake as a cause for heart failure, a short course of thiamine is appropriate.

There is some evidence to suggest that many patients with chronic heart failure have subclinical deficiencies of micronutrients and some evidence that dietary supplementation may help more generally. Trials are ongoing to assess the value of this approach in more detail.

The results of one clinical trial (GISSI-HF) suggest that omega-3 fatty acids may have modest beneficial effects in chronic heart failure.

Malnutrition as shown by, for example, low albumin is common in elderly patients and common in patients with chronic heart failure. Low serum cholesterol is also common, and a common finding in epidemiological studies is that low cholesterol is associated with a high mortality risk.

Epidemiological studies strongly suggest that cachexia is a potent adverse prognostic factor. Lesser degrees of weight loss are also important, and, conversely, a patient with mild-to-moderate obesity actually appears to have improved survival compared with patients with 'ideal' body weight.

Taken together, these features suggest that patients should be advised to maintain a healthy diet with plenty of fresh fruit and vegetables; unless a patient is morbidly obese, weight loss should not be recommended. A high intake of oily fish should be encouraged.

Dietary supplements

Although preliminary studies of multivitamin supplements are encouraging, there is no good evidence for their routine use. This does not, of course, prevent patients from using dietary supplements and 'alternative' therapies.

Some of these supplements are dangerous, particularly Chinese herbs, which can contain positive inotropic agents. Other supplements, such as *Crataegus* extract, can interact with prescribed medication.

It is good practice to take a thorough history from all patients and to advise patients appropriately about any dietary supplements they may be taking.

Salt and water manipulation

As part of the general education of patients with chronic heart failure and their carers, it is important to teach patients to help control their fluid balance. Most patients can find their ideal non-oedematous weight, weigh themselves several times a week, and can learn to manipulate diuretic therapy appropriately to keep themselves within a

kilogram or two of their ideal weight. Persuading a patient to use kilograms rather than pounds or stones is useful: 1 litre of water weighs 1 kg.

Older treatment regimes for chronic heart failure suggested that patients should be on a low-salt diet. There is little evidence that such a very unpalatable diet is beneficial, particularly with loop diuretic therapy.

A policy of not adding salt to meals is appropriate. Occasionally patients can have episodes of acute pulmonary oedema precipitated by a dietary high salt burden (particularly if a dose of diuretic has been omitted).

Replacing sodium chloride with potassium chloride (as in Lo-Salt) is not a good idea: the combination of potassium supplements together with angiotensin-converting enzyme inhibitors and possible aldosterone antagonists can cause life-threatening hyperkalaemia.

Short-term sodium restriction can occasionally help a patient with symptomatic hyponatraemia.

Formal water restriction is generally not necessary unless the patient is very oedematous and usually hospitalized. As part of a strategy for inducing diuresis and weight loss, restricting fluid intake to 1.5 L per 24 hours (or even on occasion 1 L) can be helpful.

Smoking

Although there is no formal study examining the effects of smoking in patients with chronic heart failure, all patients who continue to smoke (particularly those with underlying ischaemic heart disease) should be encouraged to stop.

Nicotine replacement therapy seems to be safe in heart failure even though it is a vasoconstrictor.

Alcohol

Those patients who are thought to have an alcoholic cardiomyopathy should be advised to abstain altogether. For other patients, there is no good evidence that alcohol is harmful, and the same guidance as applies to the general population should be followed.

Vaccination

Patients with chronic heart failure are more at risk from influenza than the normal population. Although there is no rigorous evidence to support it, patients with chronic heart failure should be offered an annual influenza vaccination.

Exercise

Older text books of cardiology recommend rest as an integral part of heart failure management. There are a few studies suggesting that prolonged bed-rest might reduce heart size, but these were conducted before the availability of modern therapy, particularly loop diuretics. There was a high risk of thromboembolic complication with this regime.

A large body of evidence has accumulated since the 1990s that, in contrast, exercise training might be beneficial for evenpatients, even those with severely symptomatic heart failure. It should be emphasized that this discussion relates to patients with chronic stable disease without fluid retention or recent cardiovascular event.

Skeletal muscle is profoundly abnormal in patients with chronic heart failure (see Chapter 2.2, Dyspnoea):

- Muscle is reduced in bulk, weaker, and with lesser endurance than normal;

Table 6.3.1 Similarities between the chronic heart failure state and detraining

	Detraining	Heart failure
Heart rate	↑	↑
Exercise capacity	↓	↓
Muscle size	↓	↓
Muscle enzymes	↓	↓
Sympathetic	↑	↑
Renin:angiotensin	↑	↑
Renin:angiotensin	↑	↑
Heart rate variability	↓	↓

- It is structurally abnormal with an increase in the proportion of type II fast twitch fibres; mitochondria are structurally abnormal
- It is functionally abnormal with early acidosis during exercise and decreased levels of some enzymes of the Kreb's cycle and oxidative chain.

Many of these changes are similar to those seen in subjects who have detrained (Table 6.3.1) and raises the possibility that training might be beneficial.

Concerns were initially raised that training might worsen left ventricular function through a rise in wall stress during exercise, but these concerns proved unfounded.

The training response (Table 6.3.2). Initial studies assessed the effects of exercise in carefully selected highly motivated patients and found increases in around of up to 20% in maximum aerobic capacity (peak oxygen consumption (VO_2)) and similar increase in anaerobic threshold (Fig. 6.3.1).

Further work has shown that training increases exercise duration at fixed loads and increases the 6-minute walk test distance.

There is a reduction in the ventilatory response to exercise.

Additional benefits include improvement in quality of life, reduction in sympathetic nervous system overactivity and improved heart rate variability.

Mechanisms of benefit. Most of the benefit from training seems to be at the level of the skeletal muscle. There is

Table 6.3.2 The training response

Well-being	↑
Exercise capacity	↑
Anaerobic threshold	↑
Cardiac output	↑
Leg muscle bulk	↑
Muscle metabolism	↑
Leg AV O_2	↑
Ventilatory response	↓
Sympathovagal balance	↓

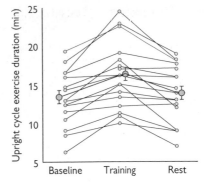

Fig. 6.3.1 The effects of training and subsequent detraining on exercise duration in 17 men with chronic heart failure. From Coats *et al.*, Controlled trial of physical training in chronic heart failure, in *Circulation*, copyright 1992.

increase in muscle bulk, strength, and endurance; mitochondria are more plentiful and more metabolically normal; the onset of acidosis is delayed. Other findings include an improvement in flow-mediated mediated vasodilation.

There are inconsistent effects on central haemodynamic function. Some studies have suggested that there may be an increase in cardiac output after training.

At least some of the beneficial effects are mediated through a decrease in the activity of the ergoreflex (see Chapter 2.2, Dyspnoea) perhaps driving the improvement in breathlessness (and reduced ventilatory response) and reduced sympathetic activity.

Type and intensity of exercise. Initial work used cycle training as this can be used to give a fairly precise exercise prescription. However, any form of aerobic exercise appears to mediate a training effect.

The usual intensity recommended is at around 70% of predetermined peak heart rate. The widespread use of beta-blockers can make peak heart rate difficult to determine. Low-intensity exercise at around 50% of peak heart rate also has a training effect.

As a rule of thumb, to have a training effect, exercise should be at a level to induce feelings of mild breathlessness and then continued for a minimum of 20 minutes, at least three times a week. Walking, jogging, cycling, and rowing are all effective.

The effect of a training regime is proportional to compliance.

Swimming causes some concern in patients as the effect of immersion is theoretically to cause a shift of blood from the periphery to the thorax, which might precipitate pulmonary oedema. However, evidence suggests that swimming is safe, even in patients with severely reduced left ventricular function.

Other concerns. Many patients with chronic heart failure are, of course, elderly and have multiple co-morbidities that may limit their ability to exercise. There is some evidence that electrical muscle stimulation may be helpful to inducing a training effect in such patients.

Although it is prudent to start a training programme under supervision, continued supervision is not necessary; a home exercise programme can be effective.

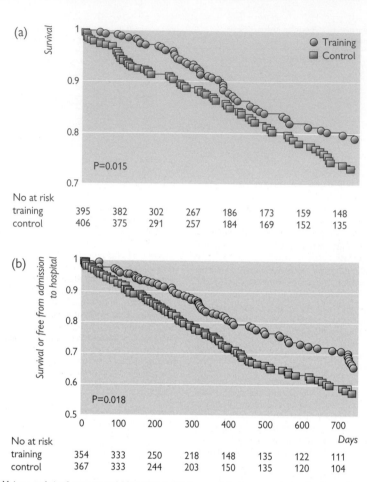

Fig. 6.3.2 Kaplan–Meier cumulative 2-year survival (a) and Kaplan–Meier cumulative 2-year survival or free from admission to hospital (b).

Effect on outcomes. Meta-analysis of early trials of exercise training suggested that there was a survival benefit from training (Fig. 6.3.2). A large-scale trial (HF-Action) randomized 2331 heart failure patients (NYHA class II–IV, left ventricular ejection fraction ≤35%) to either an exercise programme or to usual care. HF-Action demonstrated an early and sustained improvement in quality of life.

It just 'missed' its primary endpoint of all-cause mortality/hospitalization; all the secondary analyses supported the use of exercise training to increase survival. It is certainly safe, with no increase in the risk of injury.

As with all exercise trials, it is difficult to persuade patients to make long-term changes to lifestyle, and difficult to persuade motivated members of a control group from adopting the lifestyle change, diluting any effect in the study.

Practicality. Providing exercise training in some guise to the very large number of people with chronic heart failure is a major challenge to healthcare systems. Short-term rehabilitation is widely available to patients recovering from acute myocardial infarction or undergoing intervention for coronary disease, but a shift in emphasis to provide low-intensity long-term encouragement and supervision for a large number of patients remains a distant prospect.

Other forms of training

There is some evidence to suggest that very controlled training in the form of T'ai Chi may improve quality of life, decrease BNP levels and increase exercise capacity.

Respiratory muscle training specifically can help improve exercise capacity. A more interesting approach is to train patients to control respiratory rate. This has the effect of reducing the sensation of dyspnoea and increasing exercise capacity.

Taken together, these findings suggest that there may be a role for teaching ventilatory control in a manner similar to that used for chronic hyperventilation.

Acute ventilatory support

For patients with acute fulminant pulmonary oedema, intubation and ventilation can be life-saving. In small studies, non-invasive positive pressure ventilation, either with continuous or bi-level positive airways pressure (CPAP or BiPAP) appears to offer mortality benefit.

A single large-scale study with more than 1000 patients found that non-invasive ventilation induced a more rapid improvement in symptoms than standard oxygen therapy but had no effect on short-term mortality.

It seems reasonable to use CPAP or BiPAP to help relieve symptoms in patients with acute pulmonary oedema.

Home ventilatory support for CHF

A common complication of chronic heart failure is sleep disordered breathing (SDB). Periods of apnoea or hypopnoea are associated with hypoxia, in turn leading to a rise in blood pressure, increased sympathetic activity, and a predisposition to arrhythmia.

There are two main kinds of SDB:
- Obstructive sleep apnoea (OSA) is typically found in overweight middle-aged men and associated with day-time sleepiness. During sleep, the muscles of the pharynx and hypopharynx relax, leading to airway obstruction. Respiratory efforts continue with marked reduction (or complete loss of) airflow.
- Central sleep apnoea (CSA) is associated with CHF in particular, and often observed during waking hours as well as sleep. There is periodic respiration with periods of apnoea alternating with hyperventilation, often termed Cheyne–Stokes ventilation.

SDB is common in patients with chronic heart failure. The prevalence varies with the population studied, but perhaps half of patients with NYHA class III symptoms or worse have SDB. Approximately half have predominantly CSA and half OSA.

There is no doubt that the symptoms associated with OSA can be successfully treated with continuous positive airways pressure (CPAP) used overnight. However, CPAP is not effective for patients with CSA and should not be used unless there is a significant component of OSA.

More sophisticated adaptive servo-ventilators can detect and treat CSA as well as prevent OSA. Small studies have found servo-ventilators to have beneficial effects on surrogate markers for prognosis, and a definitive survival study is in progress at the time of writing.

Home oxygen therapy

Home oxygen therapy (HOT) is frequently prescribed on the model of HOT for chronic airways disease. However, patients with CHF are rarely hypoxic, and where hypoxia is detected, an alternative explanation should be sought.

HOT may help relieve symptoms in very symptomatic patients, particularly as part of providing palliative care, but there is no evidence to suggest that the oxygen itself is providing anything other than a placebo effect and there is no evidence to support its widespread use.

Enhanced external counterpulsation (EECP)

Enhanced external counterpulsation (EECP) uses cuffs inflated around the legs in sequence during diastole to imitate the effects of an intra-aortic balloon pump and to coronary perfusion pressure and flow while reducing central aortic pressure. It is effective in helping to control angina.

It is delivered as a course of an hour or so per day over several weeks. It cannot be used in oedematous patients or those with significant peripheral vascular or abdominal aortic disease.

The PEECH trial studied the effects of EECP in 187 patients with chronic heart failure (average age 63; mean left ventricular ejection fraction (LVEF) 26%) who received 35 hour-long sessions over 7–8 weeks.

There was no difference in peak VO_2 in the patients taken together between treatment and placebo groups, but some improvement in quality of life measures with EECP. There was a significant increase in peak VO_2 in the older patients.

There may thus be a role for EECP in selected patients with severe symptoms, particularly elderly patients.

Lifestyle support

Travelling is usually possible for most patients with chronic heart failure. Supplementary oxygen is usually not necessary for long haul flights if a patient can manage a flight of steps without stopping.

A patient is travelling to a hot, dry climate should be advised of the need to monitor fluid intake and output carefully. Daily weighing becomes important, and the patient may well need less diuretic than usual to maintain fluid balance.

Similarly, during an episode of diarrhoea and/or vomiting, a reduction in diuretic will be necessary to avoid excessive fluid loss.

Work. Patients should be encouraged to work where appropriate. Work requiring heavy physical exertion may be impossible, but there is reasonable evidence to suggest that patients with chronic disease who remain in work have a better prognosis than those who do not. Helping the patient to work may involve some education of the employer.

Driving. There is no limitation to driving for the patient with well-controlled chronic heart failure. Patients should not drive if so symptomatic that they cannot manage a flight of stairs in one go.

Vocational driving licences will be revoked (in the UK) if the LVEF is less than 40%.

Sexual activity often causes concern but need not be discouraged. Prophylactic use of nitrate may prevent undue breathlessness. Phosphodiesterase inhibitors, such as sildenafil may be useful in patients with erectile dysfunction (and are being studied in patients with pulmonary hypertension due to heart failure). However, a nitrate should *never* be used in conjunction with a phosphodiesterase inhibitor.

Pregnancy is occasionally an issue, particularly for women with postpartum cardiomyopathy. Pregnancy should be considered to be contraindicated in a woman with symptomatic left ventricular dysfunction, and should not be considered in a case of postpartum cardiomyopathy unless there has been complete recovery of left ventricular function.

An additional concern is that some drugs used for heart failure are strongly contraindicated in pregnancy—particularly angiotensin-converting enzyme inhibitors and angiotensin receptor antagonists.

Contraception thus may be a concern and a method offering near 100% protection, such as long-acting injection, should be used.

End of life issues

Despite modern therapy, patients with chronic heart failure still have a bleak prognosis, and may have a prolonged death.

Most patients when asked would prefer to die at home rather than in hospital. It can be difficult for those caring for a patient in hospital to know when to 'throw in the towel' and accept that death is inevitable.

Palliative care services are becoming more aware of the needs of patients with chronic heart failure. A good service is much, much more than a way of disposing of a patient for whom nothing more can be offered. The service should be engaged early rather than at the end; palliative care services can offer valuable help in managing difficult-to-control symptoms.

An important role for palliative care is to provide a link with primary care, so allowing the dying patient to get home.

Difficulties can arise over implantable defibrillators and these issues should be discussed with the patient (and his or her carers) before implantation.

Towards the end of life, repeated shocks can be very painful and serve little purpose.

Turning the defibrillator off may be appropriate, but does not equate to turning off a ventilator as some patients believe.

Further reading

Banerjee P, Caulfield B, Crowe L, Clark AL. Prolonged electrical muscle stimulation exercise improves strength, peak Vo$_2$ and exercise capacity in patients with stable chronic heart failure. *J Card Fail* 2009;**15**:319–26.

Coats AJ, Adamopoulos S, Radaelli A, *et al.* Controlled trial of physical training in chronic heart failure. Exercise performance, hemodynamics, ventilation, and autonomic function. *Circulation* 1992;**85**:2119–31.

Feldman AM, Silver MA, Francis GS, *et al.*, PEECH Investigators. Enhanced external counterpulsation improves exercise tolerance in patients with chronic heart failure. *J Am Coll Cardiol* 2006;**48**:1198–205.

Flynn KE, Piña IL, Whellan DJ, *et al.*, HF-ACTION Investigators. Effects of exercise training on health status in patients with chronic heart failure: HF-ACTION randomized controlled trial. *JAMA* 2009;**301**:1451–9.

Gray A, Goodacre S, Newby DE, *et al.*, 3CPO Trialists. Noninvasive ventilation in acute cardiogenic pulmonary edema. *N Engl J Med* 2008;**359**:142–51.

O'Connor CM, Whellan DJ, Lee KL, *et al.*, HF-ACTION Investigators. Efficacy and safety of exercise training in patients with chronic heart failure: HF-ACTION randomized controlled. *JAMA* 2009;**301**:1439–50.

Schmid JP, Noveanu M, Morger C, *et al.* Influence of water immersion, water gymnastics and swimming on cardiac output in patients with heart failure. *Heart* 2007;**93**:722–7.

Disease management programmes

Disease management programmes specifically targeting individuals who have experienced an acute hospital admission related to the syndrome chronic heart failure provide a framework to apply the following:

- Gold-standard diagnosis and evaluation (see Chapter 6.1).
- Pharmacological therapy (see Chapters 6.2 and 6.7).
- Non-pharmacological treatment (see Chapter 6.3).

Definition

Although there is considerable heterogeneity in how these programmes have been developed and subsequently applied, they can be broadly defined as 'systems of coordinated health care specifically designed to optimize the quality of management and subsequent health outcomes of patients with chronic heart failure in a cost-effective manner'.

Evidence base

Early pivotal trials comparing a dedicated approach to heart failure management (applied within a multidisciplinary framework) compared with standard care demonstrated the capacity to both reduce readmissions to hospital (Rich et al. 1995) and indeed prolong survival (Stewart et al. 1999) within 3–6 months of an index hospital admission. Subsequent systematic reviews and meta-analyses have confirmed these benefits overall with the strength of evidence still favouring programmes that apply a multidisciplinary framework (McAlister et al. 2004) with those programmes providing a face-to-face component of management (Sochalski et al. 2009) appearing to be superior to remote management involving either structure telephone care and/or more advanced physiological monitoring (Clark et al. 2007).

Applying disease management in chronic heart failure

The American Heart Association Disease Management Taxonomy Writing Group's scientific statement on categorizing disease management (with the identification of eight key domains) provides a framework for understanding the core principles and components of programmes specifically targeting patients with chronic heart failure (Krumholz et al. 2006).

Patient population

Programmes are broadly directed towards individuals in whom a confirmed diagnosis of chronic heart failure has been established. All patients with chronic heart failure are at inherent risk of recurrent hospitalization, poor quality of life and/or a premature death. However, these programmes are particularly targeted towards those patients who survive an acute hospitalization and assume some responsibility for their own care. This largely excludes patients who are discharged to a high-dependency care environment (e.g. nursing home).

There is a lack of evidence to support programmes that target inherently stable and, therefore, lower risk patients with chronic heart failure (DeBusk et al. 2004).

Alternatively, these programmes appear to benefit patients with both impaired and preserved left ventricular systolic function with associated New York Heart Association Class II, III or IV at hospital discharge. Such patients tend to be older and have multiple co-morbidities.

Recipients

Patients are the major focus for disease management with a strong component of self-care strategies promoted. However, modern programmes increasingly recognize the important role of immediate caregivers and provide specific support to improve or maintain their quality of life.

Given the complexity of management, many programmes also target a patient's usual healthcare team (e.g. their general practitioner/primary care physician) in order to indirectly update them on the gold-standard management of the syndrome.

Intervention component

There are many components inherent to this kind of programme the most important being:

- Pre-discharge planning
- Formal pathways to improve communication within the healthcare team
- Optimization of gold-standard pharmacological therapy (including up-titration of doses to evidence-based levels)
- Application of non-pharmacological strategies—including formal exercise programmes, monitoring weight, and adjusting dietary intake
- Patient (and caregiver) education
- Promotion of self-care
- Increase surveillance for impending crises.

Delivery personnel

Historically, programmes have been predominantly nurse-led or mediated with a broad remit for the nurse to coordinate healthcare activities and ensure effective communication within the healthcare team in order to provide integrated care. They also act as a patient advocate. Specific responsibilities (depending on the level of qualifications and training of the individual) include:

- Non-invasive clinical evaluation.
- Patient education/promotion of self-care activities.
- Initiation and titration of pharmacological therapy (particularly flexible diuretic regimen and up-titration of beta-blockers).

Other key personnel that can form part of a multidisciplinary approach to management include:

- Cardiologist to provide advanced diagnostic techniques and treatment
- General practitioner/primary care physician to provide day-to-day medical management
- Case manager to coordinate healthcare via an agreed plan of management (i.e. following a multidisciplinary team meeting)
- Pharmacist to optimize pharmacological therapy and patient adherence
- Dietician to individualize dietary assessment and advice
- Social worker to coordinate health services, particularly if the patient is depressed and/or has limited social support
- Exercise therapists to develop and supervise an individualized exercise programme.

Method of communication

Historically, programmes have relied on direct patient (and caregiver) contact to deliver the interventional components listed above. Two main forms of face-to-face communication (often supplemented by routine telephone calls and, more recently, electronic mail) have been applied via the following:

- Specialist heart failure clinic, usually located in a tertiary referral hospital where the bulk of the multidisciplinary heart failure team is located
- In the patient's own home with reliance of subsequent community-based contacts in a primary care clinic and local pharmacy.

However, an increasing number of programmes now rely on indirect methods of communication and monitoring (Clark et al. 2007; Inglis et al. 2008). These can incorporate information technology in the form of monitoring of single or multiple biological parameters (e.g. blood pressure, weight, 12-lead ECG, oxygen saturation and/or indices of pulmonary congestion) via the telephone or dedicated digital devices (telemonitoring). Alternatively, they can involve structured telephone contacts using touch phone technology to allow the patient to report their clinical status to a central monitoring station.

Intensity and complexity

The required intensity and complexity of any heart failure programme to achieve optimal health outcomes (relative to standard care) continues to be a point of debate (Clark et al. 2009), particularly given a recent trial from the Netherlands suggesting that neither moderate or intensive disease management in chronic heart failure offered advantages over care provided by a cardiologist with respect to reducing heart failure-related readmissions (Jaarsma et al. 2008). However, most studies focus on a programme's impact on all-cause readmissions (see Clinical outcomes) in recognition of the complexity of the syndrome. Moreover, there was a non-significant (but potentially clinically significant) survival benefit of 15% in favour of the intervention groups in this study (Jaarsma et al. 2008).

The following parameters are considered in establishing and applying a programme relative to available personnel and resources:

- Duration of intervention: most programmes offer active management for 3–6 months post hospital discharge in order to ensure that all areas of need are addressed (e.g. need to enhance a patient's ability to self-care and recognize an impending crisis).
- Frequency: face-to-face contacts are far more time-consuming and costly than telephone contacts. The need for at least one face-to-face contact appears extremely important with scheduled clinic or community visits thereafter dependent on residual issues to be addressed (e.g. need to up-titrate pharmacologic treatment).
- Complexity: the most successful programmes have been those that involve a range of interventions and involve multidisciplinary care (particularly delivered face-to-face). The threshold for applying only 'essential' components of care to achieve optimal outcomes is unknown. Therefore, most programmes apply a combination of those interventions described above.

In order to strike the right balance of intensity and complexity for any individual patient (particularly with considering when to return them to standard care) there are three key parameters to consider:

- Clinical stability: if the patient is unstable and/or readmitted to hospital during follow-up, the intensity of surveillance and contacts is usually maintained or increased.
- Risk profile: if the patient has factors that predispose them to suboptimal management (e.g. non-adherence and/or poor self-care abilities) they are more likely to require more intense management.
- Gold standard pharmacological and non-pharmacological treatments: a programme should always strive to apply gold-standard treatments (within a reasonable time-frame of 3–6 months).

Tele-monitoring techniques, while offering the chance for continuous or periodic clinical data of potential importance, pose the problem of delineation of clinically trivial versus significant (as expressed by sensitivity and specificity) information and the potential need for costly surveillance systems (human or otherwise).

Environment

Heart failure management programmes typically span the hospital setting (index event), outpatient setting (specialist heart failure clinic) to the community (either in the patient's home or via remote monitoring).

Clinical outcomes

The evidence in favour of applying these programmes is built on three key parameters and should be routinely monitored accordingly:

- All-cause mortality
- Readmission to hospital (including that specific to heart failure) both with respect to the proportion readmitted to hospital within a certain time-frame (usually 6 months) and the frequency of readmissions
- Event-free survival from hospitalization or death.

Other key parameters of importance (particularly those that are more orientated towards individual patient outcomes) include:

- Quality of life (both generic and disease specific)
- Mental health status (including depression and cognition)
- Treatment adherence and self-care abilities
- Treatment patterns relative to gold-standard guidelines
- Cost of healthcare.

Patient support: www.heartfailurematters.org (Practical heart failure information for patients, families and caregivers provided by the Heart Failure Association of the European Society of Cardiology).

Healthcare professional support: American Heart Association (www.americanheart.org) Get With the Guidelines—Heart Failure.

References

Clark AM, Savard L, Thompson DR. What is the strength of evidence for heart failure disease-management programs?. J Am Coll Cardiol 2009;54:397–401.

Clark R, Inglis S, et al. Telemonitoring or structured telephone support programmes for patients with chronic heart failure: systematic review and meta-analysis. BMJ 2007;334:942–5.

DeBusk RF, Miller NH, et al. Care management for low-risk patients with heart failure. a randomized controlled trial. Ann Intern Med 2004;141:606–13.

Inglis SC, Clark RA, et al. Structured telephone support or telemonitoring programs for patients with chronic heart failure. Cochrane Database Syst Rev 2008(3):CD007228.

Jaarsma T, van der Wal MH, et al. Effect of moderate or intensive disease management program on outcome in patients with heart failure Coordinating Study Evaluating Outcomes of Advising and Counseling in Heart Failure (COACH). Arch Int Med 2008; 168: 316–24.

Krumholz HM, Currie PM, et al. A taxonomy for disease management: A scientific statement from the American Heart Association disease management taxonomy writing group. Circulation 2006;114:1432–45.

McAlister FA, Stewart S, et al. Multidisciplinary strategies for the management of heart failure patients at high risk for admission: a systematic review of randomized trials. J Am Coll Cardiol 2004;44:810–9.

Rich MW, Beckham V, et al. A multidisciplinary intervention to prevent the readmission of elderly patients with congestive heart failure. N Engl J Med 1995;333:1190–5.

Sochalski J, Jaarsma T, et al. What works in chronic care management: the case of heart failure. Health Affairs 2009;28:179–89.

Stewart S, Marley JE, Horowitz JD. Effects of a multidisciplinary, home-based intervention on unplanned readmissions and survival among patients with chronic congestive heart failure: a randomised controlled study. Lancet 1999;354:1077–83.

Acute heart failure

Definition

Acute heart failure (AHF) is the term used to describe the rapid onset of signs and symptoms of pulmonary congestion and/or peripheral hypoperfusion due to cardiac and/or vascular dysfunction needing urgent therapy. AHF includes both acute exacerbations of chronic heart failure (acutely decompensated chronic heart failure) or appearance of signs and symptoms without a prior history of heart failure (acute *de novo* or new-onset heart failure) (Dickstein et al. 2008; Filippatos and Zannad 2007).

Classification

Many different names and classification schemes have been proposed for AHF. According to the European Society Of Cardiology's most recent guidelines (Dickstein et al. 2008), AHF includes a heterogeneous patient population classified into six distinct clinical conditions:

- Worsening or decompensated chronic heart failure: gradually increased peripheral oedema and/or pulmonary congestion in patients with chronic heart failure.
- Acute pulmonary oedema: severe and rapid pulmonary congestion with low oxygen saturation (<90%) requiring urgent pharmacologic and oxygen therapy and/or ventilatory support.
- Acute hypertensive heart failure: pulmonary congestion in the presence of high systolic blood pressure (SBP), usually in patients with preserved ejection function.
- Cardiogenic shock. pulmonary congestion accompanied by low SBP (<90 mmHg or drop of mean arterial pressure >30 mmHg) in combination with peripheral organ hypoperfusion, i.e. oliguria/anuria.
- Right heart failure: low output condition due to right ventricular dysfunction presenting with elevated systemic venous pressures in the absence of pulmonary congestion.
- AHF due to acute coronary syndromes (ACSs): evidence of pulmonary congestion and/or low cardiac output in the presence of an ACS documented by the clinical picture, ECG and/or positive biomarkers of necrosis (more than 15–20% of patients with an ACS develop heart failure and 20–30% of patients with AHF have evidence of an ACS (Nieminen et al. 2006)).

However, these conditions are not well defined and there is significant overlap among them. Moreover, different names have been proposed for similar classifications. A simple classification scheme (De Luca et al. 2007) that aims to avoid overlap is based on the systolic blood pressure (SBP) at presentation:

- Hypertensive AHF (SBP >140 mmHg): 40–50% of AHF cases; this condition usually involves elderly women with preserved left ventricular ejection fraction (LVEF) and has an in-hospital mortality of usually <5% (Adams et al. 2005).

- Normotensive AHF (SBP 90–140 mmHg): 40–50% of AHF cases; in this group are usually included patients with worsening of chronic heart failure and relatively low left ventricular ejection fraction; in-hospital mortality 8–10% (Tavazzi et al. 2006).
- Hypotensive AHF (SBP <90 mmHg): ~5% of AHF cases; this group also includes patients with cardiogenic shock; in-hospital mortality >15% (Alla et al. 2007).

Precipitating and prognostic factors

The most common factors that predispose to a new episode of AHF are summarized in below (Dickstein et al 2008). Initial evaluation and management of these factors are essential for the clinical stabilization of the patient and for the prevention of new heart failure exacerbations (i.e. surgical correction of valvulopathies, revascularization for underlying coronary artery disease).

The most important factors that predict adverse short- and long-term prognosis (mortality and rehospitalization) in AHF are advanced age, low SBP at presentation, low serum sodium, high BUN and serum creatinine, high serum troponin, and high B-type natriuretic peptide (BNP) or NT-proBNP levels (Fonarow et al. 2005; Daniels and Maisel 2007).

Precipitating factors for AHF episodes

Acute coronary syndromes.
Uncontrolled hypertension.
Arrhythmias.
Infections (e.g. pneumonia).
High output conditions (anaemia, sepsis, thyrotoxicosis).
Acute pulmonary embolism.
Renal dysfunction.
COPD, asthma.
Non-compliance with medical treatment.
Drugs (NSAIDs corticosteroids).
High-salt diet.
Valvular disease.
Acute myocarditis.
Unknown cause.

Clinical and laboratory evaluation

The three major steps of the clinical and laboratory evaluation of patients with suspected AHF are presented in below. Plasma levels of BNP <100 pg/mL and NT-proBNP <400 pg/mL can exclude cardiac causes of dyspnoea in the emergency department, whereas plasma levels of BNP >400 pg/mL and NT-proBNP >2000 pg/mL are compatible with elevated left ventricular filling pressures (Dickstein et al. 2008; Omland 2008). Unexpectedly low plasma levels of natriuretic peptides are present in the following conditions with AHF: flash pulmonary oedema, acute mitral regurgitation, acute pulmonary oedema due to severe mitral stenosis.

Clinical and laboratory evaluation of suspected AHF

Initial evaluation

History (known history of heart disease or heart failure).
Physical examination (assessment of peripheral and pulmonary congestion, evaluation of peripheral perfusion).
Abnormal ECG.
Chest X-ray for congestion.
Abnormal oxygen saturation and/or blood gasses.
Elevated plasma levels of natriuretic peptides*.

Confirmation of diagnosis

Echocardiography.
Right heart catheterization*.

Assessment of aetiology and severity and planning of treatment

Echocardiography.
Coronary angiography.
MRI.
Right heart catheterization*.
Other techniques according to the clinical suspicion.

*See text for the indications and limitations.

Use of pulmonary artery catheter measurements did not improve prognosis in randomized clinical trials but could help in the following situations (Dickstein et al. 2008): (1) for differential diagnosis between a cardiogenic and non-cardiogenic mechanism in complex patients, especially those with concurrent cardiac and pulmonary disease, (2) to guide the use of vasoactive medications in unstable patients not responding to standard therapy. Echocardiography is necessary for all patients with AHF, and especially those with ACS to exclude mechanical complications.

Management

Several agents and interventions have been used for the treatment of AHF but their use is based on expert opinion and not on large randomized trials. Additionally, no drug or intervention has improved the short- or long-term prognosis of AHF patients, although many therapeutic approaches may lead to symptomatic and haemodynamic improvement (Dickstein et al. 2008).

Although there are controversial data in the literature (Masip et al. 2005, 2008; Peacock et al. 2005) regarding the effect of non-invasive ventilation (NIV) on the short-term mortality of AHF patients with pulmonary oedema, clinical evidence suggests that early use (within the first 30 minutes) of this treatment improves symptoms and reduces the need for mechanical ventilation. Non-invasive ventilation

with a positive end expiratory pressure (PEEP) of 5–7.5 cmH$_2$O should be applied first and titrated to clinical response up to 10 cmH$_2$O. The main adverse effects of non-invasive ventilation include: (1) worsening of severe right ventricular failure, (2) drying of the mucous membranes with prolonged, continuous use, (3) CO$_2$ retention, and (4) anxiety or claustrophobia.

Morphine and its analogues should be considered early in the management of non-hypotensive AHF patients admitted with severe pulmonary congestion, especially if they have dyspnoea, anxiety and/or chest pain (Peacock et al. 2005; Dickstein et al. 2008). Intravenous morphine 2.5–5 mg may be administered to AHF patients. This dosing can be repeated if there is no initial response. Although retrospective data suggest an increase in mortality by morphine, it is particularly useful in patients with anxiety on NIV. Some important points for the safe use of this drug are that (1) respiratory efficiency should be monitored; (2) nausea or vomiting are frequent, and antiemetic therapy may be required; and (3) this agent should be avoided in patients with hypotension, bradycardia, advanced AV block or patients with history of severe respiratory disease and hypercapnia.

The dosing, indications, main adverse effects and various limitations of IV vasodilators used for the management of hypertensive and normotensive AHF patients (SBP >90 mmHg) are summarized in Table 6.5.1 (Hollenberg 2007; Dickstein et al. 2008).

Intravenous loop diuretics should be used for the alleviation of symptoms in AHF patients presenting with volume overload and congestion. These agents may cause electrolyte disturbances and hypovolaemia and should be administered carefully in patients with hypotension (<90 mmHg). Furthermore, hypotension, hyponatraemia and acidosis can cause a degree of resistance to their effects. Thus, IV diuretics should be combined with other therapies such as vasodilators or inotropes according to the underlying conditions and SBP levels (Kirk et al. 2009). Table 6.5.2 summarizes the recommended diuretics and their dosing used for the treatment of congestion in AHF.

Classical inotropic agents (beta-agonists, phosphodiesterase inhibitors) act in a cAMP-dependent manner and have been extensively used in the management of AHF exacerbations that are accompanied by low output state and marked hypoperfusion of peripheral tissues (Parissis et al. 2007; Dickstein et al. 2008). These drugs have been also used as a short-term 'bridge' to other forms of destination therapy, such as emergency cardiac operations or cardiac transplantation, or as prolonged infusions for the long-term treatment of patients with end-stage chronic heart failure resistant to conventional therapies (Parissis et al. 2007). Although this therapy usually causes a short-term symptomatic and haemodynamic improvement, accumulating evidence suggests that they may lead to an adverse long-term prognosis. Consequently, newer inotropic agents with cAMP-independent mechanisms of action, and

Table 6.5.1 Dosing, indications and adverse effects of iv vasodilators in AHF management (SBP >90 mmHg) (modified from Dickstein *et al.* 2008)

Drug	Indication	Regimen	Adverse effects	Limitations
Nitroglycerine	Pulmonary oedema Pulmonary congestion	Start with 10–20 µg/min Increase up to 200 µg/min	Hypotension Headache	Tolerance is common after 24–48 hours
Isosorbite dinitrate	Pulmonary oedema Pulmonary congestion	Initial regimen 1 mg/hour Increase up to 10 mg/hour	Hypotension Headache	Tolerance as in nitroglycerine
Nitroprusside	Acute hypertensive congestion Congestion due to acute MR	Starting 0.3 mg/kg/min Increase up to 5 mg/kg/min	Hypotension Isocyanate toxicity	Light sensitive. Arterial line is usually required for blood pressure monitoring
Nesiritide	Pulmonary oedema Pulmonary congestion	Bolus 2 µg/Kg plus continuous infusion 0.015–0.030 µg/kg/min	Hypotension	Not currently available in most European countries. Increased rate of adverse events in metaanalyses

which do not increase intracellular calcium levels have been used in AHF (Parissis *et al.* 2005; De Luca *et al.* 2008). Levosimendan is a calcium sensitizer (not approved by the US FDA), which is currently used in several countries for the treatment of patients with symptoms of low cardiac output AHF, secondary to cardiac systolic dysfunction, without severe hypotension. In clinical trials it did not improve mortality compared with dobutamine, but could be more useful than beta-agonists in the management of AHF patients who are on beta-blocker therapy at hospital admission (Mebazaa *et al.* 2007).

Potential therapeutic algorithms of AHF based on SBP levels at presentation are presented in Figs 6.5.1–3.

Table 6.5.2 Indications, dosing and adverse effects of diuretics in AHF management (modified from Dickstein *et al.* 2008)

Drug	Indication	Dosing	Adverse effects	Recommendations
Furosemide	Severe fluid retention Moderate fluid retention	40–100 mg iv bolus 5–40 mg/h (continuous infusion) 20–40 mg iv bolus	Hypovolaemia Electrolyte disturbances Worsening of renal function	Uptitrate dosing of diuretics according to clinical response Check frequently serum sodium, potassium, magnesium, BUN creatinine
Torasemide	Fluid retention	10–100 oral	Electrolyte disturbances	
Bumetanide	Fluid retention	0.5–4 mg oral or IV	Electrolyte disturbances	
Thiazides	Fluid retention refractory to loop diuretics	50–100 mg oral (combined with high doses of loop diuretics)	Severe hypokalaemia	If there is resistance to this combination consider IV inotropes and/or peripheral haemofiltration
Metolazone	Fluid retention refractory to loop diuretics	25–100 mg oral	Severe hypokalaemia	Consider this agent if the creatinine clearance is less than 30 mL/min

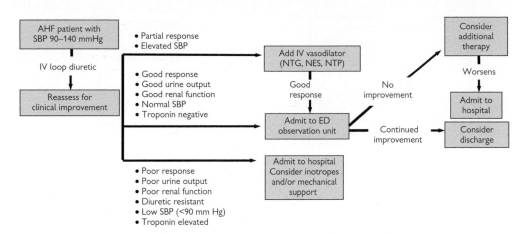

Fig. 6.5.1 Treatment algorithm for the AHF patient with systolic blood pressure 90–140 mmHg at ED. Modified from Kirk JD, et al. 2009. AHF, acute heart failure; ED, emergency department; IV, intravenous; NES, nesiritide; NTG, nitroglycerin; SBP, systolic blood pressure.

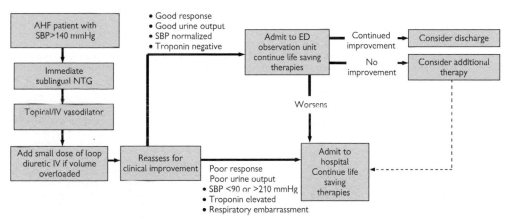

Fig. 6.5.2 Treatment algorithm for the AHF patient with elevated systolic blood pressure (>140 mmHg) at ED. Modified from Dickstein et al 2008. AHF, acute heart failure; ED, emergency department; IV, intravenous; NTG, nitroglycerine; SBP, systolic blood pressure.

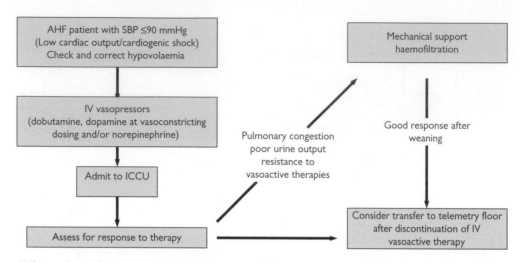

AHF, acute heart failure; ICCU, intensive cardiac care unit; IV, intravenous; SBP, systolic blood pressure.

Fig. 6.5.3 Treatment algorithm for the AHF patient with low systolic blood pressure (<90 mmHg) at ED (modified from Kirk JD et al 2009).

References

Adams KF Jr, Fonarow GC, Emerman CL, et al. ADHERE Scientific Advisory Committee and Investigators. Characteristics and outcomes of patients hospitalized for heart failure in the United States: rationale, design, and preliminary observations from the first 100,000 cases in the Acute Decompensated Heart Failure National Registry (ADHERE). Am Heart J 2005;**149**:209–216.

Alla F, Zannad F, Filippatos G. Epidemiology of acute heart failure syndromes. Heart Fail Rev 2007;**12**:91–5.

Daniels L, Maisel A. Natriuretic peptides. J Am Coll Cardiol 2007;**50**:2357–2368.

De Luca L, Fonarow G, Adams K, et al. Acute heart failure syndromes: clinical scenarios and pathophysiologic targets for therapy. Heart Fail Rev 2007;**12**:97–104.

De Luca L, Mebazaa A, Filippatos G, et al. Overview of emerging pharmacologic agents for acute heart failure syndromes. Eur J Heart Fail 2008;**10**:201–13.

Dickstein K, Cohen-Solal A, Filippatos G, et al. ESC guidelines for the diagnosis and treatment of acute and chronic heart failure 2008: the Task Force for the diagnosis and treatment of acute and chronic heart failure 2008 of the European Society of Cardiology. Developed in collaboration with the Heart Failure Association of the ESC (HFA) and endorsed by the European Society of Intensive Care Medicine (ESICM). Eur Heart J 2008;**29**:2388–2442.

Filippatos G, Zannad F. An introduction to acute heart failure syndromes: definition and classification. Heart Fail Rev 2007;**12**:87–90.

Fonarow GC, Adams KF Jr, Abraham WT, et al. Risk stratification for in-hospital mortality in acutely decompensated heart failure: classification and regression tree analysis. JAMA 2005;**293**:572–580.

Gray A, Goodacre S, Newby DE, et al., 3CPO Trialists. Non-invasive ventilation in acute cardiogenic pulmonary edema. N Engl J Med 2008;**359**:142–151.

Hollenberg SM. Vasodilators in acute heart failure. Heart Fail Rev 2007;**12**:143–147.

Kirk JD, Parissis JT, Filippatos G. Pharmacologic stabilization and management of acute heart failure syndromes in the emergency department. Heart Fail Clin 2009;**5**:43–54.

Masip J, Mebazaa A, Filippatos GS. Noninvasive ventilation in acute cardiogenic pulmonary edema. N Engl J Med 2008;**359**:2068–9.

Masip J, Roque M, Sánchez B, et al. Noninvasive ventilation in acute cardiogenic pulmonary edema: systematic review and meta-analysis. JAMA. 2005;**294**:3124–30.

Mebazaa A, Nieminen MS, Packer M, et al., SURVIVE Investigators. Levosimendan vs dobutamine for patients with acute decompensated heart failure: the SURVIVE Randomized Trial. JAMA 2007;**297**:1883–91.

Nieminen MS, Brutsaert D, Dickstein K, et al. EuroHeart Failure Survey II (EHFS II): a survey on hospitalized acute heart failure patients: description of population. Eur Heart J 2006;**27**:2725–2736.

Omland T. Advances in congestive heart failure management in the intensive care unit: B-type natriuretic peptides in evaluation of acute heart failure. Crit Care Med 2008;**36**(1 Suppl):S17–27.

Parissis JT, Farmakis D, Nieminen M. Classical inotropes and new cardiac enhancers. Heart Fail Rev. 2007;**12**:149–56.

Parissis JT, Filippatos G, Farmakis D, et al. Levosimendan for the treatment of acute heart failure syndromes. Expert Opin Pharmacother 2005;**6**:2741–51.

Peacock WHJ, Diercks D, Fonarow G, Emerman C. Morphine for acute decompensated heart failure: valuable adjunct or a historical remnant?. Acad Emerg Med 2005;**12**:97b–98b.

Tavazzi L, Maggioni AP, Lucci D, et al. Nationwide survey on acute heart failure in cardiology ward services in Italy. Eur Heart J 2006;**27**:1207–15.

Heart failure with a normal left ventricular ejection fraction

It has been realized for some time that not all patients with the symptoms and signs of heart failure have a depressed left ventricular (LV) ejection fraction. Because it was assumed that systolic function was normal it was considered the primary problem in these patients was in diastole alone and the syndrome was called diastolic heart failure or heart failure with preserved systolic function. However, it is now clear that systolic function is not entirely normal and therefore heart failure with a normal left ventricular ejection fraction (HFNEF) is the preferred term to diastolic heart failure—the term diastolic heart failure implies that the primary or dominant abnormality is in diastole alone to which therapy should be targeted, which may be misguided. Recent research suggests that there are subtle abnormalities of both systole and diastole function in HFNEF.

Epidemiology

Many recent studies have found that approximately 50% patients with a clinical diagnosis of heart failure will have a normal LV ejection fraction with a normal size LV. Patients with HFNEF typically tend to be older, female, and have a history of hypertension and other co-morbidities such as obesity, diabetes, mild coronary artery disease, renal failure, anaemia, and atrial fibrillation (Maeder and Kaye 2009). However, the prognosis of HFNEF is similar to those with heart failure and reduced EF (HFREF) (Owan et al. 2006).

Pathophysiology (Sanderson 2007)

Traditional concepts have considered increased myocardial stiffness and delayed relaxation to be critical (Westermann et al. 2008). Although these are clearly involved, newer studies have shown a more complicated picture with evidence of reduced myocardial systolic strain, reduced ventricular systolic rotation at rest (which fails to increase normally on exercise), reduced mitral annular motion in systole and diastole, and delayed ventricular untwisting associated with reduced left ventricular suction (Tan et al. 2009). Impaired atrial function on exercise may also contribute to breathlessness. Thus, HFNEF is not an isolated disorder of diastole and the normal close relation between systole and diastole is disrupted. Increased systolic ventricular and arterial stiffening, i.e. deranged ventriculo-arterial coupling, may contribute to the pathophysiology of HFNEF by exaggerating hypertensive response on exercise. Other factors such as exercise induced pulmonary hypertension, chronotropic incompetence, and renal dysfunction may also be involved. Metabolic abnormalities of the myocyte may underlie some of the abnormalities but the major pathological changes are in the extracellular matrix (ECM), with increased collagen and change in collagen type, which is stiffer (Querejeta et al. 2004). Hypertension, diabetes, and myocardial ischaemia may all affect the extracellular matrix and collagen quantity and quality. The changes in the ECM may have an important impact on ventricular rotation and untwisting, recoil, and therefore early diastolic filling and upon the important action of ventricular suction which is vital for rapid ventricular filling at higher heart rates. It is not clear if HFNEF evolves into HFREF although hypertension is a common cause of HFREF in Asia and Africa possibly because of poor treatment (Sanderson 2007).

Clinical features

There are few differences between HFNEF and HFREF except that HFNEF patients tend to be older and female. Hypertension is more common, whereas a history of myocardial infarction is more common in HFREF. The main differences between HFNEF and HFREF are shown in Table 6.6.1. The main echocardiographic difference is the presence of ventricular chamber enlargement due to remodelling in HFREF.

Diagnosis

Clinical diagnosis can be difficult in an elderly breathless individual who is also obese, diabetic, with some degree of lung disease and unfitness. The recent updated European Society of Cardiology guidelines suggest that the diagnosis of HFNEF depends on:

1 clinical symptoms and signs of heart failure
2 left ventricular ejection fraction >50%
3 a non-dilated LV (LV end-diastolic volume <97 mL/m^2)
4 abnormalities in LV diastolic function/filling (Fig. 6.6.1) (Paulus et al. 2007).

Tissue Doppler imaging can provide a non-invasive method for estimating LV filling pressures (the ratio E/e´), although recently doubt has arisen about this index in HFREF (Nagueh et al. 1997; Mullens et al. 2009). However, the simplest measure is the left atrial volume index (LAVI) as an enlarged LAVI suggests a chronically raised LV end-diastolic pressure (Lim et al. 2006). The presence of LVH

Table 6.6.1 Comparison of clinical features of HFREF and HFNEF

	Heart failure with reduced ejection fraction (HFREF)	Heart failure with normal ejection fraction (HFNEF)
Gender	M>F	F>M
Age	50–70	60–80
Aetiology	Myocardial infarction Idiopathic DCM	Hypertension Diabetes Atrial fibrillation Transient ischaemia
Clinical progress	Persistent HF	Often episodic HF
Ventricular remodelling (increased volume)	+++	0
LV hypertrophy	+/–	++
Peak mitral inflow velocity pattern	RFP	ARP
Peak mitral annular velocity	Markedly reduced	Moderately reduced
LA volume index	Increased	Increased

DCM, dilated cardiomyopathy; HF, heart failure; RFP, restrictive filling pattern; ARP, abnormal relaxation pattern.

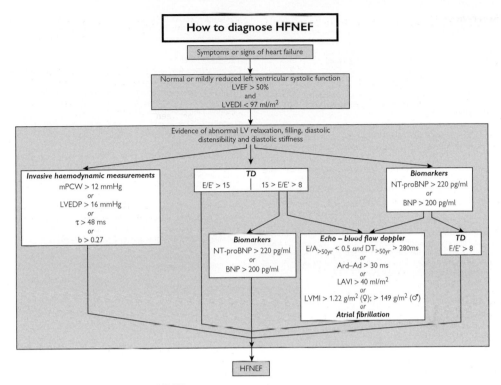

Fig. 6.6.1 Algorithm on how to diagnose HFNEF.

and an increased LAVI in a breathlessness patient strongly suggests the likelihood of HFNEF. BNP and NT-proBNP <100 and <120 pg/mL respectively are helpful to exclude the diagnosis, especially in the presence of indeterminate diastolic function based on tissue Doppler and strain echocardiography.

Treatment

Because all major therapeutic trials in heart failure were based on an entry criteria of a reduced LVEF, HFNEF patients were excluded and consequently there is very little evidence on which to base treatment. In the 'Effect of candesartan in patients with chronic heart failure and pre-served left-ventricular ejection fraction, the CHARM-Preserved Trial' it was found that the angiotensin receptor antagonist candesartan modestly reduced hospital admissions for heart failure but did not significantly affect mortality in patients with heart failure with a normal ejection fraction (Yusuf et al. 2003). Another recent study also evaluated the effect of the angiotensin receptor blocker (ARB) irbesartan on mortality and cardiovascular morbidity in 4128 patients with heart failure with a normal ejection fraction (I-PRESERVE trial) (Massie et al. 2008). It found no benefit of irbesartan over placebo in reducing mortality or morbidity from cardiovascular disease. However, a small randomized controlled trial found that diuretics alone reduced symptoms and improved quality of life significantly, but that adding ramipril or irbesartan was not more efficacious (Yip et al. 2008). These negative results are surprising.

Fibrosis of the left ventricle is increased with LV hypertrophy and hypertension. Angiotensin-converting enzyme inhibitors and angiotensin receptor blockers can block the fibrogenic action of angiotensin experimentally and have been shown to reduce fibrosis in patients with hypertension. Fibrosis and altered collagen in LV hypertrophy may have a deleterious effect on overall myocardial architecture, particularly ventricular twist and torsion. Nevertheless, the reduction of fibrosis may be an important therapeutic target, and the ongoing studies of spironolactone in heart failure with a normal ejection fraction will be interesting. In essence, treatment is therefore symptomatic with diuretics for relief of breathlessness and control of blood pressure with usually an angiotensin-converting enzyme inhibitor (ACEI) or ARB. A beta-blocker may be helpful by reducing heart rate on exercise to allow more time for filling and will obviously be indicated if there is associated angina. Calcium channel blockers (CCBs) have also be suggested as they may in theory improve myocardial relaxation but there is no good evidence for benefit in HFNEF. Diltiazem may be useful for control of ventricular rate with atrial fibrillation.

Conclusion

HFNEF appears to be a relatively common cause for heart failure especially in elderly people and has a mixture of causes and pathophysiological mechanisms involving both diastole and systole, and probably differing in individual patients. Treatment is still largely empirical.

References

Lim TK, Ashrafian H, Dwivedi G, *et al.* Increased LAVI is an independent predictor of raised serum natriuretic peptide in patients with suspected heart failure but normal LVEF: implication for diagnosis of DHF. *Eur J Heart Fail* 2006;**8**:38–45.

Maeder MT, Kaye DM. Heart failure with a normal ejection fraction. *J Am Coll Cardiol* 2009;**53**:905–18.

Massie BM, Carson PE, McMurray JJ, *et al.* Irbesartan in patients with heart failure and preserved ejection fraction. *N Engl J Med* 2008;**359**:2456–67.

Mullens W, Borowski AG, Curtin RJ, *et al.* Tissue Doppler imaging in the estimation of intracardiac filling pressure in decompensated patients with advanced systolic heart failure. *Circulation* 2009;**119**: 62–70.

Nagueh SF, Middleton KJ, Kopelen HA, *et al.* Doppler tissue imaging a non-invasive technique for evaluation of LV relaxation and estimation of filling pressures. *J Am Coll Cardiol* 1997;**30**:1527–33.

Owan TE, Hodge DO, Herges RM, Jacobsen SJ, Roger VL, Redfield MM. Trends in prevalence and outcome of heart failure with preserved ejection fraction. *N Engl J Med* 2006;**355**:251–9.

Paulus WJ, Tschope C, Sanderson JE, *et al.* How to diagnose diastolic heart failure: a consensus statement on the diagnosis of heart failure with a normal ejection fraction by the Heart failure and Echocardiography associations of the European Society of cardiology. *Eur Heart J* 2007;**28**:2539–50.

Querejeta R, Lopez B, Gonzalez A, *et al.* Increased collagen type I synthesis in patients with heart failure of hypertensive origin: relation to myocardial fibrosis. *Circulation* 2004;**110**:1263–68.

Sanderson JE. Heart failure with a normal ejection fraction. *Heart* 2007;**93**:155–8.

Tan YT, Wenzelburger F, Li E, *et al.* The pathophysiology of heart failure with normal ejection fraction: exercise echocardiography reveals complex abnormalities of both systolic and diastolic ventricular function involving torsion, untwist and longitudinal motion. *J Am Coll Cardiol* 2009;**54**:36–46.

Westermann D, Kasner M, Steendijk P, *et al.* Role of left ventricular stiffness in heart failure with normal ejection fraction. *Circulation* 2008;**117**:2051–60.

Yip GW, Wang M, Wang T, *et al.* The Hong Kong diastolic heart failure study: a randomized controlled trial of diuretics, irbesartan and ramipril on quality of life, exercise capacity, left ventricular global and regional function in heart failure with a normal ejection fraction. *Heart* 2008;**94**:573–80.

Yusuf S, Pfeffer MA, Swedberg K, *et al.*, for the CHARM Investigators and Committees. Effect of candesartan in patients with chronic heart failure and preserved left-ventricular ejection fraction: the CHARM-Preserved Trial. *Lancet* 2003;**363**:777–81.

Systolic heart failure: pharmacological treatment

Pharmacological treatment

Although there is no consensus for the exact definition of systolic or diastolic heart failure, the distinction is made on the basis of a left ventricular ejection fraction below or above 40%. The ultimate goals of treatment for systolic heart failure are to reduce symptoms, improve exercise tolerance, decrease hospitalization, and prevent mortality. The mainstay of treatment is pharmacology based although lifestyle modification, device implantation, and heart transplantation may also be needed in selected cases. Pharmacological agents can be categorized as symptomatic relief during acute decompensation or disease modification. Commonly used medications are shown in Table 6.7.1.

Symptomatic relief agents (acute decompensation)

Diuretics

- Mechanism: they interfere with the sodium retention in heart failure by inhibiting the reabsorption of sodium or chloride at specific sites in the renal tubules. This will reduce systemic vascular resistance, arterial pressure, ventricular end-diastolic pressures, cardiac work, and myocardial oxygen consumption and thus increase cardiac output and cardiac efficiency.
- Diuretics are essential treatment for symptomatic relief in patients with decompensating heart failure.
- Lower daily doses are used in maintenance therapy.

Table 6.7.1 Dosage of drugs

Drug	Doses per day	Initial dose	Target dose
Symptomatic relief			
Diuretics			
Frusemide	1–4	IV 40 mg po 40 mg	*360 mg
Metolazone	1 po	2.5 mg	*20 mg
Vasodilators			
Nitroprusside	IV infusion	5 µg/min	*200 µg/min
Nitroglycerin	IV infusion	5–10 µg/min	*400 µg/min
Inotropes			
Dobutamine	IV infusion	2.5 µg/kg/min	*15 µg/kg/min
Dopamine	IV infusion	3–10 µg/kg/min	*50 µg/kg/min
Milrinone	IV infusion	0.375 µg/kg/min	*0.75 µg/kg/min
Calcium-sensitizing agents			
Levosimendin	IV infusion	0.1 µg/kg/min	*0.2 µg/kg/min
Digitalis			
Digoxin	1 po	62.5 µg	*0.25 mg
Disease-modifying agents (po)			
Beta-blockers			
Metoprolol CR/XL	1	12.5 mg	200 mg
Bisoprolol	1	1.25 mg	10 mg
Carvedilol	2	3.125 mg	100 mg
ACE inhibitor			
Captopril	3	6.25 mg	150 mg
Enalapril	2	2.5 mg	20–40 mg
Perindopril	1	2.0 mg	8 mg
Ramipril	1 or 2	2.5 mg	10 mg
Lisinopril	1	2.5 mg	20-35 mg
Trandolapril	1	1.0 mg	4 mg
ARBs			
Candesartan	1	4 mg	32 mg
Losartan	1	50 mg	150 mg
Valsartan	2	40 mg	320 mg
Aldosterone blockers			
Spirolonactone	1 or 2	12.5 mg	50 mg
Epleronone	1	25 mg	50 mg
Hydralazine-isosorbide dinatrate			
Hydralazine	2 or 3	25 mg	225 mg
Isosorbide dinitrate	2 or 3	20 mg	120 mg

*Maximum target dosage; IV, intravenous; po, per os.

- Patient's fluid balance as well as body weight should be monitored for adjustment of dosage.
- Commonly used diuretics in systolic heart failure patients include: loop-diuretics (e.g. frusemide) and thiazide group (metolazone).
- Intravenous therapy may be required in patients not responding well to oral diuretics.
- Levels of electrolytes and renal function should be monitored because of risk of hyponatraemia, hypo/hyperkalaemia and deterioration in renal function.
- Side effects: electrolyte disturbances, hypovolaemia, hypotension, gout.

Vasodilator
- Mechanism: decrease preload and afterload leading to increased cardiac output. Increase coronary perfusion for ischemic heart disease patients.
- Commonly used drugs include nitroprusside and nitroglycerine.
- Cautious use in patients with systolic blood pressure <90 mmHg.
- Close monitoring of haemodynamics is essential
- Contraindication: hypotension.
- Adverse effects: hypotension, tolerance.

Inotropes
- Mechanism: transient increase in cardiac output by stimulating beta-1 adrenergic receptor in the heart or increase in myocardial inotropy by inhibiting degradation of cyclic AMP.
- Commonly used drugs include dobutamine, milrinone, and dopamine.
- Use in patients with systolic blood pressure <90 mmHg, have symptomatic hypotension despite adequate filling pressure, or are unresponsive to, or intolerant of, intravenous vasodilators.
- Accompanied by continuous or frequent blood pressure monitoring and continuous monitoring of cardiac rhythm.
- If symptomatic hypotension or worsening tachyarrhythmias develop during administration, discontinuation or dose reduction should be considered.
- Adverse effects: precipitate heart failure, ventricular arrhythmia.

Calcium sensitizing agents
- Mechanism: improves cardiac contractility by binding to troponin-C in cardiomyocytes. It also has vasodilatory effect mediated through ATP-sensitive potassium channel. Increases cardiac output; reduces peripheral and pulmonary vascular resistance.
- Reserved for patients with acute decompensated heart failure.
- Commonly used drug is levosimendan.
- Haemodynamic response lasts for several days.
- When systolic blood pressure is less than 100, loading dose can be omitted.
- Associated with decrease in blood pressure and increase in heart rate.
- Contraindication: hypotension, renal failure.
- Adverse effects: hypotension, tachycardia, renal impairment, arrhythmia.

Digitalis
- Mechanism: it inhibits the Na,K-ATPase pump in myocardial cells. Increased intracellular sodium promotes sodium–calcium exchange, leading to a rise in the intracellular calcium concentration. This results in improved isolated myocyte contractile performance and overall left ventricular systolic function. Parasympathetic activation for atrioventricular nodal suppression.
- Commonly used drug is digoxin.
- Clinical studies showed that digoxin may relieve symptoms but does not reduce mortality.
- In patients with concurrent atrial fibrillation, digoxin may be used as a rate controlling agent.
- For patients in sinus rhythm with refractory symptoms despite optimal disease modifying agents.
- Therapeutic serum concentration between 0.6 and 1.2 ng/mL.
- Risk of toxicity is increased in the presence of hypokalaemia.
- Contraindications: renal failure, bradyarrhythmias, Wolf–Parkinson–White syndrome.
- Adverse effects: bradycardia, heart block, confusion, nausea, anorexia, disturbance of colour vision.

Disease-modifying agents
Beta-blockers
- Mechanism: long-term activation of the sympathetic nervous system exerts deleterious effects that can be antagonized by the use of beta-blockers. Beta-blockers inhibit the adverse effects of the sympathetic nervous system, and these effects outweigh their negative inotropic effects.
- Beta-blockers are essential first-line therapy for patients with systolic heart failure.
- There are three beta-blockers with proven benefits in chronic heart failure, including metoprolol controlled release/extended release (CR/XL), bisoprolol and carvedilol.
- Treatment should be initiated only when patient is out of acute pulmonary oedema.
- For patients that are already taking beta-blockers, it should be continued during episodes of decompensation unless patient had compromised haemodynamics or systemic under perfusion.
- Treatment improves systolic function, reduced rate of hospital admission and reduces mortality by 34% when used in conjunction with other disease modifying agents.
- Contraindications: peripheral artery disease, asthma, heart block, sick sinus syndrome, sinus bradycardia.
- Adverse effects: hypotension, bradycardia, heart block, fatigue, worsening of heart failure symptoms.

Angiotensin-converting enzyme (ACE) inhibitors
- Mechanism: inhibition of the renin–angiotensin–aldosterone system by inhibiting conversion of angiotensin I to angiotensin II.
- Use of an ACE inhibitor represents the cardinal pharmacological treatment for systolic heart failure.
- Commonly used drugs include captopril, enalapril, lisinopril, ramipril, perindopril, trandolapril.
- It should be initiated once diagnosis is established and should be continued indefinitely.

- Treatment with ACE inhibitors reduces ventricular size, improves LVEF, functional class, heart failure decompensation, and mortality.
- One of the limiting side-effects is bradykinin-induced cough.
- ACE inhibitors are recommended for all patients with heart failure irrespective of cause.
- Contraindications: hyperkalaemia, renal failure, bilateral renal artery stenosis.
- Adverse effects: hypotension, worsening of renal function, hyperkalaemia, angioedema, cough.

Angiotensin receptor blockers (ARBs)
- Mechanism: inhibition of the renin–angiotensin–aldosterone system by inhibiting angiotensin II receptor without accumulation of kinins.
- The ARBs have similar efficacy as ACEI in systolic heart failure.
- Commonly used drugs include candesartan, valsartan, and losartan.
- Less cough as a side-effect, due to selective blockade of the angiotensin II receptor.
- ARBs are less well-proven than ACE inhibitors and therefore used as an alternative when patient develop intractable cough from ACE inhibitors.
- ARBs may also be used in conjunction with beta-blockers in refractory symptomatic patients.
- Contraindication: hyperkalaemia, renal failure, bilateral renal artery stenosis.
- Adverse effects: hypotension, worsening of renal function, hyperkalaemia.

Aldosterone antagonist
- Mechanism: Inhibiting renin–angiotensin–aldosterone system at the receptor for aldosterone.

- Commonly used drugs include spirolonactone, eplerenone.
- Should be considered in symptomatic patients with left ventricular ejection fraction of less than 35%.
- Reduce hospital admission for worsening heart failure and increase survival when added to existing therapy including ACE inhibitor and beta-blockers.
- Important to monitor renal function and serum potassium level.
- Contraindications: hyperkalaemia, renal failure.
- Adverse effects: worsening of renal function, hyperkalaemia, gynaecomastia (spironolactone).

Hydralazine and isosorbide dinitrate
- Mechanism: vasodilatory effect reducing preload and afterload.
- Studies have suggested that African American patients respond better to hydralazine isosorbide dinitrate than to ACE inhibitors.
- Can be used as an alternative for patients that are intolerable or contraindicated to ACE inhibitors and ARBs.
- Reduces heart failure hospitalization, improves quality of life and reduces mortality.
- Contraindications: hypotension, lupus syndrome, severe renal failure.
- Adverse effects: symptomatic hypotension(dizziness), arthalgia/muscle aches.
- Conclusions.
- Pharmacological treatment of systolic heart failure requires careful selection of patients depending on clinical condition.
- The aim of treatment should be directed at both symptomatic relief and modifying the disease process.
- The algorithm of treatment is shown in Fig. 6.7.1.

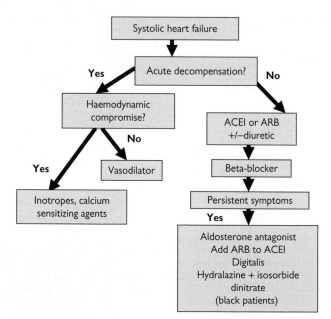

Fig. 6.7.1 Algorithm for treatment of systolic heart failure.

Further reading

Dickstein K, Cohen-Solal A, Filippatos G, et al., Task Force for Diagnosis and Treatment of Acute and Chronic Heart Failure 2008 of European Society of Cardiology. ESC Guidelines for the diagnosis and treatment of acute and chronic heart failure 2008: Developed in collaboration with the Heart Failure Association of the ESC (HFA) and endorsed by the European Society of Intensive Care Medicine (ESICM). *Eur Heart J* 2008;2388–442.

Hunt SA, Abraham WT, Chin MH, et al., American College of Cardiology Foundation; American Heart Association. 2009 Focused update incorporated into the ACC/AHA 2005 Guidelines for the Diagnosis and Management of Heart Failure in Adults A Report of the American College of Cardiology Foundation/American Heart Association Task Force on Practice Guidelines Developed in Collaboration With the International Society for Heart and Lung Transplantation. *J Am Coll Cardiol* 2009;**53**:e1–e90.

McMurray JV. Systolic heart failure. *N Engl J Med* 2010; **362**:228–38.

Acute myocarditis

Acute myocarditis is an inflammatory disease of the myocardium. It can be defined either in a strictly histological sense by a 'cellular inflammatory process of the myocardium with necrosis of cardiomyocytes' (Aretz 1987), or in a broader sense clinically as an acute onset of cardiac symptoms highly suspicious for myocardial inflammation in patients found not to have an other reason for those symptoms.

Epidemiology

The incidence of myocarditis is difficult to establish, as symptoms vary and are often unspecific. Evidence of myocarditis can be found in 1–9% of routine autopsy cases and in 17–19% of those performed for unexplained sudden cardiac death in young people, emphasizing the importance of myocarditis as a cause of sudden cardiac death. The prevalence of histological inflammation in recent-onset idiopathic dilated cardiomyopathy varies widely and has been estimated as approximately 10% of analysed endomyocardial biopsies. In a homogeneous population of young military servicemen, the incidence of myocarditis was reported 0.17 per 1000 man-years, but the real numbers are expected to be substantially higher due to the often subclinical presentation of acute myocarditis and misinterpretation of unspecific symptoms. The overall incidence of myocarditis in viral infections is estimated as 3–6%.

Aetiology

Aetiologies include viruses, protozoa, bacteria, fungi, toxins, drugs, and myocardial involvement caused by systemic autoimmune diseases, but often the underlying cause cannot be identified. Although virtually any microbial agent can cause myocardial inflammation and dysfunction, bacterial infections are rare in Western countries, and viral forms are considered the most common cause nowadays (Liu and Schultheiss 2008). Ten to 15% of virus-related myocarditis are caused by enteroviruses. Analysis of endomyocardial biopsies employing molecular biology techniques has also identified, with geographical differences and varying degrees of frequency, erythrovirus genotypes 1 and 2, human herpesvirus type 6, adenoviruses, human immune deficiency virus (HIV), cytomegalovirus (CMV), herpes simplex type 2 virus, and hepatitis C virus in the myocardium. Although viral genomes can be detected in >50% of patients with clinically suspected myocarditis, virus loads are often low and in these cases clinical importance remains doubtful.

Other infectious agents including bacteria (e.g. tuberculous perimyocarditis), protozoa (e.g. *Trypanosoma cruzi*, Chagas' disease), and fungi may account for the majority of infectious cases in non-developed areas. Chagas' disease is the most frequent non-viral myocardial infection limited to Central and South America, particularly Brazil and Argentina.

Non-infectious causes of myocarditis
Allergic/toxic
- Drugs (doxorubicin, herceptin, antibiotics (penicillin), sulphonamide, methyldopa; alcohol, cocaine)
- Vaccine related (small pox, influenza)
- Radiation.

Autoimmune and infiltrative diseases
- Systemic lupus erythematodes
- Other connective tissue diseases
- Granulomatous diseases (sarcoidosis, tuberculosis, lepromatosis)
- Vasculitis (Churg–Strauss)
- Giant cell myocarditis
- Amyloidosis (heart involvement in 6 out of 22 subtypes)
- Haemochromatosis
- Rheumatic carditis
- Haematological disorders (eosinophilic syndrome)
- Sepsis
- Kawasaki disease
- Malignancies.

Clinical approach
History: key points
A myocarditis has to be suspected in patients with a recent and sudden onset of symptoms of chest pain or heart failure, with or without arrhythmias, when other specific cardiomyopathies, other cardiac diseases, or systemic diseases with cardiac involvement are unknown. In the majority of cases the acute disease will afflict a previously healthy individual.
- Acute myocarditis may be preceded by a:
  - History of viral illness (50–60%)
  - Pulmonal or gastrointestinal infection
  - Recent intake of respective drugs
  - Vaccination.

Examination
Physical examination can reveal signs of heart failure, e.g. peripheral or lung oedema, a third heart sound, tachypnoea, dyspnoea at rest or at exercise, or signs of rhythm disturbances (tachycardia, arrhythmia, extrasystoles). A chronic cough may be present, suggestive of pulmonary venous congestion. Neck veins may be prominent, together with hepatomegaly secondary to elevated systemic venous pressure. But often, the examination remains inconclusive.

Signs and symptoms
- Clinical presentation ranges from mild 'flu-like' symptoms with no haemodynamic consequences, to congestive heart failure, ventricular dysfunction, and arrhythmias. The prevailing symptoms develop with a variable delay after the viral illness, so that fatigue, weakness, chest pain or dyspnoea are initially not recognized as symptoms of an underlying infectious heart disease.

Frequent signs and symptoms are:
- Sudden or continuous progression of heart failure due to diastolic or systolic dysfunction with fatigue, weakness, loss of appetite, dyspnoea, orthopnoea, oedema, congestion, hepatomegalia, embolic events.
- Infarction-like presentation with sudden onset of chest pain, ST-segment elevations, positive creatine kinase (CK)/CKMB and troponins with normal or regionally or globally impaired wall motion.
- Arrhythmias ranging from sinus tachycardia at rest or at exercise to ventricular extrasystoles, and ventricular

tachycardia. Bradycardia and third-degree AV block or ventricular fibrillation may cause a syncope or sudden cardiac death as first manifestation of acute myocarditis.

Investigations

At first, cardiac and systemic diseases with similar presentation need to be excluded. When myocarditis is clinically suspected because of the history and presentation, the first signs of myocardial involvement and injury, and determination of the patient's risk are obtained by ECG, echocardiography, and basic laboratory tests and continuous surveillance.

ECG-findings

Electrocardiographic abnormalities range from T-wave inversion to frank ST-segment elevation, bundle branch blocks, or ventricular tachycardia depending on the region and extent of inflammatory damage. Initial inconspicuous ECG recordings cannot exclude sudden unexpected arrhythmic events and typical presentation warrants careful monitoring.

Laboratory findings

CK and CKMB, frequently raised by a factor of 2–5, raised troponin T test, or elevated (NT)-pro-BNP also suggest myocardial cell damage and compromise but they are not always conclusive during the acute stage of the disease. Importantly, it is not possible to distinguish acute myocarditis from acute myocardial infarction, neither electrocardiographically nor chemically. Other laboratory parameters such as erythrocyte sedimentation rate (ESR), C-reactive protein, or liver enzymes are often pathologically increased. Since these parameters are not specific and caused by the underlying infection they do not allow one to draw conclusions regarding myocardial involvement. Elevated viral titres may provide evidence for certain infections but do not prove direct myocardial involvement. White and red blood cell counts, electrolytes, and creatinine, may support acute management of patients.

Echocardiogram

Ventricular contractility might be unaffected during the early stage, but regional or, less frequently, global wall motion abnormalities are found in about 50–60% of cases. Pericardial effusion points towards pericardial involvement or myocardial involvement in acute pericarditis. Increase in wall diameters (pseudohypertrophy due to increased interstitial water content) may be present during the first 2 weeks of acute myocarditis and associated with diastolic dysfunction. At later stages echocardiography is useful as a follow-up imaging modality to monitor natural history of the patient's ventricular function or response to treatment.

Facultative investigations

The MRI is the only non-invasive tool which allows indirect information on possible myocardial inflammation, fibrosis, and scar formation. T_2-relaxation parameters in cardiac magnetic imaging (CMR) characterize myocardial tissue according to water content and changes in contrast kinetics by local changes in membrane permeability, tissue oedema, and ultimately tissue fibrosis or scar formation in possible association with inflammatory events. Extracellular contrast agents such as gadolinium DTPA distributes between inflamed or scarred tissue leading to delayed enhancement on T_1-weighted images. It does, however, not allow a more specific diagnosis because neither the inflammatory cell subtypes nor a viral involvement is recognized.

24-hour electrocardiogram (ECG) is useful if rhythm disturbances are present in the ECG at rest or are clinically suspected.

Nuclear medicine techniques can demonstrate myocardial damage. Necrosis of myocardial cells can be detected using antimyosin scintigraphy, but such findings are not specific for myocarditis. Radionuclide ventriculography during exertion reveals latent myocardial damage by demonstrating significantly reduced or absent pumping reserves.

After a period of about 1–2 weeks the acute laboratory and echocardiographic changes characteristic of the early phase of the disease may have receded. Myocardial contractile dysfunction recedes at a significantly slower pace, although it does normalize in many cases. ECG findings during this follow-up phase (14 days after appearance of the cardiac symptoms) include non-specific changes in ST segments or T inversion, sinus tachycardia, or a slow normalization of the pulse following stress, supraventricular and ventricular immature beats, and conduction system abnormalities.

If the echocardiogram, ECG, and laboratory findings are normal and symptoms have rapidly receded, further intensive investigations are often not necessary. A control echocardiogram should be done after 3 and 6 months and possibly at intervals thereafter in order to exclude a slow, asymptomatic worsening of left ventricular function.

Endomyocardial biopsy

The gold standard of diagnosing acute myocarditis and its underlying cause is the histological, immunohistological and polymerase chain reaction-based analysis of endomyocardial biopsies. Approximately 10–12% of patients with cardiomyopathy of recent onset who undergo endomyocardial biopsy have this condition. The proof of inflammatory cells without myocyte necrosis account for cases described as 'borderline' myocarditis. In the histological sections low lymphocyte numbers are frequently overlooked. This procedural low sensitivity is significantly improved by immunohistological staining techniques. If myocardial biopsies are taken, they should be analysed in centres that can perform a complete diagnostic workup including histological, immunohistological, and virus analysis.

The inflammatory infiltrate, which may be mild, moderate, or severe, is typically lymphocytic but may also include eosinophilic, neutrophilic, or a mixed type of cells. In rare cases, multinucleated giant cells (GMCs) or eosinophils dominate the active inflammatory process. GMCs are associated with autoimmune diseases (20%) but may also occur as a manifestation of drug hypersensitivity. Poorly formed granulomas and myocyte necrosis in association with mixed lymphocytic infiltrates composed of lymphocytes, plasma cells, histiocytes, and eosinophiles are common. Overt myocyte necrosis is also found in idiopathic hypereosinophilic syndrome but is less frequently seen in allergic or parasite-induced eosinophilic myocarditis, in which direct drug-related toxicity and necrotizing vasculitis contribute to the pathogenesis. The infiltrates are composed of lymphocytes, histiocytes, and eosinophils but no giant cells.

Only a biopsy with the finding of lymphocytes and myocyte damage proves a myocarditis, but due to the patchy nature of both the viral infection and inflammatory cells associated with myocyte necrosis this procedure is fraught with significant problems. Despite a typical clinical history and presentation, sampling error may cause a considerable number of false negative biopsy results, especially during the early stage of the disease (<4 weeks).

The same holds true for the proof of viral involvement. Although virus-associated myocarditis is considered the most frequent cause of the disease, the unambiguous molecular biological proof of viral involvement is hampered by a number of reasons that include:

- Sampling error in cases of focal infections
- Early virus elimination by immune effector cells
- Decrease in virus load by antiviral immunity.

The best way to overcome these difficulties is to analyse a sufficient number of biopsy samples of good quality. Furthermore, it is important to interpreted all questionable or negative results in view of the features of the individual clinical case.

Specific clinical considerations

According to the clinical features at presentation, acute myocarditis can be classified as

1 fulminant myocarditis

2 acute (non-fulminant) myocarditis

3 acute myocarditis with MI-like presentation

4 allergic/eosinophilic myocarditis

5 acute myocarditis of unknown cause.

Fulminant lymphocytic myocarditis presents with fever, distinct rapid onset of symptoms, the presence of severe haemodynamic compromise, and a history of a viral illness within 2 weeks before hospitalization (Liebermann et al. 1991). Such patients present with systolic blood pressures of less than 90 mmHg (50%) or either tachycardia or bradycardia (60%).

Patients classified as having a non-fulminant acute presentation are reported to present with a distinct but longer history of symptoms of heart failure (weeks or months, instead of days) and a haemodynamically more stable heart failure which responds to low doses of vasopressors or symptomatic heart failure medication, including ACE inhibitors, beta-adrenergic drugs, or diuretics. Lymphocytic myocarditis causes left ventricular dysfunction that may be persistent or reversible. There are no clinical criteria that predict which patients will recover ventricular function and which cases will progress to dilated cardiomyopathy. While 93% of patients with fulminant myocarditis remained alive without having received a transplant after 11 years in one study, long-term survival was reduced to 45% in those with non-fulminant acute myocarditis, regardless of an active or borderline histological classification. (McCarthy et al. 2000; Aoyama et al. 2002).

Eosinophils predominate the acute inflammatory infiltrate in allergic granulomatosis, angiitis (Churg–Strauss syndrome), and hypersensitivity myocarditis to drugs or parasitic infections, or the idiopathic hypereosinophilic syndrome, the latter of which often presents with multiorgan infiltrations and >50% cardiac involvement being one major cause of morbidity and mortality. Drug-related myocarditis may occur as a dose-dependent (toxic) or dose-independent (hypersensitivity) reaction.

Necrotizing eosinophilic myocarditis is a rare condition known only from small case series and case reports. The prognosis is poor, with most cases diagnosed at autopsy. This form of eosinophilic heart disease is characterized by an acute onset and rapid progression of haemodynamic compromise. Histologically, necrotizing eosinophilic myocarditis may be identified by a diffuse inflammatory infiltrate with predominant eosinophils associated with extensive myocyte necrosis. It differs from typical hypersensitivity myocarditis in that the lesions are diffuse rather than perivascular and interstitial, and myocyte necrosis is prominent.

Giant cell myocarditis (GCM) is a rare but frequently fatal disorder. It has been associated with various autoimmune disorders (20%) but the pathogenic cause of myocardial compromise is unknown. Congestive heart failure (75%) not responding to standard treatment, sudden cardiogenic shock (5%), and development of fatal arrhythmias (15%) in previously healthy adults are highly suspicious for this condition; 90% of patients either die or undergo transplantation.

Granulomatous myocarditis is found in 25% of cases with systemic sarcoidosis. Similar to other granulomatous diseases, cardiac involvement is often associated with conductance disturbances requiring pacemaker insertion, or acute heart failure (10%). Immunosuppressive treatment may improve outcome.

Differential diagnoses

Any specific cardiac disease known to present with symptoms mimicking myocarditis.

Dilated cardiomyopathy

- Peripartum cardiomyopathy
- Takutsubo
- Tachykardiomyopathy
- ARVD/C
- Non-compaction cardiomyopathy
- End-stage HCM.

Genetic advice

Inheritance and recurrence risk

Although familial occurrence has been recognized, familial myocarditis has not yet been proven and often reported cases were acquired (virus induced). In rare cases of acute myocarditis, inheritance may be associated with:

- General immune disorders
- Autoimmune diseases
- Haemochromatosis
- ATTR-amyloidosis (FAP, autosomal dominant).

Predictive testing

Not established.

Natural history and management

The natural course of the disease includes full recovery of myocardial function, progression to chronic heart failure, or death due to arrhythmias or heart failure. Cases documented so far indicate that 12% of patients with clinically suspected myocarditis and 40% of biopsy-proven myocarditis cases develop dilated cardiomyopathy (DCM). Prospective studies have revealed a grave prognosis for myocarditis patients (biopsy proven) with a 4- to 10-year survival rate of 25–56%, mostly due to manifestation of DCM and sudden cardiac death.

In contrast to the adverse prognosis of patients with early systolic heart failure, the long-term outcome of patients with acute lymphocytic myocarditis mimicking an acute myocardial infarction (sudden-onset angina, MI-like ST segment elevations, and positive troponin I/T or CK/

CKMB) but preserved systolic function seems generally good since >80% of patients clinically recover within a few weeks of months. It is currently unknown whether such a condition predisposes to the later development of DCM.

Management of acute disease

Hospital admission is required in patients with signs of myocardial injury, severe arrhythmias, or grossly impaired myocardial function.

First-line management

This includes:

- Close monitoring of vital signs, basic laboratory parameters, haemodynamic performance, and rhythm disturbances.

- Despite aggressive haemodynamic support with high doses of intravenous vasopressors, left ventricular assist device, and antiarrhythmic therapy, early mortality exceeds 40–45% of afflicted patients. If the condition is quickly recognized and patients are given aggressive treatment, more than 90% of patients who survive the critical early phase will make a full recovery with minimal long-term sequelae and may return to normal life (McCarthy et al. 2000; Aoyama et al. 2002).

- Ventricular arrhythmia is common in patients with active myocarditis, but in most cases does not require specific therapy. If patients present with severe refractory ventricular arrhythmias, antiarrhythmic treatment with amiodarone or implantable cardioverter-defibrillators is necessary. Similarly, patients with atrioventricular block may require insertion of a temporary pacemaker. Because myocarditis may result in spontaneous remission, long-term antiarrhythmic therapy should only be given after all methods of controlling arrhythmia have proved to be unsuccessful.

- Although baseline treatment of fulminant heart failure and arrhythmias is generally supportive and does not depend on the aetiology of the disease, it is important to identify early those patients that need immediate specific medical support:

- In GCM early and intensive immunosuppression with muromonab-anti-CD3 antibodies, cyclosporine, azathioprine, and high doses of steroids improves transplant-free survival (Cooper et al. 2001; 2008).

An eosinophilic myocarditis generally responds well to rapid treatment with high doses of corticosteroids.

Myocarditis in the context of a systemic disease, such as lupus or sarcoidosis, responds to treatment with immunosuppressant agents in high doses, given for at least 6–12 months.

Management of subacute disease

If ECG, laboratory findings and echocardiogram are normal and the patient is in a stable condition, hospital admission is not mandatory. The patient should avoid excessive physical activities, but bed rest is usually not necessary. A control echo should be done after 3, 6, and 12 months in order to exclude slow progression of left ventricular dysfunction. The question of prophylactic therapy with beta-blockers or ACE-inhibitors remains controversial; to date, there exist no studies that show a benefit of such a therapy, as long as left ventricular function is not impaired.

Patients with stable heart failure are treated according to the guidelines proposed by the ACC/AHA Task Force on Practice Guidelines with ACE Inhibitors, diuretics, digitalis, and beta-blockers (Hunt et al., 2005).

Non-fulminant virus-negative myocarditis may benefit from a 6-month course with cortisone and azathioprine (Frustaci et al. 2009).

Immunosuppressive treatment of virus-positive myocarditis has been associated with adverse outcome (Frustaci et al. 2003) and should be avoided in patients without biopsy-proven exclusion of viral infectious. Subgroups of these patients respond to 6 months of treatment with interferon-β (Kühl et al. 2003). In contrast to chronic viral heart disease, data on beneficial effects of early antiviral treatment do not yet exist.

Any anti-inflammatory or antiviral treatment regiment should not be given until a specific diagnosis has been reached by endomyocardial biopsy. Specific biopsy indications have been published recently. (Cooper et al. 2007). Such therapies should be initiated in a centre specializing in inflammatory heart diseases.

Potential long-term complications

End-stage heart failure, refractory arrhythmias, SD, thromboembolic complications.

References

Aoyama N, Izumi T, Hiramori K, et al. National survey of fulminant myocarditis in Japan: therapeutic guidelines and long-term prognosis of using percutaneous cardiopulmonary support for fulminant myocarditis (special report from a scientific committee). *Circ J* 2002;**66**:133–44.

Aretz HT. Myocarditis: the Dallas criteria. *Hum Pathol* 1987;**18**: 619–24.

Cooper L, Hare JM, Tazelaar HD, et al. Usefulness of Immunosuppression for Giant Cell Myocarditis. *Am J Cardiol* 2008;**102**: 1535–9.

Cooper LT, Jr., Berry GJ, Shabetai R. Idiopathic giant-cell myocarditis—natural history and treatment. Multicenter Giant Cell Myocarditis Study Group Investigators. *N Engl J Med* 1997;**336**:1860–6.

Frustaci A, Chimenti C, Calabrese F, Pieroni M, Thiene G, Maseri A. Immunosuppressive therapy for active lymphocytic myocarditis: virological and immunologic profile of responders versus nonresponders. *Circulation* 2003;**107**:857 63.

Frustaci A, Russo MA, Chimenti C. Randomized study on the efficacy of immunosuppressive therapy in patients with virus-negative inflammatory cardiomyopathy: the TIMIC study. *Eur Heart J* 2009;**30**:1995–2002.

Hunt SA, Abraham WT, Chin MH, et al. ACC/AHA 2005 Guideline Update for the Diagnosis and Management of Chronic Heart Failure in the Adult: a report of the American College of Cardiology/American Heart Association Task Force on Practice Guidelines (Writing Committee to Update the 2001 Guidelines for the Evaluation and Management of Heart Failure): developed in collaboration with the American College of Chest Physicians and the International Society for Heart and Lung Transplantation: endorsed by the Heart Rhythm Society. *Circulation* 2005;**112**:e154–235.

Kühl U, Pauschinger M, Noutsias M, et al. High prevalence of viral genomes and multiple viral infections in the myocardium of adults with 'idiopathic' left ventricular dysfunction. *Circulation* 2005;**111**:887–93.

Kühl U, Pauschinger M, Schwimmbeck PL, et al. Interferon-beta treatment eliminates cardiotropic viruses and improves left ventricular function in patients with myocardial persistence of viral genomes and left ventricular dysfunction. *Circulation* 2003;**107**:2793–8.

Kuhl U, Schultheiss HP. Viral myocarditis: diagnosis, aetiology and management. *Drugs* 2009;**69**:1287–302.

Lieberman EB, Hutchins GM, Herskowitz A, et al. Clinicopathologic description of myocarditis. *J Am Coll Cardiol* 1991;**18**:1617–26.

Liu PP, Schultheiss HP. Myocarditis. In: *Baunwald (ed.) Heart disease*, 8th edn. Philadelphia: W B Saunders, 2008; pp. 1775–92.

McCarthy RE, 3rd, Boehmer JP, Hruban RH, et al. Long-term outcome of fulminant myocarditis as compared with acute (nonfulminant) myocarditis. *N Engl J Med* 2000;**342**:690–5.

Dilated cardiomyopathy

Dilated cardiomyopathy (DCM) is disease of the myocardium characterized by impaired function and dilation of the left ventricle in the absence of coronary artery disease, congenital heart disease, and abnormal loading conditions of sufficient severity to cause the observed myocardial dysfunction.

Epidemiology
Prevalence ranges from 14–36 per 100 000 population. DCM is one of the most common causes of heart failure and cardiac transplantation in the young.

Aetiology
Cardiomyopathies can be classified into familial and non-familial forms.

Familial DCM
Family studies suggest that 25–50% of patients with DCM have a genetic predisposition. Most cases exhibit age-dependent incomplete penetrance. Familial DCM should be suspected when more than one member of the same family has DCM or a compatible phenotype (e.g. sudden cardiac death or conduction system disease). Pedigree analysis can help determine the mode of inheritance and may give clues about the disease-causing mutation (Table 6.9.1).

Desmosomal gene mutations, classically associated with arrhythmogenic right ventricular cardiomyopathy (ARVC) have recently been shown to cause DCM characterized by a high incidence of ventricular arrhythmias and sudden cardiac death, with minimal or absent right ventricular involvement. This overlap syndrome combines the morphological features of DCM and the electrical instability of ARVC.

Table 6.9.1 Causes of familial DCM according to inheritance

Autosomal dominant	Commonest mode of inheritance. Mutations described in cardiac sarcomere, cytoskeletal, nuclear membrane, and ion channel genes. Lamin A/C mutations are associated with conduction system disease, early onset atrial fibrillation and sudden cardiac death
Autosomal recessive	Cardiac troponin I mutations cause severe, early onset DCM
X-linked	Dystrophin gene mutations (also implicated in Duchenne and Becker muscular dystrophy) can cause DCM with no clinical skeletal muscle involvement apart from increased serum levels of creatine kinase. In males, heart failure typically develops in the second and third decade of life and rapidly progresses. Female carriers are also at risk, but the disease is usually milder
Matrilineal (mitochondrial)	MELAS (mitochondrial encephalomyopathy, lactic acidosis and stroke-like episodes), Kearns–Sayre syndrome and MERFF (myoclonus epilepsy with ragged red fibres) and other mitochondrial cytopathies

Non-familial DCM
Cancer chemotherapy
- Anthracyclines (doxorubicin, daunorubicin, epirubicin): cardiac toxicity is mediated by free radical formation and is related to cumulative exposure. Female sex, extremes of age and preexisting cardiac disease are risk factors.
- High-dose cyclophosphamide: toxicity is caused by toxic metabolites and is accentuated by co-administration of anthracyclines. Cardiac dysfunction is related to the dose of an individual cycle rather than cumulative exposure, and is characterized by an acute course and significant mortality.
- Trastuzumab: this recombinant monoclonal antibody binds to human epidermal growth factor 2. The mechanism of cardiac toxicity is unknown. The risk increases with previous anthracycline and radiation treatment. Up to 11% of patients develop DCM, which is usually reversible after withdrawal of treatment.
- Tyrosine kinase inhibitors: sunitinib causes a reduction in systolic function, especially in the presence of coronary artery disease. Toxicity is probably mediated by mitochondrial damage. There is good response to withdrawal and conventional medical therapy.

Radiotherapy
- Radiation-induced DCM manifests many years after exposure and is more common in anthracycline-treated patients. Restriction, pericardial constriction, valve disease, and coronary disease are also common features.

Toxins
- Ethanol: the risk of developing DCM is proportional to the magnitude and duration of alcohol intake. However, there is wide range of exposure between affected individuals. Abstinence improves survival.
- Cocaine: direct toxicity in combination with a hyperadrenergic state contribute to the development of DCM in chronic users.
- Amphetamines: DCM is seen in chronic users and may reverse with abstinence.

Nutritional
- Selenium deficiency: a rare cause of DCM with a high incidence in some areas of China (Keshan disease). Patients on long-term parenteral nutrition are also at risk.
- Thiamine deficiency: Beriberi causes high output cardiac failure and can present acutely (Shoshin beriberi). The left ventricle is enlarged and hyperdynamic but occasionally systolic function is impaired, mimicking DCM. Malnourished and alcoholic patients are at risk.
- Zinc and copper deficiency: micronutrients are under investigation as a cause or contributor to the development of DCM.

Iron overload
- Transfusion dependent states: parenteral iron overload in transfusion-dependent states such as thalassaemia major leads to DCM that is reversible with iron chelation.
- Haemochromatosis: enhanced enteral absorption and excessive release of iron from macrophages lead to mitochondrial toxicity manifesting as DCM.

Inflammatory
- Sarcoid: cardiac involvement occurs in ~25% of patients. DCM, conduction system disease, ventricular arrhythmias, and left ventricular aneurysms are common.
- Autoimmune diseases
  - Systemic lupus erythematosus: DCM caused by lymphocytic myocarditis is uncommon. Pericardial, valvular and coronary pathology are more frequent.
  - Rheumatoid arthritis: left ventricular dysfunction mediated by small intramyocardial artery vasculitis or granulomatous myocarditis is uncommon. Pericardial and coronary artery disease are more typical.
  - Polymyositis/dermatomyositis: myocarditis, often associated with conduction system disease, is rare but is associated with high mortality.
  - Spondyloarthropathies: DCM is rare. Aortic valve and conduction system disease are typical manifestations of cardiac involvement.
  - Churg–Strauss syndrome: myocardial eosinophilic infiltration leads to systolic and diastolic dysfunction, often associated with conduction system and valvular disease.
  - Wegener's granulomatosis: DCM with regional wall motion abnormalities with a predilection for the septum is seen in up to 20% of patients.
- Giant cell myocarditis: this is characterized by acute onset heart failure secondary to DCM, associated with ventricular arrhythmias, heart block, thymoma, and autoimmune disorders. The myocardium is infiltrated by lymphocytes, eosinophils and multinucleated giant cells; prognosis is poor.

Infectious (Chapter 6.8)
- Viruses: coxsackie B, adenovirus, parvovirus B19, hepatitis C, Epstein–Barr, cytomegalovirus, HIV
- Bacteria: many bacteria can cause cardiac dysfunction during systemic infection either by direct invasion, toxin-mediated effects or the immune response. Rheumatic fever is mediated by the host's immune response after group A streptococcal tonsillitis. In Lyme disease, caused by *Borrelia burgdorferi*, DCM is rare but conduction system disease is a common.
- Protozoa: Chagas' disease (*Trypanosoma cruzi*) causes DCM after a long latent infection. Ventricular aneurysms and arrhythmias are common. It is prevalent in central and south America.

Endocrinopathies (Chapter 6.12)
- Hypo/hyperthyroidism
- Cushing's/Addison's syndrome
- Phaeochromocytoma.

Peripartum
DCM develops during the last month of pregnancy or within 5 months of delivery in previously healthy women. Advanced maternal age, multiparity, African descent and family history of DCM are risk factors but the pathogenesis is unclear. Only 50% recover completely; the remainder have a variable course and may require transplantation.

Tachycardia mediated (Tachycardiomyopathy)
Incessant atrial or ventricular tachycardia is a rare cause of DCM, which usually reverses once the tachycardia is controlled.

Idiopathic
No cause is identified following appropriate investigation for acquired and inherited forms. As further information becomes available during long term follow-up the diagnosis may be revised.

Clinical assessment
History: key points
- Symptoms of cardiac failure and arrhythmias.
- Past medical history: hypertension and associated end-organ damage; coronary disease and risk factors; thromboembolism; past treatment with chemotherapy and radiotherapy, and previous diagnosis of other systemic diseases.
- Drug therapy: prescribed, over-the-counter medication (non-steroidal anti-inflammatory drugs), oral contraceptives, and drugs of abuse.
- Family history: a three-generation family tree should be constructed. Enquire for consanguinity, pacemaker implantations, sudden cardiac death, and heart transplantation. Familial diabetes and deafness suggest mitochondrial diseases.

Examination: key points
- General examination: signs of endocrine pathology, and other systemic diseases/syndromes.
- Cardiovascular examination: presence of heart failure, murmurs and hypertension.
- Musculoskeletal examination for skeletal myopathy.
- Ophthalmological examination: ptosis, retinal pigmentation and ophthalmoplegia are associated with mitochondrial diseases.

Investigations
Echocardiography
DCM is diagnosed when the left ventricular ejection fraction is <0.45 (and/or fractional shortening <25%) with a left ventricular end-diastolic diameter >117% of the age and body surface area corrected value.

The Henry equation, $(45.3 \text{ (body surface area)}^{1/3} - 0.03 \text{ (age)} - 7.2)$ can be used to calculate the predicted left ventricular end-diastolic diameter.

Cardiac magnetic resonance (CMR) imaging
- Cardiac magnetic resonance (CMR) can used to establish or confirm the diagnosis in patients with poor echocardiographic windows.
- Late gadolinium enhancement (LGE) in the mid ventricular wall is seen in one-sixth of DCM patients. LGE may help exclude coronary artery disease since in ischaemic cardiomyopathy enhancement occurs in a coronary artery distribution and almost always involves the subendocardium. In myocardial inflammation, focal LGE associated with regional wall motion abnormalities is seen.
- T_2*-imaging can reliably assess myocardial iron content in haemochromatosis and transfusion dependent patients.

Electrocardiography/ambulatory monitoring
Evidence of conduction system disease is suggestive of LMNA disease, neuromuscular diseases, autoimmune diseases, sarcoid, and giant cell myocarditis.

Laboratory investigations
- Full blood count, renal function, thyroid function, liver function, glucose, iron studies, calcium and parathyroid

hormone, serum angiotensin-converting enzyme, inflammatory markers.

- Creatinine kinase as a screen for neuromuscular disease.
- Autoimmune screen (ANCA, dsDNA, ENA, ANA, RhF).
- Serological testing for infections.
- 24-hour urine collection for catecholamines for phaeochromocytoma or cortisol for Cushing syndrome if clinically suspected.

Chest radiography
Signs of heart failure, interstitial lung disease, sarcoid (bilateral hilar lymphadenopathy).

Coronary angiography
Excludes epicardial coronary artery disease as the cause of DCM. The presence or absence of regional wall motion abnormalities is neither sensitive nor specific for coronary artery disease.

Endomyocardial biopsy (EMB)
- The indications for EMB have been reviewed by the AHA/ACC/ESC in 2007. EMB is of limited value in DCM and best reserved for cases where giant cell myocarditis is suspected:
  - Unexplained DCM of <2 weeks' duration associated with haemodynamic compromise.
  - Unexplained DCM with new-onset heart failure of 2 weeks' to 3 months' duration with ventricular arrhythmias, Mobitz type II AV heart block, or failure to respond to conventional care.

Right and left heart catheterization
Used for assessment of pulmonary vascular resistance and reactivity for transplant assessment.

Genetic testing
The availability of genetic testing is limited and its widespread clinical application is hampered by the large number of genes involved and the heterogeneity of mutations.

Currently it may be helpful in establishing the diagnosis in neuromuscular diseases and Lamin A/C disease.

Natural history
The prognosis depends on the severity of cardiac dysfunction and aetiology (Fig. 6.9.1). DCM secondary to myocarditis, substance abuse, and connective tissue disease probably has the same outcome as 'idiopathic' DCM. Prognosis in different forms of familial DCM is less certain. Some familial forms of DCM are associated with SCD, and are examined in 'Managing special patient groups', p. 249.

Management
Pharmacological treatment (Chapter 6.2, Pharmacological therapy and Chapter 6.7, Systolic heart failure: Pharmacological treatment)
Irrespective of the cause of DCM, the treatment of heart failure is the same (see ESC guidelines on the treatment of acute and chronic heart failure 2008).

Prevention of SCD
Sudden death accounts for ~30% of mortality and is mediated primarily by complex ventricular arrhythmias. SCD is less frequent in mild DCM but accounts for a greater proportion of deaths in this subgroup.

Predictors of overall mortality, including NSVT reflect the severity of the underlying myocardial disease but are not specific markers for the risk of SCD. Electrophysiological testing is of limited value. The 2006 AHA/ACC/ESC guidelines for the prevention of sudden cardiac death provide guidelines for the use of ICDs in DCM.

Primary prevention
- ICDs should be used in patients with sustained VT and significant ventricular impairment.
- CDs improve survival in non-ischaemic DCM patients with LVEF <35%, NYHA II or III, who are receiving optimal medical therapy (SCD-HeFT trial). ICDs may also be considered in NYHA I patients.

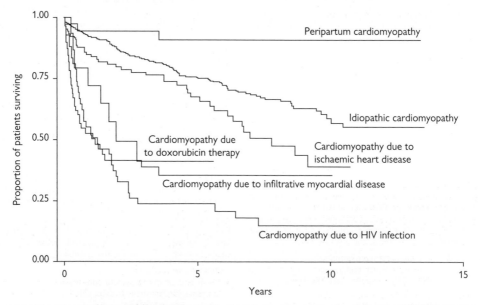

- Unexplained syncope is associated with a higher risk of SCD and ICDs may be beneficial.
- Cardiac resynchronization therapy as an adjunct to ICD can be effective for primary prevention in symptomatic patients (NYHA III-IV) and QRS ≥120 ms on optimal medical treatment (COMPANION trial).

Secondary prevention
ICDs are recommended in survivors of VF.

Prevention of systemic emboli
The annual risk of stroke ranges from 1.5–4% and is proportional to the severity of disease. Atrial fibrillation (paroxysmal/permanent/persistent) is a major risk factor and anticoagulation with warfarin (or equivalent anticoagulant) is recommended. High dose aspirin (300 mg od) is less effective and has been associated with exacerbation of heart failure.

In the presence of sinus rhythm the value of anticoagulation is less established, and anticoagulant treatment relies on an assessment of the risks and benefits for an individual patient. Anticoagulation should be considered in patients with a previous cardioembolic event and for primary prevention in patients with intracardiac thrombus, severe cardiac dysfunction/dilation or left atrial dilation.

Family screening
When personal and family history suggests familial disease, first-degree relatives should be counselled on their risk and it appropriate, offered clinical and genetic screening.

In the absence of an alternative diagnosis, cardiac abnormalities in first degree relatives are probably the expression of the same genetic defect as that affecting the proband.

European guidelines define affected relatives by the presence of one major criterion, or left ventricular dilatation >117% of predicted values and one minor criterion, or three minor criteria (Table 6.9.2). Since the expression of disease is time-dependent, screening demands long-term follow-up.

Genetic screening
If the disease-causing mutation is identified in the proband other family members can then be genetically screened. Carriers require long term clinical assessment for disease expression whereas relatives who do not carry the mutation can be reassured (if there is no reason to suspect the presence of more than one mutation in the family).

Table 6.9.2 Family screening criteria for DCM

Major criterion
Impaired left ventricular function and dilatation satisfying the conventional diagnostic criteria for DCM

Minor criteria
Supraventricular or ventricular arrhythmias, or ventricular ectopy >1000/24 hours before the age of 50 years
Left ventricular dilatation >112% of predicted
Ejection fraction <50% or fractional shortening <28%
II or III AV block, LBBB, sinus node dysfunction
Unexplained sudden death or stroke before age of 50
Unexplained regional wall motion abnormalities

Managing special patient groups
DCM secondary to Lamin A/C mutations
Lamin A/C gene (LMNA) mutations can cause an autosomal dominant form of DCM associated with:
- Early-onset atrial fibrillation or conduction system disease with a third of patients requiring antibradycardia pacing after the third decade of life.
- SCD occurs in almost half of all carriers at a mean age of 46 years.
- Preliminary data suggest that carriers with conduction system disease benefit from an ICD for the primary prevention of SCD.
- Heart failure typically develops after conduction system disease.
- Other phenotypes (with DCM) include:
  - autosomal dominant Emery–Dreifuss muscular dystrophy
  - limb-girdle muscular dystrophy type 1B.

DCM in neuromuscular diseases
Dystrophinopathies
- Mutations of the dystrophin gene on chromosome Xq21 cause Duchene or Becker muscular dystrophy.
- Prognosis depends on cardiac involvement.
- Slowly progressive DCM and heart failure are common and treated in the conventional manner.
- Conduction system disease and ventricular arrhythmias are uncommon.
- In Duchene Muscular Dystrophy annual evaluation with ECG and echocardiography is recommended.
- In Becker Muscular Dystrophy cardiac evaluation is recommended at least every 5 years.
- Female carriers are at risk of developing DCM and screening is also recommended.

X-linked Emery–Dreifuss muscular dystrophy
- Caused by PTA gene mutations on chromosome Xq28.
- Cardiac involvement determines prognosis.
- Progressive conduction system disease leads to SCD and antibradycardia pacing is recommended in asymptomatic sinus or AV node disease.
- DCM is less common.
- Female carriers are at risk and regular screening is suggested.

Myotonic dystrophy
- Type 1 myotonic dystrophy is caused by an expanding CTG trinucleotide repeat sequence in the untranslated region of a serine-threonine kinase gene on chromosome 19q13.3 (autosomal dominant with anticipation).
- Conduction system disease leads to SCD.
- DCM is less common.
- Asymptomatic mild conduction abnormalities require close monitoring. An EP study may be useful since asymptomatic patients with an HV interval >70 ms are likely to benefit from antibradycardia pacing.
- Antibradycardia pacing is recommended in third and Mobitz 2 second-degree AV block irrespective of symptoms and should be considered even in patients with first-degree heart block as conduction disease may progress unpredictably.
- Ventricular arrhythmias can cause sudden cardiac death in a minority of patients but selection criteria for ICD implantation are unclear.

Fascioscapulohumeral muscular dystrophy
- Caused by a deletion of an integral number of 3.3-kb tandem repeats from the subtelomeric region on chromosome 4q35 (autosomal dominant).
- DCM and clinically significant conduction system disease is uncommon.
- Cardiac evaluation needed at time of diagnosis and further follow-up depending on clinical situation.

Limb-girdle muscular dystrophy (LGMD)
- Genetically heterogeneous group of dystrophies with variable cardiac involvement.
- Conduction system disease is seen primarily in LGMD2 types C to F secondary to sacroglycan gene mutations.
- Cardiomyopathy is seen in LGMD2I caused by FKRP gene mutations.
- Cardiac care as for dystrophinopathies, with the exception of LGMD1B which is a laminopathy.

Acquired DCM

In addition to standard heart failure treatment, further therapeutic interventions may be required to improve cardiac function. Abstinence from drugs of abuse, modification of cancer chemotherapy and nutritional supplementation are appropriate in relevant cases. In haemochromatosis and transfusion-dependent states, venesection and iron chelators respectively are used to minimize cardiac toxicity and improve function. Immunosuppression is required to control disease activity in inflammatory DCM secondary to autoimmune disease and selected cases of myocarditis.

DCM and pregnancy

Patients with DCM are at a high risk of deteriorating during pregnancy and counselling about contraception and risks of pregnancy is essential. In the ESC guidelines on the management of cardiac conditions during pregnancy (2003) pregnancy is contraindicated, and termination advised. Pregnancy in women with previous peripartum cardiomyopathy is associated with significant morbidity and mortality especially if there is incomplete recovery.

Support groups: The Cardiomyopathy Association (www.cardiomyopathy.org).

Website

www.escardio.org/guidelines-surveys/

Hypertrophic cardiomyopathy

Hypertrophic cardiomyopathy (HCM) is a condition characterized by the presence of left ventricular hypertrophy (LVH) for which there is no or insufficient explanation (e.g. mild hypertension or mild aortic stenosis with marked LVH). In healthy young competitive athletes with mild LVH the distinction from athlete's heart may be difficult, and in some affected individuals the LVH may be mild, indeed wall thickness may even be within normal limits.

Epidemiology
In the past HCM was considered a rare disorder with a poor prognosis. However, recent population screening studies suggest a prevalence of 1 in 500 individuals.

Genetics (see also Table 6.10.1)
In adolescents and adults the disorder usually exhibits autosomal dominant inheritance and is due to a mutation in the genes coding for one of eight sarcomere proteins. However, sporadic causes account for 50% of cases. In infants and small children the phenotype is usually due to an inherited metabolic or neuromuscular disorder.

Recent data suggests that approximately 5% of males presenting with HCM over the age of 40 have Anderson–Fabry's disease, suggested by the demonstration of a reduced plasma activity of the enzyme α-galactosidase and confirmed by genetic testing. Although X-linked, females may also be affected but plasma α-galactosidase may be normal and the diagnosis in women requires genetic testing.

Pathology
Gross
- Unexplained LVH
- Usually asymmetric LVH (involving the interventricular septum (IVS))
- LVH may be concentric, localized to the apex, or may involve the right ventricle.

Histology
- Extensive disarray of myocytes and myofibrils which may be patchy
- Thickening of intramural microvessels
- Interstitial fibrosis.

Pathophysiology
The clinical features of HCM result from the underlying abnormalities:
- *Diastolic dysfunction* due to an increase in LV stiffness as a result of hypertrophy and fibrosis and to impaired LV relaxation associated with energy deficiency and ischaemia, together impairing the ability to increase stroke volume on exercise and results in a rise in LVEDP
- *Left ventricular outflow tract obstruction* occurs in 25–30% of patients as a result of hypertrophy of the IVS and anterior motion of the mitral valve during systole (SAM). The resulting pressure gradient is highly variable as is influenced by central blood volume and contractile state
- *Myocardial ischaemia* as a result of increased myocardial mass, thickening of the coronary microvessels, and a reduced transcoronary perfusion gradient (secondary to raised LVEDP)
- *Vascular instability* is present in 30% of patients and characterized by an abnormal blood pressure response to exercise. These patients have an exaggerated fall in systemic vascular resistance due to inappropriate firing of LV mechanoreceptor (stretch-sensitive) on exercise, as well as impaired vasoconstriction or paradoxical vasodilatation which may result in presyncope or syncope
- *Arrhythmias* SVTs are common in HCM (approximately 30%), with AF being the most common. NSVT occurs in 15–20% and is associated with an increased risk of sudden cardiac death. Sustained VT is rare, and may be associated with apical LV aneurysms
- *Systolic dysfunction* occurs in a small subset of patients (10–15%) due to progressive wall thinning (end-stage or burnt-out HCM).

Clinical
History
Family history is vital as 50% of cases are inherited in an autosomal dominant pattern.

Symptoms
Approximately half are asymptomatic or have minimal symptoms.
- Chest pain—may be typical angina (often worse postprandially) or atypical

Table 6.10.1 Gene mutations (sarcomere disease)

β-myosin heavy chain
Cardiac myosin binding protein C
Cardiac troponin T
Cardiac troponin I
Essential and regulatory myosin light chains
Cardiac actin
α-Tropomyosin
Non-sarcomeric disease
Metabolic
Glycogen storage disorders
Carnitine deficiency
Infants of diabetic mothers
AMP kinase gene mutations
Hurler's syndrome
Mitochondrial disorders
Anderson–Fabry's disease
Danon's disease
Syndromic disease
Noonan's syndrome
LEOPARD syndrome
Friedrich's ataxia

Table 6.10.2 Underlying cause of symptoms

Chest pain
Myocardial ischaemia

Breathlessness
Diastolic dysfunction
Outflow tract obstruction
Atrial fibrillation
Progressive LV systolic impairment

Palpitations
Paroxysmal or established atrial fibrillation/flutter

Presyncope/syncope
Outflow tract obstruction
Arrhythmia
Inappropriate vasodilation

- Shortness of breath—associated with a reduced peak oxygen consumption
- Palpitations
- Presyncope and syncope (at rest or on exertion).

For the underlying causes of symptoms see Table 6.10.2.

Clinical examination

The classic findings are described in Table 6.10.3. However, in many patients clinical examination may be entirely normal. Investigations (see also Table 6.10.4):

- *ECG*—abnormal in the majority
- *Echocardiogram*—apical HCM may be difficult to visualize. HCM can occur in the setting of normal wall thickness
- *Ambulatory ECG monitoring*—as routine risk factor stratification
- *Exercise testing*—assessment of blood pressure response as a predictor of risk of sudden cardiac death. ST segment changes are poorly predictive of underlying coronary artery disease. Profound impairment of peak oxygen consumption and early lactic acidosis raise the possibility of an underlying mitochondrial myopathy
- *Cardiac MRI*—better delineation of the pattern and magnitude of hypertrophy in patients with poor echocardiographic windows
- *Coronary angiography*—in patients with typical angina age >40
- *Aetiological testing*—for non-sarcomere disease. Routine renal function testing (patients with Anderson-Fabry disease usually have co-existing renal impairment).

Natural history

HCM is the most common aetiological cause of sudden cardiac death in young adults, but sudden death is less common than previously thought. Sudden death may be the first presentation of the disease, and the challenge is to identify the minority at high risk and reassure those patients at low risk for sudden death.

- *Sudden cardiac death (SCD)*: annual incidence of <1% in large unselected series. Risk factors are shown in Table 6.10.5
- *Progressive impairment of systolic function*: incidence of 1% per year

Table 6.10.3 Findings on clinical examination

Obstructive HCM	
Arterial pulse	'Jerky' (rapid upstroke/downstroke)
JVP	Prominent 'a' waves
	Raised in patients with heart failure
Apex beat	Sustained
	'Double impulse' (palpable atrial impulse)
	'Triple impulse' (late systolic impulse)

Ejection systolic	
Murmur	Left sternal edge
	Radiates to axilla and up the sternum (not into the neck)
	Increase in intensity with standing, amyl nitrate, Valsalva manoeuvre

Pansystolic	
Murmur	Associated mitral regurgitation
	Radiates to axilla

Non-obstructive HCM
Examination may be normal

- *Stroke:* patients with AF (either paroxysmal or permanent) have an increase risk
- *Infective endocarditis:* the risk is low (4 cases per 1000 person-years) and almost exclusively in patients with outflow tract obstruction.

Clinical management

The aims of clinical management are as follows:
- Treatment of symptoms
- Prevention of stroke in patients with AF
- Assessment and reduction of risk for SCD
- Family screening
- Genetic counselling.

Symptomatic therapy

Patients with outflow tract obstruction
- Beta-blocker (BB) monotherapy initially
- Disopyramide if still symptomatic (contraindicated in patients on amiodarone), started at low-dose and up-titrated

Table 6.10.4 Abnormalities on investigation

ECG
Atrial fibrillation
Left atrial enlargement (P-mitrale)
Repolarization abnormalities
LVH by voltage criteria
Pathological Q waves

Table 6.10.5 Established risk factors for SCD

Conventional risk factors

(1) A history of at least one sudden cardiac death in a relative aged <45 years

(2) Prior aborted cardiac arrest

(3) Unexplained syncope

(4) Maximum wall thickness >30 mm

(5) Abnormal blood pressure response during exercise

(6) The presence of non-sustained VT on 48-hour ambulatory ECG monitoring

Possible risk factors in individual patients

(1) Resting outflow tract gradient >30 mmHg

(2) Extensive late gadolinium on MRI

(3) Myocardial ischaemia

(4) Specific mutations (troponin T and I)

- Verapamil if refractory to above or BB contraindicated (cautious use as may worsen degree of obstruction in some)
- Septal myectomy if drug refractory
- Alcohol septal ablation as alternative to surgery
- Short AV delay dual-chamber pacing may reduced the outflow tract gradient in some, but data is weak

Patients without obstruction
- Calcium channel blocker (CCB) is first-line therapy, titrated up to high dose (Verapamil 480 mg)
- BB if refractory to CCB

Patients with systolic impairment
- Conventional heart failure therapy
- Systolic impairment is progressive and some may proceed to cardiac transplantation

Management of atrial fibrillation
- Amiodarone is most effective for reducing occurrence of paroxysmal AF and for maintaining sinus rhythm after DCCV after new-onset AF
- Rate control of permanent AF with BB or CCB
- AV nodal ablation and permanent pacing occasionally
- Anticoagulation in *all* with paroxysmal or permanent AF unless contraindicated

Risk stratification and risk reduction for SCD
There is general agreement that the greater the number of clinical risk factors, the higher the risk of sudden cardiac death. A single risk factors carries an annual SCD risk of 1%, whereas two or more risk factors carry an annual risk of 3–6%.
- High-risk patients (≥2 risk factors) should be considered for an ICD
- If previous averted SCD consider ICD despite absence of other risk factors
- Data for effect of amiodarone in reducing SCD is controversial
- Balance risk of SCD against risk of device-related complications in young patients
- Annual discharge rate of ICDs in HCM patients is low.

Family screening/genetic counselling
- Screening should be offered to all family members after counselling about potential insurance and employment implications
- ECG and echocardiogram
- Screening should continue into middle age in families with a pedigree of late-presentation disease
- Genetic testing not yet widely available.

Pregnancy and HCM
Serious complications are relatively rare during pregnancy and delivery.
- Symptoms may worsen
- Epidural analgesia can theoretically increase outflow tract obstruction via a reduction in systemic vascular resistance.

Key points in diagnosis
- Thorough family history
- Symptomatic status
- ECG
- Echocardiogram
- 48-hour ambulatory ECG
- Monitoring
- Assessment of blood pressure
- Response on exercise
- Aetiological testing.

Key points in treatment
- Medical therapy
  - Non-obstructive HCM: verapamil
  - Obstructive HCM: Beta-blockers with or without disopyramide; verapamil if beta-blockers contraindicated
  - Septal myectomy/alcohol: septal ablation (if drug refractory).
- Risk factor stratification
- Family screening/genetic counselling.

Support groups: Severe support groups are available for affected individuals are the families within the United Kingdom:
The Cardiomyopathy Association: www.cardiomyopathy.org
Cardiac Risk in the Young: www.c-r-y.org.uk

Further reading
American College of Cardiology/European Society of Cardiology clinical expert consensus document on hypertrophic cardiomyopathy. A report of the American College of Cardiology Foundation Task Force on Clinical Expert Consensus Documents and the European Society of Cardiology Committee for Practice Guidelines. *J Am Coll Cardiol* 2003;**42**:1687–713.

Elliott P, McKenna WJ. Hypertrophic cardiomyopathy. *Lancet* 2004;**363**:1881–91.

Elliott P, Spirito P. Prevention of hypertrophic cardiomyopathy-related deaths: theory and practice. *Heart* 2008;**94**:1269–75.

Maron BJ (ed.). Diagnosis and management of hypertrophic cardiomyopathy. Massachusetts: Blackwell Futura, 2004.

Maron BJ. Hypertrophic cardiomyopathy: a systematic review. *JAMA* 2002;**287**:1308–20.

Prasad K, Atherton J, Smith GC, *et al.* Echocardiographic pitfalls in the diagnosis of hypertrophic cardiomyopathy. *Heart* 1999;**82**(Suppl 3):III8–III15.

Restrictive and infiltrative cardiomyopathies

The definitions used in this chapter are in keeping with the 1996 WHO/ISFC classification of the cardiomyopathies (Richardson *et al.* 1996). Cardiomyopathies are defined as diseases of the myocardium associated with cardiac dysfunction and are classified as dilated (DCM), hypertrophic (HCM), restrictive (RCM), and arrhythmogenic right ventricular.

Restrictive cardiomyopathies

RCMs are characterized by restrictive filling and reduced diastolic volume of either or both ventricles with normal or near-normal systolic function and wall thickness (Table 6.11.1). Increased interstitial fibrosis may be present. RCMs should be differentiated from constrictive pericarditis (CP) (Table 6.11.2). RCM may be:
1 idiopathic
2 familial/genetic due to sarcomeric gene mutations, particularly troponin I, and may be part of the HCM spectrum (Morimoto S, 2008)
3 associated with other disease, e.g. amyloidosis, endomyocardial disease (EMD) with or without hypereosinophilia.

Clinical approach in RCM

History: key points
• Family history: enquire for familial HCM, sudden cardiac death, skeletal myopathy
• Patient history: enquire for specific geographical sites, e.g. near the equator for EMD, for neoplastic illness (e.g. multiple myeloma), for extracardiac involvement (e.g. kidney, liver, carpal tunnel, gastrointestinal disease, neuropathy, etc.).

Clinical presentations and examination: key points
Cardiac presentation may include:
• exercise intolerance, weakness, progressive dyspnoea
• right-sided heart failure with peripheral oedema, hepatomegaly, ascites, anasarca in advanced RCM
• jugular venous distention, S3, S4 or both.

Table 6.11.1 Echocardiographic Doppler features of 'restrictive filling' in RCM (Tam JW, *et al.* 2002)

Mitral inflow pattern
E/A >1.5
Deceleration time <150 ms
Isovolumic relaxation time (IVRT) <60 ms
No significant respiratory variation
Pulmonary venous (PV) flow pattern
Systolic:diastolic ratio of PV forward flow <0.4
Atrial reversal wave >35 cm/s
Pulmonary A wave/mitral A wave duration >30 ms
Mitral A wave duration/PVa duration ≤0.9
No significant respiratory variation
Hepatic venous flow
Blunted systolic forward wave
Deep atrial reversal wave

Diagnosis of RCM: key points
• ECG often shows atrial fibrillation, left ventricular hypertrophy may be present in restrictive-hypertrophic forms, in contrast to low voltage in cardiac amyloidosis
• It is important to demonstrate a restrictive filling, reduced diastolic volume of either or both ventricles with normal or near-normal systolic function and wall thickness, atrial enlargement (Tables 6.11.1 and 6.11.2) as well as exclude constrictive pericarditis (Table 6.11.2) by echocardiography, cardiac catheterization and/or cardiac magnetic resonance
• Need to exclude infiltrative forms, particularly cardiac amyloidosis (Tables 6.11.3 and 6.11.4).

Natural history and management

Prognosis in RCM is variable, usually progressive worsening of symptoms and high mortality and need for heart Tx. No specific therapy is available.

Infiltrative cardiomyopathies

Infiltrative cardiomyopathies (CMPs) are listed among the specific cardiomyopathies, defined as heart muscle diseases that are associated with specific cardiac or systemic disorders. Predominantly restrictive-infiltrative CMP include:
1 cardiac amyloidosis.
2 endomyocardial disease (EMD) with hypereosinophilia (Löffler endocarditis).
3 endomyocardial fibrosis (EMF), also known as EMD without hypereosinophilia.

In addition other systemic disorders may be associated with specific DCM, or HCM or DCM-HCM, or inflammatory CMP with a restrictive haemodynamic component and these include:
1 sarcoidosis
2 metabolic and storage disorders (haemochromatosis, fabry disease, glycogenosis, mucopolysaccharidoses, Gaucher disease) (see Chapter 6.10, Hypertrophic cardiomyopathy, and Chapter 6.9, Dilated cardiomyopathy)
3 neoplasms (carcinoid, metastatic).
4 miscellaneous (radiation, antracycline toxicity, drugs causing fibrous endocarditis, e.g. serotonin, methysergide, ergotamine, mercurial agents, busulfan) (see Chapters 6.8 and 6.9).

Cardiac amyloidosis

Amyloidosis is a syndrome caused by extracellular deposition of unique twisted beta-pleated sheet fibrils formed by various proteins using different pathogenetic mechanisms. Amyloid may be found in almost any organ, but heart involvement is seen mainly in the conditions listed in Table 6.11.3. In primary (AL) amyloidosis, amyloid is formed from portions of the immunoglobulin light chain by a monoclonal population of plasma cells related to (but usually not associated with) multiple myeloma. In reactive (secondary) amyloidosis amyloid is formed using a non-immunoglobulin protein termed AA. In familial autosomal dominant amyloidosis (ATTR) amyloid is formed of a mutant pre-albumin serum carrier protein named transthyretin (TTR). ATTR amyloidosis is four times more common in black people. In senile systemic amyloidosis, amyloid may be due to deposition of atrial natriuretic-like protein or non-mutant TTR. Cardiac amyloidosis is more frequent in men and it is rare before the age of 40.

Table 6.11.2 Differential features in RCM and constrictive pericarditis (CP) (I lancock EW, 2001; Tam JW, *et al.* 2002)

Feature	CP	RCM
Past medical history	Pericarditis, cardiac surgery, trauma, radiotherapy, connective tissue disease	These items rare
Jugular venous waveform	X and Y dips brief and 'flicking', not large positive waves	X and Y dips less brief, may have large A wave or V wave
Extra sounds in diastole	Early S3, high pitched 'pericardial knock'. No S4	Later S3, low pitched, 'triple rhythm'. S4 in some cases
Mitral or tricuspid regurgitation	Usually absent	Often present
Paradoxical pulse	Often present to a moderate degree	Rarely present
ECG	P waves: intra-atrial conduction delay. Atrioventricular (AV) or intraventricular (IV) conduction defects rare	P waves: right or left atrial hypertrophy/ overload. AV or IV conduction defects not unusual
Chest radiograph	Pericardial calcification in 20–30%	Pericardial calcification rare
M-mode echocardiography (echo)	Abrupt septal movement ('notch') in early diastole in most cases	'Notch' only occasionally
2D echo	Septal movement toward left ventricle (LV) in inspiration	Relatively little septal movement toward LV in most cases
	Slight or moderate atrial enlargement	Pronounced atrial enlargement
Doppler echo	Respiratory variation in mitral and tricuspid flow velocity >25%	Respiratory variation in mitral and tricuspid flow velocity <15%
Tissue Doppler of mitral annulus	E' ≥8 cm/s, E/E' <15	E'<8 cm/s, E/E' >15
Cardiac catheterization (CC): Equilibration of diastolic pressures in all cardiac chambers	Within 5 mmHg in nearly all cases, often essentially the same	Within 5 mmHg in a small proportion of cases
CC: dip–plateau waveform in the right ventricular (RV) pressure waveform	End diastolic pressure >1/3 of systolic pressure in many cases	End diastolic pressure often <1/3 of systolic pressure
CC or Doppler Echo: peak RV systolic pressure	Nearly always <60 mmHg, often <40 mmHg	Frequently >40 and possibly >60 mmHg
CC: respiratory variation of ventricular peak systolic pressures	Out-of-phase RV and LV peak systolic pressure variations	In-phase RV and LV peak systolic pressure variations
MR/CT imaging	Thick pericardium in most cases	Global subendocardial late gadolium enhancement in amyloidosis
Endomyocardial biopsy	Normal, or non-specific abnormalities	Amyloid or other infiltrative disease

Clinical approach

Clinical presentations: key points
- Congestive heart failure is a common presentation (50%) in AL amyloidosis, the worst prognostic factor and the most frequent cause of death
- In familial ATTR amyloidosis heart involvement is late, often dominated by conducting system disease, but death is related to heart failure or arrhythmia in 50% of cases
- Cardiac involvement in senile systemic amyloidosis varies from no functional impairment to heart failure
- Most common presentation of cardiac amyloidosis is that of RCM (see p. 256) due to amyloid infiltrates and diastolic dysfunction by circulating immunoglobulin light chains (in AL amyloidosis). Right-sided findings may dominate the presentation in ATTR amyloid
- Congestive heart failure related to systolic dysfunction is also common in late disease. There may be angina pectoris with angiographically normal coronary arteries (small-vessel disease), small but persistent troponin I release (bad prognostic marker)
- Orthostatic hypotension and exertional syncope are common. The latter is a bad prognostic feature (death within 3 months)
- Sudden cardiac death due to electromechanical dissociation or less commonly to sustained ventricular tachycardia/ ventricular fibrillation is another presentation.

Diagnosis: key points (Table 6.11.4)
- Clinical suspicion based on heart failure without cardiomegaly, or concentric left or biventricular hypertrophy with prominent valves, septal infiltration, biatrial dilation with non dilated ventricles, a 'granular sparkling' myocardial texture on 2D-Echo, absence of valve disease or hypertension, low voltages (QRS voltage ≤0.5 mV in all limbs leads, or ≤1 mV in all precordial leads), pseudo-infarct patterns and extreme axis deviation on ECG and a restrictive filling on Doppler Echo (Table 6.11.1).

Table 6.11.3 Main types of cardiac amyloidosis (Shah, *et al.* 2006; Falk, 2005)

Type	Protein	Cardiac involvement/median survival (mo)	Extracardiac features
Primary (AL)	Immunoglobulin light chain	One-third to one-half of AL patients/13 (4 months if heart failure at diagnosis), bad prognosis, affects both genders equally	Renal failure, proteinuria (30–50%), hepatomegaly autonomic dysfunction (dys), macroglossia, periorbital purpura, neuropathy, carpal tunnel, weight loss
Hereditary (ATTR)	Mutant TTR	Variable/70 months (better prognosis than AL)	Severe peripheral and autonomic polineuropathy, renal involvement rare, blindness
Senile systemic (ATTR)	Wild-type TTR	Common/75 mo (slow progression)	Extracardiac organ involvement unusual, elderly men (>70 yrs)
Isolated atrial (AANF)	Atrial natriuretic factor	Common, limited to atrium, mostly in women, may increase atrial fibrillation risk/?	None
Reactive (AA)	Serum amyloid A	<10%/heart involvement rarely clinically significant, 24 mo	Renal failure, proteinuria, hepatomegaly associated with chronic inflammatory conditions
AApoA1	Mutant apolipoprotein	Very rare/ ?	Renal failure

- Search for indirect evidence of amyloid in other organ systems: renal involvement, purpura, neuropathy, organomegaly (tongue, liver, spleen).
- Search for an associated potentially amyloidogenic disorder: serum and urine analysis for monoclonal immunoglobulin, including serum free light chain assay (99% sensitivity for combined positive serum immunofixation and abnormal κ/λ light-chain ratio in AL amyloid),

hematologic and biochemical blood profiles, 24-hour urine collection for creatinine clearance and proteinuria.
- Search direct evidence for amyloid deposition: (1) serum amyloid P component (SAP) scintigraphy; (2) apple-green birefringence on Congo red staining of a screening biopsy, e.g. rectal, gingival biopsy or abdominal subcutaneous fat aspirate (both 50–80% sensitive in AL and variant TTR amyloidosis), or of a clinically involved organ biopsy

Table 6.11.4 Diagnosis and treatment of cardiac amyloidosis (Shah *et al.* 2006; Falk, 2005)

Type	Diagnostic tools	Treatment
Primary (AL)	Serum and urine protein immunofixation electrophoresis, serum free light chain assay and κ/λ light-chain ratio, bone marrow biopsy tissue analysis revealing clonal plasma cell dyscrasia related to (but usually not associated with) multiple myeloma, and κ and λ light-chain antiserum staining on biopsy tissue	Chemotherapy with autologous stem cell replacement
Hereditary (ATTR)	ATTR antiserum staining on biopsy tissue, serum TTR isoelectric focusing, genetic testing for TTR mutations	Liver transplantation (Tx), though cardiac amyloid may progress despite Tx
Senile systemic (ATTR)	ATTR antiserum staining on endomyocardial biopsy tissue	Supportive
Isolated atrial (AANF)	Atrial natriuretic factor antiserum staining	None required
Reactive (AA)	Target organ biopsy specimen analysis, AA antiserum staining	Treat underlying inflammatory disease
AApoA1	Apo A1 antiserum staining	Liver Tx, HTx?

tissue, e.g. heart or kidney, particularly if abdominal fat is negative.

- Consult other colleagues, in particular internists, nephrologists, and haematologists, e.g. bone marrow biopsy tissue analysis revealing plasma cell dyscrasia related to (but usually not associated with) multiple myeloma.
- Definite diagnosis of amyloidosis type: (1) immunohistochemical staining of tissue containing amyloid, e.g. ATTR antiserum staining, (2) may require genetic analysis to exclude TTR mutations (or other rare genetic types), (3) rarely may require extraction and sequencing of amyloid fibril proteins.

Natural history and management: key points
- Prognosis is a function of amyloid type (Table 6.11.4).
- Mainstay of supportive therapy is the use of diuretics.
- ACE inhibitors and angiotensin II inhibitors are poorly tolerated, calcium channel blockers are contraindicated (negative inotropic effect). Anticoagulation is used if atrial fibrillation is present.
- In AL amyloidosis the advanced nature of the disease at diagnosis makes them unfit for high-dose chemotherapy with autologous stem cell replacement, or is associated with high peritreatment mortality (up to 30%). Ejection fraction <40% is an absolute contraindication to high-dose chemotherapy.
- AL amyloidosis is considered a contraindication for heart transplantation (HTx), although HTx may precede chemotherapy. Candidates for the latter approach are rare, since <5% of AL patients have exclusive cardiac involvement and extracardiac disease is a contraindication to HTx.
- Late age of onset and heart failure at diagnosis preclude liver Tx in most ATTR patients. Liver Tx should be considered at an early stage in patients with genetic diagnosis and clinical evidence of disease activity or positive abdominal fat. Amyloid deposition in the myocardium may progress if the patient has amyloid cardiomyopathy at the time of liver Tx. Few ATTR patients with cardiomyopathy has been treated with combined HTx and liver Tx or Htx only.

Endomyocardial disease (EMD) with hypereosinophilia (Löffler endocarditis)
On pathological examination there is biventricular cardiac involvement, with mural endocardial thickening of the inflow portions and the apex. Histological findings include variable extent of (1) acute eosinophilic myocarditis and endocarditis, (2) thrombosis, fibrinoid change and vasculitis of intramural coronary vessels, (3) mural thrombosis with eosinophils, (4) marked fibrotic thickening (see Chapter 6.12). The typical patient is a man in the fourth decade who lives in a temperate climate and has the hypereosinophilic syndrome (i.e. persistent eosinophilia with 1500 eosinophils/mm^3 for at least 6 months) due to (1) unknown cause, (2) leukaemia, (3) parasitic, allergic, granulomatous, hypersensitivity or neoplastic disorders.

Clinical approach
History: key points
- Patient history: enquire for neoplastic illness (e.g. multiple myeloma), for causes of inflammatory CMP or immune-mediated systemic disorders.

Clinical presentations and examination: key points
- Cardiac presentation may include:
  - Weight loss, fever, cough, rash and congestive heart failure, right, left-sided or both, pulmonary congestion, or less frequently pulmonary infiltrates
  - A murmur of mitral regurgitation is common, as well as systemic embolism, leading to neurological and renal dysfunction
  - Atrial fibrillation and conduction defects may also be present
  - Death is due to heart failure, often with concomitant renal, hepatic or respiratory dysfunction.

Diagnosis: key points
- On 2D- and Doppler Echo, there may be (1) localized thickening of the posterobasal LV wall, with limited motion of the posterior mitral valve leaflet; (2) obliteration of the apex with thrombus; (3) atrial dilation; (4) preserved systolic function, mitral regurgitation and a restrictive filling (Tables 6.11.1 and 6.11.2).
- On CC there is a restrictive filling with biventricular obliteration of the apex. EMB often confirms the diagnosis.

Natural history and management
Standard medical therapy is indicated in the early stage, palliative surgical therapy may be necessary in selected cases in the fibrotic stage. Corticosteroids and hydroxyurea may be beneficial, selected refractory cases responded to treatment with interferon.

Endomyocardial fibrosis (EMF) (or EMD without hypereosinophilia)
EMF is a common form of RCM in equatorial Africa, less frequent in South America, Asia and non-tropical countries. On pathological examination there is marked mural endocardial thickening of the subvalvular regions of one or both ventricles and the apex, leading to restrictive physiology. It is debated whether EMF and EMD with the hypereosinophilic syndrome (see paragraph above) are variants or the same disease. Pathology is similar, but EMF has its distinct geographical distribution (equatorial Africa) and affects younger patients of both sexes. Hypereosinophilia, thromboembolia and generalized arteritis are not common or distinctive features of EMF.

Clinical approach
Clinical presentations and examination: key points
- Cardiac presentation may include:
  - Congestive heart failure, right, left-sided or both
  - Atrioventricular regurgitation is common
  - Atrial fibrillation and conduction defects may also be present
  - Death is due to heart failure, and patients presenting with advanced right-sided heart failure have worse prognosis.

Diagnosis: key points
- On 2D- and Doppler Echo, there may be (1) localized thickening of the posterobasal LV wall, with limited motion of the posterior mitral valve leaflet; (2) obliteration of the apex with thrombus; (3) atrial dilation; (4) mitral and/or tricuspid regurgitation and a restrictive filling (Tables 6.11.1 and 6.11.2); (5) pericardial effusion.
- On CC there is a restrictive filling with biventricular obliteration of the apex. EMB may reveal endocardial

thickening, and fibrotic changes extending into the myocardium, but lack of acute myocarditis or coronary arteritis (see Chapter 6.7).

Natural history and management

Standard medical therapy is indicated in the early stage, palliative surgical therapy may be necessary in selected cases in the fibrotic stage.

Further reading

Falk RH. Diagnosis and treatment of the cardiac amyloidoses. *Circulation* 2005;**112**:2047–60.

Hancock WE. Differential diagnosis of restrictive cardiomyopathy and constrictive pericarditis. *Heart* 2001;**86**:343–49.

Morimoto S. Sarcomeric proteins and inherited cardiomyopathies. *Cardiovasc Res* 2008;**77**:659–66.

Richardson P, McKenna WJ, Bristow M, *et al.* Report of the 1995 World Heath Organization/International Society and federation of Cardiology task force on the definition and classification of cardiomyopathies. *Circulation* 1996;**93**:841–2.

Selvanayagam JB, Hawkins PN, Paul B, Myerson SG, Neubauer S. Evaluation and management of the cardiac amyloidosis. *J Am Coll Cardiol* 2007;**50**:2101–10.

Shah KB, Inoue Y, Mehra MR. Amyloidosis and the heart. A comprehensive review. *Arch Intern Med* 2006;**166**:1805–13.

Tam JW, Shaikh N, Sutherland E. Echocardiographic assessment of patients with hypertrophic and restrictive cardiomyopathy: imaging and echocardiography. *Curr Opin Cardiol* 2002;**17**:470–77.

Zipes DP, Libby P, Bonow RO, Braunwald E. (eds). *Braunwald's heart disease. A textbook of cardiovascular medicine.* 2004; 7th edn. Philadelphia: Elsevier.

Inflammatory cardiomyopathies: endocrine and alcohol

The definitions used in this chapter are in keeping with the 1996 WHO/ISFC classification of the cardiomyopathies (Richardson *et al.* 1996), although other scientific position papers (Maron *et al.* 2006; Elliott *et al.* 2008) have been published. Inflammatory and endocrine cardiomyopathies are listed among the specific cardiomyopathies, defined as heart muscle diseases that are associated with a specific cardiac or systemic disorder.

Inflammatory cardiomyopathies

Inflammatory cardiomyopathy is defined as myocarditis in association with cardiac dysfunction. Myocarditis is an inflammatory disease of the myocardium, diagnosed on endomyocardial biopsy (EMB). Inflammatory cardiomyopathy is involved in the pathogenesis of dilated cardiomyopathy (DCM) and other cardiomyopathies, e.g. Chagas' disease, etc. Recognized forms of inflammatory cardiomyopathy include

1 idiopathic
2 infectious
   - Bacterial: Staphylococcus, Streptococcus, Pneumococcus, Meningococcus, Gonococcus, Salmonella, *Corynebacterium diphtheriae, Haemophilus influenzae*, Mycobacterium (tuberculosis), *Mycoplasma pneumoniae, Brucella*
   - Spirochaetal: Borrelia (Lyme disease), Leptospira (Weil disease)
   - Fungal: Aspergillus, Actinomyces, Blastomyces, Candida, Coccidioides, Cryptococcus, Histoplasma, Mucormycoses, Nocardia, Sporothrix
   - Protozoal: *Trypanosoma cruzi* (Chagas's disease), *Toxoplasma gondii*, Entamoeba, Leishmania
   - Parasitic: *Trichinella spiralis, Echinococcus granulosus, Tenia solium*
   - Rickettsial: *Coxiella burnetii* (Q fever), *R. rickettsii* (Rocky Mountain spotted fever), *R. tsutsugamuschi*
   - Viral: coxsackievirus A and B, echovirus, poliovirus, hepatitis viruses, influenza A and B viruses, adenovirus, respiratory syncytial virus, mumps virus, measles virus, rubella virus, dengue virus, Chikungunya virus, yellow fever virus, Junin virus, Lassa fever virus, lymphocytic choriomeningitis virus, herpes simplex virus, varicella-zoster, human herpes virus-6, cytomegalovirus (CMV), Epstein–Barr virus, variola virus, vaccinia virus, parvovirus B19, rabies virus, human immunodeficiency virus-1 (HIV).
3 Immune-mediated due to:
   - Allergens
     - Tetanus toxoid, vaccines, serum sickness
     - Drugs: penicillin, cefaclor, colchicine, furosemide, isoniazid, lidocaine, tetracycline, sulfonamides, phenytoin, phenylbutazone, methyldopa, thiazide diuretics, amitriptyline
   - Alloantigens
     - Heart transplant rejection
   - Autoantigens
     - Idiopathic: virus-negative lymphocytic, virus-negative giant cell

   - Associated with other extracardiac autoimmune disorders, including systemic lupus erythematosus, rheumatoid arthritis, Churg–Strauss syndrome, Kawasaki's disease, inflammatory bowel disease, scleroderma, polymyositis, myasthenia gravis, type 1 insulin-dependent diabetes mellitus, thyrotoxicosis, Hashimoto thyroiditis, sarcoidosis, Wegener's granulomatosis.

4 Toxic due to
   - Drugs: amphetamines, anthracyclines, cocaine, cyclophosphamide, ethanol, fluorouracil, lithium, catecholamines, hemetine, interleukin-2, trastuzumab, clozapine
   - Heavy metals: copper, iron, lead
   - Miscellaneous causes: scorpion sting, snake and spider bites, bee and wasp stings, carbon monoxide, inhalants, phosphorus, arsenic
   - Hormones: phaeochromocytoma
   - Vitamins: beri-beri
   - Physical agents: radiation, electric shock

Inflammatory cardiomyopathy/myocarditis is a challenging diagnosis in cardiology and needs a high level of suspicion; clinical presentation is polymorphic. It may heal or lead to DCM and the pathophysiology of this progression in man is incompletely understood.

Clinical approach

History: key points
- Family history: enquire for familial DCM, other cardiomyopathy, sudden cardiac death, and for autoimmune disease
- Patient history: enquire for recent (days to 2 weeks) upper respiratory or gastrointestinal suspected viral syndrome, allergy, other autoimmune diseases, previous suspected or proven myocarditis, heavy alcohol intake, assumption of drugs and toxic substances (e.g. cocaine), vaccines, travel to places where specific cardiotropic infection is possible or endemic (e.g. Brazil, Argentina and Chile for Chagas' disease), proximity with domestic animals, conventional coronary risk factors, etc. The aim is search as well as exclude possible treatable causes (e.g. drug-related toxicity or hypersensitivity). Most patients will have 'idiopathic' or presumed viral myocarditis.

Clinical presentations and EMB correlates: key points
Clinical presentation is variable (Caforio 2007, 2008; Cooper 2007; Dennert 2008), including:
- Acute myocardial infarction-like syndrome with normal coronary arteries, frequent, particularly in the young with few or no risk factors, onset days or weeks after a presumed respiratory or gastrointestinal viral syndrome with or without increased systemic inflammatory markers and fever. Chest pain may be pleuritic if concomitant pericarditis is present, or similar to ischemic chest pain
  - EMB correlates: active lymphocytic, less frequently necrotizing eosinophilic or giant-cell myocarditis.
- Unexplained heart failure with normal-sized or dilated left ventricle with systolic dysfunction (DCM) and hemodynamic compromise, distinct onset with a viral prodrome within 2 weeks before cardiac symptoms (fulminant myocarditis)

- EMB correlates: active lymphocytic, less frequently necrotizing eosinophilic or giant-cell myocarditis.
- Unexplained heart failure with DCM and new ventricular arrhythmias, high-degree heart block, or lack to response to usual care within 1–2 weeks; onset may date back weeks or months
  - EMB correlates: most likely giant-cell myocarditis, or cardiac sarcoidosis or specific infection (Chagas' disease, *Borrelia burgdoferi*), less frequently necrotizing eosinophilic or active lymphocytic.
- Heart failure, DCM, no viral prodrome, no new ventricular arrhythmias, or high-degree heart block, onset of symptoms weeks to several months
  - EMB correlates: most likely active lymphocytic or borderline myocarditis, inflammation by sensitive immunohistological staining may be present also in Dallas negative cases and in up to 40% of cases.
- Heart failure with eosinophilia, variable onset, possible association with the hypereosinophilic syndrome (see Chapter 6.11), Churg–Strauss syndrome, cancer, parasitic, helminthic or protozoal infection, vaccines, drug-induced hypersensitivity
  - EMB correlates: most likely eosinophilic or hypersensitivity myocarditis, or eosinophilic endomyocarditis.
- Unexplained bradytachyarrhythmia and syncope, or sudden cardiac death
  - EMB correlates: active lymphocytic or giant-cell myocarditis.
- Peripartum cardiomyopathy
  - FMB correlates: most frequently active lymphocytic myocarditis.

ECG findings: key points
Variable, including
- ST-segment and T-wave changes (pericarditic or mimicking acute coronary syndromes), Q waves, atrioventricular and bundle branch blocks, supraventricular as well as ventricular arrhythmia, including ventricular tachycardia and ventricular fibrillation.

Diagnosis on EMB combines histology, immunohistology, detection of viral genome: key points
- Histological (Dallas) criteria (Aretz et al. 1985): active myocarditis is an inflammatory infiltrate of the myocardium with necrosis and/or degenerative changes of adjacent myocytes not typical of infarction; when the inflammatory cells are sparse and no myocyte necrosis is observed, no definitive diagnosis is possible and the term used is borderline myocarditis. Myocardial inflammation is qualitatively described as (1) mild, moderate or severe; (2) focal, confluent, or diffuse; (3) lymphocytic, neutrophilic, eosinophilic, giant cell, granulomatous or mixed. Follow-up EMB permits distinction into: (1) ongoing (persistent), (2) resolving (healing), or (3) resolved (healed) myocarditis. The Dallas criteria have several pitfalls including interobserver variability, low sensitivity, partly due to sampling error in focal disease, and lack of differentiation of viral from non-viral myocarditis, therefore they are no longer used in isolation.

- Immunohistochemical stains (increased number of inflammatory cells and upregulation of HLA molecules) have led to increased diagnostic accuracy (Caforio et al. 2007, Dennert et al. 2008; Kindermann et al. 2008).
- Molecular detection of viral genomes by polymerase chain amplification or in situ hybridization suggests viral aetiology (Kuhl et al. 2005).

Selective coronary angiography: key points
- Needed for exclusion of coronary artery disease.

Non-invasive cardiac imaging: key points
- Echocardiography defines morphology and biventricular function, but it is not specific. It may be normal or similar to DCM. Pericardial effusion may be present, as well as segmental wall motion abnormalities. Apical left ventricular aneurisms suggest Chagas' disease. In fulminant myocarditis there may be a slight increase in left ventricular wall thickness and a mildly dilated severely hypokinetic ventricle.
- [111]Indium antimyosin antibody and [67]gallium nuclear imaging are rarely used (limited availability of tracers, poor spatial resolution, radiation issues).
- Cardiovascular magnetic resonance (CMR) imaging defines morphology and biventricular function of the heart and provides tissue characterization. Myocardial oedema is assessed on T_2-weighted CMR images, hyperaemia/capillary leak on myocardial early gadolinium enhancement ratio (EGEr), and necrosis/fibrosis on late-gadolinium enhancement (LGE). LGE is typically subepicardial, localized in inferolateral and less frequently in anteroseptal left ventricular segments, and may be focal or diffuse in distribution. The best overall diagnostic accuracy (78%) is found by the combination of all three tissue-based CMR parameters, but correlative data with EMB are still based on low numbers. CMR does not differentiate viral from non-viral myocarditis.

Blood studies: key points
- Viral serology does not give diagnosis of certainty although raised IgM with seroconversion at the time of cardiac symptoms may suggest viral heart disease
- Elevated cardiac enzymes may or not be present, as well as raised systemic inflammatory markers
- Serum anti-heart autoantibodies may be present. Lack of viral genome on EMB with serum AHA suggests immune-mediated DCM/myocarditis (Caforio et al. 2007, 2008)
- Blood tests are available for specific forms and should be used if clinical features are suggestive (e.g. Machado–Guerreiro test in Chagas' disease; organ and non-organ-specific autoantibodies in autoimmune disorders; HIV serology; pp65 antigenaemia in CMV infection, etc).

Natural history and management
Potential long-term complications
Inflammatory cardiomyopathy/acute myocarditis of suspected viral aetiology resolves in about 50% of cases in the following 2–4 weeks, but about 25% will develop persistent cardiac dysfunction and 12–25% may acutely deteriorate and either die or progress to end-stage DCM with a need for heart transplantation. Risk stratification based on

standard clinical and diagnostic markers is poor; biventricular dysfunction at presentation has been reported as the main predictor or death or transplantation (Caforio et al. 2007; Dennert et al. 2008). Giant cell myocarditis is associated with poor prognosis (Cooper et al. 2007). Prognosis may also be worse in selected forms with multisystem involvement. The detection of selected viral genomes on EMB or of chronic inflammation by immunohistology may have independent prognostic value but further confirmation is required (Kuhl et al. 2005; Kindermann et al. 2008). Fulminant myocarditis has been associated with a good prognosis.

Standard treatment

Inflammatory cardiomyopathy should be treated in keeping with current heart failure and arrhythmia guidelines (Hunt 2005; Dickstein et 2008). Patient with fulminant myocarditis or with haemodynamic compromise in spite of optimal medical management need intravenous inotropic agents and/or mechanical circulatory support as a bridge to recovery or transplantation. Aerobic activity should be restricted for a period of months, and gradually reintroduced.

Aetiology-directed treatment

Antibiotic or antiviral therapy should be instituted if appropriate or available in specific infectious forms. Seek guidance from your infectivologist colleagues. Hypereosinophilic inflammatory cardiomyopathy often responds to withdrawal of the offending agent (e.g. drugs, toxic substances) or to treatment of the underlying cause (e.g. parasitic infection), but steroids are often needed.

Immunosuppressive/immunomodulatory therapy should be used in virus-negative giant cell myocarditis, in cardiac sarcoidosis and in inflammatory cardiomyopathy/DCM associated with other extra-cardiac autoimmune diseases. The immunosuppressive regimen should be tailored to the patient and follow-up should be in collaboration with the clinical immunologist and/or rheumatologist.

Immunosuppressive/immunomodulatory therapy may also be helpful in selected virus-negative inflammatory cardiomyopathy/DCM patients with exclusive cardiac involvement who are cardiac autoantibody positive and do not respond to standard heart failure therapy, but double-blind placebo controlled multicenter randomized studies in patients with defined viral or autoimmune CMP/DCM are not yet available.

Alcoholic cardiomyopathy

Chronic alcohol intake may be associated with congestive heart failure, hypertension, cerebrovascular accidents, arrhythmia and sudden death, as well as with alcoholic/toxic DCM. DCM may be idiopathic, familial/genetic, viral and/or immune, alcoholic/toxic or associated with recognized cardiovascular disease in which the degree of myocardial dysfunction is not explained by the abnormal loading conditions (see Chapter 6.9) (Richardson et al. 1996). Alcoholic/toxic DCM is more common in men aged 30–55 years, who have been heavy consumers of whisky, wine or beer, generally for more than 10 years. Myocardial damage may result from direct toxic effect of alcohol, nutritional factors, in particular thiamine deficiency that leads to beri-beri disease and/or to additives in the alcoholic beverage (cobalt).

Clinical approach

History: key points

- Family history: enquire for familial DCM, other cardiomyopathy, sudden cardiac death (not all alcoholics develop DCM, thus there may be genetic predisposition)
- Patient history: enquires should be made to exclude other viral and/or immune DCM causes (see previous paragraph and Chapter 6.9). A high level of suspicion should be present not to miss a history of heavy alcohol intake, even in the absence of liver disease or peripheral neuropathy.

Clinical presentations: key points

- Physical examination and clinical presentation are similar to those of idiopathic DCM, palpitation is common, especially on the weekend due to higher alcohol intake
- Atrial fibrillation and flutter and first-degree heart block are common and ECG abnormalities may disappear after cessation of alcohol consumption
- Cardiac catheterization and echocardiographic findings are those of idiopathic DCM.

Natural history and management

Alcohol cessation as early in the disease course as possible can stabilize clinical signs and symptoms and partially improve the natural history. The prognosis in those who continue to drink in poor, particularly if they have been symptomatic for a long time. Medical management except for alcohol cessation is that of an idiopathic DCM, although thiamine may be given on the assumption that beriberi may be contributing to heart failure.

Endocrine cardiomyopathies

Cardiovascular involvement and/or specific cardiomyopathy may be observed in several endocrine disorders.

Acromegaly

It is an uncommon condition, in 99% due to benign adenomas of the anterior pituitary gland, producing human growth hormone (hGH), which stimulates the synthesis of insulin-like growth factor type (IGF-1) in the liver and in other cell types. Diagnosis is based upon demonstration of high serum growth hormone levels (>5 ng/dL) and of serum IGF-1 >300 μIU/mL at 1 hour after a 100-g glucose load. The tumour is localized by magnetic resonance imaging. Therapy is resection of adenoma by trans-sphenoidal surgery. Octreotide acetate, a somatostatin analogue, is effective in lowering hGH, a hGH receptor antagonist, pegvisomant, lowers IGF-1 in the long-term and may be used in somatostatin-resistant patients.

Cardiovascular findings: key points

- Hypertension, insulin resistance, diabetes mellitus, hyperlipidaemia, cardiomegaly, congestive heart failure, non-ischaemic cardiomyopathy, cerebrovascular accidents have a major impact on survival.
- Up to two-thirds of patients have echocardiography criteria for left ventricular hypertrophy, there may be associated aortic and valve disease. ECG findings are abnormal in about 50% of patients, and include left axis deviation, septal Q waves, ST depression, conduction defects, sick sinus syndrome, supraventricular and ventricular tachycardia.
- Cardiovascular complications improve with treatment of the endocrine neoplasm, and survival is better in patients with clinical and biochemical remission.

Cushing disease

Excess cortisol secretion due to excess release of adreno-corticotropic hormone (ACTH) by a pituitary adenoma causes Cushing disease. Rarely, excess cortisol results from excess ACTH produced by neoplastic lesions in the adrenal gland (Cushing syndrome) or from ectopic ACTH production by small cell carcinoma of the lung, carcinoids, and other endocrine or haematological neoplasms. Diagnosis is based upon 24-hour urinary free cortisol test and anatomical localization of the neoplastic lesions by magnetic resonance imaging. Treatment is based upon surgical resection of the underlying cause with hormone replacement therapy as necessary.

Cardiovascular findings: key points
- Hypertension, hyperlipidaemia, chronic congestive heart failure, coronary artery disease and myocardial infarction, cerebrovascular and peripheral vascular disease due to accelerated atherosclerosis have a major impact on survival, even in minimal or subclinical degrees of Cushing syndrome. There seems to be a direct relation between cortisol production rates and PR interval.
- A monogenic autosomal dominant trait mapping to the q2 region of chromosome 17, defined as Carney complex includes Cushing syndrome, cardiac mixoma (mostly in the left atrium, but can occur anywhere in the heart, at young age, and may be multicentric), various pigmented dermal lesions (not café-au-lait).

Hyperaldosteronism

Excess aldosterone production by benign adrenal adenomas leads to primary hyperaldosteronism (Conn syndrome). Treatment is based upon surgical removal.

Cardiovascular findings: key points
Hypertension, sodium retention and renal loss of magnesium and potassium, left ventricular hypertrophy, disproportionate to that expected from hypertension alone.

Adrenal cortical insufficiency (Addison disease)

Adrenal cortical insufficiency may be due to autoimmunity, infection, haemorrhage, malignancy, inborn errors of steroid hormone metabolism, or to pituitary-dependent loss of ACTH secretion. Acute adrenal cortical insufficiency is an endocrine emergency.

Cardiovascular findings: key points
Tachycardia, hypotension, cardiovascular collapse, hyponatraemia and hyperkalaemia, reduced left ventricular end-diastolic and end-systolic dimensions. Cardiac atrophy is a response to reduced cardiac workload, but restoration of normal plasma volume with mineral corticoid and glucocorticoid replacement increases ventricular mass.

Hyperthyroidism

Cardiovascular symptoms and findings in hyperthyroidism are an integral and frequently predominant part of the clinical presentation. Diagnosis is based upon low TSH levels (<0.01–0.001 µIU/mL).

Cardiovascular findings: key points
- Haemodynamic alterations induced by hyperthyroidism include a decrease in systemic vascular resistance, increased blood volume, venous return and cardiac preload, increased cardiac output, contractility, and heart rate.
- Symptoms include palpitation, exercise intolerance, dyspnoea, anginal-like chest pain with often normal coronary arteries. Sinus tachycardia and atrial fibrillation are common features, and TSH should be measured in all new-onset unexplained atrial fibrillation/supraventricular arrhythmia cases.
- A minority of cases develop biventricular heart failure in spite of high cardiac output at rest, e.g. thyrotoxic cardiomyopathy. However, exercise intolerance may relate to skeletal muscle myopathy rather than heart failure. As a result of increased output to the pulmonary bed there is an increase in pulmonary artery pressures leading to neck vein distension, hepatic congestion and peripheral oedema similar to that observed in primary pulmonary hypertension or right heart failure.
- All symptomatic patients should receive beta-blockers, as these drugs treat the tachycardia-induced component of ventricular dysfunction and improve cardiac signs and symptoms. Definitive therapy requires iodine-131 alone or combined with an antithyroid drug.

Hypothyroidism

Cardiovascular symptoms and findings in hypothyroidism are subtler than in hyperthyroidism. Diagnosis is based upon high TSH levels (>5 µIU/mL).

Cardiovascular findings: key points
- Haemodynamic alterations induced by hyperthyroidism include an increase in systemic vascular resistance and after load, reduced blood volume, venous return and cardiac preload, reduced cardiac output, contractility and heart rate.
- Sinus bradycardia, narrow pulse pressure, diastolic hypertension, a quiet precordium and reduced intensity of the apical impulse, increased serum total and low-density lipoprotein (LDL) cholesterol are typical. Pericardial effusion is frequent, but tamponade is rare. Hypothyroid patients may be at increased risk of coronary artery disease. ECG there may be low voltage, QT prolongation that may predispose to ventricular arrhythmias. Serum creatine kinase (CK) is higher by 50% to 10-fold and is mainly of skeletal muscle origin. Replacement therapy reverses these findings.

Phaeochromocytoma

Phaeochromocytomas are primarily benign tumours originating from neuroectodermal chromaffin cells within the adrenal medulla, abdomen or within plexus of sympathetic adrenergic cells, 10% of cases are familial. It may co-exist with medullary thyroid carcinoma or hyperparathyroidism, in the multiple endocrine neoplasia (MEN) syndrome type II, due to a mutation in the RET proto-oncogene. In MEN IIB phaeochromocytomas co-exist with medullary thyroid carcinoma and mucosal neuromas on the lips and tongue. Phaeochromocytomas may also be associated with neurofibromatosis or with cerebellar or retinoangiomas in von Hippel–Lindau disease. Diagnosis requires demonstration of increased noradrenaline norepinephrine or adrenalin (epinephrine) or its metabolites in serum and blood. Quantitative 24-hour urinary metanephrines are useful. Treatment is surgical.

Cardiovascular findings: key points

• Headache, palpitation, excess sweating, chest pain, weight loss, hypertension with associated orthostatic hypertension due to episodic excess catecholamine secretion. There are case reports of cardiomyopathy, as well as autopsy reports of histological myocarditis (see Inflammatory cardiomyopathies, p. 262) in patients with previously diagnosed or undiagnosed phaeochromocytomas. ECG shows left ventricular hypertrophy and strain pattern

• Preoperative management requires 7–14 days of alpha-adrenergic blockade, usually with prazosin or phenoxybenzamine. Beta-blockade is contraindicated prior to alpha-adrenergic blockade. If necessary for control of supraventricular arrhythmia or incessant tachycardia beta-1-selective agents, such as atenolol are preferred. If surgery is not feasible, metyrosine can decrease catecholamine synthesis and improve cardiovascular signs and symptoms.

Diabetic cardiomyopathy

The higher incidence of congestive heart failure and its poorer prognosis in diabetics compared to non-diabetics has elicited the speculation that the heart muscle may be more vulnerable to ischemia. A 'true' diabetic cardiomyopathy may exist, but its prevalence, nature, and cause directly related to diabetes are debated, since other risk factors, common in diabetics, such as hypertension, coronary atherosclerosis and microvascular dysfunction can directly contribute to myocardial dysfunction. Treatment and prevention of myocardial dysfunction in diabetes requires aggressive control of hyperglycaemia as well of other associated cardiovascular risk factors in keeping with current heart failure guidelines.

References

Aretz HT, Billingham ME, Edwards WE et al. Myocarditis: a histopathologic definition and classification. Am J Cardiol Pathol 1985;**1**:1–10.

Caforio ALP, Calabrese F, Angelini A, et al. A prospective study of biopsy-proven myocarditis: prognostic relevance of clinical and aetiopathogenetic features at diagnosis. Eur Heart J 2007;**28**:1326–33.

Caforio ALP, Iliceto S. Genetically determined myocarditis: clinical presentation and immunological characteristics. Curr Opin Cardiol 2008;**23**:219–26

Caforio ALP, Mahon NG, Baig KM, et al. Prospective familial assessment in dilated cardiomyopathy. Cardiac autoantibodies predict disease development in asymptomatic relatives. Circulation 2007;**115**:76–83.

Cooper LT, Baughman KL, Feldman AM, et al. The role of endomyocardial biopsy in the management of cardiovascular disease: a scientific statement from the AHA, the American College of Cardiology, and the European Society of Cardiology. Endorsed by the HFSA and the Heart Failure Association of the ESC. J Am Coll Cardiol 2007;**50**:1914–31.

Dennert R, Crijns HJ, Heymans S. Acute viral myocarditis. Eur Heart J 2008;**29**:2073–82.

Dickstein K, Cohen-Solal A, Filippatos G, et al. ESC guidelines for the diagnosis and treatment of acute and chronic heart failure 2008: the task force for the diagnosis and treatment of acute and chronic heart failure 2008 of the European Society of Cardiology. Developed in collaboration with the Heart Failure Association of the ESC (HFA) and endorsed by the European Society of Intensive Care Medicine (ESICM). Eur J Heart Fail 2008;**10**:933–89.

Elliott P, Andersson B, Arbustini E, et al. Classification of the cardiomyopathies: a position statement from the European Society of Cardiology working group on myocardial and pericardial disease. Eur Heart J 2007;**29**:270–76.

Hunt S. ACC/AHA 2005 guideline update for the diagnosis and management of chronic heart failure in the adult: a report of the ACC/AHA Task Force on Practice Guidelines (Writing Committee to Update the 2001 Guidelines for the Evaluation and Management of Heart Failure). J Am Coll Cardiol 2005;**46**:e1–e82.

Kindermann I, Kindermann M, Kandolf R, et al. Predictors of outcome in patients with suspected myocarditis. Circulation 2008;**118**:639–48.

Kuhl U, Pauschinger M, Seeberg B, et al. Viral persistence in the myocardium is associated with progressive cardiac dysfunction. Circulation 2005;**112**:1965–70.

Maron BJ, Towbin JA, Thiene G, et al. Contemporary definitions and classification of cardiomyopathies. An American Heart Association Scientific statement from the Council on Clinical Cardiology, Heart Failure and Transplantation Committee; quality of Care and Outcome research and Functional Genomics and Translational Biology Interdisciplinary Working Groups: and Council on Epidemiology and Prevention. Circulation 2006;**113**:1807–16.

Richardson P, McKenna WJ, Bristow M, et al. Report of the 1995 World Heath organization/International Society and federation of Cardiology task force on the definition and classification of cardiomyopathies. Circulation 1996;**93**:841–2.

Zipes DP, Libby P, Bonow RO, Braunwald E, (eds). Braunwald's heart disease. A textbook of cardiovascular medicine, 7th edn. 2004. Philadelphia: Elsevier.

Cardiac cachexia

Cardiac cachexia is a complication of chronic heart failure. It is defined as:

- An unintended and progressive loss of lean body mass, fat and/or bone tissue, often accompanied by weakness, fever, nutritional deficiencies, and diarrhoea as a complication of chronic heart failure.
- Cachexia is diagnosed when there is an involuntary weight loss of more than 5% of weight within a 3- to 6-month period.
- The word cachexia originates from the Greek *kakos* meaning bad and *hexis* meaning condition.

This definition is pragmatic and has been agreed by a consensus conference on cachexia. Cachexia can be a complication of many chronic illnesses and diseases, including cancer, chronic heart failure, chronic obstructive pulmonary disease, chronic kidney disease, rheumatoid arthritis, tuberculosis, cystic fibrosis, Crohn's disease, HIV-AIDS, liver cirrhosis, and sepsis. In all these underlying conditions a similar composite of neurohormonal activation, immune and pro-inflammatory cytokine activation, and anabolic/catabolic imbalance is seen. In contrast, starvation causing weight loss is not associated with these changes.

Epidemiology and prognosis

In developed countries 1.5–2.5% of the adult population has chronic heart failure, with a new incidence of approximately 1% per year. Of patients with established heart failure 10–25% will develop cachexia per year during follow-up. Once diagnosed 1-year mortality in cardiac cachexia has been shown to be between 20% and 40% in most large series.

Classification

According to a consensus conference in 2008 (Evans 2008), a working definition of cachexia was proposed: 'cachexia, is a complex metabolic syndrome associated with underlying illness and characterized by loss of muscle with or without loss of fat mass'. The prominent clinical feature of cachexia is weight loss in adults (corrected for fluid retention) or growth failure in children (excluding endocrine disorders). Anorexia, inflammation, insulin resistance and increased muscle protein breakdown are frequently associated with cachexia. Cachexia is distinct from starvation, age-related loss of muscle mass, primary depression, malabsorption and hyperthyroidism and is associated with increased morbidity.

Cachexia can be associated with many separate chronic illnesses.

Pathophysiology (von Haehling 2007)

- Immune cytokine activation, including tumour necrosis factor (TNF)-α, interleukin (IL)-1 and IL-6
- Catabolic activation, including increased levels of cortisol
- Anabolic deficiency with reduced levels of testosterone, DHEA, and IGF-1
- Neurohormonal activation with markedly elevated levels (higher than in non-cachectic heart failure) of epinephrine (adrenaline), norepinephrine (noradrenaline), aldosterone, renin, angiotension II and aldosterone in particular

- Acquired hormonal resistance syndromes affecting growth hormone and insulin
- Intramuscular immune activation.

Clinical approach

Symptoms

- Cardiac cachexia always occurs on the background of chronic heart failure, which should have been evident to the treating doctors.
- The paramount symptoms are unintentional weight loss, muscular fatigue, exaggerated dyspnoea, anorexia, and occasionally dizziness. Diarrhoea or malabsorption can also occur.

Complications

Complications of cachexia are those of generalized and severe weight loss, and immune paresis. Cachexia itself is a complication of an underlying chronic disorder, in this case chronic heart failure.

- Death: cachexia is an ominous development. The rate of death in cardiac cachexia is two- to threefold that of general heart failure and can reach 50% per annum in severe cases.
- Immune paresis: modern thinking is that one of the triggers for cachexia development is an exaggerated cytotoxic response to repetitive immune challenge such as by repeated bacteraemia and endotoxin release into the circulation, for example by bowel wall passage of bacterial products secondary either to bowel wall oedema or ischaemia or a combination (Sandek 2009). When established, cachexia is associated with inflammatory and immune activation but a relative inefficiency of immunity leading to increased risk of sepsis.
- Falls, accidents, and fractures: the profound muscle weakness and loss of all body components including bone mass and bone calcium mean that falls are both more common and more likely to lead to fractures. As the condition occurs in heart failure, which is itself a condition predominantly of the older people, this can be a serious issue.
- Arrhythmias and sudden death: heart failure is associated with opportunistic ventricular and atrial arrhythmias and research has shown cachectic patients in particular have an exaggerated predominance of these complications. This may be related to the severe disturbances of autonomic function and cardiopulmonary reflexes that is seen in cardiac cachexia.
- Sleep disordered breathing: obstructive sleep apnoea is common in many cardiovascular disorders. In heart failure there is also an increase in central sleep apnoea so that the most common pattern seen clinically is mixed. In cardiac cachexia the severe abnormalities of cardiopulmonary reflex control makes central sleep apnoea, periodic breathing, and even Cheyne–Stokes breathing much more common. This can be a cause of both disturbed sleep and an increased risk of potentially fatal nocturnal arrhythmias.

Signs

Weight loss, whole body wasting, and muscle wasting on the background of chronic heart failure.

Investigation

Dietary and weight history

- To determine the rate and extent of weight loss, and whether intentional or not.
- To assess dietary intake of protein calories, essential fatty acids, vitamins, and other essential nutrients.
- To assess appetite, and advise of dietary and nutritional strategies and support.

Full heart failure assessment

- An assessment of the aetiology, staging, management, and progression of the underlying heart failure is essential for optimal care of the cardiac cachexia patient.

Management

- Integrated care of the cardiac cachexia patient is essential and these are frail and extremely high-risk patients requiring physician, nursing, occupational, nutritional, psychological, and palliative care variously at different points in their disease progress (Moughrabi 2007).
- Currently no approved therapies for cardiac cachexia exist. Apart from growth hormone and some appetite stimulants in acquired immunodeficiency syndrome-induced cachexia, no cachexia syndrome has an approved treatment option. Some potential candidates have been tested such as exogenous oral amino acid supplementation, hyperalimentation, and steroid derivative anabolics such as nandrolone or oxandrolone. Newer experimental therapies are being actively sought and tested now that the pathophysiology of the condition is becoming better understood (Muscaritoli 2006). This includes ghrelin (Deboer 2008), myostatin antibodies (Hoenig 2008), anti-inflammatory (Kalantar-Zadeh 2008),

nutritional (Pasini 2008), and antineurohumoral strategies (Lainscak 2006).

- Cardiac transplantation has been used in cachectic patients with no apparently worse outcome than when used for non-cachectic patients (Clark 2007).

References

Clark AL, Knosalla C, Birks E, et al. Heart transplantation in heart failure: the prognostic importance of body mass index at time of surgery and subsequent weight changes. Eur J Heart Fail 2007;**9**:839–44.

DeBoer MD. Emergence of ghrelin as a treatment for cachexia syndromes [Review]. Nutrition 2008;**24**:806–14.

Evans WJ, Morley JE, Argiles J, et al. Cachexia: a new definition. Clin Nutr 2008;**27**:793–9.

Hoenig MR. Hypothesis: myostatin is a mediator of cardiac cachexia. Int J Cardiol 2008;**124**:131–3.

Kalantar-Zadeh K, Anker SD, Horwich TB, Fonarow GC. Nutritional and anti-inflammatory interventions in chronic heart failure [Review]. Am J Cardiol 2008;**101**:89E–103E.

Lainscak M, Andreas S, Scanlon PD, et al. Ghrelin and neurohumoral antagonists in the treatment of cachexia associated with cardiopulmonary disease. Intern Med 2006;**45**:837.

Moughrabi SM. Evangelista LS. Cardiac cachexia at a glance [Review]. Prog Cardiovasc Nurs 2007;**22**:101–3.

Muscaritoli M, Bossola M, Aversa Z, et al. Prevention and treatment of cancer cachexia: new insights into an old problem. Eur J Cancer 2006;**42**:31–41.

Pasini E, Aquilani R, Dioguardi FS, et al. Hypercatabolic syndrome: molecular basis and effects of nutritional supplements with amino acids. Am J Cardiol 2008;**101**:11E–15E.

Sandek A, Anker SD, von Haehling S. The gut and intestinal bacteria in chronic heart failure. Curr Drug Metab 2009;**10**:22–8.

von Haehling S, Doehner W, Anker SD. Nutrition, metabolism, and the complex pathophysiology of cachexia in chronic heart failure [Review]. Cardiovasc Res 2007;**73**:298–309.

Cardiac surgery and left ventricular assist device

Surgery for patients in advanced heart failure aims to correct or repair many of the pathophysiological changes that are not corrected by medical treatment alone. The surgical techniques currently performed include revascularization of hibernating myocardium, ventricular restoration surgery, mitral valve repair, use of ventricular assist devices, and heart transplantation. These procedures have not been exposed to the same degree of scrutiny as medical treatment to provide the level of evidence needed to become a standard part of heart failure management. The most established operations for heart failure are heart transplantation and coronary artery bypass grafting (Hunt et al. 2005).

Revascularization of hibernating myocardium

The aims of myocardial revascularization are to correct myocardial ischaemia and hence prevent further adverse ventricular remodelling and myocardial infarctions, and to improve myocardial contractility in regions of ischaemic hibernating myocardium that have been shown to be viable.

Several non-randomized studies have reported that coronary artery bypass graft (CABG) in patients with advanced ischaemic heart failure can be performed with an acceptable risk (operative mortality of 1.7–5.3%) and improves ejection fraction by up to 40% above the baseline value. The reported 5-year survival is 60–75% (Lorusso et al. 2001). Unfortunately, complete data are not reported for many of these studies and the patient population is not uniform across the studies. Accurate reporting of ventricular function, heart failure symptoms, and NYHA functional class at late follow-up is absent from most studies. This is of importance as many of the benefits noted may not be sustained at late follow-up.

There is some evidence that recurrence of heart failure symptoms after CABG for ischaemic heart failure may be related to the severity of ventricular dilatation. Yamaguchi et al. (1997) reported a recurrence of heart failure following CABG in 69% of patients when the left ventricular end systolic volume index (LVESVI) was greater than 100 mL/m^2 compared with only 15% when the LVESVI was less than 100 mL/m^2 (P <0.01). Five-year survival was also worse when LVESVI was greater than 100 mL/m^2 (53.5% versus 85%; P <0.01). Similarly, Louie et al. (1991) reported a failure of CABG in 27% of patients with ischaemic cardiomyopathy undergoing CABG for heart failure symptoms, all of whom had a left ventricle that was significantly more dilated than those in whom CABG was successful (LV end diastolic diameter of 81 mm versus 68 mm). In these patients, it may be necessary to perform some form of ventricular restoration surgery in addition to CABG.

Ventricular restoration

The aim of ventricular restoration is to restore the size, shape, and geometry of the dilated left ventricle towards normal. Restoration of ventricular shape and geometry towards a more elliptical structure also leads to greater efficiency of ventricular systole. Ventricular restoration is achieved by resection of myocardium and reconstructing the remaining ventricle into a more elliptical shape.

Ischaemic cardiomyopathy

Surgical ventricular restoration (SVR) in ischaemic cardiomyopathy is largely done using the Dor procedure. The technique involves the resection of the akinetic or dyskinetic anterior free wall of the left ventricle. Typically, these patients have had an anterior myocardial infarction with scarring and akinesia or dyskinesia of the left ventricle anterior free wall, which may extend into the septum. This segment of non-functional myocardium is resected and an oval dacron patch is then placed which excludes the infarcted part of the septum from the rest of the ventricle. The size of the patch is tailored to the required size of the ventricle, and the shape of the patch is such that it helps restore the geometry of the left ventricle towards a more elliptical configuration. CABG is always performed at the same time. The aim is to (1) recruit hibernating myocardium and hence enhance myocardial contractility, (2) resect non-functional akinetic or dyskinetic myocardium and hence improve the efficiency of ventricular contraction, and (3) restore the left ventricle to its normal size, shape, and geometry with the benefits discussed previously.

There are no positive randomized controlled trials of SVR; the largest, the STICH trial showed no significant improvement in death or cardiac hospitalization rates (Jones et al. 2009).

Mitral valve surgery

Mitral valve surgery is an option in advanced heart failure when significant mitral regurgitation is present. The mitral regurgitation is usually functional due to failure of mitral leaflet coaptation as a result of dilatation of the left ventricle, which pulls the subvalvular mitral apparatus and the papillary muscles apart, and mitral annular dilatation. Grigioni et al. (2001) demonstrated that the presence of functional mitral regurgitation following myocardial function has an adverse effect on long-term survival (62% at 5 years versus 39%; P<0.001) and is an independent predictor of adverse survival (RR 1.88; P <0.001). Furthermore, the severity of functional mitral regurgitation also determined long-term survival. The 5-year survival of those with an effective regurgitant orifice area (ERO) of greater than 20 mm^2 was only 21% compared with 47% in those whose ERO was less than 20 mm^2 (P <0.001, RR of death of 2.23, or 1.40 per 10 mm^2 ERO increase).

There are no randomized controlled trials. The non-randomized studies report an operative mortality of between 2.3% and 11%. All of the studies show a significant improvement in NYHA functional class and ejection fraction. The reported improvement in symptoms, functional capacity, and cardiac function, which appears to be maintained for up to 3 years is encouraging. The reported actuarial survival is 58% at 5 years.

Left ventricular assist devices

Bridge-to-transplant

The use of left ventricular assist devices (LVADs) as a bridge-to-transplant in patients with decompensated chronic heart failure is well established. It has been used in more than 4000 patients worldwide. It is estimated that up to 20% of heart transplant recipients in the United States receive an LVAD prior to transplantation (Frazier and Delgado 2003). The use of LVADs in these patients improves their cardiac output, NYHA functional class, and helps reverse any end-organ dysfunction, e.g. renal and liver impairment. Their physical condition improves significantly while on LVAD support, and as many as 50% are well enough to be discharged home with an LVAD while waiting for a donor heart. The results of transplantation are improved in these patients who demonstrate a better survival at 1 year after transplantation than those who did not receive and LVAD (90% versus 67%).

Bridge to recovery
The number of patients showing sustained myocardial recovery following LVAD explantation is small, and the predictors of such patients have not been fully identified at present. The duration of heart failure prior to LVAD implantation may be important as once significant myocyte loss and myocardial fibrosis occurs, ventricular remodelling may be irreversible. It has been reported that patients who demonstrated significant myocardial recovery had a smaller left ventricular end diastolic diameter (71 ± 2 mm versus 81 ± 7 mm) and less myocardial fibrosis (24 ± 4% versus 34 ± 2%) compared with those who showed no myocardial recovery . There is also some evidence that the use of the beta-agonist clenbuterol in combination with maximal heart failure drugs may augment myocardial recovery with an LVAD in a significantly greater proportion of patients than has been reported hitherto (Birks et al. 2006).

Destination therapy
The efficacy of LVADs as permanent or destination therapy was demonstrated in the REMATCH trial (Rose et al. 2001); 129 patients with end-stage heart failure who were not eligible for transplantation were randomized to either optimal medical therapy or to treatment with a LVAD. These patients were all in NYHA class IV heart failure, had an ejection fraction of less than 25%, and were either dependent on intravenous inotropic support or had a peak oxygen consumption of less than 12 mL/kg/min. The group of patients treated with LVADs showed a highly significant 48% reduction in the risk of death at 2 years (23% survival versus 8%; P = 0.002). The most common cause of death in the LVAD group was device failure whereas in the medical group it was congestive heart failure. In addition, quality of life (SF36 scores) and NYHA functional class were significantly improved in the LVAD group (mean NYHA class II versus IV). There was more morbidity in the LVAD group in the first 30 days principally related to complications of the LVAD such as bleeding, infection, and thromboembolic complications but these had evened out by 30 days. Mortality was consistently lower in the LVAD group, both early and late.

Heart transplantation
Heart transplantation remains the most effective treatment for patients with end-stage heart failure. The reported survival following heart transplantation is 79–85% at 1 year, 75–80% at 3 years, and 69–75% at 5 years (Taylor et al. 2008).

The shortage of donor hearts limits transplantation as a universal treatment for these patients. Only 128 heart transplants were performed in the UK in 2007/8, a small decrease on 2006/7, the figure for which was 156 (UKTSSA 2008; refer to http://www.organdonation.nhs.uk/ukt/statistics/latest_statistics/latest_statistics.jsp). The contraindications to transplantation such as advanced age and other co-morbidities further limit the use of heart transplantation in many patients. There is also morbidity associated with heart transplantation such as chronic rejection and complications from the use of immunosuppressive drugs. These include an increased incidence of renal failure and graft vascular disease.

The patients who show the greatest benefit from heart transplantation are those with refractory cardiogenic shock, dependence on inotropic, or mechanical circulatory support or persistent NYHA class IV symptoms with a peak oxygen consumption less than 10 mL/kg/min (Hunt et al. 2005).

Despite all the limitations, heart transplantation remains the greatest success story for truly end-stage disease, with more than 50 000 patients now transplanted worldwide. The breadth of its impact far exceeds the actual recipients, because the lure of heart transplantation called attention to the newly defined population of advanced heart failure, whereas the restricted donor supply inspired the development of better heart failure management and of new strategies for replacement, such as mechanical cardiac devices.

References
Birks EJ, Tansley PD, Hardy J, et al. Left ventricular assist device and drug therapy for the reversal of heart failure. N Engl J Med 2006; **355**: 1873–84.

Frazier OH, Delgado RM. Mechanical circulatory support for advanced heart failure. Circulation 2003; **108**:3064–8.

Grigioni F, Enriquez-Sarano M, Zehr KJ, et al. Ischemic mitral regurgitation: long term outcome and prognostic implications with quantitative Doppler assessment. Circulation 2001;**103**:1759–64.

Hunt SA, Baker DW, Chin MH, et al. ACC/AHA 2005 Guideline update for the Diagnosis and Management of Chronic Heart Failure in the Adult—Summary Article: A report of the American College of Cardiology/American Heart Association Task Force on Practice Guidelines (Writing Committee to update the 2001 Guidelines for the Evaluation and Management of Heart Failure): Developed in Collaboration with the American College of Chest Physicians and the International Society for heart an Lung transplantation: Endorsed by the Heart Rhythm Society. Circulation 2005; **112**. 1825–52.

Jones RH, Velazquez EJ, Michler RE, et al. for the STICH Hypothesis 2 Investigators. Coronary bypass surgery with or without surgical ventricular reconstruction. N Eng J Med 2009;**309**:DOI: 10.1056/NEJMoa0900559.

Lorusso R, La Canna G, Ceconi C, et al. Long-term results of coronary artery bypass grafting procedure in the presence of left ventricular dysfunction and hibernating myocardium. Eur J Cardiothorac Surg 2001;**20**:937–48.

Louie HW, Laks H, Milgalter E, et al. Ischaemic cardiomyopathy. Criteria for coronary revascularisation and cardiac transplantation. Circulation 1991;**94**(Suppl III):III-290–III-295.

Rose EA, Gelijns A, Moskowitz AJ, et al. Long term use of a left ventricular assist device for end stage heart failure (REMATCH). N Engl J Med 2001;**345**:1435–43.

Taylor DO, Edwards LB, Aurora P, et al. Registry of the International Society for Heart and Lung Transplantation: Twenty-fifth Official Adult Heart Transplant Report—2008. J Heart Lung Transplant 2008; **27**: 943–56.

Yamaguchi A, Ino T, Adachi H, et al. Left ventricular volume predicts postoperative course in patients with ischaemic cardiomyopathy. Ann Thorac Surg 1997;**65**:434–8.

Heart transplantation

Definition, epidemiology, and approach to heart failure

Heart failure is defined as a *clinical syndrome*, in which secondary to impaired function of the heart—a performance commensurate with the metabolic needs of the body—cannot be maintained or can only be maintained at the expense of elevated filling pressures.

The number of patients with advanced heart failure is growing. This is a consequence of improved management (revascularization strategies, arrhythmia surveillance) in acute coronary syndromes) and improved longevity of the world population. The *prevalence* in industrialized parts of the world is estimated around 1%, the incidence around 0.15%.

A staged approach to *heart failure management* has been widely proposed. It includes (1) comprehensive lifestyle modification (day–night rhythm, endurance training, salt and fluid restriction, nutrition, weight log-keeping), (2) tailoring of diuretics to remove excessive fluid for optimization of preload, (3) tailoring of neurohormonal blockade for optimization of afterload and heart rate, (4) implantation of defibrillator and biventricular pacemaker (Hunt 2006), (5) evaluation of cardiac surgical options including mechanical circulatory support devices (MCSD) and heart transplantation (HTx) (Deng 2007) (Fig. 6.15.1).

Heart transplant candidacy

At *initial presentation*, it is important that (1) the team gains a basic impression of the patient as a person and the severity of his/her condition, (2) the patient and his/her relatives gain a basic impression of the nature of the management and care programme in the centre, and (3) the cornerstone of a long-term working relationship is founded.

Once it is determined that a patient is potentially an appropriate candidate for transplantation, the complete *transplant evaluation* is performed on an inpatient or outpatient basis. In patients who are unstable and require hospitalization for management of their medical condition, the entire workup is performed as an inpatient. In ambulatory patients, the majority of the workup is done as an outpatient. For stable outpatients who require continued anticoagulation (i.e. history of emboli, prosthetic valves), right heart catheter will be performed in the hospital on heparin.

Current *indications* include (1) Heart Failure Survival Score high risk (Aaronson 1997), (2) peak VO$_2$ <10 mL/kg/min after reaching anaerobic threshold, (3) NYHA class III/IV heart failure refractory to maximal medical therapy, (4) severely limiting ischaemia not amenable to interventional or surgical revascularization, and (5) recurrent symptomatic refractory ventricular arrhythmias to medical, ICD, and surgical treatment.

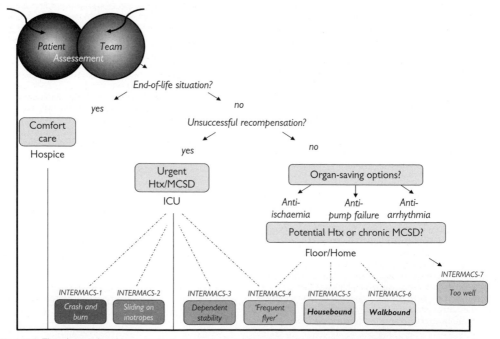

Fig. 6.15.1 The selection algorithm starts with the encounter between patient and team, and is followed by a stepwise evaluation of important issues including: (1) Is an end-of-life situation present? (2) Can the patient be recompensated? (3) After neurohormonal blockade initiation, are there organ-saving options including revascularization, contractility enhancement, and antiarrhythmia therapy? (4) Is the patient a suitable candidate for heart replacement options including mechanical circulatory support and heart transplantation? (5) If so, how urgent is heart replacement according to INTERMACS criteria? (Kirklin 2010). Adapted from Deng MC *et al.* Curr Opin Cardiol 2002;17:137, reproduced with permission from Imperial College Press (2007), from: http://ebooks.worldscinet.com/ISBN/9781860 948305/9781860948305.html.

Every condition that elevates the early and long-term postoperative risk for the patient and therefore reduces the anticipated survival and quality benefit from cardiac transplantation has to be considered a risk factor and potential *contraindication*. During the evaluation process it needs to be established whether or not this circumstance is of temporary or permanent nature. These include (1) irreversible pulmonary hypertension (pulmonary vascular resistance (PVR) >6 WU (Wood's units)), (2) active infection, (3) pulmonary infarction within the last 6–8 weeks, (4) significant chronic renal impairment with crea >2.5 or clearance <25 mL/min, (5) significant chronic hepatic impairment with bili >2.5 or ALT/AST >×2, (6) active or recent malignancy, (7) systemic diseases such as amyloidosis, (8) significant chronic lung disease, (9) significant symptomatic carotid or peripheral vascular disease, (10) significant coagulopathies, (11) recent peptic ulcer disease, (12) major chronic disabling disease, (13) diabetes with end-organ damage and/or brittle diabetes, (14) excessive obesity (e.g. >30% over normal), (15) evidence of drug, tobacco, or alcohol abuse within the last 6 months, (16) active mental illness, (17) psychosocial instability, and (18) >65–70 years.

The *listing decision* is a consequence of a recommendation on the part of the team and the acceptance of the recommendation on the part of the patient. The basis for the listing recommendation is the anticipated gain in quantity and quality of life by the intervention compared with all other established treatment options. The complexity of the evaluation process mandates a team approach for or against a listing recommendation. For the patient who has permanent contraindications against cardiac transplantation and therefore is not recommended for listing it must be emphasized that this decision is in his/her best interest because the anticipated gain in quantity and quality of life would be unacceptably low. It also must be emphasized that the advanced heart failure team in the centre offers continued care, in conjunction with the primary care physician and the local cardiologist, with the same intensity as it would offer care if the patient were a transplant candidate.

The *waiting time* naturally constitutes one of the most stressful periods of life for the heart transplant candidate and his/her family. A main focus lies on the ability of the patient to detect signs of deteriorating heart failure early. Also, patient availability in case of an organ offer must be clearly understood by the patient and communication rules, best achieved by a beeper and/or cell phone, established. A continuous update of the transplant indication with the option of delisting in case of deterioration with new contraindications or improvement is of major importance during the waiting time.

At any time during the waiting period, deteriorating heart failure may precipitate organ failure, specifically respiratory failure following left heart decompensation or renal failure following low cardiac output syndrome. The temporary *bridging of organ function*, for example with MCSD therapy, with the goal of complete recovery must be part of the rationale of caring for heart transplant candidates.

If organ dysfunction progresses to irreversible stages and the goal of recovery appears out of reach, the termination of life support must be entertained, based on the patient's and his/her family's preferences.

The heart transplantation period

The practice of heart transplantation donor acceptance criteria needs to be continuously revised in order to responsibly increase the donor pool. Specifically, scientific evidence for the survival benefit from donor organs with extended acceptance criteria for recipients with a high risk of dying from their heart failure without heart transplantation needs to be reviewed. These extended criteria include advanced donor age, donor heart dysfunction, donor resuscitation, and donor infection. The donor acceptance criteria of Columbia University Medical Center include (1) declaration of brain death with signed consent for heart donation by next-of-kin, (2) age <65 years (coronary angiography recommended for male donors >45 and female donors >50), (3) no evidence of cancer (except for low malignancy brain tumours), (4) no evidence of septicaemia, (5) no antibodies to HIV or HCV, (6) no history of prolonged low cardiac output syndrome (transitory low output, hypotension, arrhythmia does not exclude donation), (7) donors with prolonged high-dose inotrope support (dopamine/dobutamine >10 μg/kg/min) will be considered with reversal after T3 replacement, (8) normal electrocardiogram (ECG) and X-ray (neurogenic T-wave changes are acceptable), (9) normal cardiac physical examination, (10) normal cardiac enzymes, nuclear angiography, and cardiac catheter as indicated, (11) negative blood and sputum cultures, and (12) at the time of organ removal, normal cardiac structures on direct inspection (except ASD/PFO (atrial septal defect/patent foramen ovale)).

The optimal management of the multi-organ donor is critical to the successful outcome of transplantation. In order to achieve this end, a dedicated, multidisciplinary team is necessary, consisting not only of medical staff, but also support workers who organize logistics, and who play their own part in vital areas, such as transport of the donor team and organs. The coordinator's role is pivotal in bringing together, in harmony, teams from different centres.

Although standard surgical techniques have evolved from the original technique developed by Norman Shumway and Richard Lower to the bicaval anastomosis (Kirklin 2002), with an increasing fraction of patients undergoing orthotopic heart transplantation after previous cardiac surgery, intra- and perioperative operative management has become more challenging.

Patient care after heart transplantation

Post-transplantation management serves (1) the maintenance of allograft function, (2) minimization of side-effects of immunosuppressants on the recipient, (3) psychological coping with the transplantation process, and (4) complete reintegration into society.

The *physiology of orthotopic cardiac transplantation* is unique in two aspects: (1) denervation, which leads to a characteristic change in pharmacology, summarized in Table 6.15.1, and (2) allograft rejection, i.e. the transplantation of foreign tissue initiates complex inflammatory responses that are mediated by different leucocyte subsets and their cytokine mediators and usually results, in the absence of immunosuppression, in acute graft rejection and graft destruction.

Current *rejection monitoring methods* advantages and disadvantages are listed in Table 6.15.2. Survivors of haemodynamically compromising rejection episodes associated

Table 6.15.1 Effect of denervation on cardiac pharmacology

Substance	Effect on recipient	Mechanism
Digitalis	Normal increase of contractility	Direct myocardial effect
	Minimal effect on AV node	Denervation
Atropine	None	Denervation
Adrenaline	Increased contractility	Denervation hypersensitivity
	Increased chronotropy	
Noradrenaline	Increased contractility	Denervation hypersensitivity
	Increased chronotropy	
Isoproterenol	Normal increase in contractility	No neuronal uptake
	Normal increase in chronotropy	
Chinidine	No vagolytic effect	Denervation
Verapamil	AV-block	Direct effect
Nifedipine	No reflex tachycardia	Denervation
Hydralazine	No reflex tachycardia	Denervation
Beta-blocker	Increased antagonist effect	Denervation

Table 6.15.3 Commonly used immunosuppressive drugs: targets, main side-effects, and selectivity

Method	Target	Major side-effects	Selectivity
Steroids	Lymphocytes/RES	Osteoporosis Diabetes Psychosis Infection Obesity	+
Azathioprine	Lymphocytes	Marrow suppression Hepatopathy	++
Polyclonal antithymocyte globuline	T-lymphocytes	Infection Malignancies	++
Monoclonal CD3 antibodies	CD3+ T-lymphocytes	Infection Malignancies	+++
Mycophelolate	De novo purine synthesis in lymphocytes	Gastrointestinal	++++
Cyclosporine	IL-2 inhibition in T-lymphocytes	Nephropathy	++++
Tacrolimus	IL-2 inhibition in T-lymphocytes	Nephropathy	++++
Daclizumab	IL-2 receptor antibodies	None	++++

with low biopsy scores in the International Society for Heart and Lung Transplantation grading system have a significantly worse long-term outcome than survivors of episodes associated with high scores, suggesting that immunological mechanisms other than lymphocytic infiltration of the cardiac allograft are important and distinct causes of allograft dysfunction. Recently, molecular leucocyte gene expression profiling has been introduced to rule out acute cellular cardiac allograft rejection in stable heart transplant recipients without endomyocardial biopsy (Deng 2006, Pham 2010).

The degree of selectivity of *immunosuppressive therapies* determines their side-effects. The *immunsuppression and infection management* after cardiac transplantation is summarized in Tables 6.15.3 and 6.15.4.

The *early post-transplant* period is characterized by more typical surgical complications such as pump failure, bleeding, tamponade, arrhythmias, hypotension, hypertension, respiratory, renal, haematological, gastrointestinal, neurological, metabolic, musculoskeletal, and psychological dysfunction.

Long-term complications include (1) cardiac allograft vasculopathy, an unusually accelerated and diffuse form of obliterative coronary arteriosclerosis, determines long-term function of the transplanted heart. Cardiac allograft vasculopathy is a complicated interplay between immunological and non-immunological factors resulting in repetitive vascular injury and a localized sustained inflammatory

Table 6.15.2 Rejection monitoring methods

Method	Delay	Serial assessment	Costs	Indication of rejection	Sens	Spec
History	None	Yes	+	Dyspnoea, weight gain, discomfort	+	+
Physical	None	Yes	+	Arrhythmia, S3, crackles, JVD, edema	+	+
ECG	None	Yes	+	Atrial arrhythmias, low voltage	+	+
Pacemaker	Telemetry	Every night	+++	Voltage ↓ 7%	+++	+++
Echo	30 min	Yes	+++	RT↑, IVRT↓, FS↓	+++	+++
Emb	24 hour	Max 1/week	+++	Cell infiltrates, haemorrhage	+++	+++
Myosin scan	24 hour	Max 1/3 months	+++	Heart–lung ratio >1.6	+++	+++
MRI	1 hour	Max 1/Wo	+++	Signal↑ due to oedema	+++	+++
Immune monitoring	4 hour	Yes	+++	CD4/CD8↑, HLA-DR+/CD14 ↑, IL-2↑	+++	+++

Table 6.15.4 Infection treatment after heart transplantation

Organism	Test	Treatment
Cytomegalovirus	IE-Gene, PCR, IgM	Gancyclovir IV 2 × 5 mg/kg × 2–3 weeks If severe consider CMV abs 300 IE/kg/d × 5–10 days Consider reduction of immunosuppression Ganciclovir resistance: foscarnet
Herpes simplex virus	IgM	Aciclovir IV 3 × 5–10 mg/kg × 10–14 d
Varicella zoster virus	IgM	Aciclovir IV 3 × 5–10 mg/kg × 10–14 d or Aciclovir po 5 × 800 mg/d
HBV	IgM	Lamivudine po 100 mg/d
Legionella	Urine antigen patchy nodular infiltrates	Erythromycin 250–500 mg q 6–12h × 10–14 d
Mycobacterium tuberculosis	Ziehl–Neelson	Rifampicin Isoniacid Myambutol
Nocardia asteroides	Infiltrates with cavernous nodules or abscess formation	Sulfamethoxazole/trimethoprine CNS: trimethoprime IV 480–640 mg/d + Sulfamethoxazole for 6–8 weeks Maintainance dose trimethoprime po 160 mg/Tag + sulfamethoxazole for 6–12 months
Pneumocystis carinii	Diffuse infiltrates	Sulfamethoxazol/trimethoprine 160/800mg q12–24h × 10–14 d
Toxoplasma gondii	Diffuse infiltrates IFT, KBR, IgA ISAGA, IgM ISAGA	Pyrimethamine po 50–100 mg/d + Sulfadiazine po 100 mg/kg/d up to 8 g + Folic acid po 5–15 mg/d (up to 4–6 weeks after reversal of symptoms)
Candida albicans	Direct	Fluconazole IV/po 200–400 mg/dx >10 d Itroconazole
Aspergillus fumigatus	Infiltrates with cavernous nodules or abscess formation	Itroconazole Amphotericine B IV 0,3–0,5 mg/kg QID + Flucytosine po 150 mg/kg/d in 3–4 doses Total duration 3–6 weeks
Cryptococcus neoformans		CNS: itroconazole Amphotericine B IV 0,3–0,5 mg/kg QID + Flucytosine po 150 mg/kg/d in 3–4 doses Total duration 3–6 weeks or fluconazole IV/po 200–400 mg/d x 2 weeks –2 months
Listeria monozytogenes		CNS: ampicillin IV 6–10g/d in 3–4 doses for > 3 weeks + gentamycin IV 3 x 80 mg/d for 1–2 weeks

response, (2) malignancies that are encountered with a risk of 1–2% per year. This risk is 10- to 100-fold higher than the risk in an age-matched control population. Malignant tumours of the skin and lymphomas are the most frequent types, but any solid organ tumour may occur. The incidence of lymphoproliferative diseases with a cyclosporine-based immunosuppressive regimen is estimated to be around 2–4%, and (3) hypertension, respiratory, renal, haematological, gastrointestinal, neurological, metabolic, musculoskeletal, and psychological dysfunction.

Heart transplantation and society

The 5- and 10-year survival rates are in the range of 70% and 50–60%, respectively, after heart transplantation. In the official Heart Transplantation Registry of the International Society for Heart and Lung Transplantaiton (ISHLT) (www.ishlt.org) more than 100 000 thoracic organ transplantation procedures have been registered.

Cardiac transplantation serves only a very limited fraction of the rapidly increasing numbers of heart failure patients. It is playing a paradigmatically important rather than a quantitatively important role in the management of advanced heart failure. This role varies among societies. Practice of cardiac transplantation has developed heterogeneously in industrialized societies, societies with economies in transition, and non-industrialized societies. High technology medicine constitutes a challenge for defining new boundaries. This requires a contemporary role of the physician/team within an adequate framework of the patient–physician encounter (Deng 2001).

References

Aaronson KD, Schwartz JS, Chen TMC, *et al.* Development and prospective validation of a clinical index to predict survival in ambulatory patients referred for cardiac transplant evaluation. *Circulation* 1997;**95**:2660–7.

Deng MC, Eisen HJ, Mehra RM, *et al.*, for the CARGO Investigators. Non-invasive detection of rejection in cardiac allograft recipients using gene expression profiling. *Am J Transplant* 2006;**6**:150–60.

Deng MC, Naka Y. *Mechanical circulatory support therapy for advanced heart failure.* Imperial College Press, London 2007.

Deng MC, Scheld HH. An international perspective towards cardiac transplantation. In: Shelton W (ed). *The ethics of organ donation and transplantation.* JAI Press 2001.

Hunt SA, Abraham WT, Chin MH, *et al.*, American College of Cardiology; American Heart Association Task Force on Practice Guidelines; American College of Chest Physicians; International Society for Heart and Lung Transplantation; Heart Rhythm Society.

ACC/AHA 2005 Guideline Update for the Diagnosis and Management of Chronic Heart Failure in the Adult: a report of the American College of Cardiology/American Heart Association Task Force on Practice Guidelines (Writing Committee to Update the 2001 Guidelines for the Evaluation and Management of Heart Failure): developed in collaboration with the American College of Chest Physicians and the International Society for Heart and Lung Transplantation: endorsed by the Heart Rhythm Society. *Circulation* 2005;**112**:e154–235.

Kirklin JK, Naftel DC, Kormos RL, *et al.* Second INTERMACS annual report: more than 1,000 primary left ventricular assist device implants. *J Heart Lung Transplant* 2010;**29**:1–10.

Kirklin JK, Young JB, McGiffin DC. *Cardiac Transplantation.* Churchill-Livingstone New York 2002.

Pham MX, Teuteberg JJ, Kfoury AG, *et al.*, IMAGE Study Group. Gene-expression profiling for rejection surveillance after cardiac transplantation. *N Engl J Med* 2010;**362**:1890–900.

Cardiac resynchronization therapy

Cardiac resynchronization therapy (CRT), also known as atriobiventricular or just biventricular pacing, is a treatment designed for use in patients with a dilated and poorly contracting left ventricle to improve cardiac function in order to improve symptoms of heart failure, prognosis, or both (Cleland et al. 2005). It is highly effective in patients who are in sinus rhythm and who have a markedly prolonged QRS duration, which is thought to be a marker of cardiac dyssynchrony. However, there is no group of patients with heart failure where there is substantial evidence for a lack of efficacy (Cleland et al. 2007). Understanding how CRT works, and in whom, is a rapidly evolving field of research. CRT may be combined with other technologies including a defibrillator (CRT-D) that can be used to treat ventricular, and potentially supraventricular, arrhythmias, or telemonitoring, which can be used to interrogate remotely not only the device but patients clinical status (Braunschweig et al. 2008). Features of cardiac dyssynchrony are (Cleland et al. 2007):

1 Prolonged atrioventricular conduction: delayed activation of the ventricles will lead to diastolic mitral regurgitation, delayed onset of systole, and hence a delay in the onset of diastole in the next cardiac cycle.

2 Interventricular mechanical delay: usually delayed activation of the free wall of the left ventricle, leading to contraction of the right ventricle and interventricular septum prior to the left ventricular free wall. Coordination of diastolic relaxation may be similarly affected.

3 Intraventricular dyssynchrony: meaning that segments of the left ventricle are contracting and relaxing at different times, which is mechanically inefficient. This leads to a shorter left ventricular ejection time but longer isovolumic contraction and relaxation times.

4 Some segments may reach peak contraction either before or after the aortic valve has closed, which impairs diastolic function and is wasted energy. Theoretically almost all segments could have peak contraction after aortic valve closure. In such a case, intersegmental left ventricular dyssynchrony is not severe but overall cardiac dyssynchrony is very severe.

5 Incoordinate activation of papillary muscles may result in functional mitral regurgitation.

Dyssynchrony is even more complex than the above picture suggests, since it may vary according to the degree of cardiovascular stress (posture, exercise, etc.) and vary over time (QRS duration increases progressively in heart failure) (Cleland et al. 2009). It is little wonder that imaging studies have so far been unable to identify useful dyssynchrony criteria by which to select patients for CRT.

An alternative imaging approach is to use cardiac magnetic resonance imaging to assess cardiac synchrony and the amount of myocardial scar. Transmural myocardial scar from myocardial infarction should not respond to either pharmacological or device therapy and patients with extensive transmural scar probably have a poor outcome regardless of treatment. However, outcome with treatment and response to it are different concepts. A patient who has an excellent intrinsic prognosis may have an excellent outcome with therapy, even though they have no response to it. A patient with a very poor prognosis may have an excellent response but still have a poor outcome

that would have been even worse had they not got the treatment (Cleland et al. 2009).

Delivery of cardiac resynchronization

Currently, CRT is delivered by means of a pacemaker that, in addition to the conventional right atrial and right ventricular leads, has a third lead placed via the coronary sinus into an epicardial coronary vein overlying the left ventricular free wall. In addition to the usual risks associated with standard pacing, there is a risk of coronary sinus dissection during placement of the left ventricular lead, but this is rarely fatal. Placement of the left ventricular lead is the most challenging aspect of delivering CRT. There is a strongly held belief supported by some evidence that positioning of this lead is important in order to deliver effective CRT. Pacing in a posterolateral left ventricular vein is recommended. Measurement of cardiac function or, as a surrogate, systolic blood pressure during the procedure is often advocated, because an acute response might indicate a better long-term response. Left ventricular lead displacement is common but reduced by modern lead technologies. Diaphragmatic and phrenic nerve pacing are other common problems that can often be detected and corrected at the time of implantation.

After CRT device implantation atrioventricular pacing should be programmed to the shortest atrioventricular delay that does not impede the atrial filling wave on Doppler echocardiography. There is little evidence to support using any other interventricular pacing delay than zero, although ensuring that all left ventricular segments have peak contraction before the aortic valve closes seems intuitively obvious. The timing of CRT impulses should be repeated after 3 months and probably again after 12 months, as the optimal settings may change as the heart changes in response to CRT and or disease progression. More research is required into how to optimize the timing of CRT impulses for the individual patient.

Who should be considered for CRT?

CRT can be used to improve symptoms or prognosis or both. The goals of treatment will help determine patient selection. CRT is a rapidly evolving area but experts and guidelines agree about the benefits for the following patients:

1 A dilated left ventricle (left ventricular end-diastolic dimension >30 mm per metre in height) with left ventricular ejection fraction <35% despite pharmacological treatment.

2 Moderate or severe symptoms of heart failure despite pharmacological treatment.

3 ECG showing sinus rhythm and QRS duration >150 ms.

Although guidelines generally recommend consideration for patients with QRS >120 ms, most patients in trials have had a QRS >150 ms and therefore not all experts agree. However, the choice of any QRS interval threshold is arbitrary. Recent data, not yet considered by guidelines, suggest that CRT can improve cardiac function, delay worsening of heart failure and reduce mortality in patients who have few or no symptoms (Linde et al. 2008; Cleland et al. 2009b) and with a left ventricular ejection fraction up to 40%. When the objective of CRT is to improve prognosis, it is no longer appropriate to exclude patients with few or no symptoms. Some advocate the use of biventricular pacing in patients with atrial fibrillation, usually with atrioventricular node ablation to ensure ventricular capture. The results of relevant trials are awaited. There is no agreement on the value of dyssynchrony imaging. Of the imaging measures of dyssynchrony, only interventricular mechanical delay appears useful, although even it is a poor marker of response (Richardson et al. 2007; Cleland et al. 2008; Ghio et al. 2009). Age is not an important criterion for selection for CRT, but older patients may have less to gain from CRT-D.

Who should be considered for CRT-D

Adding a defibrillator to a CRT device may save an extra one or two lives per year by preventing sudden death (Yao et al. 2007), although clinical trials have yet to prove that CRT-D is superior to CRT alone. A recent study showed that CRT-D was superior to ICD alone in patients with heart failure and ischaemic heart disease (Coletta 2008) and CRT alone reduces the risk of sudden death (Cleland et al. 2006). The effect of CRT-D compared with CRT might be larger in patients who have already experienced an haemodynamically unstable arrhythmia. The rates of appropriate, unnecessary and inappropriate shocks in the trials of CRT-D reported so far have been large (24% per year overall (Saxon et al. 2006)) and have an adverse effect on patients' psychological state and quality of life and may damage myocardium. The incremental cost per quality-adjusted life-year for CRT compared with medical therapy alone is about ~7500 but the incremental cost-effectiveness of CRT-D compared with CRT is ~48 000 (Yao et al. 2007). For these reasons, only selected patients who require CRT should have CRT-D. Patients with few co-morbidities who would be expected to live a long time (10 or more years) if death from heart failure or arrhythmias are prevented should generally receive CRT-D. Patients with a life expectancy <5 years should generally have CRT only. Clinical judgement and informed patient choice should guide the use of CRT-D in those with an intermediate prognosis. Age is an important determinant of longevity due to the common occurrence of life-limiting co-morbid disease and must influence judgement. Patients aged >70 years should generally receive CRT rather than CRT-D. There is little evidence that risk stratification for sudden death prior to CRT implantation is useful but patients with milder symptoms probably have a low risk of dying of heart failure and therefore proportionately higher risk of dying suddenly.

On the other hand, CRT should always be included at the time of an ICD implantation if the patient has a dilated left ventricle with an ejection fraction ≤40% and QRS >120 ms. Indeed, since QRS increases over time, there is an argument for ignoring QRS duration in this selection process (Cleland et al. 2008).

Expected benefits

CRT may improve cardiac function instantaneously when it corrects moderate or severe mitral regurgitation. These patients often also feel better immediately, sometimes even before the procedure is over. For many patients, CRT will result in a substantial reduction in left ventricular volume and a rise in ejection fraction over the ensuing 6–12 months. These effects are greater in patients with dilated cardiomyopathy than in those with ischaemic heart disease (Ghio et al. 2009). However, the effect of CRT on prognosis is similar in patients with or without ischaemic

heart disease (Wikstrom et al. 2008). Blood pressure rises, which in the context of heart failure is a good thing (Cleland et al. 2005). Although improvement in ventricular function is a good sign after CRT, it does not explain all (or perhaps much) of the effects of treatment on prognosis (Cleland et al. 2008).

Most of the improvement in symptoms occurs within 3 months of implantation. It is associated with improved quality of life, largely due to improved physical functioning (Cleland et al. 2009c). In the longer term, CRT reduces the rate of worsening symptoms and of the need for hospitalization for worsening heart failure (Cleland et al. 2005). As with all treatment, all patients do not respond equally well. There is no effective means of identifying responders, although a good clinician will often be able to judge the likely outcome by looking a issues such as co-morbidity (stroke, renal failure, respiratory disease). Patients with a low systolic blood pressure, moderate mitral regurgitation and marked interventricular mechanical delay who do not have extensive myocardial scar may identify a population who have a very rewarding response to therapy. There must be some patients who do not respond or get worse because of CRT but this may be a small population (<10%) when care is taken with device programming (Cleland et al. 2009a). Patients who deteriorate despite CRT may do so because the underlying disease is progressing. These patients deteriorate even faster when CRT is turned off (Cleland et al. 2009a).

CRT reduces overall mortality by about 10% due to a reduction in death from worsening heart failure and of sudden death. The latter effect is similar to that observed with a defibrillator. It seems likely that CRT-D can reduce sudden death compared with CRT but the only large comparative trial showed no difference in overall survival (Bristow et al. 2004). There is no evidence that CRT reduces the risk of developing atrial fibrillation (Hoppe et al. 2006).

Advances in technology

Wireless myocardial stimulators that can be inserted into the left ventricular endocardium via catheters are being developed. There is evidence that endocardial may be superior to epicardial left ventricular stimulation and that the position of the endocardial stimulator may not be very important (e.g. apical versus left ventricular free wall).

Technologies have been developed to try to automate device programming and remote communication. Their value has not been adequately tested. A variety of features have been introduced including the ability to monitor patient physical activity, sleep patterns, heart rate variability, and electrical bioimpedance to try and improve medical management of patients but the value of these are not yet proven.

References

Braunschweig F, Ford I, Conraads V, et al. Can monitoring of intrathoracic impedance reduce morbidity and mortality in patients with chronic heart failure? Rationale and design of the Diagnostic Outcome Trial in Heart Failure (DOT-HF). Eur J Heart Fail 2008;**10**:907–16.

Bristow MR, Saxon LA, Boehmer J, et al. Cardiac-resynchronization therapy with or without an implantable defibrillator in advanced chronic heart failure. New Engl J Med 2004;**350**:2140–50.

Cleland JG, Coletta AP, Clark AL, Cullington D. Clinical trials update from the American College of Cardiology 2009: ADMIRE-HF, PRIMA, STICH, REVERSE, IRIS, partial ventricular support, FIX-HF-5, vagal stimulation, REVIVAL-3, pre-RELAX-AHF,

ACTIVE-A, HF-ACTION, JUPITER, AURORA, and OMEGA. *Eur J Heart Fail* 2009b;**11**:622–30.

Cleland JG, Freemantle N, Ghio S, et al. Predicting the Long-Term Effects of Cardiac Resynchronisation Therapy on Mortality from Baseline Variables and the Early Response: A Report from CARE-HF (Cardiac Resynchronisation in Heart Failure). *J Am Coll Cardiol* 2008;**52**:438–45.

Cleland JG, Tavazzi L, Daubert J-C, Freemantle N. Cardiac resynchronization therapy. Are modern myths preventing appropriate use? *J Am Coll Cardiol.* 2009a;**53**:608–11.

Cleland JG, Coletta AP, Clark L, Cullington D. Clinical trials update from the American College of Cardiology 2009: ADMIREHF, PRIMA, STICH, REVERSE, IRIS, partial ventricular support, FIX-HF-5, vagal stimulation, REVIVAL-3, pre-RELAX-AHF, ACTIVE-A, HF-ACTION, JUPITER, AURORA, and OMEGA. *Eur J Heart Fail* 2009b;**11**:622–30.

Cleland JG, Calvert MJ, Verboven Y, Freemantle N. Effects of cardiac resynchronisation therapy on long-term quality of life, length of hospital stay and survival (The "Patient Journey"). An analysis from the CARE-HF Study. *Am Heart J* 2009c;**157**:457–66.

Cleland JG, Daubert J-C, Erdmann E, et al. Longer-term effects of cardiac resynchronization therapy on mortality in heart failure (the Cardiac Resynchronization–Heart Failure (CARE-HF) trial extension phase). *Eur Heart J* 2006;**27**:1928–32.

Cleland JG, Daubert J-C, Erdmann E, et al. The effect of cardiac resynchronization on morbidity and mortality in heart failure. *New Engl J Med* 2005;**352**:1539–49.

Cleland JGF, Nasir M, Tageldien A. Cardiac resynchronization therapy or atriobiventricular pacing–what should it be called?. *Nat Clin Pract Cardiovasc Med* 2007;**4**:90–101.

Cleland JGF, Tageldien A, Maarouf N, Hobson N. Patients with heart failure who require an implantable defibrillator should have cardiac resynchronisation routinely. *Heart* 2008;**94**:963–6.

Coletta AP. ESC 2008. *Eur J Heart Fail* 2009;**11**:214–9.

Ghio S, Freemantle N, Serio A, et al. Long term left ventricular reverse remodelling with cardiac resynchronization therapy. Results from the CARE-HF trial. *Eur J Heart Fail* 2009;**11**:480–8

Hoppe UC, Casares JM, Eiskjaer H, et al. Effect of Cardiac Resynchronization on the Incidence of Atrial Fibrillation in Patients With Severe Heart Failure. *Circulation* 2006;**114**:18–25.

Linde C, Abraham WT, Gold MR, et al. Randomized Trial of cardiac resynchronization in mildly symptomatic heart failure patients and in asymptomatic patients with left ventricular dysfunction and previous heart failure symptoms. *J Am Coll Cardiol* 2008;**52**:1834–43.

Richardson M, Freemantle N, Calvert MJ, et al. Predictors and Treatment Response with Cardiac Resynchronisation Therapy in Patients with Heart Failure Characterised by Dyssynchrony: A Predefined Analysis from the CARE-HF Trial. *Eur Heart J* 2007;**28**:1827–34.

Saxon LA, Bristow MR, Boehmer J, Krueger S, et al. Predictors of sudden cardiac death and appropriate shock in the comparison of medical therapy, pacing, and defibrillation in heart failure (COMPANION) trial. *Circulation* 2006;**114**:2766–72.

Wikstrom GB, Lundqvist CB, Andren B, et al. The effects of aetiology on outcome in patients treated with cardiac resynchronization therapy in the CARE HF trial. *Eur Heart J* 2009;**30**:782–8.

Yao G, Freemantle N, Calvert M, et al. The long-term cost-effectiveness of cardiac resynchronization therapy with or without an implantable cardioverter-defibrillator. *Eur Heart J* 2007;**28**:42–51.

Valvular heart diseases

Infective endocarditis

Definition

Infective endocarditis (IE) is an infection of the endocardium of one or more valves or valvular prostheses or pacemaker/defibrillator leads. Rarely, it involves the mural endocardium.

IE requires a collaborative approach, involving cardiologists, cardiac surgeons, infectious disease specialists, microbiologists, and often also neurologists, neurosurgeons, pathologists, and others.

Epidemiology

Annual incidence: 36 per million inhabitants (range 3–224).

Despite improvements in healthcare, the incidence of IE has not changed over the last decades because of changes in risk factors: rheumatic heart disease has become rare; there are more elderly people with valve sclerosis, more patients with valvular prostheses, more patients exposed to nosocomial disease or to haemodialysis, more intravenous drug users.

Major increase with age: <50 years: ≤5/million; >65 years: ≥15/million.

Male–female ratio: 2:1.

Classification

- According to localization of infection and presence or absence of intracardiac material
  - Left-sided native valve IE
  - Left-sided prosthetic valve IE (early, <1 year; late, >1 year)
  - Right-sided IE
  - Device-related IE (pacemaker, defibrillator)
- According to mode of acquisition
  - Health-care associated IE
- Nosocomial IE: IE developing in a patient hospitalized >48 hours prior to the onset of signs/symptoms consistent with IE
- Non-nosocomial IE: signs/symptoms of IE starting <48 hours after admission in a patient with health care contact (home-based nursing or IV therapy; haemodialysis or IV chemotherapy <30 days before the onset of IE; hospitalized in an acute care facility <90 days before the onset of IE; resident in a nursing home or long-term facility)
  - Community-acquired IE: signs/symptoms of IE starting <48 hours after admission in a patient not fulfilling the criteria for healthcare associated infection
  - Intravenous drug use-associated IE.

Microbiology

- IE with positive blood cultures: 85% of IE; mainly streptococci, enterococci and staphylococci
  - Streptococci: oral (viridans) streptococci: *S. sanguis, S. mitis, S. salivarius, S. mutans, Gemella morbillorum*; members of the 'S. milleri' or 'S. anginosus' groups: *S. anginosus, S. intermedius, S. constellatus*; nutritionally variant 'defective' streptococci: *Abiotrophia* and *Granulicatella*; group D streptococci: 'S. bovis/S. equinus' complex
  - Enterococci: *E. faecalis, E. faecium, E. durans*
  - Staphylococci: *S. aureus*, coagulase-negative staphylococci

- IE with negative blood cultures because of prior antibiotic treatment
- IE with frequently negative blood cultures: usually due to fastidious microorganisms: nutritionally variant streptococci, bacilli of the HACEK group (*Haemophilus, Actinobacillus, Cardiobacterium, Eikenella, Kingella*), *Brucella*, fungi
- IE with always negative blood cultures: 5% of IE; caused by intracellular bacteria: *Coxiella burnetii, Bartonella, Chlamydia, Tropheryma whipplei.*

Pathophysiology

- Endothelial damage
- Deposition of fibrin and platelets
- Bacteraemia, bacterial adherence and infection.

Diagnosis

- Presentation: acute, rapidly progressive infection, or subacute or chronic disease with low-grade fever and non-specific symptoms
- Variety of very different clinical situations
- High clinical suspicion if
  - New valve lesion or regurgitant murmur
  - Embolic event of unknown origin
  - Sepsis of unknown origin
  - Fever + intracardiac prosthetic material, previous IE, congenital heart disease, predisposition and recent intervention with recent bacteraemia, heart failure, new conduction disturbance, positive blood cultures with typical IE causative microorganism or positive serology for *Coxiella burnetii*, vascular or immunological phenomena (embolic event, Roth spots, splinter haemorrhages, Janeway lesions, Osler's nodes), neurological symptoms/signs, pulmonary embolism, or peripheral abscess
- Echocardiography +++: for diagnosis and follow-up during medical treatment
  - Major criteria: vegetation, abscess, new dehiscence of a prosthetic valve
  - Transthoracic echo: always; transoesophageal echo in almost all cases (not indicated if good quality transthoracic echo and low clinical suspicion of IE)
- Microbiology: blood cultures +++; serology; polymerase chain reaction; pathological examination of resected tissue or embolic fragments.

Complications

- Frequent and severe
- Cardiac complications
  - Heart failure (50–60% of IE overall)
  - Valve dysfunction (acute regurgitation; rarely valve stenosis)
  - Perivalvular extension (abscess, pseudoaneurysm, fistula, periprosthetic dehiscence, ventricular septal defect, third degree atrioventricular block, acute coronary syndrome)
  - Myocarditis, pericarditis
  - Transoesophageal echocardiography is more sensitive and specific than transthoracic echocardiography

- Early surgery needed in most cases
- Non cardiac complications
  - Embolic events: frequent (20–50% of patients with IE); totally silent in 20% of patients with IE; mainly spleen and brain; lungs in right-sided IE and device-related IE; systematic imaging in all patients with IE; most potent predictors of embolic events: size and mobility of vegetations; risk of embolism is highest during the first days and then decreases rapidly
  - Neurologic complications (20–40% of patients with IE); mainly ischaemic stroke (embolism); haemorrhagic stroke
  - Infectious aneurysm, acute renal failure, rheumatic complications (peripheral arthritis, spondylodiscitis), splenic abscess

Prognosis

- Median in-hospital mortality rate: 16% (range 10–26)
- Predictors of poor short-term prognosis
  - Patient characteristics: prosthetic IE, insulin-dependent diabetes mellitus, co-morbidities
  - Presence of complications of IE: heart failure, renal failure, stroke, septic shock
  - Microorganism: *S. aureus*, fungi, Gram-negative bacilli
  - Echocardiographic findings: periannular complications, severe left-sided valve regurgitation, premature mitral valve closure, low left ventricular ejection fraction, pulmonary hypertension, large vegetation

Antibiotic treatment

- Bactericidal therapy, synergistic combination, high doses, long duration
- Oral streptococci and group D streptococci
  - Penicillin-susceptible streptococci (minimal inhibitory concentration <0.125 mg/L)
  - Standard treatment (4 weeks): penicillin G, 6 × 2 3 million U/day IV or amoxicillin, 100 mg/kg/day IV in six doses or ceftriaxone, 2 g once a day IV or IM
  - Two-week treatment: penicillin G or amoxicillin (same doses) + gentamicin, 3 mg/kg once a day IV or IM; or ceftriaxone (same doses) + netilmicin, 4–5 mg/kg once a day IV
- Penicillin-resistant streptococci (minimum inhibitory concentration (MIC) >0.5 mg/L): penicillin G, 6 × 3 million U/day IV or amoxicillin, 200 mg/kg/day IV in six doses, 4 weeks; + gentamicin, 3 mg/kg once a day IV or IM, 2 weeks
- Beta-lactam allergic patients: vancomycin, 2 × 15 mg/kg/day IV, 4 weeks
- Staphylococci
- Native valves
- Methicillin-susceptible staphylococci: (flu)cloxacillin or oxacillin, 6 × 2 g/day IV, 4–6 weeks; + gentamicin (optional), 3 mg/kg/day IV or IM in 2–3 doses, 3–5 days
- Patients allergic to penicillins: cefazolin, 3 × 2 g/day IV, 4–6 weeks; + gentamicin (optional), 3 mg/kg/day IV or IM in 2–3 doses, 3–5 days; patients allergic to beta-lactam: vancomycin, 2 × 15 mg/kg/day IV, 4–6 weeks
- Methicillin-resistant staphylococci: vancomycin, 2 × 15 mg/kg/day IV, 4–6 weeks
- Prostheses

- Methicillin-susceptible staphylococci: (flu)cloxacillin or oxacillin, 6 × 2 g/day IV, ≥6 weeks; + rifampin, 2 × 600 mg/day IV or PO, ≥6 weeks; + gentamicin, 3 mg/kg/day IV or IM in 2–3 doses, 2 weeks
- Methicillin-resistant staphylococci or patients allergic to penicillins: vancomycin, 2 × 15 mg/kg/day IV, ≥6 weeks; + rifampin + gentamicin, same doses, same duration as above
- Enterococci
  - Beta-lactam and gentamicin-susceptible enterococci: amoxicillin, 200 mg/kg/day IV in six doses or ampicillin, 6 × 2 g/day IV, 4–6 weeks; + gentamicin, 3 mg/kg/day IV or IM in 2–3 doses, 4–6 weeks
  - Beta-lactam allergic patients: vancomycin, 2 × 15 mg/kg/day IV, 6 weeks; + gentamicin, 3 mg/kg/day IV or IM in 2–3 doses, 6 weeks
- Antibiotic treatment of blood culture negative IE
  - *Coxiella burnetii*: doxycycline (2 × 100 mg/day) + hydroxychloroquine (3 × 200 mg/day) or doxycycline + quinolone, >18 months
  - *Brucella*: doxycycline (2 × 100–200 mg/day) + rifampin (300–600 mg/day) + cotrimoxazole (2 × 960 mg/day), ≥3 months
  - *Legionella, Mycoplasma*: macrolide + rifampin, or newer fluoroquinolones, >6 months
  - *Bartonella*: ceftriaxone or ampicillin or amoxicillin + gentamicin or netilmicin (2 weeks) or doxycycline, ≥6 weeks
  - *Tropheryma whipplei*: cotrimoxazole, or beta-lactam + aminoglycoside, long-term
- Empirical treatment
  - Native valves, prostheses >12 months: amoxicillin-clavulanate or ampicillin-sulbactam, 4 × 3–4 g/day IV, 4–6 weeks; + gentamicin, 3 mg/kg/day IV or IM in 2–3 doses, 4–6 weeks
  - Beta-lactam allergic patients: vancomycin, 2 × 15 mg/kg/day IV, 4–6 weeks; + gentamicin, 3 mg/kg/day IV or IM in 2–3 doses, 4–6 weeks; + ciprofloxacin, 2 × 500 mg/day PO or 2 × 400 mg/day IV, 4–6 weeks
  - Prostheses <12 months: vancomycin, 2 × 15 mg/kg/day IV, 6 weeks; + rifampin, 2 × 600 mg/day PO; + gentamicin, 3 mg/kg/day IV or IM in 2–3 doses, 2 weeks
- Monitoring of serum gentamicin and vancomycin concentrations
  - Gentamicin, once a day: pre-dose (trough) concentration <1 mg/L; post-dose (peak; 1 hour after injection) concentration 10–12 mg/L
  - Gentamicin, three doses a day: trough concentration <1 mg/L; peak (1 hour after injection) concentration 3–4 mg/L
  - Vancomycin: trough concentration 10–15 mg/L; peak (1 hour after infusion is completed) concentration 30–45 mg/L

Surgical treatment

- In approximately half of patients
- Rarely needed in right-sided IE; can be considered in case of large vegetations and recurrent pulmonary emboli, fungi, or other virulent microorganisms unresponsive to antibiotic treatment, or severe heart failure despite medical treatment

- Indications for surgical treatment (emergent: within 24 hours; urgent: a few days; or elective)
- Native IE
  - Heart failure: aortic or mitral IE
    - with severe acute regurgitation or obstruction, or with fistula into a cardiac chamber or pericardium, causing refractory pulmonary oedema or cardiogenic shock: emergent
    - with severe acute regurgitation or obstruction and persisting heart failure or signs of poor haemodynamic tolerance (early mitral closure or pulmonary hypertension): urgent
    - with severe regurgitation and heart failure easily controlled with medical treatment: elective
- Uncontrolled infection
  - Persisting fever and positive blood cultures >5–7 days: urgent
  - Locally uncontrolled infection (abscess, false aneurysm, fistula, enlarging vegetation): urgent
  - Infection caused by fungi or multiresistant microorganisms: urgent/elective
- Vegetations
  - Left-sided IE with large vegetation (>10 mm) following one or more embolic episodes or with large vegetation (>10 mm) and other predictors of complicated course (heart failure, persistent infection, abscess): urgent
  - Very large vegetation (>15 mm): urgent
  - IE relapse caused by microorganisms other than oral streptococci: elective
- Prosthetic IE
  - Same as above, +
  - Severe prosthetic dysfunction (dehiscence or obstruction)
    - causing refractory pulmonary oedema or cardiogenic shock: emergent
    - and persisting heart failure: urgent
    - and heart failure easily controlled with medical treatment: elective
  - Infection caused by fungi or multiresistant microorganisms, by staphylococci or Gram-negative bacteria (most cases of early prosthetic IE): urgent
  - Recurrent embolic despite appropriate antibiotic treatment: urgent
  - IE relapse: elective
- Two primary objectives of surgery: removal of all infected tissues and reconstruction of cardiac morphology

- Intraoperative transoesophageal echocardiography recommended in all cases
- Excised material must be sent to the microbiology; if culture is positive, a full course of antibiotic treatment must be given.

Specific situations

- Prosthetic valve IE
  - 20% of all cases of IE
  - In-hospital mortality: 20–40%
  - Diagnosis is more difficult than in native IE: echocardiography and blood cultures are negative more often
  - Transoesophageal echocardiography is mandatory
- Device-related IE
  - Main mechanism: local contamination during device implantation
  - Clinical presentation frequently misleading
  - Complete device removal is always required; percutaneous extraction is feasible in the majority of patients.

Prophylaxis

- Good oral hygiene in everybody
- No scientific evidence of the efficacy of antibiotic prophylaxis
- NICE recommendations: no antibiotic prophylaxis in anybody
- European Society of Cardiology (American Heart Association: very similar) recommendations:
- Antibiotic prophylaxis:
  - In patients with previous IE, prosthetic valve, or cyanotic congenital heart disease
  - When they have dental procedures with manipulation of the gingival or periapical region of the teeth or perforation of the oral mucosa or respiratory tract procedures with incision of the mucosa
  - Single dose 30–60 minutes before procedure; amoxicillin or ampicillin, 2 g po or IV; if allergy to penicillin or ampicillin, clindamycin, 600 mg po or IV
- No antibiotic prophylaxis for other procedures nor for other patients.

Further reading

European Society of Cardiology. Guidelines on the prevention, diagnosis and treatment of infective endocarditis. *Eur Heart J* 2009;**30**:2369–413.

Moreillon P, Que YA. Infective endocarditis. *Lancet* 2004;**363**:139–49.

Nishimura RA, Carabello BA, Faxon DP, *et al.* American College of Cardiology/American Heart Association 2008 guideline update on valvular heart disease: focused update on infective endocarditis. *J Am Coll Cardiol* 2008;**52**:676–85.

Acute rheumatic fever

Definition

Acute rheumatic fever (ARF) results from an autoimmune response to infection with group A beta-haemolytic streptococci (GABHS). Although the acute illness causes considerable morbidity and some mortality, the major clinical and public health effects derive from the long-term damage to heart valves and is known as rheumatic heart disease (RHD).

Incidence and epidemiology

- ARF is an important public health problem affecting about 500 000 people in the world annually.
- It is mainly a disease of the developing world, affecting as many as 100/100 000 people in the endemic areas and less than 1/100 000 in developed countries.
- The first attacks of ARF usually occur between the ages of 5 and 15 years. Recurrent attacks are seen in adolescent and young adults.

Aetiopathogenesis

All three components of the classical epidemiological triad interact with each other to result in the development of disease.

Agent

- GABHS pharyngitis if left untreated, results in ARF in 0.3–3% cases (primary attack rate).
- Out of more than 100 serotypes of GABHS, the mucoid strains which adhere well to the pharyngeal tissue appear to be rheumatogenic.

Host

- Those with previous history of ARF are more likely (5–50%) to develop ARF after an untreated GABHS pharyngitis (secondary attack rate).
- Frequency of rheumatic recurrences following streptococcal infection is consistently greater in those with RHD than in those who escaped cardiac injury during prior attacks.
- Tendency to suffer recurrences of ARF following streptococcal infection declines with the passage of years since the preceding attack.

Environment

- Overcrowding, poor living conditions and limited access to healthcare facilities are related to the development of ARF.

Molecular mimicry theory: several epitopes of GABHS mimic several host tissues (heart, synovia, skin, and brain). Antibodies formed after GABHS infection cross-react with these host tissues and this autoimmune reaction results in the syndrome of ARF. RHD usually results from the cumulative damage of recurrent episodes of ARF, although initial attacks can lead directly to RHD.

Clinical features

The disease usually has an acute febrile onset and variable combinations of arthritis/arthralgia, carditis, chorea, and skin manifestations. No single clinical feature is diagnostic of ARF. However, a diagnosis of ARF can reliably be made using a combination of different clinical and laboratory manifestations. Currently, revised Jones criteria (1992) and WHO criteria (2002–3) are commonly used for the diagnosis of ARF (Table 7.2.1).

- In regions of world where ARF is endemic and where risk associated with missed diagnosis outweigh the consequences of over-diagnosis, the revised Jones criteria might not be sufficiently sensitive.
- The WHO criteria specified less stringent requirement for the diagnosis of recurrent ARF in patients with established RHD and should probably be adopted in such a situation.

Arthritis

- Migratory polyarthritis is the most frequent (occurs in up to 75% patients) and the earliest manifestation (occurs within 2–3 weeks of onset of ARF). In about one third to half of the patients, it may be the only apparent manifestation.
- The large joints of the extremities are most frequently affected, but any joint can be involved. Knee and elbow joints are most frequently affected followed by wrist, elbows, shoulders, and hips, whereas small joints of the hands, feet, and spine are rarely affected.
- Migratory involvement is characteristic but inflammation of several large joints at one time is not unusual.
- Characteristically, each joint is involved for about 1–2 weeks. Polyarthritis as a whole resolves within a month without any sequelae or residual deformity with a rare exception of Jaccoud's arthritis.
- Mono-articular arthritis is recognized to be important in populations where ARF is common.
- Dramatic response to salicylates (within 24 hours) is a characteristic of ARF polyarthritis.

Table 7.2.1 Diagnostic criteria of acute rheumatic fever

Revised Jones criteria	WHO criteria
Major manifestations	**First episode**
1 Carditis	As Jones criteria
2 Arthritis	
3 Chorea	**Recurrent episode**
4 Erythema marginatum	1 In a patient without established rheumatic heart disease: as first episode.
5 Subcutaneous nodules	
Minor manifestations	
1 Arthralgia	2 In a patient with established rheumatic heart disease: requires two minor manifestations, plus evidence of prior group A streptococcal infection.
2 Fever	
3 Raised ESR or CRP	
4 ECG: prolonged PR interval	
Diagnosis of rheumatic fever	
Two major/one major and two minor manifestations plus	
Evidence of prior group A streptococcal infection	Evidence of prior group A streptococcal infection as per Jones criteria, but with addition of recent scarlet fever.
(Positive throat culture or rapid antigen test for group A streptococcus or raised/rising streptococcal antibody titre)	
Chorea and indolent carditis do not require evidence of prior group A streptococcal infection	Chorea and indolent carditis do not require evidence of prior group A streptococcal infection
Recurrent episode requires only one major or several minor manifestations, plus evidence of prior group A streptococcal infection	

- Arthritis frequently overlaps with the onset of carditis. Severities of both these manifestations are inversely related to each other.
- Arthritis is almost always associated with raised anti-streptolysine O (ASO) titre.

Carditis

- Rheumatic carditis is 'pancarditis' and involves all three components of heart; pericardium, myocardium, and valves. Characteristic signs and symptoms are mentioned in Table 7.2.2.
- About 70% of patients who develop carditis do so within the first week of the disease, 85% within the first 12 weeks of the disease, and almost all within 6 months from the onset of the ARF episode.
- It is the single most important component of the disease which determines the prognosis. About 40–60% episodes of ARF result in RHD. Its clinical manifestations may vary widely from difficult to detect subclinical carditis to life-threatening heart failure.
- Carditis typically manifests after about 2–3 weeks of the onset of ARF with either pain of pericarditis or symptoms of heart failure.
- Neither myocarditis nor pericarditis can occur without valvulitis. If evidence of valvulitis is not present, alternative causes should be considered.
- Rheumatic carditis is almost always associated with significant cardiac murmurs.
- Ventricular function is rarely affected, and heart failure is almost always the result of acute valvular regurgitation.
- Recurrent carditis occurs with very high frequency in subsequent episodes of ARF ('mimetic' carditis). A definitive clinical diagnosis of recurrence of carditis can be made if one or more of the following can be demonstrated:
  - Appearance of a new murmur or change in the character of the pre-existing organic murmur
  - Pericardial friction rub or pericardial effusion
  - Unexplained congestive heart failure
  - Definite increase in the heart size.

Chorea (Sydenham's chorea)

It is a neurological disorder characterized by rapid involuntary, purposeless movements associated with muscular weakness, and emotional lability. The movements are neither purposeful nor repetitive but abrupt and erratic and disappear during sleep. Central nervous system stimulants exacerbate and sedatives suppress choreiform activity.

- It is an uncommon manifestation and occurs in less than 10% patients.
- It is a delayed manifestation of ARF and the latent period may be as long as several months after the initiating streptococcal infection. Arthritis always subsides before the appearance of chorea. Carditis is sometimes discovered for the first time when the presenting feature of ARF is chorea.
- Like arthritis, it also does not result in any residual neurological deficit.

Rheumatic nodules

- Firm, painless, pea-sized nodules situated over bony prominence. Characteristic locations are the extensor tendons of hands and feet, elbows, margins of patellae, scalp, scapulae, and over the spinous processes of vertebrae.
- Characteristically they occur in crops.
- Because skin over them is not inflamed and they are situated over bony prominences, they may easily be missed if not carefully sought on physical examination.
- It is an uncommon manifestation and occurs in less than 10% patients.
- They are invariably associated with carditis and typically appear 6 weeks after the streptococcal infection.
- Like other non cardiac manifestations, they also resolve completely within weeks to 1 or 2 months.

Erythema marginatum

- It is an erythematous, non-pruretic, non-indurated rash with clear centre and round or surpeginous margins. It blanches on pressure and may be brought out by a warm bath.
- It typically occurs on the trunk and proximal parts of extremities, never on the face.
- The rash tend to be very evanescent and may disappear within hours and then may reappear.
- It is an extremely uncommon manifestation and may be difficult to detect in dark-skinned patients.
- It typically occurs in conjunction with carditis and unlike subcutaneous nodules, may last for months or years.

Investigations

Streptococcal antibody test

- ASO titres are elevated in about 85% patients of ARF.
- Titres increase within 7–10 days of streptococcal pharyngitis, peak at 2–3 weeks and drop steadily thereafter.
- Titres of more than 240 in adults and 320 in children are considered to be abnormal.
- Increased titres do not reflect rheumatic activity per se, and their rate of decline is independent of the course of the rheumatic attack.
- Baseline antibody levels in the normal population are influenced by age, geographic location, socioeconomic status, and seasonal variations. So, mere elevation of ASO titres in the presence of non-specific symptoms should not be labelled as ARF and penicillin prophylaxis should not be started on this basis. In such cases demonstration of rising titres in a repeat sample taken after 1 week may be helpful in making the diagnosis.

Table 7.2.2 Signs and symptoms of carditis

Pericarditis
Pericardial chest pain
Pericardial friction rub
Myocarditis
Disproportionate tachycardia
Soft first sound
Gallop rhythm
Valvulitis
Apical holosystolic murmur of MR (common)
Apical mid-diastolic murmur (Carey Coomb's murmur); may be transient
Basal early diastolic murmur of AR (less common)

- Other streptococcal antibodies such as antistreptozyme, anti-DNase B, or antihyaluronidase can be used to improve sensitivity. Combination of these tests with ASO can improve the sensitivity to more than 95%.
- Streptococcal antibody levels may be normal if the interval between the streptococcal pharyngitis and diagnosis of ARF is more than 2 months, a condition which occurs in patients presenting with chorea and subclinical carditis. Except in these two instances, one should be reluctant to make the diagnosis of ARF in the absence of serological evidence of recent streptococcal infection.

Throat culture

The presence of a positive throat cultures alone is of limited value, because many individuals are carriers, whereas a negative culture may be secondary to antibiotic administration, elimination of GABHS by immune response and due to difficulty in isolation by single culture.

Rapid streptococcal antigen testing

Rapid detection of streptococcal antigen from throat swabs using latex agglutination or enzyme immunoassay is a practical alternative to the throat swab. It has a sensitivity of 60–90% and a specificity of 95%.

Acute-phase reactants

- Both erythrocyte sedimentation rate (ESR) and C-reactive protein (CRP) are significantly elevated in ARF except in patients presenting with chorea.
- They are reliable markers for the severity of the inflammatory activity and their time course of elevation generally correlates with disease activity.
- Unlike ESR, CRP levels are not affected by presence of heart failure or anaemia.

ECG

- Prolonged PR interval occurs in about 25% cases of ARF.
- During sinus tachycardia the PR interval usually shortens and even modest prolongation is abnormal in the face of tachycardia.
- It is neither specific nor diagnostic of serious cardiac involvement.
- Other non-specific ECG changes are also commonly seen.

Echocardiography

Its role in the diagnosis of ARF is controversial. However, it avoids over-diagnosis of ARF, by excluding flow murmurs and congenital heart disease in up to 20% of suspected cases. Similarly, subclinical acute rheumatic carditis as well as indolent carditis can be diagnosed by echocardiography. Echocardiography offers several clues to support the diagnosis of ARF (Table 7.2.3). One should be careful to differentiate pathological from physiological valvular regurgitation. Discrete posteriorly directed mitral regurgitation (MR) jet, holosystolic flow, significant turbulence in MR jet and MR jet seen in orthogonal planes are the important clues suggesting rheumatic aetiology for MR. However, inclusion of patients with 'silent carditis' or 'echocarditis' has been thought to result in over-diagnosis of ARF.

Differential diagnosis

- Over-diagnosis of ARF is quite common. A number of clinical conditions mimic ARF (Table 7.2.4).
- Unless ill-defined febrile illness is clearly associated with a major manifestation of ARF, the diagnosis of ARF should not be made.

Table 7.2.3 Echocardiographic findings suggestive of acute rheumatic fever

Mitral valve
Thick leaflets
Restricted mobility of posterior mitral leaflet
Rheumatic nodules (small nodules on leaflet margins)
Flail leaflet
Thickened subvalvular apparatus
Varying grades of mitral regurgitation

Aortic valve
Thick leaflet margins
Reduced mobility of aortic cusps
Varying grades of aortic regurgitation

Tricuspid valve
Rarely involved in the first episode

Pericardial effusion
Does not produce large pericardial effusion, cardiac tamponade or pericardial constriction

- A common error is the premature administration of salicylates/steroids before the signs and symptoms of ARF are clearly expressed. In the absence of a curative agent, one should not suppress the signs and symptoms of ARF.

Treatment

- Most of the patients currently are treated on an outpatient basis.
- Bed rest is advisable for patients presenting with carditis (for 4 weeks or at least during the symptomatic stage).
- Antimicrobial therapy for eradication of pharyngeal streptococcal infection is mandatory. A single dose of benzathine penicillin is ideal. Other agents can also be used (Table 7.2.5).
- Once the ARF manifests, the treatment algorithm varies, depending upon the major manifestation.

Table 7.2.4 Differential diagnosis of acute rheumatic fever

Polyarthritis	**Chorea**
Septic arthritis	Systemic lupus erythematous
Reactive arthritis	*Drug intoxication*
Connective tissue and other autoimmune diseases	Anticonvulsants
Viral arthropathy	Antidepressants
Infective endocarditis	Metoclopramide
Leukaemia, lymphoma	Wilson's disease
Lyme's disease	Post encephalitic
Sickle cell anaemia	Atypical seizures
Gout and pseudo gout	Intracranial tumours
'Growth pains' in children	Familial chorea—Huntington
Carditis	Lyme disease
Innocent murmur	*Hormonal*
Mitral valve prolapse syndrome	Oral contraceptives
Congenital heart disease	Pregnancy
Infective endocarditis	Hyperthyroidism
Myocarditis	Hypoparathyroidism
Pericarditis	

Table 7.2.5 Treatment of group A beta-haemolytic streptococcal pharyngitis

Antibiotic	Dose and duration
Benzathine penicillin G	1.2 million units IM × single dose (600000 units if body weight <27 kg)
Penicillin V	500 mg bid × 10 days
Amoxicillin	500 mg tid × 10 days
First-generation cephalosporin or erythromycin (only if allergic to penicillin)	Varies by drug × 10 days

Arthritis

- Salicylates are the first line therapy. Aspirin should be used in doses of 100 mg/kg/day in children and 6–8 g/day in adults (in 4–5 divided doses). After 2 weeks the dose should be decreased to 60–70 mg/kg/day for an additional 3–6 weeks.
- Any other non-steroidal anti-inflammatory agents (NSAID) can be used in patients allergic to aspirin.
- Steroids are typically not used, because they do not offer any advantage and sometimes may mask illnesses causing arthritis like lupus or may exacerbate some illnesses like infective arthritis.
- Anti-inflammatory agents provide only symptomatic relief and do not alter the natural course of the disease.

Carditis

- Patients of rheumatic carditis with heart failure should be treated by steroids.
- They rapidly relieve symptoms and facilitate early recovery. Many believe that they can be life saving in acute severe carditis, although there is little objective evidence.
- Like salicylates which are used for arthritis, steroids also do not alter the natural history of ARF and subsequent development of RHD.
- Prednisone (1–2 mg/kg/day, to a maximum of 80 mg/day given once daily or divided doses) is the drug of choice. After 2–3 weeks of therapy, dose should be decreased by 25% each week. During steroid tapering, an overlap with aspirin should be done to prevent rebound. Typically, 4–6 weeks of steroid therapy is sufficient.
- Weekly test of CRP and ESR are useful in following the healing process at the time of steroid tapering.
- Patients with severe heart failure require the usual supportive treatment.

Table 7.2.6 Secondary prophylaxis

Antibiotic	Dose and frequency
Benzathine penicillin G	1.2 million units IM every 3–4 wk (600000 units if body weight <20 kg)
Penicillin V	250 mg po bid
Erythromycin (alternative for penicillin-allergic patients)	250 mg po bid
Sulfadiazine (alternative for penicillin-allergic patients)	1 g po daily

Table 7.2.7 Duration of secondary prophylaxis

Duration of secondary prophylaxis
No carditis
5 years since last episode or 18 years of age (whichever is longer)
Mild carditis
10 years since last episode or age 25 years (whichever is longer)
Severe carditis or valve surgery or balloon mitral valvotomy
Ideally lifelong or at least up to the age of 40 years of age

- When severe carditis is complicated by marked valvular regurgitation leading to refractory heart failure, valve replacement is life-saving and should not be delayed by trials of anti-inflammatory medication. Valve repair is not advisable because of the possibility of recurrence of mitral regurgitation from ongoing inflammation.

Chorea

- Chorea is a benign and self-limiting disease.
- Mild cases need no treatment.
- NSAID and steroid have no role.
- Supportive measure like rest in a quite room along with medication such as valproic acid, carbamazepine, haloperidol, and diazepam may provide symptomatic relief in patients with moderate to severe symptoms.
- Pimozide is a new drug reported to be effective.

Prevention

Primary prevention

A course of effective antibiotic therapy started within 10 days of onset of streptococcal pharyngitis almost completely eliminates the risk of ARF. The antibiotic regimens are same as those listed for the eradication of pharyngeal streptococcal infection during the episode of ARF (Table 7.2.5).

Secondary prevention

Patients with documented ARF should receive continuous antibiotic prophylaxis for secondary prevention (Tables 7.2.6 and 7.2.7). Benzathine penicillin injection every 3–4 weeks is most effective in this regard. Oral penicillin can be used in very thin patients and for patients on oral anticoagulant therapy when deep intramuscular injections are undesirable. Only penicillin allergic patients should be offered alternative antibiotic regimen.

Further reading

Carapetis J, McDonald M, Wilson NJ. Acute rheumatic fever. *Lancet* 2005;**366**:155–68.

Guidelines for the diagnosis of rheumatic fever. Jones Criteria, 1992 update. Special writing group of the committee on rheumatic fever, endocarditis, and Kawasaki disease of the council on cardiovascular disease in the young of the American Heart Association. *JAMA* 1992;**268**:2069–73.

Kumar RK. Acute rheumatic fever. In: Shah SN (ed.). *API textbook of medicine: The Association of Physicians of India.* Volume I, 8th edn. Mumbai, India: The Association of Physicians of India: 2008, 478–84.

Raju BS, Turi ZG. Rheumatic fever. In: Libby P, Bonow RO, Mann DL, Zipes DP (eds) *Braunwald's heart disease; a textbook of cardiovascular medicine,* 8th edn. Philadelphia: WB Saunders, 2008: pp. 2079–86.

Rheumatic fever and rheumatic heart disease: Report of a WHO expert panel, Geneva 29 October–1 November. Geneva: WHO, 2004.

Mitral regurgitation

Mitral regurgitation accounted for 31.5% of cases of valve disease in the Euro Heart Survey (Iung 2003). The mitral apparatus consists of the leaflets, the annulus, chordae, papillary muscle, and the adjacent myocardium. Dysfunction of any or all of these can cause mitral regurgitation. The causes are listed below.

Organic (i.e. involvement of the valve)
- Degenerative disease with prolapse
- Rheumatic
- Endocarditis
- Rare: lupus, radiation, the anorectic drugs phentermine and fenfluramine
- Hypertrophic cardiomyopathy can cause mitral regurgitation as a result of both abnormal papillary muscle function and an abnormally long anterior leaflet.

Functional
Acute ischaemic
- Papillary muscle rupture.

Chronic
- Posterior wall motion abnormality
- Left ventricular (LV0 dilatation (ischaemic heart disease, dilated cardiomyopathy, chronic aortic valve disease).

The most common causes leading to surgery are ischaemic regurgitation, prolapse, and endocarditis. Ischaemic regurgitation implies acute regurgitation as a result of papillary muscle rupture. Functional regurgitation describes chronic mitral regurgitation from LV dilatation of which myocardial infarction is one cause.

Natural history
- The mortality in severe mitral regurgitation of all aetiologies with and without symptoms is around 5% per year (Delahaye et al. 1991).
- The natural history of mitral regurgitation secondary to left ventricular dysfunction largely reflects the underlying condition. However, the presence of moderate or severe regurgitation may independently worsen the prognosis thus justifying repair (Chen et al., 1998).
- Severe functional mitral regurgitation worsens adverse remodelling leading to a downward spiral in LV dysfunction.
- Chronic severe mitral regurgitation as a result of primary valve dysfunction causes dilatation and hyperactivity of the left ventricle. Long-term volume load induces myocardial fibrosis with a consequent deterioration in contractile function. However, because the left ventricle empties partly into the left atrium, which is at a lower pressure than the aorta, the left ventricular ejection fraction or fractional shortening is apparently normal until the terminal stages (Corin et al., 1995).
- Left atrial enlargement secondary to the mitral regurgitation is associated with paroxysmal or sustained atrial arrhythmias and if these are present there is an increased risk of thromboembolism for which anticoagulation with warfarin is indicated.
- Chronic mitral regurgitation is the underlying substrate in between 20% and 30% of cases of infective endocarditis (Otto 1999).

Clinical approach
Symptoms
- Severe mitral regurgitation may be asymptomatic (Delahaye et al., 1991) or may cause exertional breathlessness and orthopnoea. Exercise testing should be considered in any patient who claims to be asymptomatic or in whom the history is unclear.

Signs (Leatham 1975)
- Murmur: there is a pansystolic murmur at the apex radiating to the axilla. The amplitude is approximately related to the grade of regurgitation (Desjardins et al., 1996). If the regurgitation is mild and caused by prolapse, there may be a late systolic murmur sometimes preceded by a systolic click. A musical or 'seagull' quality to the murmur occurs if there is a perforation or fluttering of a flail leaflet segment.
- Diastolic sound: the diastolic sound is composed of a third heart sound sometimes succeeded by a mid-diastolic murmur caused by functional mitral stenosis as a result of high flow. This is more specific for differentiating severe mitral regurgitation than the amplitude of the murmur.
- Wide splitting of the second sound is caused by early cessation of systole leading to an early aortic closure sound and is specific for severe mitral regurgitation.
- Other signs: the radial pulse is usually normal although in severe chronic regurgitation there may be atrial fibrillation. The blood pressure may be low and the carotid upstroke of low volume in advanced disease, but these signs are not specific. The jugular venous pulse is usually normal since severe pulmonary hypertension leading to right ventricular dysfunction is rare. There may be a parasternal impulse as a result of left atrial enlargement (Basta et al. 1973) and in severe regurgitation the apex is displaced laterally.

Investigations
Echocardiography
The aetiology is determined from the appearance of the mitral valve and the anatomy and function of the LV.
- Appearance of the valve: organic regurgitation is recognized by abnormalities of the anatomy or movement of the valve. These include prolapse (Chapter 7.5), rheumatic changes as for mitral stenosis (Chapter 7.4), endocarditis (vegetation or perforation) or generalized thickening as in systemic lupus erythematosus (SLE) or exposure to radiation or to the anorectic drugs fenfluramine/phentolamine.
- Functional regurgitation causes tenting of the leaflets which may be either symmetrical (causing a central jet of regurgitation) or asymmetrical usually with relatively more restriction of the posterior leaflet (causing a posteriorly directed jet).
- Grading regurgitation: regurgitation causes reversed systolic flow in the left atrium. The severity is graded by a combination of primary factors derived from the size of the LV portion of the jet (Table 7.3.1), the pattern of flow in the pulmonary veins, the density and shape of the continuous wave signal and the size and activity of the left ventricle.

Table 7.3.1 Grading mitral regurgitation

	Mild	Moderate	Severe
Neck width (mm)	<3	3–6.9	>7.0
Flow convergence zone	Absent	Moderate	Large
PISA EROA (mm^2)	<20	20–40	>40
PISA reg volume (mL)	<30	30–60	>60

PISA, proximal isovelocity surface area; EROA, effective regurgitant orifice area; Reg, regurgitant.

- In severe regurgitation the continuous wave signal is dense and there is systolic flow reversal in a pulmonary vein distant from the axis of the jet. In torrential mitral regurgitation there is rapid depressurization of the continuous wave signal giving it a 'dagger-shape'.
- Left ventricle size: in severe organic mitral regurgitation, the left ventricle tends to be dilated in diastole and hyperdynamic. The left ventricle changes in shape to become more rounded so size should be assessed from volumes using the biplane Simpson's rule as well as using linear dimensions at the base of the heart.
- LV function: In functional mitral regurgitation there is an associated abnormality of wall motion. Asymmetrical tenting is usually associated with inferoposterior akinesis and symmetrical tenting with anterior akinesis or generalized LV dilatation.
- Other valves: aortic valve disease is common and may require surgery at the same time as the mitral valve. It may be difficult to assess aortic stenosis in the presence of low forward flow (see Chapter 7.7).
- The right heart: A PA pressure >50 mmHg at rest in the absence of symptoms is a criterion for surgery.

Chest X-ray
- There may be an increase in cardiothoracic ratio and evidence of a dilated left atrium.
- Decompensated chronic severe mitral regurgitation is associated with signs of chronic raised left atrial pressure, upper lobe blood diversion, and interstitial oedema including Kerley B and A lines (Ruttley 1995).

ECG
- There may be the signs of old myocardial infarction in functional mitral regurgitation.

Stress testing
- This is not routine, but hand-grip and exercise testing should be considered in patients with apparently mild regurgitation at rest, but either exertional symptoms or a dilated LV.
- The grade of regurgitation worsens on exercise in about one-third of patients with a symmetrically tented mitral valve.
- Surgery is indicated for a PA pressure >60 mmHg on stress.

Cardiac catheterization
- This is necessary for assessment of the coronary arteries before surgery.
- LV contrast injection is no longer a routine method of assessing the grade of regurgitation, which can be judged

from the density and speed of opacification within the left atrium.
- The height of the V wave on the pulmonary wedge pressure trace is also a guide, but is non-specific since it also occurs in conditions associated with delayed left atrial emptying (Fuchs *et al.*, 1982). Rapid depressurization of the continuous wave trace on echocardiography correlates with a large V wave on the wedge trace.

Management
- The ACC/AHA and ESC guidelines for surgery are listed in full in Table 7.3.2.
- For chronic mitral regurgitation, the criteria for surgery are more complex than for other valve disease because the LV size thresholds for organic disease cannot be applied for functional regurgitation. Furthermore mitral valve surgery can be performed as a primary procedure for regurgitation whether organic or functional or as a secondary procedure at the time of coronary artery bypass grafting.
- Patients often have mixed disease and may require surgery for moderate mitral regurgitation if combined with stenosis or with moderate aortic valve disease.

Criteria for surgery: acute severe mitral regurgitation
- Acute severe regurgitation as a result of papillary muscle rupture, chordal rupture or endocarditis requires urgent surgery if necessary after a period of stabilization including mechanical ventilation, diuretics, inotropes and an intra-aortic balloon pump.

Chronic organic mitral regurgitation
- For organic severe mitral regurgitation there is an argument for immediate repair (Enriques-Sarano 2005) even in the absence of symptoms provided that repair is very likely and can be performed at low risk, <1%. By contrast 'watchful waiting' with surgery performed at the onset of symptoms or of LV dilatation has also been shown to be

Table 7.3.2 Indications for surgery in mitral regurgitation (data sourced from Bonow 2006; Vahanian 2007)

Symptoms and acute severe MR	Class I
Chronic severe regurgitation and symptoms and preserved LV	Class I
Asymptomatic and severe regurgitation and LVSD > or equal 40 mm (ESC 45 mm) or EF 30 60%	Class I
Asymptomatic and no symptoms with LVSD <40 mm if repair very likely	Class IIa
PA >50 mmHg at rest or 60 mmHg on exercise	Class IIa
Organic MV disease and EF < 30% or end-systolic > 55 if repair highly likely	Class IIa
Patients with moderate functional MR undergoing CABG if repair is feasible class	Class IIa (ESC only)
Functional MR with EF < 30% if viability and having CABG	Class IIa (ESC only)
Functional MR with EF > 30%	Class IIb (ESC only)
Functional MR with EF < 30% with failure of full medical therapy inc CRT	Class IIb (ESC only)

safe (Rosenhek 2006). As a rule surgical risk is low below age 70 in the absence of co-morbidities and should be considered for repairable valves at an end-systolic diameter of 40 mm (Wisenbaugh et al., 1994; Bonow et al. 2006).

- When the fractional shortening falls to about 29% or the ejection fraction to about 60%, both at the lower limit of normal, myocardial fibrosis is already at an advanced stage and full recovery after surgery does not occur (Enriquez-Sarano et al. 1994).

Chronic functional mitral regurgitation

- An independent effect on outcome is seen for moderate as well as severe mitral regurgitation. Mitral repair should therefore be considered at the time of coronary artery bypass grafting (CABG) for moderate or worse regurgitation. Where surgery is not primarily indicated for coronary disease, the decision for mitral surgery rests on the presence of symptoms, the possibility of repair, whether LV function is severely impaired (EF <30%) and whether recovery of LV function is likely (e.g. as a result of coronary artery bypass graft (CABG) in the presence of viability).
- The decision is hardest in patients with a dilated cardiomyopathy with EF <30%. Medical therapy and cardiac resynchronization therapy (CRT) should be tried initially (Bax 2006). If still unresponsive, the use of a small annuloplasty ring has been reported to give 80% survival at 1 year and 70% survival at 2 years (Bolling et al. 1995; Szalay et al. 1998).

Transcatheter intervention

- These are experimental still. The mitral E-clip produces a double orifice valve and also reduces the annulus size with a consequent reduction in the grade of regurgitation. It is suitable for tented valves and prolapse without a flail segment and without excessive valve thickening.
- The mitral coronary sinus band allows a reduction in mitral annulus size. It is possible, but not yet investigated, that a combination of the two techniques might be useful.

Medical management

- In organic regurgitation there is preliminary evidence that beta-blockers may reduce the rate of progression to surgery (Stewart 2008). There is contradictory evidence for the prophylactic use of angiotensin-converting enzyme (ACE) inhibitors (Carabello 2008).
- Patients with organic regurgitation and symptoms should usually be considered for surgery, but if the risk is high because of coexistent pathology, palliative medical treatment may be given as for patients with functional mitral regurgitation using angiotensin converting enzyme (ACE) inhibitors, diuretics and beta-blockers (Lancellotti 2008).
- Antibiotic prophylaxis before dental work is no longer routinely indicated except for patients who have previously had endocarditis (Nishimura 2008). Regular dental checks to treat early decay are essential.

References

Basta LL, Wolfson P, Eckberg DL, Abboud FM. The value of left parasternal impulse recordings in the assessment of mitral regurgitation. *Circulation* 1973;**48**:1055–65.

Bax JJ, Poldermans D. Mitral regurgitation and left ventricular dyssynchrony: implications for treatment. *Heart* 2006;**92**:1363–4.

Bolling SF, Deeb GM, Brunshing LA, et al. Early outcome of mitral valve reconstruction in patients with end-stage cardiomyopathy. *J Thorac Cardiovasc Surg* 1995;**109**:676–82.

Bonow RO, Carabello BA, Chatterjee K, et al. ACC/AHA 2006 guidelines for the management of patients with valvular heart disease. *JACC* 2006;**48**:e1–148.

Carabello BA. The current therapy for mitral regurgitation. *JACC* 2008;**52**:319–26.

Chen FY, Adams DH, Aranki SF, et al. Mitral valve repair in cardiomyopathy. *Circulation* 1998;**98**(Suppl II):124–7.

Corin WJ, Sutsch G, Murakami T, Krogmann ON, Turina M, Hess OM. Left ventricular function in chronic mitral regurgitation; preoperative and postoperative comparison. *JACC* 1995;**25**:113–21.

Delahaye JP, Gare JP, Viguier E, et al. Natural history of severe mitral regurgitation. *Eur Heart J* 1991;**12**(Suppl B):5–9.

Desjardins VA, Enriquez-Sarano M, Tajik AJ, et al. Intensity of murmurs correlates with severity of valvular regurgitation. *Am J Med* 1996;**100**:149–56.

Enriquez-Sarano M, Tajik AJ, Schaff HV, et al. Echocardiographic prediction of survival after surgical correction of organic mitral regurgitation. *Circulation* 1994;**90**:830–7.

Enriquez-Sarano M, Avierinos J-F, Messika-Zeitoun D, et al. Quantitative determinants of the outcome of asymptomatic mitral regurgitation. *N Engl J Med* 2005;**352**:875–83.

Feldman T, Wasserman HS, Herrmann HC et al. Percutaneous mitral valve repair using the edge-to-edge technique. *JACC* 2005;**46**:2134–40.

Fuchs RM, Heuser RR, Yin FC, Brinker JA. Limitations of pulmonary wedge V waves in diagnosing mitral regurgitation. *Am J Cardiol* 1982;**49**:849–54.

Iung B, Baron G, Butchart EG, Delahaye F, et al. A prospective study of patients with valvular heart disease in Europe: The Euro Heart Survey on valvular heart disease. *Eur Heart J* 2003;**24**:1231–43.

Lancellotti P, Marwick T, Pierard LA. How to manage ischaemic mitral regurgitation. *Heart* 2008;**94**:1497–1502.

Leatham A. *Auscultation of the heart and phonocardiography*, 2nd edn. Churchill Livingstone, 1975.

Nishimura RA, Carabello BA, Faxon DP, et al. AVV/AHA 2008 guideline update on valvular heart disease: focused update on infective endocarditis. *Circulation* 2008;**118**:887–96.

Otto CM. *Vavular heart disease*. WB Saunders, 1999: p. 421.

Rosenhek R, Rader F, Klaar U, et al. Outcome of watchful waiting in asymptomatic severe mitral regurgitation. *Circulation* 2006;**113**:2238–44.

Stewart RAH, Raffel OC, Kerr AJ, et al. Pilot study to assess the influence of beta-blockade on mitral regurgitant volume and left ventricular work in degenerative mitral valve disease. *Circulation* 2008;**118**:1041–6.

Szalay ZA, Civelek A. Hohe S, et al. Mitral annuloplasty in patients with ischemic versus dilated cardiomyopathy. *Eur J Cardiothocic Surg* 1998;**23**:567–72.

Wisenbaugh T, Skudicky D, Sareli P. Prediction of outcome after valve replacement for rheumatic mitral regurgitation in the era of chordal preservation. *Circulation* 1994;**89**:191.

Zoghbi WA, Enriquez-Sarano M, Foster E, et al. Recommendations for evaluation of the severity of native valvular regurgitation with two-dimensional and Doppler echocardiography. *J Am Soc Echo* 2003;**16**:777–802.

Mitral stenosis

Mitral stenosis accounts for about 10% of valve disease in the West (Hostkotte et al. 1991; Iung et al. 2003). It is most frequently rheumatic in origin, although 12.5% in the Euro Heart Survey had degenerative stenosis (Iung et al. 2003). Elderly patients particularly with renal failure can develop heavy annular calcification, which may extend along the leaflets and cause significant obstruction. There are rare congenital causes (e.g. parachute, double-orifice mitral valve). SLE, Whipple's disease, Fabry's disease, and amyloid may occasionally cause mitral stenosis.

Natural history

- Rheumatic involvement usually follows untreated recurrent rheumatic fever in childhood. In the absence of subsequent prophylaxis with penicillin and aspirin, progressive fibrosis and calcification occurs.
- The normal mitral orifice is 4–5 cm^2 in area and symptoms do not occur until the orifice area falls to below about 2.0 cm^2. The rate of haemodynamic progression may be slow in two-thirds of patients, but in those with more calcified and deformed valves, the decrease in orifice area may be as high as 0.3 cm^2 per year (Gordon et al., 1991).
- In one study, symptoms developed 16 years after the acute illness and become severe after a further 9 years (Horstkotte et al. 1991). The 5-year survival with severe symptomatic mitral stenosis was 44% without surgery (Horstkotte et al., 1991).
- Pulmonary pressures are raised in mitral stenosis initially by passive back pressure and reactive vasoconstriction. Ultimately histological changes occur similar to those seen in primary pulmonary hypertension and these are irreversible (Otto et al. 1993).
- The left ventricle is protected since it is downstream from the valve lesion. However, the right ventricle is under threat as pulmonary artery pressure rises. Established right heart failure as a result of pulmonary hypertension may cause a reduction in breathlessness as a result of lowered left atrial filling pressures. However, this apparent improvement is spurious and a sign of end stage and usually inoperable disease.
- Symptoms may be precipitated by intercurrent illness, pregnancy or the development of atrial fibrillation.

Clinical approach

History

- The main symptoms are exertional breathlessness as a result of raised left atrial pressure and fatigue as a result of low cardiac output (Rowe et al. 1960). Exertional breathlessness is usually of slow onset so that the patient may claim to be asymptomatic. If there is any doubt, the patient should be exercised either formally or by simply walking with him or her in a hospital corridor.
- Orthopnoea and paroxysmal nocturnal dyspnoea are caused by increased venous return on lying down leading to higher left ventricular filling pressures and stiffening of the lungs.
- The risk of thromboembolism in the presence of atrial fibrillation and mitral stenosis is 18 times that of age-matched subjects (Wolf et al. 1978) and stroke may be the presenting symptom.

- Complications of chronically raised pulmonary venous pressure are recurrent chest infections (Wood, 1954) and haemoptysis.
- Right-sided signs: ankle-swelling and ascites may develop as a result of right ventricular failure.
- Other: dysphagia as a result of compression from a large left atrium and hoarseness from recurrent laryngeal nerve palsy.

Signs (Leatham 1975)

- Murmur: with the patient on the left side and using the bell, there is a mid-diastolic murmur. If you suspect the diagnosis but cannot hear anything abnormal, ask the patient to perform sit-ups and then listen again. In severe mitral stenosis, the left atrial pressure is high and exceeds left ventricular pressure allowing the mitral valve to open early. The murmur then begins soon after aortic closure and lasts until the end of diastole on a long cycle. In fast atrial fibrillation the murmur of even mild mitral stenosis may fill diastole. In patients still in sinus rhythm there is presystolic accentuation of the murmur.
- Opening snap: if the mitral valve is still mobile there is an opening snap. This sounds like a tiny hammer blow but more usually like a more than usually discrete start to the murmur. A palpable opening snap causes the 'tapping' apex.
- Pulmonary hypertension: wide splitting of the second sound is caused by delay of pulmonary closure. The sign is the same as for mitral regurgitation but the mechanism is different. A malar flush as a result of chronic pulmonary hypertension is no longer common. Pulmonary hypertension may also cause a right ventricular impulse, and the basal pansystolic murmur and systolic waves of tricuspid regurgitation. A basal immediate diastolic murmur, louder on inspiration (Graham Steele murmur), may occur as a result of pulmonary regurgitation, but may be confused with the similar murmur from aortic regurgitation.
- Other signs: the pulse is often irregular as a result of atrial fibrillation. The jugular venous pressure may be high and, if there is tricuspid regurgitation, there will be prominent venous systolic waves shown as large amplitude waves timed with the central pulse. As for mitral regurgitation, the carotid upstroke and blood pressure are not specific. The apex beat may be displaced if there is right ventricular dilatation, but there should be a still region between the right and left ventricular impulses. In mitral stenosis uncomplicated by right ventricular dilatation, the apex beat is not displaced.

Investigations

Echocardiography

- Appearance of the valve: the rheumatic aetiology is confirmed by thickening of the tips of the leaflets extending down the chordae and the presence of commissural fusion. Valvotomy is contraindicated (Wilkins et al. 1988) if there is:
  - Heavy chordal thickening and matting
  - Calcium at the commissures
  - Thickening and immobility of the valve

- More than mild mitral regurgitation
- Thrombus on transoesophageal echocardiography (usually in the left atrial appendage)
- Coronary disease requiring coronary artery bypass graft (CABG)
- Significant disease of the aortic or tricuspid valves requiring surgery.
- Grading the stenosis: this is by a combination of planimetry and measures derived from the continuous wave signal (Table 7.4.1) (Baumgartner et al. 2009).
  - Planimetry of the orifice requires careful angulation of the probe and can be more accurate using three-dimensional echocardiography.
  - The pressure half-time is a measure of depressurization of the left atrium and can be used to estimate a haemodynamic orifice area from the empirical Hatle formula: orifice area = 220/pressure half-time. Planimetered (or geometric) orifice area and haemodynamic orifice area are often similar but there may be discrepancies as a result of co-existent mitral or aortic regurgitation or left ventricular dysfunction.
  - Mean gradient is calculated using the on line software.
- Pulmonary artery pressure: from the modified Bernoulli formula the pressure difference across the tricuspid valve is $4 \times v^2$ where v is the peak velocity of the tricuspid regurgitant signal. To this must be added an estimate of right atrial pressure which can be obtained from the degree of contraction of the inferior vena cava during inspiration. This is usually >50% giving an estimated right atrial pressure of 5–10 mmHg. If the inferior vena cava is engorged and non-contractile, the right atrial pressure is taken as 20 mmHg.
- Other signs: involvement of the aortic and tricuspid valves and right ventricular size and function must be assessed. Left atrial size determines the need for anticoagulation if in sinus rhythm.

Chest X-ray
- Left atrial dilatation causes prominence of the appendage just below the left pulmonary artery, widening of the carina and a double atrial shadow.
- Signs of pulmonary hypertension are enlargement of the pulmonary arteries and peripheral pruning.
- Early signs of chronic raised left atrial pressure are upper lobe blood diversion, and interstitial oedema including Kerley B and A lines. In long-established pulmonary venous hypertension, pulmonary haemosiderosis causes diffuse nodular shadowing 1–2 mm in diameter mainly in the mid- and lower zones. Bone formation in chronic oedema is more common in men and causes nodules up to 10 mm in diameter in the mid and lower zones (Ruttley 1995).

Table 7.4.1 Grading mitral stenosis

	Mild	Moderate	Severe
Planimetry (cm²)	>1.5	1.0–1.5	<1.0
Pressure half-time (ms)	<150	150–220	>220
Mean gradient (mmHg)	<5	5–10	>10
PA systolic pressure (mmHg)	<30	30–50	>50

ECG
- Atrial fibrillation is the most common abnormality and is dependent more on age than grade of stenosis. In one study it was present in 17% aged 21–30 years, 45% aged 31–40, 60% aged 41–50 and 80% aged >51 (Deverall et al. 1968).
- P-mitrale may accompany left atrial dilatation but is non-specific.
- The signs of pulmonary hypertension (right-axis deviation, P-pulmonale, dominant R and widened QRS complex in lead V1) may occur.

Stress testing
- This is not routine, but exercise testing (or even walking with the patient to the echocardiography laboratory to reveal breathlessness) should be considered in apparently asymptomatic patients with severe stenosis.
- Stress echocardiography is indicated for patients with symptoms despite apparently only moderate stenosis. Severe stenosis is indicated if the mean gradient increases above 18 mmHg or the PA pressure >60 mmHg.

Cardiac catheterization
- This is necessary for assessment of the coronary arteries before surgery or balloon valvotomy.
- Catheterization is also necessary for the measurement of pulmonary vascular resistance if the PA pressure is high on echocardiography.
- There is a delay between left atrial and pulmonary wedge pressure trace leading to overestimation of the degree of stenosis from a PA catheter-derived pressure.

Management
Surgery
- The indications for valve replacement (Bonow et al. 2006; Vahanian et al. 2007) are
  - Class I: moderate or severe mitral stenosis and symptoms:
    - Class IIa: PA systolic pressure >60 mmHg at rest
- Symptoms are often underestimated in mitral stenosis and exercise testing should be considered to reveal symptoms.
- Patients often have mixed disease and may require surgery for only moderate mitral stenosis if there is also moderate mitral regurgitation or moderate aortic valve disease. The grade of associated aortic stenosis may be underestimated as a result of low flow (see Chapter 7.7).
- The Cox maze procedure should be considered at the time of mitral valve replacement to maintain sinus rhythm.

Balloon valvotomy
- This is indicated in patients with suitable valve morphology for (Bonow et al. 2006):
  - Class I: moderate or severe mitral stenosis and symptoms
  - Class II: asymptomatic moderate or severe MS and PA pressure >50 mmHg at rest or >60 mmHg on exercise.
- It is also indicated palliatively in a patient with non-ideal valve morphology in whom the surgical risk is high.
- Procedural success is defined by a rise in area to >1.5 cm².

- Major complications (Vahanian 2007) are death 0.5–4%, haemopericardium (0.5–10%), embolism (0.5–5%), severe regurgitation (2–10%).

Medical

- Rate control: digoxin should be used in atrial fibrillation usually with the addition of a beta-blocker to control the ventricular rate on exercise
- Pulmonary congestion: in patients not suitable for balloon valvotomy or surgery, exertional symptoms will require a diuretic in addition to ventricular rate control
- Anticoagulation with warfarin is essential to an international normalized ratio (INR) 2–3 if there is atrial fibrillation. It is also recommended in the presence of sinus rhythm and severe mitral stenosis for
  - Prior thromboembolism
  - Thrombus shown in left atrium
  - Left atrial dimension >50 mm (Vahanian et al. 2007) (or 55 mm AHA) (Bonow et al. 2006).
  - Spontaneous contrast in the LA.
- Antibiotic therapy: secondary prevention is necessary to the age of 40 in the presence of valvulopathy. Antibiotic prophylaxis before dental work is no longer routinely indicated except for patients who have previously had endocarditis (Nishimura et al. 2008). Regular dental checks to treat early decay are essential.
- Monitoring: a clinical visit with echocardiography for the grade of stenosis, associated valve disease, pulmonary pressure and left atrial size should usually be performed 6 monthly for severe stenosis and annually for moderate mitral stenosis. In unequivocally mild mitral stenosis a visit every 2–3 years is sufficient.

Further reading

Baumgartner H, Hung J, Bermejo J, et al. Echocardiographic assessment of valve stenosis: EAE/ASE recommendations for clinical practice. *Eur J Echo* 2009;**10**:1–25.

Bonow RO, Carabello BA, Chatterjee K, et al. ACC/AHA 2006 guidelines for the management of patients with valvular heart disease. *J Am Coll Cardiol* 2006;**48**:e1–148.

Delahaye JP, Gare JP, Viguier E, et al. Natural history of severe mitral regurgitation. *Eur Heart J* 1991;**12** (Suppl B):5–9.

Deverall PB, Olley PM, Smith DR, et al. Incidence of systemic embolism before and after mitral valvotomy. *Thorax* 1968;**23**:818–28.

Enriquez-Sarano M, Tajik AJ, Schaff HV, et al. Echocardiographic prediction of survival after surgical correction of organic mitral regurgitation. *Circulation* 1994;**90**:830–7.

Gordon SP, Douglas PS, Come PC, Manning WJ. Two-dimensional and Doppler echocardiographic determinants of the natural history of mitral valve narrowing in patients with rheumatic mitral stenosis: implications for follow-up. *JACC* 1991;**19**:968–73.

Horstkotte D, Niehues R, Strauer BE. Pathomorphological aspects aetioloy and natural history of acquired mitral valve stenosis. *Eur Heart J* 1991;**12**(Suppl):55–60.

Iung B, Baron G, Butchart EG, et al. A prospective study of patients with valvular heart disease in Europe: The Euro Heart Survey on valvular heart disease. *Eur Heart J* 2003;**24**:1231–43.

Leatham A. *Auscultation of the heart and phonocardiography*, 2nd edn. Churchill Livingstone 1975.

Nishimura RA, Carabello BA, Faxon DP, et al. AVV/AHA 2008 guideline update on valvular heart disease: focused update on infective endocarditis. *Circulation* 2008;**118**:887–96.

Otto CM, Davis KB, Reid CL, et al. Relation between pulmonary artery pressure and mitral stenosis severity in patients undergoing balloon mitral commissurotomy. *Am J Cardiol* 1993;**71**:874–8.

Otto CM. *Valvular heart disease*. WB Saunders 1999, p. 421.

Rowe JC, Bland EF, Sprague HB, White PD. The course of mitral stenosis without surgery: ten and twenty year perspectives. *Ann Intern Med* 1960;**52**:741–9.

Ruttley MST. Radiology. In: Acar J, Bodnar E (eds) *Textbook of acquired heart valve disease*. ICR publishers. 1995: pp. 249–80.

Vahanian A, Baumgartner H, Bax J, et al. Guidelines on the management of valvular heart disease. *Eur Heart J* 2007;**28**:230–68.

Wilkins GT, Weyman AE, Abascal VM, et al. Percutaneous balloon dilatation of the mitral valve: an analysis of echocardiographic variables related to outcome and the mechanism of dilatation. *Br Heart J* 1988;**60**:299–308.

Wolf PA, Dawber TR, Thomas HE, Kannel WB. Epidemiologic assessment of chronic atrial fibrillation and risk of stroke: the Framingham study. *Neurology* 1978;**28**:973–7.

Wood P. An appreciation of mitral stenosis. *Br Med J* 1954;**1**:1054.

Mitral prolapse

Mitral prolapse is defined as either:
- Systolic movement of part of the mitral leaflet at least 2 mm behind the plane of the annulus in any echocardiographic view other than the four-chamber view

or

- Displacement of the point of coaption at least 2 mm behind the plane of the annulus in the four-chamber view.

This definition has evolved with our understanding that the mitral annulus is saddle-shaped and that buckling of the mitral leaflets behind the plane of the annulus is normal in the four-chamber view. Earlier, less strict definitions identified prolapse in up to a third of the population and the current definition still includes variations of normal. A separate group has degenerative mitral valve disease characterized by prolapse associated with valve thickening, annulus dilatation, and abnormal chordae. The chordae are abnormally prone to stretching and rupture and may be deficient particularly at the commissures or the middle scallop of the posterior leaflet. Degenerative disease is caused by myxomatous infiltration or fibroelastic deficiency and the degree of histological abnormality varies (Pellerin et al. 2002). Myxomatous infiltration causes irregular thickening of the leaflets on the echocardiogram which may be described as 'floppy'. Prolapse associated with myxomatous degeneration has a genetic component and is more frequent in Marfan syndrome and Ehlers–Danlos syndrome Type IV. Fibroelastic deficiency is more common in elderly people. Prolapse including normal variants occurs in around 2% of the adult population (Freed et al. 1999) and may be associated with tricuspid prolapse in 10% of cases (Marks et al. 1989) and rarely with aortic valve prolapse.

Clinical approach

Symptoms
- Mitral prolapse only has symptoms arising from any associated mitral regurgitation if this is severe (see Chapter 7.3) or from atrial or ventricular arrhythmias.
- Earlier descriptions of a mitral prolapse syndrome consisting of anxiety, autonomic dysfunction, and atypical chest pain arose from referral bias compounded by over-diagnosis based on auscultatory findings alone or nonspecific echocardiographic findings.

Complications
Complications probably occur only in the presence of myxomatous degeneration and not normal variant prolapse. Studies of the natural history of mitral prolapse do not usually separate these groups.
- Stroke. There is no convincing association between mitral prolapse and stroke (Gillon et al. 1999) unless there is associated atrial fibrillation. Myxomatous valves could cause platelet aggregation or possibly thrombus formation (Chesler et al. 1983) although this remains uncertain.
- Endocarditis. The risk of endocarditis is about five times that of the general population particularly in the presence of a murmur when the risk is one case in 1400 patient-years (MacMahon et al. 1987).

- Mitral regurgitation occurs in about 7% with prolapse. The grade of regurgitation depends on the degree of leaflet thickening and prolapse and is worse with ruptured chordae leading to flail or partially flail leaflet segments. In these the mean 10-year survival without heart failure is only 37% (Ling et al. 1996). Severe regurgitation causes gradually progressive LV and atrial dilatation, but rapid deterioration can occur as a result of new chordal rupture, the development of endocarditis or atrial fibrillation.
- Arrhythmias and sudden death. The incidence of atrial fibrillation depends on LA size. The mean 10-year risk of atrial fibrillation is 30% with severe regurgitation as a result of a flail or partially flail leaflet (Ling et al. 1996). There is a 1–2.5% risk of sudden death (Farb et al. 1992).

Signs
- Mid-systolic clicks associated with prolapse are both insensitive and non-specific unless associated with a murmur.
- Murmur: mild regurgitation is associated with a late crescendo murmur which may be accentuated by manoeuvres that reduce the size of the LV, e.g. standing up, a GTN spray, a valsalva manoeuvre. Moderate or severe regurgitation causes a pansystolic murmur but this may be maximal in areas other than the mitral area. It may be best heard at the base of the heart or the 'aortic' area with an anteriorly directed jet in posterior prolapse or in the back with a posteriorly directed jet in anterior prolapse (Antman et al. 1978).

Investigation

Echocardiography
- Presence and site of prolapse: the Carpentier classification is most commonly used which divides the leaflets into three equal segments (A1, A2, and A3 and P1, P2, P3) with segment 1 adjacent to the lateral commissure, segment 3 adjacent to the medial commissure and segment 2 in the middle. The site of prolapse is usually obvious on conventional transthoracic echocardiography but may be better defined by 3D echocardiography especially if commissural or bileaflet. Transoesophageal echocardiography is not routinely needed unless image quality is poor.
- The grade of mitral regurgitation (see Chapter 7.3): a particular problem for prolapse is that the jet may not be holosystolic so that a moderate width jet developing only in the latter half of systole may still equate to only mild regurgitation.
- LV size and function: as for mitral regurgitation of any aetiology, surgery is indicated for early LV systolic dilatation (see Chapter 7.9).
- LA size: enlargement is an indirect relatively nonspecific guide to the presence of severe regurgitation.
- The right heart: pulmonary hypertension is an indication for surgery even in asymptomatic severe mitral regurgitation. Tricuspid regurgitation may occur secondary to pulmonary hypertension or because of associated tricuspid valve prolapse.

- Stress studies: non-holosystolic regurgitation may become holosystolic on exercise and it is easy to test for this by an acute increase in afterload using hand-grip. If there are symptoms despite mild or moderate regurgitation or if the LV appears disproportionately large then exercise echocardiography should be considered.

ECG and chest X-ray

- The ECG may show non-specific inferior T wave changes. There may be atrial fibrillation or ventricular or supraventricular ectopics.
- The chest X-ray appearances are of the associated mitral regurgitation (see Chapter 7.3).

Management

- Severe regurgitation as a result of degenerative disease is usually repairable, but the timing remains controversial.
- For organic severe mitral regurgitation there is an argument for immediate repair (Enriques-Sarano et al. 2005) even in the absence of symptoms provided that the patient has no co-morbidity. It is crucial to this approach that the surgeon is a high-volume specialist in valve repair.
- By contrast 'watchful waiting' with surgery performed at the onset of symptoms or of LV dilatation has also been shown to be safe (Rosenhek et al. 2006). Watchful waiting remains the more common approach in Europe and surgery should be considered in low-risk patients if the LV end-systolic diameter rises to 40 mm. It is crucial to this approach that there is careful observation every 6 months with an expert echocardiographer and ideally a cardiologist specialising in valve disease.
- Antibiotic prophylaxis before dental work is no longer routinely indicated except for patients who have previously had endocarditis (Nishimura et al. 2008). Regular dental checks to treat early decay are essential.

References

Antman EM, Angoff GH, Sloss LJ. Demonstration of the mechanism by which mitral regurgitation mimics aortic stenosis. *Am J Cardiol* 1978;**42**:1044–8.

Chesler E, King RA, Edwards JE. The myxomatous mitral valve and sudden death. *Circulation* 1983;**67**:632–9.

Enriquez-Sarano M, Avierinos J-F, Messika-Zeitoun D, *et al.* Quantitative determinants of the outcome of asymptomatic mitral regurgitation. *N Engl J Med* 2005;**352**:875–83.

Farb A, Tang AL, Atkinson JB, *et al.* Comparison of cardiac findings in patients with mitral valve prolapse who die suddenly to those who have congestive heart failure from mitral regurgitation and to those with fatal noncardiac conditions. *Am J Cardiol* 1992;**70**:234–9.

Freed LA, Levy D, Levine RA, *et al.* Prevalence and clinical outcome of mitral-valve prolapse. *N Engl J Med* 1999;**341**:1–7.

Gillon D, Buonanno FS, Joffe MM, *et al.* Lack of evidence of an association between mitral valve prolapse and stroke in young patients. *N Engl J Med* 1999;**341**:8–13.

Ling LH, Enriquez-Sarano M, Seward JB *et al.* Clinical outcome of mitral regurgitation due to flail leaflet. *N Engl J Med* 1996;**335**:1417–23.

MacMahon SW, Hickey AJ, Wicken DE, *et al.* Risk of infective endocarditis in mitral prolapse with and without precordial systolic murmurs. *Am J Cardiol* 1987;**59**:105–8.

Marks AR, Choong CY, Sanfilippo AJ, *et al.* Identification of high-risk and low-risk subgroups of patients with mitral-valve prolapsed. *N Engl J Med* 1989;**320**:1031–6.

Nishimura RA, Carabello BA, Faxon DP, *et al.* AVV/AHA 2008 guideline update on valvular heart disease: focused update on infective endocarditis. *Circulation* 2008;**118**:887–96.

Pellerin D, Brecker S, Veyrat C. Degenerative mitral valve disease with emphasis on mitral valve prolapsed. *Heart* 2002;**88**(Suppl IV):iv20–iv28.

Rosenhek R, Rader F, Klaar U, *et al.* Outcome of watchful waiting in asymptomatic severe mitral regurgitation. *Circulation* 2006;**113**:2238–44.

Aortic regurgitation

Incidence

Aortic regurgitation (AR) of moderate or greater severity has been estimated to occur in 0.5% of the population, and the overall incidence of AR has been reported to be 4.9% (Framingham study). AR becomes more frequent with advancing age and its incidence peaks in the fourth to sixth decades of life.

Aetiology

Malfunction of the aortic valve leaflets, dilatation of the aortic root and annulus or a combination of these factors can lead to AR (Table 7.6.1).

Bicuspid aortic valve and degenerative disease (including annuloaortic ectasia) are the most common causes of AR in Western Europe and North America, whereas a rheumatic aetiology continues to be very common in developing countries.

Haemodynamic consequences of AR

- Left ventricular (LV) volume overload
- Increase in total LV stroke volume (sum of effective stroke volume plus regurgitant volume)
- Increased pulse pressure, with low arterial diastolic and increased systolic blood pressure
- Increased LV end-diastolic pressure
- Increased LV end-diastolic volume
- LV ejection fraction (EF) initially normal, decreases over time
- Eccentric myocardial hypertrophy
- Drop in LVEF and increase in LV volume may precede onset of symptoms.

An increase in LV end-diastolic volume is the main compensatory mechanism to maintain an adequate effective

Table 7.6.1 Aetiology of aortic regurgitation

Leaflet disorders	
Rheumatic	
Congenital	Bicuspid aortic valve
	Outlet supracristal ventricular septal defect
	Discrete subaortic stenosis
Degenerative	
Endocarditis*	
Other inflammatory disorders	
Traumatic leaflet rupture*	
Secondary AR	
Aortic root dilatation	
Aortic dissection*	Dilatation or damage to aortic annulus
	Prolapsing intimal flap with intact leaflets and annulus

*Disorders leading to acute AR.
From Maurer G. Aortic regurgitation. *Heart* 2006;92:994–1000. Reproduced with permission.

stroke volume. LVEF is initially normal, however, LV end-diastolic pressure rises. Ultimately, LV end-diastolic volume continues to increase and LVEF drops; these changes may take place before the development of clinical symptoms.

Acute versus chronic AR

Acute AR causes a sudden severe haemodynamic burden and can be life-threatening. Compensatory mechanisms, such as LV dilatation and hypertrophy cannot develop rapidly enough to avoid haemodynamic deterioration. A regurgitant volume that would be well tolerated in chronic AR can lead to marked increases in LV end-diastolic pressure and a drop in effective stroke volume. This can lead to pulmonary oedema, hypotension, and even cardiogenic shock.

Aortic versus mitral regurgitation

Both AR and mitral regurgitation (MR) result in LV volume overload. In AR there is also an increase in afterload and therefore of systolic wall stress. In MR, systolic wall stress is normal or even low, since the regurgitant blood is ejected into the left atrium, which is a low-pressure chamber. Thus, surgical correction of AR results in a decrease in afterload and frequently also an improvement of EF, while surgery for MR results in an increase in afterload and commonly in worsening of EF. The differences in afterload between the two disorders could also explain why vasodilator therapy has been thought, at least in theory, to be beneficial in AR but not in MR.

AR and the aortic root

Aortic root and annular dilatation of various aetiologies may cause AR even when the valve leaflets are normal. In the presence of a bicuspid aortic valve, the aortic root is frequently dilated, due to an abnormality of the aortic wall, which may also explain the increased incidence of aortic dissection in patients with bicuspid aortic valves. Aortic root dilatation may be independent of haemodynamics and can progress further even after valve surgery.

Clinical presentation

Patients with chronic AR can remain asymptomatic for many years, with symptoms developing only in the late stages. The most common symptom is shortness of breath, initially occurring during exercise, later also at rest. Other symptoms include sinus tachycardia that can already occur at minimal exertion, as well as palpitations due to ventricular or supraventricular arrhythmias. In some instances angina can be experienced even in absence of coronary artery disease. In addition patients may be aware of a prominent, bounding heart beat.

The severity of symptoms is largely determined by the degree of regurgitation and by the effectiveness of adaptive mechanisms, particularly that of the left ventricular function.

Physical examination

A characteristic high-pitched, blowing decrescendo diastolic murmur can be heard.

The left ventricular apical impulse is hyperdynamic, broadened and is displaced laterally and inferiorly.

Pulse pressure is widened, with low diastolic and increased systolic blood pressure. Normal or increased diastolic blood pressure is a useful sign to clinically exclude haemodynamically significant AR.

The following classical signs are variable, but can be found, particularly with more severe AR:

- Prominent arterial pulses (Waterhammer pulse, Corrigan's pulse)
- Traube sign: booming systolic and diastolic sounds heard over the femoral artery
- Duroziez sign (systolic murmur heard over the femoral artery when compressed proximally)
- Quincke sign (capillary pulsations seen when exerting pressure on the tip of a fingernail)
- DeMusset sign (head bobs with each heartbeat).

Diagnostic evaluation

ECG
ECG may be normal in mild AR. In more severe AR, LV hypertrophy with or without strain pattern can be seen.

Chest X-ray
Chest X-ray shows evidence of LV enlargement. Dilatation of the ascending aorta and aortic knob may be seen. Aneurysmal dilatation of the aorta can be present, particularly in patients in whom the AR is related to primary disease of the aortic wall.

Echocardiography
Echocardiography is the primary tool for diagnosis and evaluation of AR severity as well as for serial follow-up. Colour Doppler provides visualization of the regurgitant jet and is highly sensitive and specific for detecting AR. Continuous and pulsed wave Doppler offer important haemodynamic information and aid quantitation. 2D-echo provides evaluation of LV size and function as well as visualization of valve morphology and of the aorta. Three-dimensional echocardiography may play an increasing role in obtaining more precise measurements of ventricular volumes and may offer enhanced images of valve morphology.

Cardiac catheterization
Cardiac catheterization is primarily used to assess the coronary arteries; however, aortic root angiography can offer clarification about regurgitant severity and aortic root morphology.

Magnetic resonance imaging
Magnetic resonance imaging (MRI) is an increasingly important alternative imaging technique, particularly in instances when echocardiography is technically impossible or limited. MRI has the potential to provide precise information about regurgitant volume and regurgitant fraction.

Natural history
Severe AR results in significant increases in mortality and morbidity. With conservative management approximately half the surviving patients develop heart failure after 10 years and almost all others require valve surgery. Patients who become symptomatic are at increased risk and particularly the highly symptomatic ones (NYHA III-IV) have been noted to have high mortality rates (approximately 25% per year).

A diminished LVEF is associated with poor prognosis even in asymptomatic patients. Importantly, LV dysfunction of short duration is, in most instances reversible with valve surgery. Serial evaluation of LVEF is therefore indicated in these patients, and surgery should be considered as soon as a decrease in EF occurs. Marked LV enlargement in and of itself also constitutes an indication for surgery.

Clinical management
When managing the patient with AR the goal, in addition to relief of symptoms, is to provide optimal long-term outcome with regard to mortality and morbidity. In order to preserve LV function some patients may require surgery before the onset of symptoms. Criteria for early detection of myocardial damage focus on the evaluation of ventricular size and function. AR patients have an increased risk for developing endocarditis and should therefore be considered for antibiotic prophylaxis.

AR can be managed conservatively as long as the patient remains asymptomatic and no LV dysfunction or marked LV enlargement is present. Patients with moderate to severe AR often receive vasodilator therapy, particularly when the ventricle is already dilated. Nevertheless, the use of vasodilators in AR remains controversial, as evidence from clinical trials is conflicting.

Surgical management (Table 7.6.2)
For patients who have an indication for surgery on the aortic valve, lower thresholds can be used for combining surgery on the ascending aorta.

Aortic valve replacement
Valve replacement, using either a mechanical or a biological prosthesis continues to be the mainstay of surgical therapy.

Table 7.6.2 Indications for surgery in aortic regurgitation (From Vahanian A, Baumgartner H, Bax J, et al. Guidelines on the management of valvular heart disease. The task force on the management of valvular heart disease of the European Society of Cardiology. *Eur Heart J* 2007;28:230–268. Reproduced with permission)

	Class
Severe AR	
Symptomatic patients (dyspnoea, NYHA class II, III, IV, or angina)	IB
Asymptomatic patients with resting LVEF <50%	IB
Patients undergoing CABG or surgery of the ascending aorta, or on another valve	IC
Asymptomatic patients with resting LVEF >50% with severe LV dilatation	IIaC
End-diastolic dimension >70 mm or ESD >50 mm (or >25 mm/m² BSA)*	
Whatever the severity of AR	
Patients who have aortic root disease with maximal aortic diameter†	
>45 mm for patients with Marfan's syndrome	IC
>50 mm for patients with bicuspid valves	IIaC
>55 mm for other patients	IIaC

Severity is defined from clinical and echocardiographic assessment.
In asymptomatic patients, repeated and high-quality measures are necessary before surgery.
AR, aortic regurgitation; BSA, body surface area; CABG, coronary artery bypass grafting; ESD, end-systolic dimension; EF, ejection fraction; LV, left ventricular.
*Patient's stature should be considered. Indexing is helpful. Changes in sequential measurements should be taken into account.
†Decision should take into account the shape and thickness of ascending aorta as well as the shape of the other parts of aorta.

The use of homografts or pulmonary autografts is limited by concerns about their durability.

Aortic valve repair

Valve repair is being performed in selected patients, particularly in those with prolapsing bicuspid aortic valves and eccentric jets, but outcomes have generally been less favourable than for mitral valve repair.

In patients with significant AR in whom surgery is not indicated, meticulous serial clinical and echocardiographic evaluation is required. In stable patients 1-year follow-up intervals may be appropriate as LV dysfunction developing over 12–14 months has been shown usually to be reversible.

References

Bonow RO, Rosing DR, Maron BJ, et al. Reversal of left ventricular dysfunction after aortic valve replacement for chronic aortic regurgitation: influence of duration of preoperative left ventricular dysfunction. Circulation 1984;**70**:570–9.

Bonow RO, Picone AL, McIntosh CL, et al. Survival and functional results after valve replacement for aortic regurgitation from 1976 to 1983: impact of preoperative left ventricular function. Circulation 1985;**72**:1244–56.

Carabello BA. Vasodilators in aortic regurgitation–what is the evidence of their effectiveness? N Engl J Med 2005;**353**:1400–2.

Dujardin KS, Enriquez-Sarano M, Schaff HV, Bailey KR, Seward JB, Tajik AJ. Mortality and morbidity of aortic regurgitation in clinical practice: a long-term follow-up study. Circulation 1999;**99**:1851–7.

Enriquez-Sarano M, Tajik AJ. Clinical practice. Aortic regurgitation. N Engl J Med 2004;**351**:1539–46.

Klodas E, Enriquez-Sarano M, Tajik AJ, et al. Aortic regurgitation complicated by extreme left ventricular dilatation: longterm outcome after surgical correction. J Am Coll Cardiol 1996;**27**:670–7.

Klodas E, Enriquez-Sarano M, Tajik AJ, et al. Optimizing timing of surgical correction in patients with severe aortic regurgitation: role of symptoms. J Am Col Cardiol 1997;**30**:746–52.

Maurer G. Aortic regurgitation. Heart 2006;**92**:994–1000.

Vahanian A, Baumgartner H, Bax J, et al. Guidelines on the management of valvular heart disease. The task force on the management of valvular heart disease of the European Society of Cardiology. Eur Heart J 2007;**28**:230–68.

Zoghbi WA, Enriquez-Sarano M, Foster E, et al. American Society of Echocardiography. Recommendations for evaluation of the severity of native valvular regurgitation with two-dimensional and Doppler echocardiography. J Am Soc 2003;**16**:777–802.

Aortic stenosis

Aortic valve thickening or 'sclerosis' occurs in 25% of people in the West aged over 65 years (Stewart et al. 1997). Mild aortic stenosis is differentiated by a peak transaortic velocity >2.5 m/second on echocardiography (Baumgartner et al. 2009). Severe aortic stenosis occurs in about 3% aged over 75 tears (Stewart et al. 1997) and is the most common valve disease in the West, accounting for 43% of cases in the Euro Heart Survey (Iung et al. 2003).

The most common cause of aortic stenosis in the West is degenerative disease, although a bicuspid aortic valve occurs in 2% of the population. Rheumatic aortic valve disease is now uncommon in the West.

Degenerative aortic valve disease is now known to be an active process. The earliest histological lesions resemble those of coronary atherosclerosis and the risk factors for aortic stenosis are similar: diabetes, smoking, hypercholesterolaemia, hypertension (Stewart et al. 1997). There is also an association between coronary disease and aortic valve thickening. Progressive stenosis remains an active process sustained by inflammation and vascular calcification associated with the synthesis of extracellular matrix proteins. Neoangiogenesis, T-cell infiltration, adhesion molecules, and heat shock protein gene expression indicate an active immune-mediated process even in severe aortic stenosis immediately before surgery.

Clinical approach

History: key points

- Exertional chest pain or breathlessness are indistinguishable from angina as a result of coronary disease. However, patients may restrict exertion to avoid symptoms so it is important to ask about avoidance of previously commonplace activities or a 'slowing-down'.
- Exertional dizziness or syncope are less common. They occur as a result of a fall in blood pressure sometimes leading to a brady- or tachyarrhythmia.
- About 5% of patients having aortic valve replacement still present in heart failure.
- Chest pain at rest suggests an alternative cause including coronary disease. Presyncope or syncope at rest also suggest an alternative cause including conduction tissue disease as a result of calcium invasion from the annulus (Lev's disease).
- Ask about chronic obstructive pulmonary disease (COPD), coronary disease and other causes of exertional symptoms that could complicate your assessment of the effect of aortic stenosis.
- Ask about co-morbidities especially lung disease, cerebrovascular disease, and chronic renal failure that may affect the risk of surgery.
- Ask about the patient's attitude to surgery. Psychological problems might need to be addressed during the monitoring of asymptomatic severe aortic stenosis.

Examination (Leatham 1975)

- Murmur: an ejection systolic murmur is common in normal subjects and if it is soft and short (finishing well before the second sound) with a normal second sound and if the patient is symptom free, echocardiography is not usually necessary.

- All other patients should have echocardiography since the examination is not a reliable indicator of grade. However, a combination of a long ejection systolic murmur, soft or absent second sound and a slow-rising carotid is highly suggestive of severe aortic stenosis.
- A systolic click suggest the presence of a bicuspid aortic valve.
- A narrow pulse pressure is rare: this sign was described in young patients with rheumatic disease and most patients in the West are now older. About one-half have systemic hypertension.
- General: look for signs suggesting high surgical risk, e.g. kyphosis, general frailty.

Investigations

Echocardiography

- This is the mainstay and provides information about the aortic valve, the left ventricular (LV) and the rest of the heart.
- The minimum dataset for the aortic valve is peak velocity, mean gradient and effective orifice area using the continuity equation
- EOAi, effective orifice area indexed to body surface area; V_{max}, peak transaortic velocity.
- Grading stenosis (Table 7.7.1) may be difficult since the grades according to each threshold may be inconsistent. It is frequent for aortic stenosis to be moderate by gradient but severe by EOA. This may be because the cut-point for EOA is unrealistically high, particularly if the patient has a low body surface area (BSA), and this situation can be detected from the indexed EOA. The discrepancy can also arise if there is relatively low flow.
- Low flow is obvious if the LV ejection fraction is reduced. It can also occur with a small LV cavity when a low stroke volume may be associated with a normal ejection fraction. The situation can be diagnosed from a low subaortic velocity integral and a calcified immobile aortic valve. If in doubt consider stress echocardiography.
- In bicuspid aortic valve, check the ascending aorta for dilatation and the descending thoracic aorta for coarctation.
- The minimum dataset for the LV comprises standard LV dimensions, estimated ejection fraction, and the subaortic velocity integral.

Table 7.7.1 Grading aortic stenosis (adapted from Baumgartner et al. 2009)

	Mild	Moderate	Severe
Transaortic V_{max} (m/s)	2.6–3.0	3.0–4.0	>4.0
Mean gradient (mmHg)	<20	20–40 (50)	>40 (50)
Effective orifice area (cm²)	>1.5	1.0–1.5	<1.0
EOAi (cm²/m²)	>0.85	0.6–0.85	<0.6
Velocity ratio	>0.5	0.25–0.5	<0.25

- Right ventricular function and PA pressure must be estimated since these affect surgical risk.
- The anatomy and function of the mitral valve.

Stress echocardiography
- Low-dose dobutamine is infused starting at 5 and increasing to 10 µg/kg/min dobutamine (occasionally 15 then 20 µg/kg/min, especially if there is prior beta-blockade). This requires medical supervision because of the risk of cardiac arrhythmia although the risk is not great at low infusion rates.
- The infusion can be stopped if the subaortic velocity integral (VTI1) rises >20% or if the heart rate increases.
- Severe aortic stenosis is defined by a rise in mean gradient above 40 mmHg at any time during the infusion (Baumgartner et al. 2009).
- Contractile reserve is defined by a rise in stroke volume, EF, or velocity integral by >20%. Mortality at surgery is substantially lower with contractile reserve, about 5%, than 35% in its absence. Contractile reserve identifies those in whom the LV ejection fraction recovers early after surgery, although long-term recovery now appears to be similar with or without contractile reserve (Quere et al. 2006).

Exercise testing
- Treadmill testing is now accepted as indicated for patients with moderate or severe aortic stenosis (Carabello 2002; Vahanian et al. 2007) who appear asymptomatic with normal exercise capacity. In up to one-half patients with EOA <1.3 cm^2 symptoms will be revealed by exercise testing (Das et al. 2005)

Coronary angiography
- This is needed before aortic valve surgery but the valve should almost never be crossed. The risk of death, stroke, or pulmonary oedema is about 7% crossing the valve compared with about 3% for coronary angiography alone (Chambers et al. 2004).
- Catheter- and Doppler-derived gradients are related but different and not directly comparable.

Multislice CT and cardiac magnetic resonance (CMR)
- CT can image the anatomic orifice but produces no information similar to EOA and gradient on echocardiography. It is better than echocardiography for quantifying the calcium within the valve and aorta.
- Cardiac magnetic resonance provides anatomic orifice area and can produce haemodynamic information from flow mapping.
- Both CT and CMR provide better anatomical information than echocardiography about the aorta. CT of the aorta is used in some centres in planning transcatheter implantation of aortic valves. Both CT and CMR produce better estimations of LV mass for research studies than using 2D echocardiography, although they are only better than 3D echocardiography if echocardiographic windows are suboptimal. Neither technique is used in routine clinical practice.

B-type natriuretic peptide
- Levels of BNP or NT-BNP are raised according the grade of aortic stenosis and the degree of LV hypertrophy. They are raised further if there is diastolic or systolic dysfunction and further still if there are symptoms (Gerber et al. 2003).
- A high BNP level predicts the onset of symptoms in an asymptomatic subject. The BNP is not yet used routinely but may guide the decision for aortic valve replacement in moderate stenosis with symptoms.

Natural history
- Around 16% of patients with sclerosis progress to stenosis within 7 years (Cosmi et al. 2002; Horstkotte and Loogen 1988). The rate of progression varies, but the average reduction in orifice area is 0.1 cm^2 each year (Otto et al. 1997).
- Severe AS remains asymptomatic for many years and the risk of death is then <1% per year. Once spontaneous symptoms develop, mortality rises sharply and the median survival is 4.5 years with exertional chest pain, 2.6 years with exertional dizziness and 1 year with overt heart failure (Horstkotte and Loogen 1988). Survival is particularly poor, 20% at 3 years, in the presence of NYHA III or IV symptoms and an impaired left ventricle.
- The mortality is not linear and is about 10% in the first 6 months after the start of symptoms. Prophylactic surgery should therefore be considered in patients who are likely to develop symptoms soon.

Management
Consensus indications for surgery
- A full list of indications for surgery based on AHA and ESC guidelines (Bonow et al. 2006; Vahanian et al. 2007) is given in Table 7.7.2. These can be summarized as:
  - Severe aortic stenosis and symptoms
  - Moderate or severe aortic stenosis who require other types of cardiac surgery
  - Severe aortic stenosis with high risk signs.

Asymptomatic severe aortic stenosis
- A reduction in exercise capacity is taken as a criterion for surgery (Otto et al. 1997). In those who appear to have normal exercise capacity, exercise testing may reveal symptoms.
- In those who are proved to be asymptomatic after exercise testing, prophylactic surgery may still be performed if symptom onset is likely to be soon since 3–4% die soon after the onset of symptoms and sudden death may be the first symptom. The AHA and ESC criteria allow for surgery if the peak transaortic velocity (V_{max}) >5.0 m/s provided that the surgical risk is around 1%. They also allow surgery if the rate of increase in V_{max} is >0.3 m/s p.a. in the presence of heavy aortic valve calcification (Rosenhek et al. 2000).

Low flow aortic stenosis
- Pressure overload causes LV remodelling then hypertrophy and ultimately cavity dilatation. A low LV ejection

Table 7.7.2 Criteria for surgery in aortic stenosis (adapted from Bonow *et al.* 2006; Vahanian *et al.* 2007)

Severe AS with symptoms	Class I
Severe AS undergoing other cardiac surgery, e.g. CABG	Class I
Severe AS and EF <50%	Class I
Asymptomatic AS with symptoms on exercise testing	Class I (ESC only)
Moderate AS undergoing CABG or aortic surgery	Class IIa
Asymptomatic AS with abnormal physiology on exercise testing	Class IIb (IIa by ESC)
Asymptomatic severe AS with rapid progression	Class IIb (IIa by ESC)
Asymptomatic severe AS where surgery might be delayed after the onset of symptoms	Class IIb
Asymptomatic very severe (Vmax >5.0 m/s) and operative risk <1%	Class IIb
Patients with mild AS undergoing CABG if rate of progression likely to be fast	Class IIb
Asymptomatic severe AS and LVH >15 mm unless due to hypertension	Class IIb (ESC only)

fraction (EF) need not imply a 'poor' LV. The LV with a low EF is using its energy to overcome the resistance of the aortic valve rather than to eject a normal volume of blood at normal flow rates. The EF is expected to return towards normal after aortic valve replacement.

- If the Vmax >3.5 m/s or mean gradient >40 mmHg even if the EF is low, surgery is indicated.
- If the mean gradient <40 mmHg, there is either severe AS causing LV systolic dysfunction or moderate AS with another cause of LV dysfunction (e.g. myocardial infarction or alcoholic cardiomyopathy). These can be differentiated using low-dose dobutamine stress echocardiography.

Symptoms despite only moderate AS

- Sometimes the patient has symptoms despite the AS being moderate even taking into account the secondary factors of waveform shape, valve appearance and indexed EOA. There may often be other possible causes for the exertional breathlessness including coronary disease, obesity, lung disease, or anaemia.
- The most helpful test is stress echocardiography to reveal LV wall motion abnormalities and to test the compliance of the aortic valve. Compliance means the ability of the valve to open as flow increases during exercise. Most moderately stenotic valves open relatively well, but some do not and become effectively severely stenotic during stress. Stressors used are recumbent bicycle, treadmill and dobutamine up to 20 µg/kg/min.
- The difference between peak and baseline mean gradient divided by the difference in flow gives the pressure drop-flow slope. A slope >0.2 mmHg/mL/second is severe, but an easier guide is an increase in the mean gradient by >18 mmHg during stress (Lancellotti *et al.* 2005).

- A high B-type natriuretic peptide level also suggests that the heart is the source of breathlessness.

Combined aortic stenosis and mitral regurgitation

- Severe AS is often associated with mitral regurgitation. Mitral surgery is usually needed at the same time as aortic valve replacement if there is severe functional mitral regurgitation or moderate regurgitation as a result of organic mitral valve disease.

Patients unfit for surgery

- For patients who have severe AS and significant symptoms, but also co-morbidities that preclude conventional surgery, transcatheter valve implantation is developing rapidly (Descoutures *et al.* 2008). This can be performed via the femoral artery or, if the arteries are too narrow, through the apex of the left ventricle. The technique is more expensive than conventional surgery and still has a significant morbidity and mortality, but results are encouraging with haemodynamic results as good as those obtained by conventional surgery.

Medical management

Monitoring

- Patients with no symptoms require monitoring annually if there is moderate stenosis and every 6 months if there is severe stenosis ideally in a specialist valve clinic.

Medication

- Hypertension may increase the rate of progression and should be treated with an angiotensin-converting enzyme (ACE) inhibitor. Although previously contraindicated, there is good evidence that these drugs improve the LV response to pressure overload. They may also improve symptoms and exercise time in patients unable to have surgery (Chockalingam 2004).
- Lipid lowering is not effective at slowing the rate of progression of moderate or severe AS (Rossebo 2008).
- Nitrates should be used with caution in patients with aortic stenosis and angina to prevent the occurrence of orthostatic hypotension and syncope and beta-blockers are avoided because the patient may be critically sensitive to a small fall in contractility in the presence of tight AS.
- Antibiotic prophylaxis before dental work is no longer routinely indicated except for patients who have previously had endocarditis (Nishimura *et al.* 2008). Regular dental checks to treat early decay are essential.

References

Baumgartner H, Hung J, Bermejo J, *et al.* Echocardiographic assessment of valve stenosis: EAE/ASE recommendations for clinical practice. *Eur J Echo* 2009;**10**:1–25.

Bonow RO, Carabello BA, Kanu C, *et al.* ACC/AHA 2006 guidelines for the management of patients with valvular heart disease: a report of the American College of Cardiology/American Heart Association Task Force on Practice Guidelines (writing committee to revise the 1998 Guidelines for the Management of Patients With Valvular Heart Disease). *Circulation* 2006;**114**:e84–231.

Carabello BA. Clinical practice. Aortic stenosis. *N Engl J Med* 2002;**346**:677–82.

Chambers J, Bach D, Dumesnil J, *et al.* Crossing the aortic valve in severe aortic stenosis: no longer acceptable?. *J Heart Valve Disease* 2004;**13**:344–6.

Chetlin MD, Alpert JS, Armstrong WF, *et al.* ACC/AHA/ASE Guideline update for the clinical application of echocardiography: summary article. *Circulation* 2003;**108**:1146–62.

Chockalingam A, Venkatesan S, Subramaniam T, *et al.* Safety and efficacy of angiotensin-converting enzyme inhibitors in symptomatic severe aortic stenosis: Symptomatic Cardiac Obstruction-Pilot Study of Enalapril in Aortic Stenosis (SCOPE-AS). *Am Heart J* 2004;**147**:L1–8.

Cosmi JE, Tunick PA, Rosenzweig BP, *et al*. The risk of development of aortic stenosis in patients with 'benign' aortic valve thickening. *Arch Int Med* 2002;**162**:2345–7.

Das P, Rimington H, Chambers J. Exercise testing to stratify risk in aortic stenosis. *Eur Heart J* 2005;**26**:1309–13.

Descoutures F, Himbert D, Lepage L, *et al*. Contemporary surgical or percutaneous management of severe aortic stenosis in the elderly. *Eur Heart J* 2008;**29**:1410–7.

Gerber IL, Stewart RA, Legget ME, *et al*. Increased plasma natriuretic peptide levels reflect symptom onset in aortic stenosis. *Circulation* 2003;**107**:1884–90.

Horstkotte D, Loogen F. The natural history of aortic valve stenosis. *Eur Heart J* 1988;**9**(Suppl E):57–64.

Iung B, Baron G, Butchart EG, *et al*. A prospective study of patients with valvular heart disease in Europe: The Euro Heart Survey on valvular heart disease. *Eur Heart J* 2003;**24**:1231–43.

Lancellotti P, Lebois F, Simon M, *et al*. Prognostic importance of quantitative exercise Doppler echocardiography in asymptomatic valvular aortic stenosis. *Circulation* 2005;**112**(Suppl 9):1377–82.

Nishimura RA, Carabello BA, Faxon DP, *et al*. AVV/AHA 2008 guideline update on valvular heart disease: focused update on infective endocarditis. *Circulation* 2008;**118**:887–96.

Otto CM, Burwash IG, Legget ME, *et al*. Prospective study of asymptomatic valvular aortic stenosis. Clinical, echocardiographic, and exercise predictors of outcome. *Circulation* 1997;**95**:2262–70.

Pellikka PA, Sarano ME, Nishimura RA, *et al*. Outcome of 622 adults with asymptomatic, hemodynamically significant aortic stenosis during prolonged follow-up. *Circulation* 2005;**111**:3290–5.

Quere J-P, Monin J-L, Levy F, *et al*. Influence of preoperative left ventricular contractile reserve on postoperative ejection fraction in low-gradient aortic stenosis. *Circulation* 2006;**113**:1738–44.

Rossebo AB, Pedersen TR, Allen C, *et al*. Intensive lipid lowering therapy with simvastatin and ezetimibe in aortic valve stenosis. *N Engl J Med* 2008;**359**:1343–56.

Rosenhek R, Binder T, Porenta G, *et al*. Predictors of outcome in severe, asymptomatic aortic stenosis. *N Engl J Med* 2000;**343**:611–7.

Stewart BF, Siscovick D, Lind BK, *et al*. Clinical factors associated with calcific aortic valve disease: Cardiovascular Health Study. *J Am Coll Cardiol* 1997;**29**:630–4.

Vahanian A, Baumgartner H, Bax J, *et al*. Guidelines on the management of valvular heart disease: The Task Force on the Management of Valvular Heart Disease of the European Society of Cardiology. *Eur Heart J* 2007;**28**:230–68.

Tricuspid and pulmonary valve disease

The right-sided heart valves, tricuspid and pulmonary, are much less affected by acquired pathology than the left-sided valves, mitral, and aortic. However, the tricuspid valve is frequently secondarily involved in left-sided pathology, especially that of the mitral valve; so-called functional tricuspid regurgitation, although some believe that in these cases tricuspid regurgitation may be at least partly organic, especially in rheumatic patients (Chiappini et al. 2006). Acquired pulmonary valve disease is very rare and seldom constitutes a dilemma over the appropriate surgical management.

Tricuspid stenosis

Tricuspid valve stenosis occurs in about 15–20% of rheumatic cases and is characterized by fusion of the commissures with or without thickening and retraction of the leaflets. It is usually accompanied by variable degrees of regurgitation and is rarely found in isolation, most patients presenting also with mitral and, often, aortic valve disease (Keefe et al. 1970).

Another aetiology of tricuspid stenosis is the carcinoid syndrome. Carcinoid tumours, especially of the intestine, are associated with heart valve disease in approximately 50% of the cases. In most patients, the pulmonary valve is also involved, but the disease may also affect the mitral and aortic valves, especially in lung carcinoid tumours. Serotonin and bradykinin, the substances released by these tumours and that are related to the syndrome, are inactivated by the liver and the lungs, which determines the valves involved (Chiappini et al. 2006). Tricuspid valves affected by the carcinoid syndrome are generally far more distorted than those of rheumatic origin.

Radiation injury and systemic lupus erythematosus are other, much rarer, causes for tricuspid disease, especially stenosis.

Generally, tricuspid stenosis is clinically silent and well tolerated until a critical valve orifice is reached, after which signs of congestive heart failure and low cardiac output develop. Symptoms are usually confounded by co-existing left heart valve disease. Dilated and pulsatile jugular veins, with prominent a-waves, pulsatile hepatomegaly, ascites, and peripheral oedema progressively ensue finally indicating the need for surgical intervention.

Tricuspid regurgitation

Organic tricuspid regurgitation, with or without some degree of stenosis, may occur as a consequence of the pathologies described above. But in approximately 80% of cases, the regurgitation is judged functional, resulting from elevation of the pulmonary artery pressure secondary to mitral and/or aortic valve disease. Functional tricuspid regurgitation is, in most cases, of rheumatic aetiology but may also be associated with degenerative mitral valve disease or with senile aortic stenosis. It is, however, possible that dilatation of the annulus may be a consequence of weakening directly caused by the rheumatic process (Phillips 2005).

This situation is characterized by an enlarged right ventricle and atrium and dilated tricuspid annulus. There may be prolapse of the leaflets because of elongation, or occasionally rupture, of the chordae tendineae, but incompetence of the valve is most often caused by tethering of the leaflets caused by the dilatation and remodelling of the ventricle, which causes the walls to pull the papillary muscles apart.

Patients show signs of progressive congestive heart failure with dilated veins, hepatomegaly, ascites, and peripheral oedema. By contrast with tricuspid stenosis, significant regurgitation is poorly tolerated from an early stage, although symptoms may be relatively well controlled by antifailure therapy. However, when the right ventricle fails, the situation can only be reversed by surgery of the tricuspid valve.

It was previously believed that functional tricuspid regurgitation would regress with correction of the left heart valve disease but this does not always happen and cannot be easily predicted. Especially when there is significant dilatation and dysfunction of the right ventricle, tricuspid regurgitation tends to progress even after adequate repair of the left-sided valves (Antunes and Barlow 2007). Incomplete correction of the left-sided valve disease is an important factor for progression or recurrence of functional tricuspid regurgitation. As discussed below, late tricuspid regurgitation is becoming more frequent, years after a previous left heart valve operation. Hence, intervention on the tricuspid valve during surgery primarily directed at the mitral and aortic valves is currently more aggressively recommended.

Pulmonary valve disease

With the exception of carcinoid disease, which may cause pulmonary stenosis and regurgitation, the pulmonary valve is rarely affected by acquired heart valve disease, including rheumatic disease and infective endocarditis. Pulmonary regurgitation is the most frequent pathology and may occur in severe cases of dilatation and dysfunction of the right ventricle secondary to mitral valve disease and severe pulmonary hypertension (Waller et al. 1995). It results from dilatation of the annulus; the leaflets usually being normal. Since moderate degrees of pulmonary stenosis and regurgitation are well tolerated, surgery is seldom required (see p. 309).

Infective endocarditis of right-side heart valves

Infective endocarditis of the tricuspid and pulmonary valves is rare. Isolated tricuspid valve endocarditis accounts for only about 3% of the cases, and occurs in association with mitral and or aortic valve endocarditis in a similar percentage of cases. Pulmonary valve infection is even rarer.

Most cases of tricuspid and pulmonary valve endocarditis occur in intravenous drug addicts and often lead to extensive destruction of the leaflets resulting in free regurgitation. Staphylococcal infection is the most common, but fungal infection is also frequent and associated with a poor prognosis. In these cases, the infection occurs commonly in structurally normal valves. Although the infecting agents are virulent, aggressive antibiotic therapy is often successful and only one quarter of the patients eventually require surgery (Chan et al. 1989). Continued sepsis and uncontrolled heart failure are the main indications for surgery. However, recurrence is common, since patients usually return to the drug habit, which may require a specific surgical approach, as discussed below.

Traumatic tricuspid and pulmonary regurgitation

The tricuspid and pulmonary valves may be damaged by both blunt and penetrating chest trauma. The extent of damage depends on the type and intensity of the trauma. Penetrating instruments or weapons may perforate or tear the cusps and damage chordae and papillary muscles. As these lesions occur simultaneous with perforation of the atrial, ventricular, or vascular walls that usually require emergency life-saving surgery, the intracardiac lesions often pass unnoticed until late in their clinical course.

Blunt trauma of the tricuspid valve may cause rupture and/or dehiscence of the cusps, chordae tendineae, or papillary muscles. This pathology occurs most frequently in the setting of multi-organ involvement which masks the heart pathology, since tricuspid and pulmonary regurgitation are usually well tolerated. Hence, similarly to penetrating lesions, the diagnosis is usually also made late after the trauma (van Son et al. 1994).

Indications for, and type of treatment depend on the magnitude of the regurgitation and of the symptoms. In the more serious cases patients may present with signs of severe congestive cardiac failure, similar to those of other causes of chronic tricuspid regurgitation. Surgery is then indicated and most often is constituted of valve repair with reconstitution of the leaflets, chordae tendineae, and papillary muscles.

Surgery

Pulmonary valve

Except in extreme circumstances, the pulmonary valve affected by acquired disease rarely requires surgery as moderate degrees of both stenosis and regurgitation are usually well tolerated. When surgery is required, especially in regurgitant valves, replacement is often required, which can be performed with either mechanical or biological prostheses. The choice follows basically the same rules as for mitral and aortic valves. Right-side mechanical prostheses are more prone to thrombosis; hence, bioprostheses have generally been preferred. However, in more recent times, thrombolysis has been shown to be very effective without significant complications and mechanical prostheses are now used more frequently, especially in young patients (Cáceres-Lóriga et al. 2006).

An excellent alternative for pulmonary valve replacement is the homograft. Used initially for congenital heart surgery, homografts are very easy to implant and usually last for over 10 years. They are very resistant to infection and their use may thus be preferable for drug addicts (Saito et al. 2008). Reoperation for substitution of homografts in the pulmonary position is relatively simple but new methods of transcatheter valve implantation may obviate the need for repeat surgery in the future (Nordmeyer et al. 2006). This may also be the case with bioprostheses.

Tricuspid valve

Similar to the pulmonary valve, tricuspid valves rarely need replacement as a first intervention. Only extensively destroyed valves, as in endocarditis and in carcinoid syndromes may require substitution. The choice of substitute follows the same lines indicated above for the pulmonary valve, but the use of homografts for tricuspid valve replacement, advocated by some, has not gained wide acceptance.

Annuloplasty is, thus, the procedure of choice. Suture annuloplasties were developed in the early 1960s by Paneth, Reed and others, but the De Vega annuloplasty and its many modifications were, and still are, the most used methods. This procedure is based on the observation that dilatation of the tricuspid annulus occurs mostly in its anterior and posterior sections and that the septal portion is usually unaffected (Deloche et al. 1973). The procedure is simple and easily reproducible even by relatively inexperienced surgeons and has excellent long-term results. In my view, it should be used in all patients with more than mild 'functional' tricuspid regurgitation, since it adds little, if any, additional risk to surgery and improves long-term prognosis, as discussed above. Recent evidence may suggest that it should be used 'prophylactically' even in the absence of significant regurgitation in patients with annular dilatation (Dreyfus et al. 2005).

Prosthetic rings and bands can also be used and are preferred by many. The Carpentier–Edwards ring is the most used device. It is a rigid annuloplasty ring which has the advantage of reshaping the annulus, thus potentially providing better coaptation of the tricuspid leaflets. Better long-term results have been claimed but, in my experience, the ring is essentially indicated in patients with organic rheumatic disease when commissurotomy is also required. The latter technique should only be performed when the valve orifice is very small, and only the commissures bordering the septal leaflet should be opened.

Surgery for tricuspid valve endocarditis carries special decision problems, particularly in drug addicts, because of the risk of reinfection. Localized lesions may be treated by excision of vegetations and/or portions of the leaflets, with reconstitution of the valve continuity. Partial substitution by homograft tissue has been used in selected cases. When the tricuspid valve is completely destroyed, the whole valve apparatus needs to be removed. A couple of decades ago, simple excision without replacement was advocated by Arbulu et al. (1991), but the long-term results were poor and this approach has largely been abandoned. However, in extreme cases, valvectomy alone may be performed, followed by delayed replacement after cure of the infection by antibiotics. Homografts may have here their best indication in tricuspid valve pathology, but the results have been less than satisfactory.

Late-onset tricuspid regurgitation after left-side valve surgery

As indicated above, tricuspid regurgitation may occur or recur late after a previous surgery for the mitral and/or aortic valves, a problem which surgeons are being confronted with more frequently, as it develops in 5–10% of patients (Antunes and Barlow 2007).

Unrecognized right ventricular dysfunction is the probable mechanism. There are many factors for persisting, worsening or recurrent tricuspid regurgitation after mitral valve surgery without surgery to the tricuspid valve. Perhaps the most important is persisting or recurring mitral valve disease, especially after valve conservation procedures. On the other hand, the more severe the unrepaired tricuspid regurgitation at the initial procedure, the more likely it is to persist or increase late. Mild tricuspid regurgitation rarely persists or progresses, whereas moderate or severe regurgitation may do so. Tricuspid regurgitation may also be the direct consequence of longstanding, perhaps irreversible right ventriclular dilatation, secondary to pulmonary vascular disease. Thus, tricuspid regurgitation that does not disappear or improve considerably with intensive decongestive therapy preoperatively is more likely to persist postoperatively if not repaired. These mechanisms have been well described by Barlow et al. (1987) as 'the restrictive dilatation syndrome', which results from a vicious circle involving all the above-mentioned factors.

In these cases, surgery may be a first or a repeat tricuspid valve operation, either in isolation or simultaneously with other valve procedures. Re-do heart surgery, of any description, carries a higher operative risk, which is magnified by the number of times it takes place, and tricuspid valve replacement in patients who have had prior cardiac surgery is a very high risk procedure, with hospital mortality of up to 35% (Bernal et al. 2005). Re-entry through the sternum is one of the causes of the high morbidity and a right thoracotomy may be the preferred access route, especially for isolated tricuspid surgery. Cardiopulmonary bypass may be established in the classical way (vena cavae–ascending aorta), but the femoral vessels may be used for either arterial return or as a femoral vein–femoral artery circuit.

Even after successful surgery, long-term prognosis is relatively poor in these patients and may be explained by the chronic right ventricular dysfunction that is not fully reversed by correction of the tricuspid regurgitation, which raises the dilemma of the appropriateness of recommending surgery to these patients (Staab et al. 1999).

References

Antunes MJ, Barlow JB. Management of tricuspid valve regurgitation. Heart 2007;**93**:271–6.

Arbulu A, Holmes RJ, Asfaw I. Tricuspid valvulectomy without replacement. Twenty years' experience. J Thorac Cardiovasc Surg 1991;**102**:917–22.

Barlow JB, Pocock WA, Meyer TE. Conditions relevant to assessment or function of the mitral valve. 2. Tricuspid valve disease. In: Barlow JB (ed). Perspectives on the mitral valve. Philadelphia: FA Davis Co, 1987; pp. 338–59.

Bernal JM, Morales D, Revuelta C, et al. Reoperations after tricuspid valve repair. J Thorac Cardiovasc Surg 2005;**130**:498–503.

Cáceres-Lóriga FM, Pérez-López H, Morlans-Hernández K, et al. Thrombolysis as first choice therapy in prosthetic heart valve thrombosis. A study of 68 patients. J Thromb Thrombolysis 2006;**21**:185–90.

Chan KM, Zakkar M, Amirak E, Punjabi PP. Tricuspid valve disease: pathophysiology and optimal management. Prog Cardiovasc Dis 2009;**51**:482–86.

Chan P, Ogilby JD, Segal B. Tricuspid valve endocarditis. Am Heart J 1989;**117**:1140–6.

Chiappini B, Noirhomme P, Verhelst R, El Khoury G. Quadruple valve involvement in a patient with severe carcinoid heart disease. J Card Surg 2006;**21**:599–600.

Deloche A, Guerinon J, Fabiani JN, et al. Anatomical study of rheumatic tricuspid valve diseases: Application to the study of various valvuloplasties. Ann Chir Thorac Cardiovasc. 1973;**12**:343–9.

Dreyfus G, Corbi PJ, John Chan KM, Bahrami T. Secondary TR or dilatation: which should be the criteria for surgical repair? Ann Thorac Surg 2005;**79**:127–32.

Keefe JF, Wolk MJ, Levine HJ: Isolated tricuspid valvular stenosis. Am J Cardiol 1970;**25**:252–7.

Nordmeyer J, Coats L, Bonhoeffer P. Current experience with percutaneous pulmonary valve implantation. Semin Thorac Cardiovasc Surg 2006;**18**:122–5.

Phillips BJ. Tricuspid valve disease: a few points regarding right-sided heart failure. Internet J Thorac Cardiovasc Surg 2005;**7**:1.

Saito A, Motomura N, Kakimi K. Vascular allografts are resistant to methicillin-resistant Staphylococcus aureus through indoleamine 2,3-dioxygenase in a murine model. J Thorac Cardiovasc Surg 2008;**136**:159–67.

Staab ME, Nishimura RA, Dearani JA. Isolated tricuspid valve surgery for severe tricuspid regurgitation following prior left heart valve surgery: analysis of outcome in 34 patients. J Heart Valve Dis 1999;**8**:567–74.

van Son JA, Danielson GK, Schaff HV, Miller Jr FA. Traumatic tricuspid valve insufficiency experience in thirteen patients. J Thorac Cardiovasc Surg 1994;**108**:893–8.

Waller BF, Howard J, Fess S. Pathology of pulmonic valve stenosis and pure regurgitation. Clin Cardiol 1995;**18**:45–50.

Cardiac surgery

Introduction

The indications for valve surgery have been the subject of detailed review with evidence-based guidelines published in Europe (Vahanian *et al.* 2007) and North America (Bonow *et al.* 2006). Surgical techniques have developed rapidly with a trend towards earlier intervention, the use of complex valve reparative procedures, and implantation of prostheses that offer improved durability and enhanced haemodynamic performance.

Timing of valve surgery

Optimal decision-making requires an accurate assessment of the severity of valve lesions using the integration of clinical (symptoms and signs), non-invasive (elecrocardiogram, chest X-ray, echocardiography, functional testing, computed tomography, and magnetic resonance imaging), and invasive (cardiac catheterization) techniques (see Chapters 7.3–7.8). Judgement about the relative indication of surgery is based on determining the balance between the risks associated with the natural history of the condition and those related to surgical correction. The latter is complex and multivariate and can be estimated with the use of Euroscore calculations (Roques *et al.* 2001). Final decisions are best made in the context of multidisciplinary discussions and following careful counselling of the patient.

Types of operation and prosthesis

- Valve preservation techniques are increasingly undertaken to restore a haemodynamically efficient valve that avoids the need for anticoagulation and has a low risk of future thromboembolism, infective endocarditis, and reoperation.
- Bioprostheses include xenografts (stented or stentless), homografts, and autografts. These valves do not require anticoagulation in the absence of other indications but are susceptible to structural valve deterioration especially in younger patients.
- Mechanical valves include ball and cage valves, single tilting disc, and bileaflet prostheses. All require long-term anticoagulation, may be haemodynamically inefficient but provide durability.
- There is no difference in survival between patients receiving mechanical and bioprosthetic valves when age and risk factors are taken into account (Lund and Bland 2006).
- Decisions about prosthesis selection in individual patients must take into account the age and wishes of the patient, the risk of anticoagulation, and the likely risks of re-do valve surgery due to structural valve deterioration.
- Bioprosthetic valves are usually offered to elderly people (>65 years) or those with limited life expectancy, patients with contraindications to anticoagulation, and young women contemplating pregnancy.
- Mechanical valves are usually offered to younger patients (<65 years), those with other mechanical valves or indications for anticoagulation, and those in whom re-do surgery would be high risk.

Aortic valve surgery

Surgery is undertaken through a median sternotomy, which may be partial for minimally invasive techniques.

Operative mortality for isolated aortic valve replacement (AVR) is 1–5% but the majority of patients have other cardiac lesions, most commonly coronary artery disease (CAD), with the mortality of 6–7% for AVR and coronary artery bypass grafting (CABG). When there is an aneurysm of the proximal aorta, surgery also comprises replacement of the root and/or ascending aorta. In young patients with aortic stenosis, pulmonary valve autotransplantation (Ross procedure) may be considered to allow for growth of the autograft but this is a complex procedure that may necessitate future re-do surgery on the implanted pulmonary homograft. There are no data that clearly show long-term advantage of one type of aortic valve operation over another or for any individual prosthesis over another in patients with aortic valve disease.

Aortic stenosis

In patients with symptomatic aortic stenosis, there is a striking mortality benefit from AVR compared with conservative treatment (Schwartz *et al.* 1982). In asymptomatic severe aortic stenosis, surgery is justifiable in high-risk individuals (Vahanian *et al.* 2007). High-risk markers include the presence of left ventricular (LV) dysfunction (ejection fraction (EF) <50%) unless due to another cause, an abnormal exercise test with symptoms, fall in blood pressure, or complex ventricular arrhythmias, excessive LV hypertrophy (>15 mm) unless this is due to hypertension, and moderate-to-severe valve calcification and a rate of peak velocity progression of >0.3 m/second. In patients undergoing CABG or other cardiac operations, concomitant AVR is advisable in the presence of moderate (valve area 1.0–1.5 cm^2) and severe aortic stenosis (Vahanian *et al.* 2007). Decisions are difficult when low gradient (<40 mmHg) aortic stenosis is associated with LV dysfunction but AVR can be justified in the presence of preserved contractile reserve manifest by an increase in EF of >20% during dobutamine infusion (Monin *et al.* 2003). Age is not a contraindication to surgery in aortic stenosis and good results have been described in patients in their eighties and nineties, especially in the absence of other co-morbidites. In patients who are at high risk for conventional surgery, other techniques may be considered including transcatheter aortic valve implantation (TAVI) (see Chapter 7.10) or implantation of an LV to the descending aorta valve conduit.

Aortic regurgitation

In acute aortic regurgitation, urgent surgery is indicated. In chronic severe aortic regurgitation, timing of surgery is determined by the presence or absence of symptoms, assessment of LV size and function and the dimensions of the aortic root and ascending aorta (Vahanian *et al.* 2007). Surgery is indicated once symptoms develop but also in asymptomatic individuals when there is resting LV dysfunction (EF <50%) and/or LV dilatation (LV end-diastolic diameter >70 mm or end-systolic diameter >50 mm). Mild and moderate aortic regurgitation may be associated with dilatation of the aortic root and ascending aorta. Under these circumstances the appropriateness and timing of surgery is usually governed by aortic dimensions. In aortic dilatation, the threshold for surgical intervention is lower in patients with Marfan's syndrome (>45 mm) and with bicuspid aortic valves (>50 mm) than in others (>55 mm) and in those with rapid expansion (>5 mm/year) and with a family history of dissection (Vahanian *et al.* 2007).

Mitral valve surgery

Conventional mitral valve (MV) surgery is performed through a median sternotomy while minimally invasive techniques including thoracoscopic video- and robotic-assisted MV surgery are undertaken through smaller thoracotomy access. There is an increasing trend towards valve-conserving operations, with valve replacement only undertaken when repair cannot effectively be achieved.

Mitral repair

Mitral repair is increasingly the operation of choice for patients with mitral regurgitation (MR) secondary to degenerative valve disease and ischaemic heart disease and carries a mortality risk of 1.5–2%. This is a complex procedure that requires considerable expertise to achieve good results and comprises a combination of elements, including resection of unsupported leaflet structures, transfer of chordae, or insertion of artificial chordae to support unstable areas as well as stabilization of the size and shape of the mitral annulus using the implantation of an artificial ring. Mitral repair reduces the risk of surgery for MR and improves long-term outcome as compared with mitral valve replacement (MVR). Successful repair obviates the need for anticoagulation for those in sinus rhythm and reduces the risk of future thromboembolism, infective endocarditis, and LV dysfunction.

Mitral valve replacement

MVR is the operation of choice for patients with rheumatic valve disease where pathological changes often affect the subvalvar apparatus as well as the valve leaflets. MVR may also be necessary in patients with complex degenerative mitral valve disease that is not suitable for repair and carries a mortality risk of 5.4–6.4%. Mechanical or bioprostheses may be implanted (see p. 312). Retention of the subvalvar apparatus helps preserve left ventricular function and improves long-term results.

Mitral regurgitation

In patients with severe, symptomatic organic MR, early surgical correction is indicated (Vahanian et al. 2007). Even in the presence of heart failure and left ventricular dysfunction contraindications are rare when MR is severe. In the absence of symptoms, surgery is recommended in severe organic MR when there is evidence of LV dysfunction (EF <60% and/or LV end diastolic dimension >45 mm), atrial fibrillation, or pulmonary hypertension (Vahanian et al. 2007; Bonow et al. 2006). Given the excellent long-term results of successful mitral valve repair, surgery may be considered in patients with severe MR and suitable pathology even in the absence of symptoms and with preserved LV function provided the operation is undertaken at low risk by an expert (Vahanian et al. 2007; Enriquez-Sarano et al. 2009). In patients undergoing CABG, MR should be corrected when it is moderate or severe (Vahanian et al. 2007).

Mitral stenosis

MVR should be considered in symptomatic patients with significant mitral stenosis (MS; valve area <1.5 cm²) in whom percutaneous mitral commissurotomy is contraindicated (Vahanian et al. 2007). In asymptomatic patients, surgery is not usually recommended. Stress testing may be helpful in defining impaired functional capacity that may lead to consideration of earlier surgical intervention. especially when pulmonary hypertension (systolic pulmonary pressure >50 mmHg) is present.

Tricuspid valve disease

Isolated tricuspid valve (TV) surgery for organic TV disease is rare and usually necessitates valve replacement when leaflet anatomy is severely abnormal (Vahanian et al. 2007). TV surgery is most commonly undertaken, however, to correct tricuspid regurgitation (TR) at the time of left-sided valve surgery in the presence or absence of pulmonary hypertension. Tricuspid annuloplasty with implantation of a rigid prosthetic ring gives superior results to suture annuloplasty. Persistent TR after MVR is associated with functional impairment and reoperation is associated with high risk so that the detection and correction of TR at the time of initial surgery is recommended (Groves et al. 1991). Annuloplasty should be considered when functional TR is severe and when moderate TR is associated with a dilated tricuspid annulus (> 40 mm) (Vahanian et al. 2007).

Late complications after valve surgery

Late complications after valve surgery include structural valve deterioration, non-structural dysfunction (including inappropriate sizing and tissue in-growth around the valve), valve thrombosis or embolism, bleeding, and operated valvular endocarditis (Groves 2001). Valvular dysfunction may present with a variety of symptoms including dyspnoea, fatigue, and angina and may lead to haemolysis, sudden death, or need for reoperation. To avoid and detect these complications, careful clinical surveillance is required with optimal management of anticoagulation (see Chapter 7.11) and precautions against infective endocarditis (see Chapter 7.12) mandatory.

References

Bonow RO, Carbello BA, Kanu C, et al. ACC/AHA 2006 guidelines for the management of patients with valvular heart disease: a report of the American College of Cardiology/American Heart Association Task Force on Practice Guidelines (writing committee to revise the 1998 Guidelines for the Management of Patients with Valvular Heart Disease): developed in collaboration with the Society of Cardiovascular Anaesthesiologists: endorsed by the Society for Cardiovascular Angiography and Interventions and the Society of Thoracic Surgeons. *Circulation* 2006;**114**.e84–231.

Enriquez-Sarano M, Akins CW, Vahanian A. Mitral regurgitation. *Lancet* 2009;**373**:1382–94.

Groves PH, Lewis NP, Ikram S, et al. Reduced exercise capacity in patients with tricuspid regurgitation after successful mitral valve replacement for rheumatic mitral valve disease. *Br Heart J* 1991;**66**:295–301.

Groves PH. Surgery of valve disease: late results and late complications. *Heart* 2001;**86**:715–21.

Lund O, Bland M. Age and risk corrected impact of mechanical versus biological valves on long-term mortality after aortic valve replacement. *J Thorac Cardiovasc Surg* 2006;**132**:20–6.

Monin JL, Quere JP, Monchi M, et al. Low gradient aortic stenosis: operative risk stratification and predictors for long-term outcome—a multicenter study using dobutamine stress hemodynamics. *Circulation* 2003;**108**:319–24.

Roques F, Nashef SAM, Michel P. The EuroSCORE Study Group. Risk factors for early mortality after valve surgery in Europe in the 1990s: lessons from the EuroSCORE pilot program. *J Heart Valve Dis* 2001;**10**:572–8.

Schwartz F, Baumann P, Manthey J, et al. The effect of aortic valve replacement on survival. *Circulation* 1982;**66**:1105–10.

Vahanian A, Baumgartner H, Bax J, et al. Guidelines on the management of valvular heart disease: the Task Force on the Management of Valvular Heart Disease of the European Society of Cardiology. *Eur Heart J* 2007;**28**:230–68.

Percutaneous intervention

The last decade has seen substantial progress in the development of percutaneous therapies for structural heart disease.

Transcatheter aortic valve implantation

Many patients who could benefit from aortic valve replacement are treated conservatively because of their high operative risk. Balloon valvuloplasty does not provide sustained clinical benefit or improve survival and is only considered as a bridge to surgery in selected cases. The introduction of transcatheter aortic valve implantation (TAVI), however, will alter our threshold for intervention.

Procedure

Currently two devices, the Edwards SAPIEN valve (Edwards Life Sciences, Irving, CA) and Corevalve (Medtronic, Minneapolis, MN) have the CE mark and are the subject of clinical trials. Other devices have early human data or are in preclinical investigation.

The Edwards SAPIEN device is a bovine pericardial valve mounted inside a balloon expandable stainless steel stent (length, 16 mm; diameter, 23/26 mm). Implantation is performed under general anaesthesia. A retrograde approach, via femoral artery cut down, is preferred as it avoids transseptal puncture and potential damage to the anterior mitral valve. The calcified valve is pre-dilated and the device delivered using a steerable catheter (22/24F). Fluoroscopy, aortography, and transoesophageal echocardiography (TOE) are used to assess position. Left ventricular flow is then briefly arrested by rapidly pacing the right ventricle (200 bpm) and the device is deployed. A transapical approach, via an anterolateral thoracotomy, can be considered for individuals with poor peripheral access.

Corevalve is a trileaflet porcine pericardial valve mounted inside a self-expandable nitinol stent (length, 50 mm; maximum diameter, 22/26 mm). The stent is considerably longer than the Edwards device and is shaped to sit in the aortic root, with the lower portion providing the tensile strength to displace the calcified valve. Importantly, the current device and delivery system are 18F, avoiding the need for surgical cut down or formal vascular repair. In addition the procedure can be performed without right ventricular pacing.

Indications and patient selection

At present, TAVI is limited to patients with critical aortic stenosis who are deemed inoperable or at high surgical risk. Life expectancy, symptomatology, and co-morbidity influence individual suitability and assessment by a multidisciplinary team is fundamental. TOE or computerized tomography should be used to assess the aortic root and annular dimensions. Detailed imaging of the iliofemoral vessels is also recommended. Percutaneous coronary intervention is feasible after TAVI, but again management should be individualized.

Follow-up and complications

Initially, TAVI was associated with high procedural mortality (>25%). Device malposition led to embolization, mitral valve damage, or coronary obstruction. Paravalvular leaks were frequent though reduced by oversizing the device. As with surgery, heart block requiring permanent pacemaker implantation may occur. Operator experience, avoidance of antegrade delivery, and lower profile systems have improved results. Peripheral vascular occlusion or perforation remains a concern but less so with the lower profile Corevalve system. Patient–prosthesis mismatch in the long-term is a theoretical possibility. In a high-risk population, procedural success with the Edwards SAPIEN valve is reported at 86% with 30-day all-cause mortality at 12% (Webb et al. 2007). The trans-apical approach has comparable results but fewer strokes or arterial injuries. Similarly, Corevalve has an acute success rate of 88% with 30-day mortality at 12% (Grube et al. 2007). 'Valve in valve' implantation and deployment into a degenerated bioprosthesis have been performed with Corevalve. Improvement in left ventricular function following TAVI has been shown, with valve function and clinical benefit demonstrated to 3 years. Randomization against conventional surgery in symptomatic patients (≥NYHA Class II) with critical aortic stenosis (mean gradient ≥40 mmHg, velocity ≥4.0 m/second or valve area ≤0.8 cm^2) and annulus size 16–24 mm is the subject of the PARTNER trial due to report in 2014.

Percutaneous balloon mitral valvuloplasty

Percutaneous balloon mitral valvuloplasty (PBMV) is well established as the preferred treatment for symptomatic patients with moderate–severely stenosed mitral valves.

Procedure

Right heart catheterization is performed under sedation or general anaesthesia from a femoral approach. Trans-septal puncture is carried out using a standard Brockenbrough technique often with TOE guidance. Heparin is administered. A coiled tip guidewire is passed into the left atrium over which the Inoue catheter (Toray, Tokyo, Japan) is advanced, looped, and passively passed into the left ventricle. The Inoue catheter is 12F and consists of a polyvinylchloride balloon with coaxial lumen. The distal portion of the balloon is inflated and pulled back until resistance against the mitral valve is felt. Subsequently the proximal portion inflates causing the less compliant middle waist to dilate the stenosed valve. If the atrioventricular pressure gradient fails to fall, the balloon size is increased by 1-mm increments until it does or mitral regurgitation worsens. Success depends on appropriate balloon selection, best quantified by direct echocardiographic measurement of the mitral annulus during mid to end-systole.

An alternative approach is a double-balloon technique, using a multitrack catheter. Although more technically demanding, this approach splits the commissures with less stress to the leaflets. However, equivalent efficacy is achieved with the Inoue balloon and without the risk of perforating the left ventricular apex.

Indications and patient selection

PBMV should be considered for patients with symptomatic moderate or severe mitral stenosis (valve area ≤1.5 cm^2). Anatomic suitability is determined by echocardiography and qualified by the Wilkins score (Table 7.10.1). A valve scoring 8 or 9 is most suitable.

Contraindications include severe mitral regurgitation, left atrial (appendage) thrombus, major or bicommissural calcification and severe coexistent aortic or tricuspid valve disease or coronary artery disease requiring surgery. In asymptomatic patients, PBMV may be considered if there is a high embolic risk such as atrial fibrillation, pulmonary

Table 7.10.1 Wilkins score

Grade	1	2	3	4
Leaflet mobility	Tips restricted	Normal mid and basal leaflet	Valve moves forward in diastole	No forward movement in diastole
Leaflet thickness	Near normal (4–5 mm)	Thickened margins (5–8 mm)	Thickening of entire leaflets (5–8 mm)	Marked thickening (8–10 mm)
Valve calcification	Single area of echo brightness	Scattered brightness at margins	Brightness extends to mid leaflet	Brightness throughout leaflet
Subvalvular apparatus	Minimal thickening	Thickened chords (proximal)	Thickened chords (distal)	Thickening extends to papillary muscles

hypertension, or pregnancy. Exercise testing should be utilized to unmask subclinical disease.

Follow-up and complications
Successful PBMV can double the mitral valve area and improve symptoms. Age >50 years, previous commissurotomy and pre-existing regurgitation predict poor immediate outcome, which is itself the best indicator for long-term prognosis. Freedom from severe symptoms or reintervention is around 90% at 5 years and 70% at 10 years (Nobuyoshi et al. 2009). When severe mitral regurgitation complicates PBMV, the outlook is poor and surgery should be considered. In pregnancy, PBMV is safe if performed after the first trimester by experienced operators with minimum radiation exposure. Trans-septal puncture creates an iatrogenic left-to-right shunt, which is rarely haemodynamically significant but may persist for several years. Haemopericardium due to perforation by the Brockenbrough needle, guidewire or Inoue catheter occurs in less than 2%. Thromboembolism remains a risk despite screening with TOE. Severe mitral regurgitation has an incidence of 1–9% (Nobuyoshi et al. 2009).

Percutaneous mitral valve repair

Surgical repair is currently the treatment of choice for severe degenerative mitral regurgitation. The complex anatomy of the valve requires a wide-ranging approach that usually includes annuloplasty as well as various leaflet and chordal repair techniques. Trans-catheter technology aims to emulate surgical strategies with several devices now subject to clinical trials.

Procedure: leaflet repair
The MitraClip (Evalve, Menlo Park, CA) is a percutaneous device that mimics the double orifice repair described by Alfieri. It is delivered via a trans-septal approach using a 24F steerable catheter. Once in the left atrium, it is aligned perpendicular to the coaptation point of the mitral valve and advanced across it. In the left ventricle, the clip is opened, pulled back so as to grasp the edges of the anterior and posterior leaflets and closed. The procedure is performed with TOE guidance. The clip can be repositioned provided final deployment has not occurred. MitraClip has European regulatory approval but remains investigational in the United States.

Procedure: annuloplasty
Placement of devices in the coronary sinus has been a popular approach to percutaneous annuloplasty, on account of the technical ease, but with little evidence of clinical benefit to date. Performed via a transjugular or subclavian approach under fluoroscopic guidance, the aim is to manipulate the geometry of the posterior mitral annulus and reduce functional mitral regurgitation. The course of the circumflex coronary artery should be identified, either by contrast injection or computerized tomography, prior to device deployment. A variety of devices including Carillon (Cardiac Dimensions, Kirkland, WA), Monarc (Edwards Life Sciences, Irving, CA), and Viacor (Viacor, Wilmington, MA) have been tested clinically. Direct annuloplasty via a retrograde approach from the left ventricle has also been tested. Early human feasibility has been shown with the Mitralign system (Mitralign, Tewksbury, MA), which uses sutures to cause annular cinching. The QuantumCor device (QuantumCor, Bothell, WA) utilizes radiofrequency to pursue a similar outcome remains experimental.

Indications and patient selection
The MitraClip is designed for patients with a conventional clinical indication for mitral valve repair: at least moderate mitral regurgitation with symptoms and with left ventricular dysfunction if asymptomatic. In addition, the mitral valve leaflets must have a coaptation length ≥2 mm and the regurgitant jet must originate from the central two-thirds of the valve orifice. Typically, therefore, patients with mitral valve prolapse or functional regurgitation with normal leaflets prove most suitable. Annuloplasty techniques are also aimed at patients with normal valve leaflets and functional mitral regurgitation that is not ischaemic in origin.

Follow-up and complications
The EVEREST-I study reported successful implantation of the MitraClip in 88% of patients. Safety and feasibility were shown with no major complications at the time of implantation and a 30-day adverse event rate of 7–9% (Feldman et al. 2005). Mitral stenosis was not reported. A significant reduction in mitral regurgitation was achieved in most with an average hospital stay of less than two nights. The placement of a clip did not influence subsequent surgery. The MitraClip is now subject to randomization against conventional surgery in the EVEREST-II trial. Enrolment has completed and the study will report in 2015. The annuloplasty devices are at various stages of investigation. Safety and feasibility of the Carillon device was demonstrated in the multicentred AMADEUS study and led to subsequent European regulatory approval. Clinical outcomes and quality of life will be the subject of the forthcoming TITAN trial. The main concern with coronary sinus devices is the proximity of the circumflex artery with myocardial infarction a reported complication.

Trans-catheter pulmonary valve implantation

Trans-catheter pulmonary valve implantation (TPVI) extends the life of dysfunctional right ventricular to pulmonary artery conduits in patients with repaired congenital heart disease, reducing the need for reoperation. The commercially available device (Melody, Medtronic. Minneapolis, MN) has regulatory approval in Europe and Canada and is the subject of a feasibility study in the United States.

Procedure

Melody is a bovine jugular venous valve mounted inside a balloon expandable platinum–iridium stent. Implantation is performed under general anaesthesia, via a right femoral venous approach. Right heart pressure assessment and biplane angiography are used to determine the anatomy and haemodynamics of the implantation site. The device is hand-loaded onto the balloon-in-balloon delivery system (24 French) and advanced over a stiff guidewire under fluoroscopy. When in position, the valve is uncovered; contrast is injected to confirm position; and the inner balloon inflated to partially deploy the device. The outer balloon is then inflated to complete deployment. In heavily stenosed conduits, pre-dilatation with a high-pressure balloon and placement of a bare stent may improve outcome.

Indications and patient selection

Indications include significant pulmonary regurgitation and/or stenosis associated with symptoms, exercise impairment, right ventricular dysfunction, or arrhythmia. Underlying conditions include tetralogy of Fallot, Rastelli repair, Ross operation, or conduit placement for common arterial trunk. Occasionally dysfunctional native outflow tracts, such as after the arterial switch, may be treated. Assessment should be carried out in a centre experienced in managing congenital heart disease and should include exercise testing, echocardiography, and magnetic resonance. Melody is only suitable for outflow tracts between 16 and 22 mm in diameter. The Edwards SAPIEN valve has been suggested for slightly larger outflow tracts but experience is limited. This will be the subject of the COMPASSION Trial, which is expected to complete in 2013.

Follow-up and complications

TPVI is minimally invasive and provides an alternative to repeat open-heart surgery. It improves symptoms and cardiopulmonary exercise capacity, reduces right ventricular size, and increases resting cardiac output. Procedural mortality and morbidity are similar to surgery (around 1–2%) with specific complications of conduit rupture, coronary artery compression, and device instability (Lurz et al. 2008). Long-term valve competency appears excellent though longevity remains unknown due to limited follow-up. Stent fractures occur in approximately 20% though most are clinically silent. Stringent X-ray follow-up permits early detection and expectant management with repeat percutaneous intervention where appropriate.

References

Feldman T, Wasserman HS, Herrmann HC, et al. Percutaneous mitral valve repair using the edge-to-edge technique: Six-month results of the EVEREST phase I clinical trial. *J Am Coll Cardiol* 2005;**46**:2134–40.

Grube E, Schuler G, Buellesfeld L, et al. Percutaneous aortic valve replacement for severe aortic stenosis in high-risk patients using the second- and current third-generation self-expanding CoreValve prosthesis: device success and 30-day clinical outcome. *J Am Coll Cardiol* 2007;**50**:69–76.

Lurz P, Coats L, Khambadkone S, et al. Percutaneous pulmonary valve implantation: impact of evolving technology and learning curve on clinical outcome. *Circulation* 2008;**117**:1964–72.

Nobuyoshi M, Arita T, Shirai S, et al. Percutaneous Balloon Mitral Valvuloplasty: A Review. *Circulation* 2009;**119**:e211–9.

Webb JG, Pasupati S, Humphries K, et al. Percutaneous transarterial aortic valve replacement in selected high-risk patients with aortic stenosis. *Circulation* 2007;**116**:755–63.

Antithrombotic therapy for valvular diseases

Thrombosis, embolism, and bleeding remain significant issues in the management of patients with valvular heart disease, particularly after valve replacement.

Three important factors that contribute to the pathogenesis of thromboembolism are abnormal surface of the valve (or vascular wall), abnormal regional blood flow, and abnormal constituents of the blood (Virchow's triad).

In clinical practice, a lot of thrombogenic risk factors should be taken into consideration when planning antithrombotic therapy:

- increasing age
- past history of thromboembolism
- nature of the valvular lesion (e.g. rheumatic mitral stenosis is the most thrombogenic lesion)
- type, design, and location of the prosthetic valve (e.g. a ball and cage valve in the mitral position is more thrombogenic than others)
- co-existing cardiac pathology (e.g. atrial fibrillation, heart failure, enlarged left atrium)
- co-existing non-cardiac diseases (e.g. hypertension, diabetes mellitus, hyperlipidaemia, malignancy, deranged coagulation, liver failure)
- others, e.g. smoking, contraceptives.

Antithrombotic agents

Anticoagulant agents

Warfarin

Wafarin has been the most commonly used oral anticoagulant since it was first introduced nearly 60 years ago. Its anticoagulation effects result from inhibiting vitamin K-dependent production of clotting factors II, VII, IX and X, and proteins C and S.

Warfarin is not fully effective in the first few days of its administration and rapid induction of anticoagulation with high loading doses should be avoided. In patients with high thromboembolic risk, immediately acting anticoagulants (e.g. heparin, fondaparinux, or thrombin inhibitors) should be used until warfarin therapy has achieved its desired anticoagulant effect.

Warfarin should not be given to patients with active bleeding, active peptic ulceration, known coagulation defects, thrombocytopenia, recent haemorrhagic stroke, or to those unable to comply with appropriate international normalized ratio (INR) monitoring. However, all contraindications are relative to thrombotic risk.

Warfarin should be withheld for 4–6 weeks in patients with non-cerebral haemorrhagic events, but longer in those with cerebral haemorrhagic events.

Heparin

Heparin has a rapid onset of action. Its anticoagulation effect is mediated by antithrombin III activation, leading to deactivation of clotting factors Xa and IIa. Unfractionated heparin has variable anticoagulation effects due to variable absorption and pharmacokinetics. Low-molecular-weight heparin has superior absorption and more consistent and predictable effects.

Heparin should not be used in patients with major bleeding within the previous 2 weeks, with heparin-induced thrombocytopenia, or with renal failure.

Fondaparinux

Fondaparinux is a synthetic compound composed of the essential pentasaccharide sequence; it mediates its effects indirectly through antithrombin III. Fondaparinux is not recommended for patients with reduced platelet count, with renal dysfunction, with obesity, or weighing less than 50 kg. It should not be used in patients receiving dialysis and is relatively contraindicated in patients with a creatinine clearance less than 30 mL/min. Fondaparinux reduces the risk of ischaemic events in coronary artery disease but whether it is a suitable anticoagulant for valvular disease has not been validated.

Direct thrombin inhibitors

The direct thrombin inhibitors inhibit both free and fibrinbound thrombin and have predictable anticoagulation effects. This class includes hirudin, bivalirudin, argatroban, and the more recently developed lepirudin, melagatran, ximelagtran, and dabigatran. The clinical efficacy of this class in valvular heart disease has yet to be validated.

Antiplatelet drugs

Aspirin

Aspirin (acetylsalicylic acid) inhibits the production of thromboxane A2 by inactivating cyclooxygenase-1, leading to diminished platelet aggregation and vasoconstriction. The effect of platelet inhibition occurs within the hour of aspirin ingestion but enteric coating delays its effect.

Clopidogrel

Clopidogrel inhibits platelet aggregation by irreversibly modifying the platelet adenosine diphosphate (ADP) receptor and blocking the pro-aggregatory effects of ADP.

Both aspirin and clopidogrel provide permanent antiplatelet effects which last for the duration of the platelet lifespan, normally 7 days.

Dipyridamole

Dipyridamole inhibits platelet aggregation by multiple mechanisms. Its effect is short lasting, probably for 24 hours only.

Glycoprotein IIb/IIIa antagonists

The primary mechanism of glycoprotein (GP) IIb/IIIa antagonists is inhibition of the final common pathway of platelet aggregation: fibrinogen or von Willebrand factor binding to the GP IIb/IIIa complex. They are mainly used in the setting of coronary interventions. They can be given intravenously (e.g. abciximab, tirofiban, and eptifibatide) or orally (e.g. xemilofiban, orbofiban, sibrafiban, and lotrafiban). Their efficacy and safety have yet to be fully validated in valvular heart disease.

Antithrombotic therapy

Antithrombotic therapy is indicated in all patients with valvular heart diseases if they have one or more thromboembolic risk factors, such as atrial fibrillation, left atrial dilatation with or without spontaneous contrast, intracardiac thrombus, dilated left ventricle with poor systolic function, recurrent transient ischaemic attacks (TIAs), or prior ischaemic stroke.

Anticoagulation therapy with warfarin is monitored by the INR, which is calculated by dividing the patient's prothrombin time (PT) by the mean normal PT. The INR should be measured at least 16 hours after the dose of warfarin. Steady-state INR values are not reached for up to 3 weeks following a dose adjustment.

The efficacy of heparin therapy is monitored by the activated partial thromboplastin time (aPTT), with the therapeutic level being twice the normal control value.

Native valve diseases

Rheumatic mitral valve disease

In rheumatic mitral valve disease, particularly mitral stenosis, even in the absence of any thromboembolic risk, warfarin is recommended and the INR maintained at 2.5 (2.0–3.0). If embolic events have occurred or if left atrial thrombus has developed, aspirin should be added to warfarin. On the other hand, if the patient is in sinus rhythm and the left atrium is normal in size, aspirin alone may suffice.

Mitral valve prolapse

Mitral valve prolapse alone dose not require antithrombotic therapy. But in the presence of suspected TIA, aspirin is recommended. If there are recurrent TIAs despite aspirin therapy, warfarin is recommended maintaining the INR at 2.5 (2.0–3.0).

Mitral valve or annulus calcification

Aspirin is recommended in the absence of previous TIA or ischaemic stroke. If the patient is in AF or has had a previous ischaemic stroke or recurrent TIAs, warfarin should be prescribed with the INR maintained at 2.5 (2.0–3.0).

Aortic valve calcification

No antithrombotic therapy is needed. But aspirin should be prescribed if the patient suffers from TIA or ischaemic stroke and no other related causes are identified.

Percutaneous valvuloplasty

In mitral stenosis, antithrombotic therapy is required, using warfarin before and after the procedure, and heparin during the procedure.

In aortic stenosis, heparin should be given during the procedure but no other antithrombotic therapy is needed before or after the procedure, unless other thromboembolic risks are present.

Surgical mitral valve repair

Warfarin should be given for up to 3 months after mitral valve repair in the absence of thromoembolic risks.

Bioprosthetic valves

In patients with bioprosthetic valves, long-term antiplatelet therapy is recommended if they are in sinus rhythm and do not have any other thromoembolic risk factors. In this patient group, some guidelines recommend warfarin therapy for the first 3 months postoperatively (INR 2.5), particularly for mitral bioprostheses. If there are associated thromoembolic risk factors, lifelong anticoagulation therapy with warfarin should be considered (INR 2.5).

Mechanical valves

Patients with mechanical valves require lifelong antithrombotic therapy with warfarin. Immediately after the mechanical valve replacement, heparin is given until a stable INR has been maintained for 2 days. Thereafter, warfarin is continued and the target INR maintained at a level determined by the design and position of the valve:
- INR 2.0–3.0 for a bileaflet or tilting disk valve in the aortic position;
- INR 2.5–3.5 for a bileaflet or tilting disk valve in the mitral position;
- INR 2.5–3.5 for a caged ball or caged disk valve regardless of position;
- INR 2.5–3.5 for all those with thromboembolic risk factors regardless of valve design or position.

A higher target INR level should be achieved if patients suffer from systemic embolism despite a previous therapeutic INR. Alternatively, aspirin could be added to the warfarin therapy.

Special patient groups

Minor non-cardiac procedures

For minor non-cardiac operations including dental procedures, arthrocentesis, cataract surgery, or diagnostic endoscopy, most patients do not require any changes to their ongoing anticoagulation therapy. However, it is advisable to adjust the INR to 1.5–2.0.

Major non-cardiac procedures

For major non-cardiac procedures, anticoagulation therapy should be discontinued a few days before the operation, and, instead, a therapeutic dose of intravenous heparin given. Effective anticoagulation should be resumed as soon as possible after the operation.

Cardiac catheterization or percutaneous cardiac procedures

For cardiac catheterization or percutaneous cardiac procedures, anticoagulation therapy should be modified to an INR <2.0. A radial artery approach will allow a higher INR.

Pregnant women

For pregnant women with prosthetic valves, adequate antithrombotic therapy is important as there is an increased incidence of thromboembolism. Warfarin increases miscarriage, embryopathy, and fetal death. Therefore, it should be replaced with subcutaneous heparin twice daily until delivery. Aspirin can be added to warfarin in women with a high risk of thromboembolism.

References/further reading

Bates SM, Weitz JI. New anticoagulants: beyond heparin, low-molecular-weight heparin and warfarin. *Br J Pharmacol* 2005;**144**:1017–28.

Bonow RO, Carabello BA, Chatterjee K, *et al.* American College of Cardiology/American Heart Association Task Force on Practice Guidelines. 2008 focused update incorporated into the ACC/AHA 2006 guidelines for the management of patients with valvular heart disease: a report of the American College of Cardiology/American Heart Association Task Force on Practice Guidelines (Writing Committee to revise the 1998 guidelines for the management of patients with valvular heart disease). Endorsed by the Society of Cardiovascular Anesthesiologists, Society for Cardiovascular Angiography and Interventions, and Society of Thoracic Surgeons. *J Am Coll Cardiol.* 2008;**52**:e1–142.

Busuttil WJ, Fabri BM. The management of anticoagulation in patients with prosthetic heart valves undergoing non-cardiac operations. *Postgrad Med J* 1995; **71**:390–2.

Dunn AS, Turpie AG. Perioperative management of patients receiving oral anticoagulants: a systematic review. *Arch Intern Med* 2003;**163**:901–8.

Goldsmith I, Turpie AG, Lip GY. Valvar heart disease and prosthetic heart valves. *BMJ* 2002;**325**:1228–31.

Hirsh J. *Antithrombotic and thrombolytic therapy: American College of Chest Physicians Evidence-Based Clinical Practice Guidelines,* 8th edn. Hamilton: BC Decker, 2008: pp. 1–149.

Toohey M. Clinical experience with warfarin sodium. *Br Med J* 1958; **2**: 892–93.

Vahanian A, Baumgartner H, Bax J, *et al.,* Task Force on the Management of Valvular Heart Disease of the European Society of Cardiology; ESC Committee for Practice Guidelines. Guidelines on the management of valvular heart disease: The Task Force on the Management of Valvular Heart Disease of the European Society of Cardiology. *Eur Heart J* 2007;**28**:230–68.

Website

http://www.icsi.org/antithrombotic_therapy_supplement_guideline_14045/antithrombotic_therapy_supplement__guideline_.html

Antibiotic prophylaxis in valvular heart disease

Antibiotic prophylaxis to prevent infective endocarditis (IE) in patients with high-risk cardiac lesions undergoing invasive procedures has been a tenet of cardiac and dental practice for over half a century. However, the evidence in its favour is limited.

Many cases of IE now arise in those without known pre-existing valvular heart disease, often with no clear preceding invasive medical or dental procedure. *Staphylococcus aureus* is the most common organism (frequently a hospital-acquired infection or secondary to intravenous drug use), with fewer cases due to oral streptococci.

The lack of evidence to support antibiotic prophylaxis and changing clinical profile of IE, coupled with increasing concerns relating to antibiotic-induced anaphylaxis and antimicrobial resistance, has led international organizations including the National Institute for Health and Clinical Excellence (NICE), the American Heart Association (AHA), and the European Society of Cardiology (ESC) to significantly update their guidelines in the past few years.

A careful approach is required in explaining these changes to patients, many of whom have taken antibiotic prophylaxis for years and have previously been warned of the dangers of IE.

The lack of evidence
- Traditional practice based on three-part theory:
  1 valvular disease + bacteraemia can lead to IE
  2 invasive procedures can lead to bacteraemia
  3 in animal models, antibiotic prophylaxis reduces risk of IE.
- Relevance of animal models to humans is questionable.
- Benefit of antibiotic prophylaxis never shown in randomized trials.
- Surgical repair is currently the treatment of half of cases of IE are in patients without previously documented valvular disease.
- Chewing and tooth brushing cause transient bacteraemia with a cumulative annual exposure 10^3–10^6 times greater than single tooth extraction.
- Direct link between dental work and IE never proven, although many anecdotal cases.
- The Cochrane Review (Oliver *et al.* 2004) concluded no evidence supporting penicillin prophylaxis.

American Heart Association Guidelines (2007) (Table 7.12.1)
- Antibiotic prophylaxis only for patients with high-risk cardiac disorders.
- No longer indicated for native valve disease.
- No longer indicated for any gastrointestinal or genitourinary procedures.

Table 7.12.1 AHA Guidelines (2007)

High-risk patients	Previous IE
	Prosthetic valve
	Unrepaired or incompletely repaired cyanotic congenital heart disease
	Congenital heart disease repaired with prosthetic material (for 6 months after the procedure)
	Valve disease in cardiac transplant recipients
Procedures requiring prophylaxis	Dental procedures involving manipulation of gingival tissue, the periapical region of teeth, or perforation of the oral mucosa
	Invasive procedures of the respiratory tract needing incision or biopsy of the mucosa

National Institute for Health and Clinical Excellence Guidelines (2008) (Table 7.12.2)
- Suggest an end to antibiotic prophylaxis altogether.
- No longer indicated for dental or respiratory procedures.
- Only indicated for gastrointestinal and genitourinary procedures where there is suspicion of pre-existing infection.

European Society of Cardiology Guidelines (2009) (Table 7.12.3)
- Antibiotic prophylaxis only for those with the highest risk of IE undergoing the highest risk procedures.
- No longer indicated for native valve disease.
- No longer indicated for respiratory, gastrointestinal or genitourinary procedures.

Table 7.12.2 NICE Guidelines (2008)

High-risk patients	Previous IE
	Prosthetic valve
	Acquired valvular heart disease with stenosis or regurgitation
	Structural congenital heart disease, including surgically corrected or palliated structural conditions. Excluding: • Isolated ASD • Fully repaired VSD/PDA • Endothelialized closure devices • HOCM
Procedures requiring prophylaxis	Gastrointestinal and genitourinary procedures where there is suspected pre-existing infection

Table 7.12.3 ESC Guidelines (2009)

High-risk patients	Previous IE
	Prosthetic valve or prosthetic material used for valve repair
	Cyanotic congenital heart disease (without surgical repair or with residual defects, palliative shunts or conduits)
	Congenital heart disease repaired with prosthetic material (for six months if complete repair, indefinite if residual defect)
Procedures requiring prophylaxis	Dental procedures requiring manipulation of the gingival or periapical region of the teeth or perforation of the oral mucosa

Antibiotic regimens (Table 7.12.4)
- Single dose to be given 30–60 minutes before procedure.
- Guidelines from the AHA and ESC for prophylaxis before dental procedures (local antibiotic guidelines and guidelines for other procedures may differ).

Risks of antibiotic use
- Fatal anaphylaxis from penicillins affects ~15–25 people per million.
- Non-fatal side-effects usually minor with single-dose administration.
- Antibiotic resistance, although less likely with single doses.

Non-antibiotic prevention of infective endocarditis
- In patients with high-risk cardiac lesions, the risk of IE can be reduced by simple measures:
- Meticulous skin and dental hygiene.

Table 7.12.4 Antibiotic regimens

	Oral	Intravenous or intramuscular
Penicillin tolerant	AHA: Amoxicillin 2 g	AHA: Ampicillin 2 g or cefazolin 1 g or Ceftriaxone 1 g
	ESC: Amoxicillin 2 g or ampicillin 2 g	ESC: Amoxicillin 2 g or ampicillin 2 g
Penicillin allergic	AHA: Cefalexin* 2 g or clindamycin 600 mg or azithromycin 500 mg or clarithromycin 500 mg	AHA: Cefazolin* 1 g or ceftriaxone* 1 g or clindamycin 600 mg
	ESC: Clindamycin 600 mg	ESC: Clindamycin 600 mg

*Should not be used in patients with a history of anaphylaxis, angioedema, or urticaria with penicillins.

- Avoidance of unnecessary invasive procedures (including intravenous cannulae and urinary catheters).
- Institutional hygiene.

In patients at risk, early diagnosis is assisted by a high index of suspicion and ensuring that blood cultures are taken before antibiotic therapy is commenced in any clinical scenario where IE is suspected.

Key points
- IE remains a dangerous disease, particularly for those with high-risk cardiac lesions.
- Skin and dental hygiene are the most important preventative measures.
- Previous practice recommended antibiotic prophylaxis, but this was without robust evidence.
- New guidelines from international organizations (including NICE, AHA, and ESC) suggest a significant reduction in the practice of antibiotic prophylaxis.
- Dentists are likely to follow these guidelines as any departure could put them at medico-legal risk.
- Cardiologists may choose not to comply with the guidelines in individual cases. Here, it is important that the patient receives a clear and consistent message from all professional groups.

References
Habib G, Hoen B, Tomos P, et al. Guidelines on the prevention, diagnosis, and treatment of infective endocarditis (new version 2009): the Task Force on the Prevention, Diagnosis, and Treatment of Infective Endocarditis of the European Society of Cardiology (ESC). *European Heart Journal* 2009;**30**:2369–412.

NICE Short Clinical Guidelines Technical Team. *Prophylaxis against infective endocarditis: antimicrobial prophylaxis against infective endocarditis in adults and children undergoing interventional procedures.* London: NICE, 2008.

Oliver R, Roberts GJ, Hooper L. Penicillins for the prophylaxis of bacterial endocarditis in dentistry. *Cochrane Database Syst Rev* 2004,(2).CD003813.

Prendergast BD. The changing face of infective endocarditis. *Heart* 2006;**92**:879–85.

Roberts GJ, Jaffray EC, Spratt DA, et al. Duration, prevalence and intensity of bacteraemia after dental extractions in children. *Heart* 2006;**92**:1274–7.

Wilson W, Taubert KA, Gewitz M, et al. Prevention of Infective Endocarditis. Guidelines From the American Heart Association. A guideline from the American Heart Association Rheumatic Fever, Endocarditis, and Kawasaki Disease Committee, Council on Cardiovascular Disease in the Young, and the Council on Clinical Cardiology, Council on Cardiovascular Surgery and Anesthesia, and the Quality of Care and Outcomes Research Interdisciplinary Working Group. *Circulation* 2007;**116**:1736–54.

Chapter 8

Pulmonary vascular diseases

Primary pulmonary hypertension

Primary pulmonary hypertension (PPH) is a progressive disorder characterized by a sustained elevation of pulmonary artery pressure with pathological changes in precapillary pulmonary arteries. According to the US National Institute of Health (NIH) Registry, PPH is defined as:

- A mean pulmonary-artery pressure >25 mmHg at rest, or >30 mmHg with exertion
- In the absence of heart disease, chronic thromboembolic disease, underlying pulmonary disorder, or other secondary causes.

Since 1998, PPH has been classified as one of the causes of pulmonary arterial hypertension (PAH) by the World Health Organization (WHO) (Table 8.1.1).

Epidemiology
PPH is an uncommon condition with significant morbidity and mortality. The disease may present at any age, but most commonly at the third decade, with a female to male ratio of 1.7–3.5:1.

Table 8.1.1 WHO classification of pulmonary arterial hypertension

Pulmonary arterial hypertension
Sporadic
Familial
Related to:
• Collagen vascular disease
• Congenital systemic-to pulmonary shunts
• Portal hypertension
• HIV infection
• Drugs/toxins (appetite suppressants, toxic rapeseed oil, persistent pulmonary hypertension of the neonate

Pulmonary venous hypertension
Left-side atrial or ventricular heart disease
Left-sided valvular heart disease
Extrinsic compression of central pulmonary veins
Fibrosing mediastinitis
Adenopathy/tumours

Pulmonary hypertension associated with disorders of the respiratory system and/or hypoxaemia
Chronic obstructive pulmonary disease
Interstitial lung disease
Sleep-disordered breathing
Alveolar hypoventilation disorders
Chronic exposure to high altitude
Neonatal lung disease
Alveolar-capillary dysplasia

Pulmonary hypertension due to chronic thrombotic and/or embolic disease
Pulmonary embolism
In situ thrombus
Sickle cell disease

Pulmonary hypertension due to disorders directly affecting pulmonary vasculature
Inflammatory (schistosomiasis, sarcoidosis, other)
Pulmonary capillary haemangiomatosis

Clinical approach
Diagnosis is often delayed due to the non-specific nature of symptoms, which may overlap with those of more common diseases. PPH is a diagnosis of exclusion (Fig. 8.1.1).

History: key points
- Symptoms: shortness of breath is usually the earliest symptom. Other symptoms include fatigue, chest pain, syncope and near-syncope, ankle swelling, and palpitation
- Concomitant medical history: HIV infection, cirrhosis with portal hypertension, collagen vascular diseases, pulmonary diseases (e.g. interstitial lung disease, pulmonary embolism), and autoimmune thyroid disorders
- Drug history: use of appetite suppressants (e.g. aminorex, fenfluramine, and dexfenfluramine), illicit drugs (e.g. cocaine)
- Family history of PPH, etc.

Examination: key points
- The presence of clinical signs depends on the severity of the disorder, which are more prevalent as right heart failure develops.
- If signs suggestive of systemic disease associated with pulmonary hypertension are present, PPH may be ruled out.
- Typical signs of PPH:
  - Increased pulmonary component of second heart sound
  - Right ventricular S3 or S4 gallop
  - Tricuspid regurgitation
  - Parasternal heave.
- Signs of significant significant right ventricular decompensation:
  - Elevated jugular venous pressure with prominent 'a' (due to a non-compliant right ventricle) and 'v' waves (due to tricuspid regurgitation)
  - Hepatomegaly
  - Ascites
  - Peripheral oedema.
- Signs suggestive of secondary causes of PAH:
  - Signs of scleroderma: cutaneous telangiectasia, scelrodactyly
  - Presence of congenital heart disease: clubbing, cyanosis, tachycardia, heart murmurs
  - Concomitant lung diseases: clubbing, cyanosis, end-expiratory crackles which do not shift with cough
  - Autoimmune thyroid diseases: goitre, tremor, ocular signs (e.g. lid lag and retraction, extraocular muscle weakness), etc.

Investigations
Routine blood tests
- Laboratory investigations are non-specific
- Interpreted with the history and physical findings, relevant tests can be considered to exclude secondary causes of PAH:
  - Tests for HIV-1 antibody
  - Liver and thyroid function tests
  - Selected rheumatological screening antibodies
- It should however be noted that PPH patients may be tested positive for antinuclear antibodies of low titre without other evidence of rheumatologic disorders.

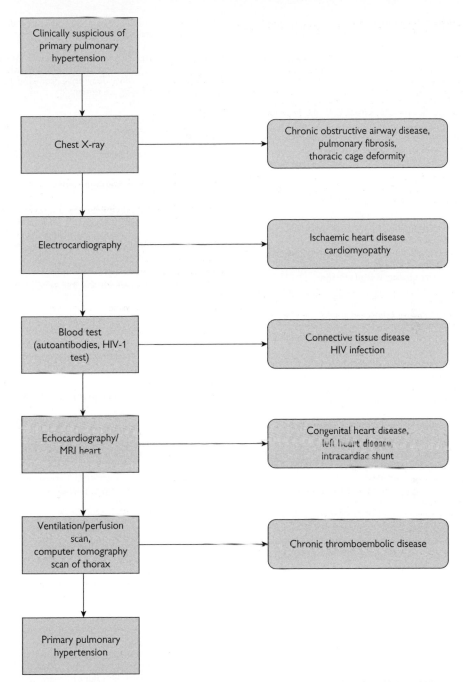

Fig. 8.1.1 Algorithm for investigation of suspected primary pulmonary hypertension. Reproduced from Gaine SP, Rubin LJ, Primary pulmonary hypertension. *Lancet* 352:719–25, copyright (1998) with permission from Elsevier.

Chest radiography
- Typical findings of pulmonary hypertension:
  - Prominent main pulmonary arteries
  - Cardiomegaly (due to right atrial and ventricular dilatation)
  - Clear lung fields.

Electrocardiography
- Right axis deviation (electrical QRS axis between +90 and +180)
- Prominent P waves (≥2.5 mm) in inferior leads
- R waves greater than S waves in lead V1
- Right-ventricular strain pattern (e.g. T wave changes).

Echocardiography
- Echocardiography is the best non-invasive test for initial screening and follow-up of PPH patients by means of assessing the following parameters:
  - Right-ventricular function and size
  - Cardiac output
  - Pulmonary artery systolic pressure (from tricuspid regurgitant jet velocity)
  - Pulmonary capillary wedge pressure.
- Valvular, congenital, and left-sided heart disease can also be detected.
- Transoesophageal echocardiography is more sensitive than that of transthoracic approach in terms of assessing intracardiac defects, e.g. patent foramen ovale, interventricular shunt.

Ventilation/perfusion lung scintigraphy
- The test provides the most reliable means of distinguishing PPH from chronic thromboembolic pulmonary hypertension, which is a major differential diagnosis of PPH
- PPH: normal or mottled patterns
- Chronic thromboembolic disease: major defects would be present.

Pulmonary function tests
- The tests are useful for the exclusion of parenchymal lung and airway disorders.
- Results are often normal but may sometimes reveal slightly reduced lung volumes and mildly to moderately reduced carbon monoxide diffusing capacity.

Arterial blood gases
- Hypoxemia with respiratory alkalosis may be detected in the presence of right-to-left shunt or ventilation–perfusion mismatch.

Right heart catheterization
- This investigation is indicated to confirm suspected PPH.
- The procedure is the most important test for assessing pulmonary hypertension as it:
  - Provides full assessment of right and left haemodynamics
  - Detects presence of shunts
  - Assesses vasoreactivity in acute drug trials (with short-acting vasodilators, e.g. nitric oxide, prostacyclin, and adenosine) which is important for patient management

- The test also has important implications on disease severity and prognosis as significant right heart failure is associated with poor survival.
- In the acute vasodilator test, short-acting titratable agents are used to minimize any possible risks and adverse effects which may arise from the tested agents. The following are tested:
  - Inhaled nitric oxide
  - Intravenous prostacyclin
  - Intravenous adenosine
  - Catheterization is generally safe but may rarely give rise to serious complications such as hypotension and death.

Natural history and management
Complications
In most cases of untreated PPH, the disorder is rapidly progressive which will lead to the development of right failure and subsequently death. New York Heart Association functional class remains a strong predictor of survival.

Management strategy
Current therapies target on the following pathogenic mechanisms:
- Pulmonary vasoconstriction
- Imbalance between vasoconstrictive or proliferative substances and vasodilator or antiproliferative agents in the lung vasculature
- Thrombin deposition associated with a procoagulant state.

Lifestyle measures
- As pulmonary arterial pressure in PPH drastically increases on exertion, patients should be cautious when participating in activities requiring significant physical demand
- Fluid restriction (1 L per day) should be practised, especially for patients with signs and symptoms suggestive of heart failure
- Supplementary oxygen may be administered for patients with hypoxemia at rest or with physical activity.

Drug treatments
General treatments
1 Anticoagulation
  - Anticoagulant therapy has been widely advocated for all patients with PPH as thrombin deposition is present in the pulmonary circulation
  - Evidence supporting the approach, however, does not arise from rigorous, well-designed trials.
2 Digoxin
Digoxin may be considered for:
  - Reversing neurohumoural activation in patients with right-heart failure
  - Counteracting the negative inotropic effect of calcium-channel blockers
  - The use of digoxin in PPH remains controversial.

3 Diuretics
- Diuretics are useful in controlling oedema, which may arise from:
  - Increased intravascular volume in patients with advanced right heart failure
  - Drug-induced oedema in patients receiving high-dose calcium channel blockers
  - Spironolactone is a useful adjunct to loop diuretics in the presence of ascites.

Specific treatments
1 Calcium channel blockers
- Acute vasodilator testing should be done before administration to identify responders.
- The commonest agents being used are nifedipine and diltiazem. Newer agents including amlodipine and nicardipine may also be considered.
- Long-term therapy with calcium channel blockers has shown sustained improvements in symptoms, exercise tolerance, cardiopulmonary haemodynamics and survival. Thrombin deposition is present in the pulmonary circulation.
- Only a small proportion of patients show favourable outcome, thus limiting the use of calcium channel blockers. Moreover, the drugs have created numerous side-effects in non-responders.

2 Phosphodiesterase Inhibitors
- The inhibitors exert their effect by blocking the effect of phosphodiesterase, which is responsible for hydrolysis of cGMP, thus potentiating the effect of nitric oxide in lowering pulmonary arterial pressure as well as inhibiting pulmonary vascular growth.
- Sildenafil (oral phosphodiesterase-5 inhibitor) acts selectively in the pulmonary vasculature with promising effects of improving exercise capacity, lowering mean pulmonary arterial pressure from initial studies.

3 Endothelin-1 receptor antagonists
- Endothelin-1, a potent vasoconstrictor, mitogen, and profibrotic agent, is proposed as a possible pathogenic agent.
- Common agents used include bosentan and sitaxentan.
- The use of non-selective endothelin receptor antagonist bosentan was shown to improve exercise tolerance, functional class and pulmonary haemodynamics in patients with PAH.

- Requires regular monitoring of liver function parameters due to its major adverse effects on the liver.

4 Prostacyclin (PGI_2) and analogues
- Effects of PGI_2 are mediated mainly through vasodilation and potent inhibition of platelet aggregation by increasing platelet cAMP concentrations.
- The drug is indicated in patients with New York Heart Association functional class III or IV and are unresponsive to other therapies.
- Continuous (due to short half-life) intravenous PGI_2 (epoprostenol):
- Improvements in exercise tolerance, pulmonary haemodynamics and survival independent of acute vasodilator response have been shown.
- Side-effects are generally well tolerated.
- Main problems arise from the delivery system which include complications including exit site infections and bleeding, paradoxical embolism, bacteraemia, or sepsis, delivery malfunction resulting in sudden, and sometimes fatal, decompensation.
- In the light of significant problems with epoprostenol, new PGI_2 analogues, e.g. beroprost, iloprost, treprostinil have been introduced with promising results.

Surgical treatments
1 Heart–lung transplantation
- At present, this is the only curative therapy for patients with PPH.
- Indications:
  - New York Heart Association functional class III/IV despite optimum medical therapy
  - Cardiac index less than 2 L/min/m2
  - Right atrial pressure greater than 15 mmHg
  - Mean pulmonary artery pressure greater than 55 mmHg
  - Complications: ventilation/perfusion mismatch, development of obliterative bronchiolitis (chronic rejection).

2 Atrial septostomy
- Blade-balloon atrial septostomy decreases right heart pressures and is used in patients who do not respond to medical therapy while heart–lung transplant is not available
- Oxygen desaturation will occur, which should be offset by improvement of cardiac output.

Side-effects and contraindications (Table 8.1.2)

Table 8.1.2 Side-effects and contraindications

Drug name	Common side-effects	Contraindications
Epoprostenol	Sepsis Anxiety Headache Tachycardia Nausea Vomiting Jaw pain	Known hypersensitivity Congestive heart failure from severe left ventricular dysfunction Development of pulmonary oedema during dose ranging
Iloprost	Vasodilatation Hypotension Headache Increased cough	Known hypersensitivity Severe coronary disease events (e.g. severe artery disease, angina or recent myocardial infarction) Recent cerebrovascular events (e.g. stroke) (Not recommended) patients with unstable pulmonary hypertension who have advanced right ventricular heart failure
Bosentan	Headache Flushing Abnormal liver function Leg oedema Anaemia	Known hypersensitivity Hepatic impairment (including aminotransferases of more than three times the upper limit of normal) On ciclosporin Pregnancy (Not recommended) women with child-bearing potential should not receive bosentan unless they are using a reliable contraceptive
Sitaxentan	Headache Peripheral oedema Nasal congestion Constipation Flushing Muscle cramp	Similar to that of bosentan
Sildenafil	Headache Flushing Dyspepsia Diarrhoea Limb pain	Known hypersensitivity Severe hepatic impairment Recent history of stroke or myocardial infarction Severe hypotension at initiation (Not recommended) use with nitric oxide-producing treatment or nitrates

Treatment targets

As PPH is progressive in nature with significant morbidity and mortality, treatment aims would therefore include:

- Symptomatic relief
- Improving cardiac output
- Preventing or slowing-down disease progression, hence improving long-term survival.

In addition to electrocardiography, the cardiopulmonary stress test (a standard 6-minute walk test) is especially useful in:

- Assessing exercise performance
- Monitoring response to therapy
- Predicting prognosis.

References

Colleen LB, Richard NC, Lewis JR. A new era in the treatment of primary pulmonary hypertension. *Heart* 2001;**85**:251–2.

Gaine SP, Rubin LJ. Primary pulmonary hypertension. *Lancet* 1998;**352**:719–25.

Lewis JR. Primary pulmonary hypertension. *N Engl J Med* 1997;**336**:111–17.

Nazzareno G, Alessandra M, Luca N, *et al*. A meta-analysis of randomized controlled trials in pulmonary arterial hypertension. *Eur Heart J* 2009;**30**:394–403.

Rich S, Dantzker DR, Ayres SM, *et al*. Primary pulmonary hypertension: a national prospective study. *Ann Intern Med* 1987;**107**:216–23.

Rich S, Kaufmann E, Levy PS. The effect of high doses of calcium-channel blockers on survival in patients with primary pulmonary hypertension. *N Eng J Med* 1992;**327**:76–81.

Runo JR, Loyd JE. Primary pulmonary hypertension [Review]. *Lancet* 2003;**361**:1533–44.

Pulmonary embolism

Pulmonary embolism (PE) is one of the leading causes of death. It affects from 23 to 69 cases per 10 000 population, with an average fatality rate of 11% in the first 2 weeks after diagnosis. PE and deep vein thrombosis (DVT) are two manifestations of the same disease. Clots usually form in the veins of the calf and tend to extend to popliteal and femoral veins. In a minority of cases clots originate from abdominal or pelvic veins, or from the veins of the arm. The severity of disease ranges from completely asymptomatic events, incidentally discovered, to cases of sudden death. Diagnosis is sometimes difficult, and it is not unusual to find patients with symptoms lasting several days.

Clinical approach

History: key points
- Common symptoms are dyspnoea (either on rest or on exertion, sudden or progressive), chest pain, cough, palpitations, faintness
- Haemoptysis and pleuritic pain suggest a pulmonary infarction
- Syncope or cardiac arrest are other possible presentations
- Symptoms of DVT of the legs may be associated
- Ask for risk factors: family history, previous venous thromboembolism, known thrombophilia, surgery, or trauma in the last 3 months, cancer, immobilization, acute medical disease (stroke, heart failure, respiratory insufficiency, sepsis, etc.), oral contraceptives, hormone replacement therapy.

Examination: key points
- Arterial blood gas analysis: hypoxaemia and hypocapnia
- Hypotension (PE at high risk of mortality)
- Distended jugular veins, systolic murmur of tricuspid regurgitation, accentuated P2 are signs of right ventricular dysfunction
- Pulmonary exam may be normal; sometimes pleural rub if pleural effusion
- Leg swelling, pain, warmth
- Electrocardiogram (ECG): heart rate 100 bpm, SI QIII TIII, T-wave inversion in V1 trough V4, new onset right bundle branch block
- Chest X-ray: usually normal, possible platelike atelectasis, elevation of hemidiaphragm, pleural effusion

Special investigations
- Validated clinical prediction scores (Wells score or Geneva score, see Table 8.2.1) are available for assessing pre-test probability
- D-dimer: screening test, with high negative predictive value
- CT angiography (multidetector CT scan) reveals thrombi in pulmonary artery, segmental, and subsegmental vessels
- Ventilation-perfusion scanning: high sensitivity. Cardiopulmonary diseases other than PE reduce test accuracy
- Pulmonary artery angiography: gold standard, but rarely performed
- Echocardiogram may be normal; signs of right ventricular dysfunction

- Troponin I and BNP may be elevated with right ventricular dysfunction
- Combined diagnostic approach
- Low or intermediate pre-test probability (Wells score): test D-dimer. If negative, it is possible to rule out PE. If positive, perform multidetector CT scan. In high pre-test probability, directly perform multidetector CT scan without D-dimer False-positive D-dimer results may

Table 8.2.1 Wells score and revised Geneva score

Canadian (Wells) prediction score

Variables	Score
DVT symptoms and signs	3.0
PE as likely as or more likely than alternative diagnosis	3.0
Heart rate >100 bpm	1.5
Immobilization or surgery in previous 4 weeks	1.5
Previous DVT or PE	1.5
Haemoptysis	1.0
Cancer	1.0
Total score	
<2.0 low pre-test probability	
2.0–6.0 moderate pre-test probability	
>6.0 high pre-test probability	
Dichotomized Wells score	
<4 PE unlikely	
>4 PE likely	

Revised Geneva score

Variables	Score
Age >65 years	1
Previous DVT or PE	3
Surgery or lower limb fracture in previous week	2
Active cancer	2
Unilateral lower limb pain	3
Haemoptysis	2
Heart rate 75–94 bpm	3
Heart rate >95 bpm	5
Pain on leg palpation	
or unilateral oedema	4
Low probability category: 0 to 3 points	
Intermediate probability category: 4 to 10 points	
High probability category: ≥11 points	

occur in elderly people, in cancer patients, in pregnant women and in other conditions.

Natural history and management

Severity of pulmonary embolism

Stratify patients according to expected early mortality risk. High risk (>15% at 1 month): patients with persistent hypotension or shock.

Non-high risk (<15%): Further stratify in: intermediate risk (3–15%) if right ventricular dysfunction is present or myocardial injury markers are elevated; low risk (<1%), if all cited prognostic factors are absent.

Management strategy: acute treatment

- The mainstay of the treatment of PE is anticoagulant therapy.
- If clinical suspicion of PE is high, initiate anticoagulant treatment while awaiting the results of diagnostic tests.
- In non-high-risk PE, acute treatment is based on short-term subcutaneous low-molecular-weight heparin (LMWH), or intravenous unfractioned heparin (UFH), or fondaparinux, followed by long-term vitamin K antagonists (VKAs) monitoring INR levels, with a therapeutic range 2.0–3.0. LMWH, UFH or fondaparinux should be continued for at least 5 days and until INR is > 2.0 for at least 24 hours.
- Monitoring aPTT is essential in UFH-treated patients; dosage of LMWH and fondaparinux should be reduced in severe renal failure.
- Give adequate oxygen support if hypoxia is present.
- In patients with a major contraindication to anticoagulant therapy, such as concomitant active bleeding, consider placement of an inferior vena cava filter; adequate anticoagulation should be initiated as soon as bleeding resolves.
- In high risk PE, thrombolysis is the first choice. In case of contraindications, consider interventional catheterization techniques or pulmonary embolectomy. Use resuscitation, vasopressor therapy, intubation, as appropriate.
- Thrombolysis may be considered also in highly selected patients with intermediate risk (right ventricular dysfunction without haemodynamic instability).
- Home-treatment of PE has not been properly studied.

Management strategy: long-term treatment

- The optimal duration of secondary prevention is unknown. In patients with a PE provoked by transient risk factors, three months of VKAs are suggested.
- In patients with idiopathic PE, PE provoked by a permanent risk factor, or with previous venous thromboembolic event, long-term secondary prevention should be considered, periodically assessing benefits and risks of continuing VKAs.

Special patient groups

- Patients with cancer: LMWH is preferred over VKAs in the first 3–6 months
- Pregnant women: D-dimer is often positive during pregnancy; use proper precautions for radiation risks.

Table 8.2.2 Geneva prognostic score

Cancer	2
Hypotension (<100 mmHg)	2
Heart failure	1
Prior DVT	1
Hypoxaemia (PaO2 <8KPa)	1
Ultrasound proven DVT	1
Low-risk category: 0	2
High-risk category: 3	8

Use LMWH instead of VKAs. VKAs are contraindicated in the first three months (teratogenic) and near delivery (for bleeding risk). Delivery should be programmed in order to timely stop LMWH. Continue anticoagulation for at least 6 weeks after delivery.

Prognosis

Prognosis of PE largely depends on the severity of clinical presentation and on underlying diseases. As described above, initial prognostic stratification relies on clinical assessment of haemodynamic status (blood pressure), markers of right ventricular dysfunction (echocardiography, brain natriuretic peptide), and markers of myocardial injury (cardiac troponins). Pre-existing patient-related risk factors are useful for optimal risk stratification. Several prognostic risk scores are available such as the Geneva prognostic score (Table 8.2.2).

Potential long-term complications

Chronic thromboembolic pulmonary hypertension (CTPH) can occur in 0.5–4.0% of patients with previous PE. Severe CTPH is associated with high mortality rates and requires thromboendoarterectomy of pulmonary arteries. Data about long-term complications of patients with asymptomatic PE are lacking; post-thrombotic syndrome of the legs can develop in patients with concomitant DVT.

Primary prevention

PE is a potentially preventable disease. Pharmacological or mechanical prevention is strongly recommended in every hospitalized surgical and medical patient at risk for venous thromboembolism.

References

Kearon C, Kahn SR, Agnelli G, et al. Antithrombotic therapy for venous thromboembolic disease: American College of Chest Physicians practice guidelines, 8th edn, 2008. ACCP

Kostantinides S. Clinical practice. Acute pulmonary embolism. N Engl J Med. 2008;**359**:2804–13.

Tapson VF. Acute pulmonary embolism. N Engl J Med 2008;**358**:1037–52.

The task force for the diagnosis and management of acute pulmonary embolism of the European Society of Cardiology (ESC). Guidelines on the diagnosis and management of acute pulmonary embolism. Eur Heart J 2008;**29**:2276–315.

Cor pulmonale

Cor pulmonale was defined by the World Health Organization expert committee in 1963 as right ventricular hypertrophy (RVH) resulting from diseases affecting the function and/or structure of the lungs, but has come to be known as the cardiopulmonary–renal syndrome seen in patients with excess fluid associated with hypoxic (and hypercapnic) lung disease such as:

1 Chronic obstructive pulmonary disease (COPD)
2 Interstitial lung disease, e.g. idiopathic pulmonary fibrosis (IPF)
3 Obstructive sleep apnoea (OSA)
4 Neuromuscular disorders, e.g. inflammatory myopathy or inherited muscular dystrophies.
5 Obesity hypoventilation
6 Extra-thoracic restriction e.g. kyphoscoliosis.

Epidemiology

The most common cause is COPD with a prevalence of 10–30% in patients with at least one previous hospital admission. It is also common in patients with IPF (30–85% depending on the course of disease) and OSA (20–40%).

Pathogenesis

Pulmonary hypertension (PH)

Hypoxic vasoconstriction
- Hypoxia increases pulmonary artery smooth muscle tone resulting in vasoconstriction.
- Initially reversible with oxygen therapy.

Pulmonary vascular remodelling
Chronic hypoxia induces structural changes in all three layers of the pulmonary arterial wall leading to obliteration of the vessel lumen.
  Other contributing factors are infections, cigarette smoke, and hyperinflation.
  Once pulmonary vascular remodelling becomes established, pulmonary vascular resistance is irreversibly elevated. This increases right ventricular afterload leading to right ventricular dysfunction and ultimately right ventricular failure.

Renal sodium and water retention

Fluid retention develops as a consequence of right heart failure but many patients with advanced COPD and peripheral oedema have normal right atrial pressures. This is due to renal retention of sodium and water mediated by the following mechanisms (Naeije and MacNee 2002):

1 Repeated stretching of right atrium during periods of raised pulmonary artery pressures (PAP) at exercise or nocturnal desaturation→activation of the sympathetic nervous system (SNS)→activation of the renin–angiotensin–aldosterone (RAA) system.
2 Hypercapnic acidosis
  - Directly increases proximal tubular reabsorption of sodium along with bicarbonate to compensate for acidosis.
  - Activates the SNS→activates the RAA system.

Clinical approach

History: key points

- Related to PH: increased shortness of breath, fatigue, exertional chest pain, or syncope
- Related to fluid retention: peripheral oedema, ascites

- Fluid retention commonly precipitated by worsened hypoxaemia ±with or without hypercapnia during acute exacerbations of the underlying lung disease
- Symptoms of the underlying lung disease.

Examination: key points

- Central cyanosis
- Signs of RVH: left parasternal heave
- Signs of PH: loud P_2 with or without split second heart sound, right ventricular fourth heart sound, pan-systolic murmur of tricuspid regurgitation (TR) at the left sternal edge with or without early diastolic murmur of pulmonary regurgitation.
- Signs of fluid retention: raised jugular venous pressure (large 'a' wave in RVH and large 'v' wave in TR), peripheral pitting oedema, pulsatile hepatomegaly, ascites.
- Signs of the underlying lung disease may mask the signs of PH.

Investigations

Full blood count
Raised haematocrit or frank polycythaemia.

Arterial blood gases
Hypoxaemia with or without hypercapnia (usually).

Electrocardiogram
- Characteristic changes are p pulmonale, RVH with strain pattern, right axis deviation and right bundle branch block
- High specificity but low sensitivity for PH
- The presence of ECG changes is a poor prognostic factor.

Chest X-ray
- Enlarged pulmonary arteries
- Signs of the underlying lung disease.

Lung function test
- A disproportionately low diffusing capacity for carbon monoxide in association with an obstructive and/or restrictive defect.

Doppler echocardiography
- Images may be suboptimal in COPD patients with hyperinflated chest or obese patients.
- Useful as a screening test to estimate pulmonary artery systolic pressure.

Computed tomography (CT)
- High-resolution CT of chest to assess the severity of lung disease.
- CT pulmonary angiogram to exclude acute pulmonary embolism during episodes of acute decompensation.

Cardiac magnetic resonance imaging
- Allows non-invasive assessment of right heart structure and function.

Exercise tests
- Six-minute walk distance predicts survival.
- Useful in monitoring functional exercise capacity.
- Useful in detecting exercise-induced arterial deoxygenation in patients with preserved resting oxygen saturation.

Sleep studies
- Useful in identifying OSA in patients with suggestive symptoms.

Right heart catheterization
- Gold standard for diagnosing PH.
- Reserved for patients with evidence of significant PH from non-invasive tests.

Natural history and management

The elevation of PAP related to chronic lung disease is usually modest (mean PAP <40 mmHg).

The rate of progression of PH is slow in COPD patients with mild to moderate hypoxaemia (incidence of 25% after a follow-up period of 6 years) (Kessler *et al.* 2001).

The risk of developing PH at rest is higher among patients with raised PAP during exercise at the outset.

Based on data from COPD patients, the presence of PH worsens prognosis (Weitzenblum *et al.* 1981). The 5-year survival for COPD patients who develop peripheral oedema is approximately 3 years.

General measures
It is essential to optimize treatment of the underlying lung disease, e.g. by the use of bronchodilators, inhaled corticosteroids and pulmonary rehabilitation in COPD.

Diuretic therapy is the mainstay of treatment for fluid overload.

Patients with severe polycythaemia despite long-term oxygen therapy may require venesection.

Other specific treatment strategies are as follows.

Long-term oxygen therapy (for at least 15 hours per day)
It is the only treatment that has been shown to reduce PAP (although the reduction is small) and improve survival in COPD patients with severe hypoxaemia (PaO$_2$ <8 kPa) (BTS 2004).

Non-invasive ventilation
It reduces mean PAP in patients with chronic hypercapnic respiratory failure due to thoracic restriction (Schonhofer *et al.* 2001).

Continuous positive airways pressure ventilation
It reduces mean PAP and the pulmonary vascular reactivity to hypoxia after 3–6 months of treatment in patients with OSA (Sajkov and McEvoy 2009).

Vasodilator therapy (prostacyclins, endothelin receptor antagonists, phosphodiesterase inhibitors)
The data on the efficacy of vasodilatory agents in this group of patients are limited. They may potentially cause harm by worsening gas exchange. Therefore, they should only be used if recommended by a PH centre.
- Intravenous epoprostenol worsens gas exchange by increasing ventilation/perfusion mismatch in COPD (Archer *et al.* 1996).
- Bosentan has no benefit on exercise capacity in patients with IPF (King *et al.* 2008).

- Sildenafil produces preferential pulmonary vasodilatation and improves gas exchange in IPF (Ghofrani *et al.* 2002).

Lung transplantation
It improves long-term survival of patients with end-stage COPD/IPF and PH.

COPD with severe PH

This is a subset of COPD patients with mean PAP >40 mmHg, similar to levels seen in idiopathic pulmonary arterial hypertension (IPAH). They have the following distinct clinical characteristics (Chaouat *et al.* 2005):
- Mild to moderate air flow obstruction
- Severe hypoxaemia
- Hypocapnia
- Very low diffusing capacity for carbon monoxide.

The pathogenesis of PH is this subset of patients is thought to be different to those with mild PH. Pre-existing genetic predisposition may increase the susceptibility of the pulmonary circulation to alveolar hypoxia, resulting in extensive pulmonary vascular remodelling, to the extent seen in IPAH. To date, there is no data from randomized controlled trials to support the routine use of vasodilator therapy. However, there is a growing body of opinion that these patients should be given a trial of vasodilator therapy, e.g. sildenafil based on their similarities to IPAH patients.

References

Archer SL, Mike D, Crow J, *et al.* A placebo-controlled trial of prostacyclin in acute respiratory failure in COPD. *Chest* 1996;**109**:750–5.

British Thoracic Society (BTS). Managing stable COPD. *Thorax* 2004;**59**:i39–130.

Chaouat A, Bugnet AS, Kadaoui N, *et al.* Severe pulmonary hypertension and chronic obstructive pulmonary disease. *Am J Respir Crit Care Med* 2005;**172**:189–94.

Ghofrani HA, Wiedemann R, Rose F, *et al.* Sildenafil for treatment of lung fibrosis and pulmonary hypertension: a randomised controlled trial. *Lancet* 2002;**360**:895–900.

Kessler R, Faller M, Weitzenblum E, *et al.* 'Natural history' of pulmonary hypertension in a series of 131 patients with chronic obstructive lung disease. *Am J Respir Crit Care Med* 2001;**164**:219–24.

King TE, Jr., Behr J, Brown KK, *et al.* BUILD-1: a randomized placebo-controlled trial of bosentan in idiopathic pulmonary fibrosis. *Am J Respir Crit Care Med* 2008;**177**:75–81.

Naeije R, MacNee W. Pulmonary circulation. In: Calverley P, MacNee W, Pride P *et al.* (eds) *Chronic obstructive pulmonary disease.* London: Arnold Health Sciences, 2003: pp. 228–42.

Sajkov D, McEvoy RD. Obstructive sleep apnea and pulmonary hypertension. *Prog Cardiovasc Dis* 2009;**51**:363–70.

Schonhofer B, Barchfeld T, Wenzel M, *et al.* Long term effects of non-invasive mechanical ventilation on pulmonary haemodynamics in patients with chronic respiratory failure. *Thorax* 2001;**56**:524–8.

Weitzenblum E, Hirth C, Ducolone A, *et al.* Prognostic value of pulmonary artery pressure in chronic obstructive pulmonary disease. *Thorax* 1981;**36**:752–8.

Vasculitides

The vasculitides are a group of multi-system disorders characterized pathologically by inflammation and destruction of the blood vessel, leading to subsequent organ dysfunction. These conditions have been defined and classified according to the size of the vessel involved (Jennette *et al.* 1994). The conditions causing pulmonary vasculitis are primarily small vessel diseases with inflammation at the level of the capillaries, venules and arterioles, as seen in the anti-neutrophil cytoplasmic antibody (ANCA), associated vasculitides (Wegener's granulomatosis (WG), microscopic polyangiitis (MPA), and Churg–Strauss syndrome (CSS)). However, it is important to consider the large vessel diseases of Takayasu's arteritis (TA) and giant cell arteritis (GCA), Behçet's syndrome, and the primary immune complex disease Henoch–Schönlein purpura (HSP), all of which may involve the pulmonary vessels.

Polyarteritis nodosa (PAN), a medium vessel vasculitis, affecting mainly visceral arteries such as renal and coronary arteries, spares the lungs. Vasculitis resulting from one of the connective tissue diseases such as systemic lupus erythematosus (SLE) is considered to be secondary and are is covered in Chapter 12.12.

The aetiology of vasculitis is poorly understood but is likely to be multifactorial and include gene expression (including HLA), gender, ethnicity, and environmental factors (including infections, UV light and smoking. status) (Watts and Scott 2002). The exact pathophysiological role of autoantibodies is still not fully defined but interactions between ANCA and its target antigens on the surface of neutrophils are thought to cause direct injury to vessels in WG.

ANCA-associated vasculitis (ANCA-AV) is rare, with a frequency within the UK general population of 20 per million population. The most common disease, WG, has an annual incidence in Europe of 2-10/million (Watts *et al.* 2000).

In patients with suspected vasculitis, a systematic assessment including a careful history and thorough examination is the key to making the diagnosis. Below are important clinical features that may alert the clinician to the diagnosis and a strategy for investigation. Each disease is then considered individually before returning to the principles of disease management.

Clinical alerts to vasculitis

History

Unexplained respiratory symptoms including cough, shortness of breath, haemoptysis, and pleuritic chest pain in the presence of a multi-system illness with constitutional symptoms of weight loss, fevers, and malaise may point to an underlying vasculitic process. Occasionally the diagnosis is made following an incidental finding of pulmonary infiltrates, nodules, or cavities on a chest X-ray. Indeed 30% of vasculitis patients with pulmonary involvement are asymptomatic at presentation. At the other end of the clinical spectrum diffuse alveolar haemorrhage (DAH) can present with life-threatening acute respiratory failure and haemoptysis.

Extra-pulmonary features include:
- Upper respiratory tract: hearing loss, new onset otitis media, chronic sinusitis, nasal crusting, and discharge. ENT features are most marked in WG. Subglottic involvement (occurring in approximately 20% of WG) can cause voice changes, dyspnoea and stridor.
- Renal disease: active urinary sediment characterized by haematuria, proteinuria, and red cell casts, with an elevated serum creatinine may indicate glomerular involvement. The term pulmonary–renal syndrome refers to patients with both DAH and rapidly progressive glomerulonephritis (RPGN) and the differential diagnosis includes ANCA-AV, in particular MPA, Goodpastures. syndrome, and SLE.
- Cutaneous: look for nailfold infarcts and a purpuric rash: a palpable, purplish rash often involving the lower limbs and pressure areas, for example, the elbows. Nodular lesions and ulcers are also described.
- Peripheral neuropathy: glove and stocking type or mononeuritis multiplex (MNM) occur with varying frequencies depending on the diagnosis. Clinicians should be alert to complaints of pain, numbness and dysthesia involving two or more peripheral nerves.
- Constitutional symptoms: weight loss, fevers, arthralgias, myalgias, and malaise are commonly found in all systemic vasculitides.

Examination

A full examination is required paying close attention to the skin (vasculitic rashes), eyes (scleritis), upper airway (nasal crusting or saddle nose deformity), respiratory system (fine inspiratory crackles), abdominal system (abdominal pain), peripheral nerves (e.g. foot or wrist drop), and peripheral pulses (absent/reduced pulses or bruits in TA).

Special investigations

- Bloods: routine laboratory blood tests including full blood count (FBC) (with white cell differential as eosinophilia may point to CSS); urea and electrolytes (U+E), an increase in serum creatinine and urea may indicate RPGN, RPGN; inflammatory markers (ESR and CRP) erythrocyte sedimentation rate (ESR) and C-reactive protein (CRP) are usually elevated in active vasculitis, but excluding infection with a full septic screen is mandatory.
- Immunology screen should include an autoantibody profile including antinuclear antibody (ANA), rheumatoid factor (RF), ANCA and anti-GBM (antiglomerular basement membrane). If SLE is suspected, in addition to ANA, check for dsDNA, ENAs (extractable nuclear antigens), anticardiolipin antibodies, and complement levels. Check for the presence of cryoglobulins (with hepatitis B and C serology), particularly in the context of purpuric rash, arthralgias, and neuropathy.
- ANCA: these are antibodies directed against antigens within the cytoplasm of neutrophils. Indirect immunofluorescent (IIF) staining reveals three distinct patterns: cytoplasmic (cANCA), perinuclear (pANCA), and atypical. Each pattern is found in association with specific antibodies against intracellular antigens detectable by

ELISAs (enzyme-linked immunosorbent assays). Anti-proteinase 3 (PR3) is found in association with cANCA and is most strongly associated with WG (>85% sensitivity with generalized Wegener's). The commonest target antigen of pANCA staining is myeloperoxidase (MPO) and is found in association with CSS and MPA. Other pANCA antigens are not specific for vasculitis.

- Urinalysis is essential in all patients. Those patients with red cell casts and/or significant proteinuria should be referred to a renal physician for consideration of a renal biopsy.
- Radiology: a chest X-ray is an essential baseline investigation; 30% of patients with an ANCA-associated vasculitis are found to have evidence of pulmonary disease on X-ray. Radiographic changes include nodules, which may contain cavities, fleeting focal shadows (a feature of alveolar haemorrhage), and interstitial infiltrates (suggestive of pneumonitis). High-resolution computerized tomography (HRCT) scanning will more accurately delineate the findings seen on X-ray and can reveal abnormalities not seen on chest X-ray. CT sinus may be helpful if there are upper respiratory tract features suggestive of localized WG.
- Pulmonary function testing: flow volume loops are useful for investigation of stridor (airflow is reduced in both inspiration and expiration) and an increase in gas transfer by more than 30% is strongly suggestive of pulmonary haemorrhage.
- Bronchoscopy: this can be helpful if haemorrhage or opportunistic infection (e.g. *Pneumocystis jiroveci*) is suspected.
- Histology: this is the gold standard diagnostic test. Areas of high diagnostic yield include the upper respiratory tract and kidneys. The presence of necrotizing vasculitis with granulomatous inflammation is characteristic of WG. These findings along with an eosinophilic-rich extra-vascular inflammatory infiltrate are supportive of CSS. MPA has the hallmark necrotizing vasculitis of the ANCA-AV but no granulomata. Renal biopsy of the ANCA-AV reveal a pauci-immune, focal, segmental GN. Immunofluorescence should be performed on tissue as IgA deposition suggests HSP and complement deposition is a feature of SLE. Transbronchial biopsy tends to have a low diagnostic yield and if lung tissue is required open or video-assisted thoracoscopic biopsy may be necessary to gain tissue for histology.

Specific diseases
ANCA associated vasculitides
Wegener's granulomatosis
Classically described as a triad of ENT, renal, and pulmonary features histologically characterized by small and medium vessel necrotizing granulomatous vasculitis. Upper respiratory tract involvement can be severe enough to cause perforation of the nasal septum (leading to saddle nose deformity) and laryngeal and tracheal involvement can lead to airway stenosis and stridor. RPGN occurs in 50–90% of patients. Ocular involvement affects up to half of all patients and includes sight-threatening uveitis. Constitutional features are prominent and include arthralgias and myalgias. Pulmonary disease affects 50% of patients at presentation and ultimately 85% will have some lung involvement although a third of these are asymptomatic despite radiological evidence of disease. cANCA/PR3 is positive by ELISA in 85% with generalized disease.

Microscopic polyangiitis
MPA is characterized by a long prodrome of constitutional symptoms and followed, almost universally, by RPGN. Biopsy reveals necrotizing vasculitis with a mixed inflammatory infiltrate without granuloma. Pulmonary involvement is less common (10–30%) but when it occurs is most often alveolar haemorrhage. Arthralgias and peripheral nerve involvement are seen in up to half of all patients. Unlike WG, ocular involvement is rare.

Churg–Strauss syndrome
CSS is characterized by a triad of late onset asthma, hypereosinophilia and necrotizing, granulomatous vasculitis. DAH and RPGN occur but much less frequently than the other ANCA-associated diseases. The diagnosis is often considered in those patients with steroid-dependent asthma who develop constitutional symptoms and musculoskeletal complaints. Cardiac (conduction delay, coronary artery disease, pericardial effusions) and gastrointestinal involvement (in particular intestinal haemorrhage, perforated viscus) are common.

Large vessel vasculitides
Takayasu's arteritis
This idiopathic large vessel vasculitis affects the aorta and its major branches, including coronary and pulmonary arteries, leading to arterial stenosis, and less commonly post stenotic dilatation and aneurysm formation. It has a predilection for young females and patients present with features of vascular occlusion (absent pulses, bruits, ischaemic limb pain) and constitutional features. Hypertension is an almost universal finding and occurs mostly as a result of renal artery involvement. Pulmonary disease can present with dyspnoea, haemoptysis and pleuritic chest pain, mimicking pulmonary embolism. Inflammation and stenosis of the pulmonary artery can lead to pulmonary hypertension. There are no specific diagnostic laboratory tests although ESR and CRP are often elevated. MRA and high-resolution ultrasound are useful investigations and can demonstrate a range of vessel involvement from early wall thickening to stenosis (Andrews and Mason 2009).

Giant cell arteritis
This granulomatous arteritis particularly affects the extracranial branches of the carotid arteries giving rise to symptoms of headache, scalp tenderness, jaw claudication, and potentially sight-threatening visual disturbances. The aorta and other large arteries can also be involved (subclavian particularly) and as with TA the main pulmonary arteries can be involved and a similar spectrum of symptoms can occur.

Other primary vasculitides
Behçet's syndrome
This disease, whose pathogenesis is unclear, was originally described as a triad of uveitis with oral and genital ulceration. However, its widespread clinical manifestations demonstrate it to be a true multi-organ disease. The vascular component is unusual in its involvement of both arteries and veins. Arteritis of the pulmonary vasculature can result in both occlusion and large aneurysm formation; hence haemoptysis, pulmonary haemorrhage, pulmonary infarction and pulmonary hypertension have all been described. This is seen most commonly in young men of Middle Eastern decent.

Henoch–Schönlein purpura (HSP)

HSP is a systemic vasculitis, most commonly seen in young children (75% of cases occurring in patients under 10 years of age). It is widely considered to be as a result of IgA immune deposits in the walls of small vessels. The clinical triad of palpable purpura, arthritis, and abdominal pain is well known; however, renal involvement is the most serious manifestation of the disease. Both pulmonary haemorrhage and interstitial lung disease have been described.

Pseudo-vasculitic syndromes

In particular cardiac myxomas, sarcoid, neoplasms, and infection, including HIV and bacterial endocarditis, should be considered as potential diagnoses in the context of vascular inflammation, raised inflammatory markers and constitutional features.

Management

Treatment is tailored to the severity and extent of the under-lying organ involvement, age and medical co-morbidities of the patient. The overall aim of therapy is to suppress active inflammatory disease while minimizing potentially life-threatening, drug-related complications. Prior to the introduction of oral cyclophosphamide and steroids in the 1970s, untreated systemic necrotizing vasculitis had a 2-year mortality rate of 90% (Walton 1958). This is now significantly improved to almost 90% 2-year survival (Jayne and Gaskin 1999).

For ANCA-AV remission-induction is usually in the form of pulsed intravenous cyclophosphamide every two to three weeks and high dosehigh-dose glucocorticoids (1 mg/kg/day), with most patients achieving remission by 3-6 months. This remission is then maintained by milder agents such as methotrexate, azathioprine, and mycophenolate alongside a reducing course of oral corti-costeroids. The optimum duration of maintenance therapy is between 2 and 5 years but is guided by the clinical course. Severe pulmonary disease in the form of alveolar haemorrhage is treated with high-dose methyl prednisolo-ne and plasma exchange, an approach also applied to those with RPGN (Brown 2006). Novel therapies for those patients unresponsive to aggressive cytotoxic therapy include the use of biologic agents such as rituximab, inflixi-mab, and antithymocyte globulin (Mukhtyar *et al.* 2009). Close monitoring of the patient including regular blood testing and assessment for intercurrent infection is essen-tial throughout the clinical course. Many features of the large vessel vasculitides (TA and GCA) can be managed with steroids alone, initially in high dose, though additional immunosuppressants may be necessary to reduce risk of steroid toxicity.

Support group Stuart Strange Vasculitis Trust www.vasculitis-uk.org, Tel: 01332 521595.

Treatment protocols: www.vasculitis.org.uk

References

Andrews J, Mason JC. Takayasu's arteritis-recent advances in imaging offer promise. *Rheumatol* 2009;**46**:6–15.

Brown KK. Pulmonary vasculitis. *Proc Am Thorac Soc* 2006;**3**:48–57.

Jayne D, Gaskin D, for EUVAS. Randomized trial of cyclophospha-mide versus azathioprine during remission in ANCA-associated vasculitis (CYCAZAREM). *J Am Soc Nephrol* 1999;**10**:105A.

Jennette JC, Falk RJ, Andrassy K, *et al.* Nomenclature of systemic vasculitides. Proposal of an International Consensus Conference. *Arthritis Rheum* 1994;**37**:187–92.

Mukhtyar C, Guillevin L, Cid MC, *et al.* EULAR recommendations for the management of primary small and medium vessel vasculitis. *Ann Rheum Dis* 2009;**68**:310–7.

Walton EW. Giant-cell granuloma of the respiratory tract (Wegner's Granulomatosis). *BMJ* 1958;**2**:265–70.

Watts RA, Lane SE, Bentham G, *et al.* Epidemiology of systemic vas-culitis: a ten-year study in the United Kingdom. *Arthritis Rheum* 2000;**43**:414–19.

Watts RA, Scott DGI. Epidemiology of Vasculitis. In: Ball GV, Louis Bridges S Jr (ed.) *Vasculitis*. Oxford: Oxford Press, 2002: pp. 211–26.Fig. 8.3.1 The pathogenesis of cor pulmonale.

Chapter 9

Pericardial diseases

Pericarditis

Pericarditis is an inflammation of the pericardium, a mesothelial cell layer overlying the heart, and usually presents with chest pain, a pericardial friction rub, and electrocardiographic changes. Patients with pericarditis may go on to develop pericardial constriction or pericardial effusions.

The aetiology has been classified as follows:

1 Idiopathic: this can account for anything between 26–84% of cases. As there are no specific clinical features to differentiate idiopathic from viral pericarditis, many may have a viral aetiology. There is seasonal variation with most cases occurring in spring and autumn.

2 Viral: proven viral pericarditis accounts for up to 10% of cases. Many viruses have been implicated, but coxsackie B and influenza viruses are probably the most common. The condition may be associated with myocarditis. HIV infection rarely causes pericarditis unless the condition is advanced.

3 Bacterial: purulent pericarditis is fortunately rare, and can be caused by many bacteria including anaerobic bacteria, particularly in children. Spread may occur from infective endocarditic lesion. Patients are often very unwell at presentation, and the mortality can be high.

4 Mycobacterium: the incidence depends upon the current prevalence of mycobacterium agents in the population. In the developed world mycobacterium pericarditis is commoner in the elderly population. It often progresses to pericardial constriction.

5 Inflammatory conditions: this includes a wide range of autoimmune disorders including rheumatoid arthritis, systemic lupus erythematosus (SLE), and scleroderma. Rheumatic fever, which is now very rare in the developed world, used to be a common cause.

6 Metabolic disorders: particularly renal failure and hypothyroidism.

7 Myocardial 'trauma': underlying damage to the heart can produce pericarditis and cause include acute myocardial infarction, cardiac contusion, Dressler's syndrome (postpericardiotomy syndrome), and aortic dissection.

8 Neoplasia: this is commonly lung tumours including mesothelioma, breast cancer, and haematological malignancies.

9 Iatrogenic: includes, percutaneous cardiac interventions, adverse drug reactions, and complications of radiation therapy.

Clinical approach
History
- Chest pain is almost universal and can be described as sharp, but it is not uncommon for the pain to be undistinguishable from ischaemic type cardiac pain. The pain may be exacerbated by movement and respiration, and can be relieved by sitting forward.
- Shortness of breath is common and would require exclusion of pericardial effusion and tamponade.
- Fever is less usual unless there is purulent pericarditis.

Examination
- A pericardial friction rub, if heard, is pathogonomic of pericarditis.

- The patient may have to be moved into various positions to reveal the rub, which is best heard using the diaphragm of the stethoscope, and has been likened to the sound made by rubbing hair between fingers.
- Fever, tachycardia, and tachypnoea may be present.
- Kussmaul's sign, a rise in the JVP on inspiration, and pulsus paradoxus, an exaggeration of the normal fall in blood pressure on inspirations, are not features of uncomplicated pericarditis and suggest pericardial constriction or cardiac tamponade due to pericardial effusion respectively.

Special investigations
Electrocardiogram
Is the most useful diagnostic test is acute pericarditis. There are J-point ST segment elevations, which are usually described as concave or 'saddle-shaped' and T-wave changes. In contrast to the regional changes suggestive of myocardial ischaemia, these changes are usually widespread affecting the majority of limb and chest leads. The changes will evolve over time with the ST segments becoming isoelectric, and the T waves inverting, before returning to normal usually over a few days.

Blood tests
- Markers of myocardial damage, such as troponin may be elevated if there is concomitant myocarditis.
- Virological, microbiological, biochemical, and autoimmune studies should be performed as indicated by the clinical history or examination.

Echocardiography
Is usually performed to exclude concomitant pericardial effusion, but is rarely abnormal unless there is some myocardial or endocardial cause for the pericarditis.

Radionuclide scanning
With agents that identify inflammation such as gallium-67 or MRI scans with gadolinium are rarely used in the diagnosis.

Chest radiography
Is usually normal unless there is a pericardial effusion or a pulmonary cause for the pericarditis.

Treatment
- Oxygen and cardiac monitoring should be provided.
- It is important to rule out other life-threatening causes of chest pain, such as myocardial infarction or aortic dissection.
- Monitoring should continue if there is any evidence of haemodynamic instability.
- Treatment for specific causes of pericarditis is directed according to the underlying cause. For patients with idiopathic or viral pericarditis, therapy is directed at symptom relief. Non-steroidal anti-inflammatory drugs (NSAIDs) are the mainstay of therapy, with relief of chest pain in about 85–90% of patients within a few days of treatment.
- Ibuprofen has the advantage of few adverse effects and increased coronary flow.

- Indomethacin has a poor adverse effect profile and reduces coronary flow, and should be avoided in patients with post-myocardial infarction pericarditis.
- Aspirin is recommended for treatment of pericarditis after STEMI.
- Colchicine, in combination with NSAIDs can be considered in the initial treatment to prevent recurrent pericarditis. Colchicine, alone or in combination with NSAIDs, can be considered for patients with recurrent or continued symptoms beyond 14 days.
- Corticosteroids should not be used for initial treatment of pericarditis unless it is indicated for the underlying disease, the patient has no response to NSAIDs or colchicine, or both drugs are contraindicated.
- Once the diagnosis is confirmed and the patient is haemodynamically stable, it is safe to discharge the patient and review on an outpatient basis.
- The absence of continued fever, immunosuppression, trauma, oral anticoagulation therapy, myopericarditis, severe pericardial effusion, and cardiac tamponade are good prognostic signs.

Complications and follow up

Outpatient follow-up should ideally be within one month, and should assess the patient for complications which include:

- A significant risk of recurrent pericarditis, which can cause significant morbidity secondary to pain. The patient should be warned that this may occur.
- Pericardial effusions leading to a risk of cardiac tamponade.
- Pericarditis, especially if recurrent, leads to a significant risk of constrictive pericarditis, or a combination of effusive and constrictive pericarditis.

Prognosis

- The prognosis depends on the aetiology.
- Idiopathic and viral aetiologies usually have a self-limited course.
- Purulent, tuberculous, and neoplastic pericardial involvement have a more complicated course with worse outcomes.

Special considerations

- NSAIDs and corticosteroids should be used with caution in patients with pericarditis secondary to acute myocardial infarction, as they may interfere with ventricular healing and remodelling.
- Pericarditis can be difficult to distinguish from acute myocardial infarction and repolarization in patients who present with chest pain and ST-segment elevation on an ECG. A careful and thorough history and physical examination, together with the fact that the repolarization does not progress through stages, and is uncommonly associated with PR depression, will help to differentiate the conditions (Figure 9.1.1).
- Serial monitoring of ECGs in young patients with chest pain helps differentiate early repolarization from acute pericarditis.
- The ST segment in acute myocardial infarction is usually convex, bowing upward with reciprocal changes, as opposed to concave ST segments without reciprocal changes observed in acute pericarditis and repolarization.
- Children may present with abdominal pain.
- The classic feature of chest pain and dyspnoea with pericarditis may be subtle and can be confused with other diagnoses, particularly in elderly people.

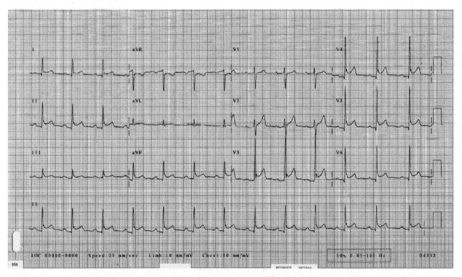

Fig. 9.1.1 Typical electrocardiographic changes in acute pericarditis including diffuse concave upward ST segment elevation, except in aVR where there is ST segment depression. The T waves are upright in the leads with ST elevation, and the PR segment deviates opposite to P-wave polarity.

Chronic constrictive pericarditis

Chronic constrictive pericarditis (CCP) is a clinical constellation that includes a thickened and rigid or semi-rigid pericardium with fusion of the visceral and parietal layers associated with impaired cardiac filling and elevated ventricular filling pressures and which presents with signs and symptoms of heart failure, most notably an elevated jugular venous pressure, dyspnoea, peripheral oedema, hepatomegaly, and ascites.

Worldwide the leading causes are as sequelae to acute pericarditis especially tuberculous. In the developed world constriction as a complication of cardiac surgery or mediastinal radiation is more common. Pericardial fibrosis and calcification may be idiopathic. A major clinical challenge is to determine the relative contribution of pericardial restraint and underlying myocardial dysfunction in determining the signs and symptoms.

Pathophysiology
Characteristic pathophysiological features of chronic constrictive pericarditis include:
- Fibrosis, fusion and usually thickening of visceral parietal pericardium
- Pericardial calcification can result in the formation of calcified plaques (eggshell appearance)
- Myocardium classically not involved but can be in radiation induced CCP, or if an underlying pericarditis involves the myocardium.

Aetiology
Causes of chronic constrictive pericarditis include:
- Tuberculosis
- Post-viral pericarditis
- Post-mediastinal radiotherapy
- Neoplastic pericardial infiltration
- Other infective pericarditides
- Post-Dressler's syndrome
- Connective tissue diseases with chronic pericarditis
- Chronic renal failure.

Prognosis
- Depends upon the underlying aetiology
- Pericardial resection can be curative
- Clinical approach.

History
Typical presentation is with features of right heart failure:
- Dyspnoea
- Dizziness or syncope
- Oedema
- Ascites.

Examination
- Raised jugular venous pressure, especially with Kussmaul sign (ordinarily the JVP falls with inspiration. Kussmaul's sign suggests impaired filling of the right ventricle due to either fluid in the pericardial space or a poorly compliant myocardium or pericardium) but this does not differentiate from tamponade.
- Signs of right heart failure such as peripheral oedema, ascites, hepatomegaly.

Special investigations
Chest radiography
- Increased cardiothoracic ratio is common, but not universal.
- Pericardial calcification can occur but is neither diagnostic nor essential.

Blood testing
- BNP may be low despite signs and symptoms of heart failure.

Echocardiography and Doppler (see also Dal-Bianco 2009)
- Thickened pericardium (may be regionalized). Transoesophageal echo is more reliable in estimating pericardial thickness than transthoracic two-dimensional echo. M-mode is intermediate. Note that the presence of an echo-free space between the visceral and parietal pericardium suggests pericardial effusion.
- Mitral inflow Doppler shows increased early diastolic filling velocity followed by rapid deceleration, with a shortened overall filling period.
- Early mitral inflow deceleration time usually <160 ms.
- Can be differentiated from restrictive cardiomyopathy by detection of dynamic changes with respiration: reduced early diastolic mitral inflow and prolonged isovolumic relaxation time with inspiration, shortened isovolumic relaxation time and increased early diastolic mitral inflow (typically >25%) velocity on expiration.
- Sensitivity and specificity of Doppler assessment of respiratory changes in confirming CCP diagnosis reported to be as high as 85% to 90% (Hancock 2001).
- Inferior vena cava (IVC) dilatation.
- Increased tricuspid regurgitant jet velocity from onset to peak inspiration can.
- Displacement of the interatrial septum toward the left atrium during inspiration.

Other imaging techniques
- Computed tomography and magnetic resonance imaging can help in detecting an abnormal pericardium.

Invasive haemodynamics
- The classical haemodynamic changes of CCP are attributed to a relatively fixed end-diastolic ventricular volume and isolation of the cardiac chambers from intrathoracic respiratory pressure changes.
- Normally respiratory changes in intrathoracic pressure affect pulmonary and systemic veins entering the heart and the intracardiac chambers relatively equally. In CCP the intracardiac chambers are protected from these respiratory pressure swings leading to characteristic changes.
- The pressure gradient between the pulmonary veins and the left atrium decreases with inspiration in CCP, producing a reduction in diastolic pulmonary vein flow and left atrial and filling.
- The rigid, noncompliant constricted pericardial sac couples both ventricles and hence an increase in filling on one side impedes filling on the other (ventricular interdependence). The inspiratory reduction in left atrial and left ventricular filling is therefore associated with

increased diastolic right ventricular filling and a shift in the septum towards the left ventricle, with the opposite pattern being seen in the expiratory phase.

- This haemodynamic pattern causes characteristic changes in the jugular venous and right atrial pressure waveforms. The elevated mean filling pressures produce a prominent 'a' wave, the sharp 'y' descent reflects rapid early diastolic RV filling due to the shift in the septum reducing RV pressures, and a preserved 'x' descent due to accelerated atrial relaxation. The RV haemodynamic waveform with a dip-and-plateau (commonly called the square root pattern) reflects rapid ventricular relaxation, with a subsequent sharp increase in filling pressure as the expanding ventricle is impeded by the rigid pericardium.
- At end-diastole right atrial, right ventricular, pulmonary wedge and LV pressures are equal and elevated.
- These haemodynamic consequences of the pathophysiological effects of pericardial constriction account for the clinical, and echocardiographic findings in CCP.

Treatment

- The management of CCP depends upon the aetiology and clinical state of the patient.
- Treat tuberculous cases with standard antituberculosis drugs for 6 months: neoplastic or connective tissue disease requires specific therapy for these conditions.
- Surgical pericardiectomy is the definitive treatment, depending on the underlying aetiology.

Further reading

Dal-Bianco JP, Sengupta PP, Mookadam F, et al. Role of echocardiography in the diagnosis of constrictive pericarditis. *J Am Soc Echo* 2009;**22**:24–33.

Hancock EW. Differential diagnosis of restrictive cardiomyopathy and constrictive pericarditis. *Heart* 2001;**86**:343–9.

Hurrell DG, Nishimura RA, Higano ST, et al. Value of dynamic respiratory changes in left and right ventricular pressures for the diagnosis of constrictive pericarditis. *Circulation* 1996;**93**;2007–13.

Pericardial effusion

Pericardial effusion is defined as the presence of an abnormal amount of pericardial fluid. There is normally between 10 and 50 mL of an ultra-filtrate of plasma ('pericardial lubrication') within the pericardial space. There is significant overlap of the causes of pericardial effusion with those of pericarditis (see Chapter 9.1). Pericardial effusions, however, are more likely to be caused by malignant disease, myocardial trauma (including iatrogenic causes and acute myocardial infarction), bacterial or mycobacterium infections, or renal failure. Pericardial effusions can be acute or chronic, and the rate of fluid accumulation has a major impact on development of the patient's symptoms. The treatment of pericardial effusion varies, from watchful waiting to emergency pericardiocentesis, and is directed at both removal of the pericardial fluid and alleviation of the underlying cause, which usually is determined by a combination of fluid analysis and correlation with co-morbid illnesses.

Physiology and pathophysiology

In health the pericardium:
- Acts as a restraint to right heart dilatation maintaining diastolic pressure, and is responsible for most of the pressure in the right atrium and ventricle.
- Evenly distributes forces across the heart to ensure uniform contraction of the myocardium.
- Stretches to accommodate small amounts of fluid without significant change in intrapericardial pressure (pericardial compliance).

When excessive pericardial fluid is produced:
- The pressure–volume curve becomes steep.
- Slow increases in volume cause increased pericardial compliance and lessen the increase in intrapericardial pressure.
- Clinical manifestations are highly dependent upon the rate of accumulation of fluid in the pericardial sac.
- During inspiration increased intrapericardial pressure is transmitted to the right heart. This leads to the shifting of the atrial and ventricular septa to the left, reducing left heart diastolic volumes and causes a fall in cardiac output.
- As intrapericardial pressures rise, this effect becomes pronounced, leading to the development of pulsus paradoxus and the signs of cardiac tamponade (Figure 9.3.1).

Clinical approach

History
- Chest pain is common and similar to pericarditis pain
- Palpitation
- Cough
- Hiccoughs.

As the patient develops tamponade the symptoms are those of reduced cardiac output:
- Dyspnoea
- Presyncope or syncope
- Confusion.

Examination
- The classical Beck's triad of hypotension, muffled heart sound and a raised jugular venous pressure is specific, but not sensitive for a diagnosis of pericardial effusion, as they are signs of incipient tamponade.
- Pulsus paradoxus is an exaggeration of the normal fall in blood pressure (normally less than 10 mmHg) on inspiration. The reason that it is termed paradoxical is that in extreme cases the peripheral pulses will disappear but on auscultation the heart continues to beat.
- A pericardial friction rub that is pathognomic of pericarditis may disappear with development of an effusion.
- Tachyopnoea and cyanosis usually indicates the development of tamponade.
- Ewart's sign: dullness to percussion in the left subscapular region due to compression of the right lung.
- Peripheral oedema and hepatosplenomegaly are unusual with acute pericardial effusion and usually occur with constrictive pericarditis or rarely with chronic effusions.

Special investigations

Echocardiography
This is the mainstay of the diagnosis of pericardial effusions.
- The presence of an echo-free space between the visceral and parietal pericardium is pathognomic for pericardial effusion.
- Pericardial effusions are usually best imaged via the sub-xiphisternal approach with the patient supine or with the back slightly elevated.
- The effusion may be localized and may require other views to exclude loculated fluid.

Signs suggestive of cardiac tamponade (which is a predominantly clinic diagnosis) include:
- Early diastolic collapse of the right ventricular free wall.
- Late diastolic collapse/compression of the right atrium.
- Swinging of the heart in the pericardial sac.
- A greater than 40% relative inspiratory augmentation of right side (tricuspid) flow.
- A greater than 25% relative inspiratory decrease of left sided (mitral) flow.

It is important to exclude pleural effusions, pericardial thickening and mediastinal lesions which may be confused with pericardial fluid.

ECG
- Often non-specific in the absence of acute pericarditis. Sinus tachycardia is common particularly with incipient tamponade. There may be low voltage QRS complexes and electrical alternans, which are due to swinging of the heart within the pericardial sac.

Chest radiography
- May show an enlarged cardiac silhouette, but may be normal when the effusion is small or of acute onset.

Pericardial fluid
- The type of pericardial fluid produced depends upon the underlying aetiology.
- Transudative fluids result from obstruction of fluid drainage, which occurs through lymphatic channels.
- Exudative fluids occurs secondary to inflammatory, infectious, malignant, or autoimmune processes within the pericardium.

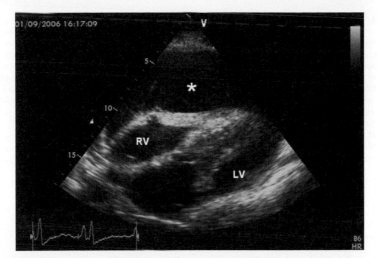

Fig. 9.3.1 A subxiphisternal view of a large pericardial effusion. A large echo-free space is seen (asterisk). The right ventricle (RV) and left ventricle (LV) are compressed.

Pericardial fluid can be analysed:
- To assess if it a transudate or exudates using protein and lactate dehydrogenase (LDI I) levels.
- Haemoglobin and white cell count to assess haemorrhagic or purulent effusions.
- Cytological examination for malignancy.
- Viral, bacterial and mycobacterium cultures.

Blood testing
- To look for myocardial damage, metabolic, endocrine, and autoimmune disorders.

Treatment
- The management of pericardial effusion depends upon the aetiology and clinical state of the patient.
- If the effusion is related to a major cardiovascular catastrophe such as aortic dissection or myocardial rupture then urgent referral for a cardiac surgical opinion is required.
- If the effusion is related to an interventional cardiac procedure and the patient is in the cardiac catheterization laboratory, urgent pericardiocentesis can be performed.
- If the patient is stable with no clinical symptoms or signs of tamponade, and there is no evidence of an infective cause which requires pericardial fluid for culture, then pericardiocentesis can be deferred.
- If the patient presents with or develops signs of cardiac tamponade then a therapeutic pericardiocentesis should be performed.
- Chronic pericardial effusion (defined as being present for greater than 6 months) has a good prognosis, is usually well tolerated, and has a higher risk to benefit ratio for pericardiocentesis.

Pericardiocentesis
- Preprocedure transthoracic echocardiography is strongly recommended unless the procedure is a life-saving emergency. This will allow appropriate patient positioning and needle length selection.

- The patient should have continuous ECG monitoring.
- Ideally the procedure should be performed in a cardiac catheterization laboratory or in a pacing room where there is access to X-ray screening if required.
- The usual approach is subxiphisternal with the patient supine, but with the back raised at about 30°.
- A sterile field is prepared and local anaesthetic is infiltrated pointing toward the left shoulder. The needle is advanced on a syringe with mild traction on the plunger and once fluid is encountered, a guidewire is passed into the pericardial space. A pigtail catheter or sheath is inserted and fluid is removed for analysis and then therapeutically is left to drain.
- Some operators use an echocardiographic guided technique from the left intercostal space, using echocardiography to identify the location and depth of the maximal fluid accumulation.
- Once the fluid is no longer draining, and the effusion is absent on echocardiography, the catheter can be removed.
- Complications of pericardiocentesis include arrhythmias, cardiac or coronary artery perforation and pneumothorax.

Recurrent or malignant pericardial effusions
- If pericardial effusion recur or are of a known malignant aetiology, then percutaneous balloon pericardiotomy or formal surgical pericardial window either using a subxiphisternal incision, or video-assisted thoracoscopic (VAT) approach should be considered.
- All these techniques make a connection between the pericardial space and the abdomen where the effusion is absorbed via the lymphatic drainage. Percutaneous balloon pericardiotomy, which is performed under local anaesthesia with sedation, is associated with the best success rates and shortest hospital stays, but if pericardial tissue is require for histology a surgical approach is necessary.

Prognosis
- Depends upon the underlying aetiology.
- Pericardial effusion associated with significant cardiovascular disease, such as aortic dissection or myocardial rupture following myocardial infarction, have very poor prognoses and require emergency referral for a cardiac surgical opinion.
- Patients with malignant pericardial effusion have a poor prognosis consistent with a diagnosis of disseminated malignancy. Since these patients are more likely to have recurrent effusions, treatment with percutaneous balloon pericardiotomy may be considered as an initial procedure, to reduce the time spent in hospital.

Special considerations
- Failure to consider pericardial effusion either as a primary or secondary diagnosis may lead to rapid deterioration and death secondary to cardiac tamponade.
- Patients with dilated or congestive cardiomyopathy may present acutely with symptoms and signs similar to cardiac tamponade. Echocardiography is mandatory in these patients to distinguish the two conditions.

Chapter 10

Peripheral vascular diseases

Carotid artery disease

Carotid artery disease is a major cause of cerebrovascular accidents (CVAs) (stroke), which is the third leading cause of death in Western countries accounting for 10–12% of all deaths.

The highest risk for stroke is with stenosis of the internal carotid arteries, with most common site of atherosclerosis being the carotid bifurcation.

CVA can be of two types: thrombotic or hemorrhagic. Thrombotic type is due to large vessel occlusion, small vessel occlusion, or embolization.

Risk factors
Same as those for coronary artery disease:
- Smoking
- Diabetes mellitus
- Male gender
- Hypertension
- Dyslipidaemia.

For patients with carotid stenosis on ultrasound who remain asymptomatic, the best indicator for CVA risk is the percentage of carotid stenosis, progression of stenosis on subsequent ultrasounds, and the presence or absence of carotid ulceration.

Clinical approach
History
- The majority of patients with carotid stenosis remain asymptomatic; the presence of bruit may be detected on physical examination.
- In all patients, enquire about transient ischaemic attack (TIA) symptoms: difficulty swallowing, visual field effects, motor and sensory loss, etc.
- Be careful to differentiate findings from vertebrobasilar disease: bilateral visual field loss, ataxia, dysarthria, diplopia.
- Symptoms due to carotid occlusion involve contralateral face and body. Hemicranial headache may occur.
- Internal carotid artery dissection triad consist of neck/retro-orbital pain, Horner's syndrome, and contralateral sensory or motor deficits.

Physical examination
- Auscultate for carotid bruit.
- Correlate with symptoms in symptomatic patients with carotid stenosis.

Special investigations
- Duplex ultrasound is the initial investigation of choice, with 90% sensitivity and specificity. First investigation in patient suspected of carotid artery disease. In patients with less than 50% stenosis, serial ultrasound on a yearly basis is suggested.
- Contrast-enhanced magnetic resonance angiography (MRA) is especially useful in patients with suboptimal ultrasound results. It allows brain imaging to assess any ischaemic events and to rule out other pathologies (vascular malformations, tumours) before endovascular treatment.
- Computed tomography angiography is useful in patients who are not candidates for MRA.
- Angiography is the gold standard; use in patients when ultrasound/MRA yield inconclusive results.

Management
The emphasis is on risk factor modification (similar to coronary artery disease):
- Control of hypertension
- Smoking cessation
- Proper glycaemic control in diabetic patients
- Lowering of lipids: statins
- Antiplatelet therapy: aspirin or clopidogrel or aspirin/diphyridamole.
- Symptomatic patients with >60% carotid stenosis require medical therapy with antiplatelet medication and risk factor modification. These patients are candidates for carotid revascularization.
- Carotid endarterectomy is indicated in asymptomatic patients, but with more than 70% internal carotid artery stenosis.
- Carotid stenting is performed in patients at high risk for carotid surgery.

Further reading
Gurm HS, Yadav JS, Fayad P, et al. Long-term results of carotid stenting versus endarterectomy in high risk patients. N Engl J Med 2008;**358**:1572–9.

Mohler ER, Jaff MR. Peripheral arterial disease, 2007. American College of Physicians.

Mohler ER. Carotid stenting for atherothrombosis. Heart 2007,

Rajagopalan S, Mukherjee M, Mohler ER. Manual of vascular diseases, 2004. Lippincott Williams and Wilkins.

Peripheral arterial disease

The term peripheral arterial disease (PAD) encompasses all stenotic, occlusive, and aneurismal diseases of the aorta and its branches (exclusive of coronary arteries); however, as in this chapter, it is commonly used to denote atherosclerotic disease of the lower extremities. The following is largely based on recent management guidelines (ACC/AHA 2005; TASC II 2007).

Haemodynamic definition: resting and/or post-exercise ankle–brachial index (ABI) ≤0.9 (and >1.3, if supported by other tests, e.g. toe–brachial index (TBI), duplex).

Prevalence of PAD: depends on age and increases from 3% to 10% (general population) to 15–20% (persons >70 years). The *incidence* of critical limb ischaemia (CLI) is estimated at 500–1000 new cases per 1 million Western population.

Clinical presentation
- Most PAD patients (75–80%) are asymptomatic.
- *Intermittent claudication:* refers to muscle discomfort (i.e. fatigue, aching, numbness, pain), reproducibly induced by exercise and relieved by rest (<10 minutes).
- *CLI* (1–3% of PAD patients): critical perfusion deficit with ischemic rest pain and/or ischaemic lesions for >2 weeks plus ankle pressure <50 mmHg (70 mmHg if non-healing lesion) or toe pressure <30 (50) mmHg.
- *Classification* according to Fontaine (I–IV) or Rutherford (0–6): asymptomatic (I, 0); mild claudication (IIa, 1); moderate (2) to severe (3) claudication (IIb); ischaemic rest pain (III, 4); minor (5) to major (6) tissue loss (IV).

Note that all PAD patients are at high risk for cardiovascular events, including a three- to sixfold increased cardiovascular mortality. Thus, they depend on early identification for secondary preventive therapy regardless of local symptoms.

Patients at risk for PAD
These characteristics should trigger evaluation for PAD:
- Age <50 years with diabetes and one other atherosclerosis risk factor
- Age 50–69 years with history of smoking or diabetes
- Age ≥70 years
- Exertional leg symptoms (claudication)
- Abnormal pulse examination
- Known coronary, carotid, or renal artery disease.

Risk factors
Presence of PAD was consistently related with these factors in epidemiological studies (odds ratio (OR)):
- Smoking (OR 3–4)
- Diabetes (OR 3–4)
- Age (per 10 years) (OR 2–3)
- Elevated C-reactive protein (OR 2–3)
- Chronic renal insufficiency (OR 1.5–2.5)
- Arterial hypertension (OR 1.5–2)
- Dyslipidaemia (OR 1.5–2)
- Race (non-white) (OR 1.5–2)
- Hyperhomocysteinaemia (OR 1–3)
- Male gender (only in younger patients) (OR 1–2).

Deterioration of PAD toward CLI is associated with other factors: diabetes (OR 4); persistent smoking (OR 3); ABI (<0.7, OR 2; <0.5, OR 2.5); age (>65 years, OR 2) and hypertriglyceridaemia (OR 2). Rapid decrease of ABI or baseline ABI <0.5 seem to be the best predictors of development of CLI (TASC II).

Clinical approach
History: key points
- Cardiovascular risk factors and previous management
- Ask for initial claudication distance/absolute walking distance. Does it consistently resolve with rest? Specific lifestyle limitations?
- Association of rest pain with position (predominant in recumbent position/at night?)
- Poorly healing/non-healing wound/gangrene of legs/feet?
- Medical history: Particularly symptoms of coronary heart disease (CHD) or cerebrovascular disease; but also renal insufficiency and varicosis (venous conduit).
- Surgical history including earlier vascular interventions.

Examination: key points
- Document peripheral pulses as 0 (absent); 1 (diminished); 2 (normal); 3 (bounding).
- Auscultation of carotid arteries, abdomen/flank, femoral and popliteal arteries for presence of bruits.
- Inflow (aortoiliac) disease likely with gluteal or thigh claudication plus femoral pulse diminuation/bruits.
- Outflow (femoropopliteal/tibial) disease characterized by calf/foot claudication plus diminished distal pulses.
- Palpation of abdomen for aortic aneurysm (AAA, prevalence in symptomatic PAD is >10%).
- Inspection of limbs including feet to evaluate colour, temperature, integrity of skin, and trophic skin changes.
- Search for any signs of local infection, in particular in skin lesions. Probe-to-bone for osteomyelitis.

Special investigations
- ABI at rest and, if normal, after exercise (or TBI, if incompressible tibial arteries (i.e. ABI >1.3)).
- Segmental limb systolic pressure measurement and plethysmographic pulse volume recording for non-invasive localization of significant occlusive lesions.
- Standardized treadmill test (to quantify claudication).
- Imaging (to characterize lesion morphology according to TASC II if revascularization is considered): duplex-ultrasound (velocity, wave form analysis), computed tomography (CT) or magnetic resonance (MR) angiography, diagnostic angiography (if immediate intervention is considered), ultrasound mapping of superficial veins, X-ray or MR for suspected osteomyelitis.
- Thorough evaluation of cardiopulmonary/renal function.

Diagnoses to consider for claudication
- Spinal stenosis or nerve root compression
- Osteoarthrosis/-arthritis
- Arteritis and rheumatological diseases
- Peripheral emboli (e.g. from popliteal aneurysm)
- Thromboangiitis obliterans (Buerger's disease)
- Baker's cyst or popliteal entrapment.

Natural history and management
Presence of PAD predicts a similar risk for cardiovascular events as CHD; 40–60% of PAD patients have co-existent CHD and/or cerebrovascular disease, and 25–40% have

renal artery disease. Overall, 80% of deaths are cardiovascular, and there is a strong inverse correlation between value of ABI and mortality/non-fatal events.

- Aggressive risk factor modification/secondary prevention (as in national treatment guidelines), antiplatelet therapy and best medical care (co-existent cardiovascular disease) are all crucial for patients with PAD.
- Diabetes: 5- to 10-fold risk of major amputation (sensory neuropathy/decreased resistance to infection). Consider ABI-screening for PAD every 5 years in diabetics.

Claudicants

Stable clinical course of intermittent claudication in most cases: only 25% will ever deteriorate significantly (7–9% in first year after diagnosis, 2–3% per year thereafter); and only 1–3.3% will need a major amputation over next 5 years (compared to an annual mortality of 5%).

- Best medical treatment including supervised exercise is the recommended primary approach.
- Indication for revascularization is based on life-style limiting claudication and not on limb salvage.
- Before evaluating for revascularization, other diseases must be excluded that would likely limit activity, even if claudication was improved (e.g. heart failure, chronic obstructive pulmonary disease (COPD)).
- Recent randomized evidence shows additional benefit of endovascular intervention over supervised exercise (MIMIC). Endovascular first is the preferred revascularization strategy if lesion morphology is favourable
- Growing body of randomized evidence for beneficial effect of primary stenting of complex, long and calcified in- and outflow lesions (TASC II, ABSOLUTE).

Patients with CLI

PAD does not follow a steady progress through increasingly severe claudication to CLI, but CLI often appears independent of earlier symptoms. Prognosis of CLI is much worse than that of intermittent claudication and is similar to that of some malignancies:

- After 1 year 25% of patients have died, 25% have been amputated and 50% are alive with their limb, half of them without symptomatic improvement.
- After below knee amputation, only 40% achieve full mobility and 30% require above knee reamputation.
- Primary treatment goals are pain relief, limb salvage by revascularization and improved function/quality of life.
- Early specialist referral and multidisciplinary evaluation seem to be crucial for those treatment goals.
- Primary palliative amputation may be the best option, if revascularization is impossible (25%).
- BASIL trial randomized CLI patients to surgery-first or angioplasty-first strategies and found broadly similar results over 3 years in terms of amputation-free survival, early and mid-term mortality, and quality of life.

Revascularization

- Inflow disease should be addressed first before revascularization of outflow disease is considered.
- In the infrainguinal position, venous grafts yield all better results than prosthetic materials, and should be anastomosed distally to the least diseased artery with best continuous run-off to the foot.
- As opposed to surgical revascularization (dedicated reporting standards established by Rutherford), results of evolving endovascular techniques are very difficult to compare due to variable outcome measures: therefore, the DEFINE initiative suggested uniform reporting standards to improve future investigations.
- Endovascular and surgical strategies seem increasingly to yield similar results, each with distinct advantages. They should be used complementary/selectively.
- Decision-making needs also to be tailored to patient preference and local availability of facilities/know-how.

Follow up

After any revascularization procedure, patients require long-term care and vascular follow-up to detect recurrence of disease or remote development of new disease. Follow-up should include interval history (new symptoms), resting, and post-exercise ABI, and duplex ultrasound to evaluate long-term patency. Suggested intervals include 3, 6, and 12 months and then annually.

Further reading

ACC/AHA. 2005 Practice Guidelines for the management of patients with peripheral arterial disease: Executive summary. *J Am Coll Cardiol* 2006;**47**:1239–12.

Adam DJ, Beard JD, Cleveland T, et al. BASIL: Bypass versus angioplasty in severe ischaemia of the leg (BASIL): multicentre, randomised controlled trial. *Lancet* 2005;**366**:1925–34.

Diehm N, Baumgartner I, Jaff M, et al., DEFINE. A call for uniform reporting standards in studies assessing endovascular treatment for chronic ischaemia of lower limb arteries. *European Heart Journal* 2007;**28**:798–805.

MIMIC-Trial Participants. The adjuvant benefit of angioplasty in patients with mild to moderate intermittent claudication (MIMIC) managed by supervised exercise, smoking cessation advice and best medical therapy. *Eur J Vasc Endovasc Surg* 2008;**36**:680–88.

Rutherford RB, Baker JD, Ernst C, et al. Recommended standards for reports dealing with lower extremity ischemia: revised version. *J Vasc Surg* 1997;**26**:517–38.

Schillinger M, Sabeti S, Dick P, et al. ABSOLUTE: Sustained benefit at 2 years of primary femoropopliteal stenting compared with balloon angioplasty with optional stenting. *Circulation* 2007;**115**:2745–9.

TASC II: Norgren L, Hiatt WR, Dormandy JA, et al. Inter-Society Consensus for the Management of Peripheral Arterial Disease (TASC II). *J Vasc Surg* 2007;**45**:Suppl 5A–67A.

Thoracic aortic aneurysm

Thoracic aortic aneurysm (TAA) is defined as dilatation of the aorta of greater than 150% of its normal diameter for a given segment. The underlying pathology is from smooth muscle cell drop-out and fibrosis with elastic fibre degeneration in the aortic wall, termed cystic medial degeneration (CMD) (Schlatmann and Becker 1977). This process leads to weakening of the aortic wall with dilation and aneurysm formation. Other causes are from inflammatory states such as in atherosclerosis, syphilis, and arteritis. For the thoracic aorta, a diameter greater than 3.5 cm is generally considered dilated, whereas more than 4.5 cm would be considered aneurysmal. There are two major types of aneurysm morphology: fusiform, which is symmetrical and uniform dilatation, that involves the entire circumference of the aortic wall; and saccular, which is a focal out pouching of only a portion of the aortic wall. Thoracic aortic aneurysm (TAA) is an important disease process to recognize and treat in the patient population with an incidence of approximately 10.4 per 100 000 person years (Clouse et al. 2004). Close follow-up and in some instances surgical planning may retard the long-term sequela such as aortic dissection and severe aortic regurgitation.

TAA can be classified into four general anatomic categories; however, some aneurysms may involve more than one segment (Isselbacher 2005).

- Ascending aortic aneurysms (60%) arise from the aortic valve to the innominate artery
- Aortic arch aneurysms (10%) include any thoracic aneurysm that involves the brachiocephalic
- Descending aortic aneurysms (40%) are distal to the left subclavian artery
- Thoracoabdominal aneurysms (10%) involve the descending aorta, extend through the diaphragm and into the abdominal aorta.

Clinical approach
History: key points
- Many patients are asymptomatic and TAA are incidentally found.
- Owing to the inflammatory nature of TAA there is often a history of coronary artery disease and peripheral vascular disease including stroke.
- Heart failure symptoms may be present from underlying aortic valve insufficiency.
- Chest, back, or flank pain may be present from compression on adjacent structures including the coronary arteries.
- Hoarseness due to compression of left vagus or left recurrent laryngeal nerve.
- Distal embolization may occur from aneurysm thrombus formation
- Family history of TAA: 19% of patients with TAA with no collagen vascular disorder have a family history (Coady et al. 1999).

Examination: key points
- Difference in arm blood pressure from brachial artery/innominate artery compression.
- Findings of aortic regurgitation, e.g. wide pulse pressure, diastolic murmur, water-hammer pulse, etc.

- Evidence of underlying connective tissue disease, e.g. laxity of joints, chest wall deformities, arched palate, etc.

Secondary causes of TAA to consider
Marfan syndrome: a condition characterized by long limbs, laxity of joints, tall stature, chest wall deformity and aortic root enlargement. Caused by mutation on chromosome 15q affecting on of the genes for fibrillin-1.

Ehlers–Danlos syndrome: a heterogeneous group of heritable connective tissue disorders arising from a defect in the synthesis of collagen, characterized by articular (joint) hypermobility, skin extensibility, tissue fragility, and aortic enlargement.

Bicuspid aortic valve (BAV): dilation of the aorta is a frequent finding in patients with BAV. The dilation of the aorta is likely from an underlying inflammatory or degenerative process with compensatory remodelling since aortic dilation has been identified in association with BAV even in the absence of haemodynamically significant aortic valve stenosis or regurgitation (Nkomo et al. 2003).

Inflammatory aortitis: inflammation of the aorta occurring in many disease processes such as syphilitic aortitis, Wegener's granulomatosis, Takayasu arteritis, rheumatoid arthritis, psoriatic arthritis, ankylosing spondylitis, reactive arthritis, and giant cell arteritis.

Special investigations
Imaging
- Chest radiograph: many TAAs are identified incidentally on chest X-ray. The aneurysm produces a widened mediastinal silhouette or enlargement of the aortic knob. However, the sensitivity and specificity for diagnosing TAA is quite low and differentiating TAA from a tortuous aorta is difficult.
- Transthoracic echocardiography (TTE): TTE is a reliable test to evaluate for aortic root disease as well as aortic valve pathology. Its sensitivity is limited in diagnosing aneurysms which involve the upper root or aortic arch. A transoesophageal echocardiogram may be indicated to evaluate the arch in more detail when ruling out aortic dissection.
- CT and MRI: CT and MRI are accurate imaging modalities that can interrogate the entire aorta and give additional information such as aneurysmal size, presence of thrombus, aneurysm extent and co-existing vessel involvement.

Screening
The United States Preventive Services Task Force (USPSTF) recommends a one-time screening ultrasound for abdominal aortic aneurysms in male smokers >65 years of age and makes no recommendations to screen for TAA.

Natural history and management
Potential long-term complications
Dilated TAAs are prone to catastrophic rupture and dissection with the incident risk directly related to increased aneurysm size. Dilated TAAs can also cause significant aortic regurgitation with adverse left ventricular remodelling and the development of heart failure.

Medical management
- Blood pressure control should be initiated to slow the progression of aorta dilation. Beta-blockers are effective medications and are thought to act by decreasing left ventricular contractility (dp/dt) and shear stress.
- Although there is no literature regarding statin therapy and TAA, statins may have an anti-inflammatory and protective role in patients with atherosclerotic disease since some evidence exists that statin therapy slows abdominal aneurysm growth (Nkomo *et al.* 2003; Schouten *et al.* 2006).

Indications for surgical management
- Rupture.
- Ascending dissection or descending dissection with subacute rupture, vital organ ischaemia, or impending rupture.
- Rapid aneurysm growth (≥10 mm per year) in TAA <5.0 cm.
- Absolute size (5.5 cm for ascending aortic aneurysm, 6.0 cm for descending aortic aneurysm; in patients with Marfan syndrome, 5.0 cm for ascending aortic aneurysm, 6.0 cm for descending aortic aneurysm).
- An aortic aneurysm >45 mm in diameter at the time of aortic valve surgery (Baliga *et al.* 2007; Ramanath *et al.* 2009).

References

Baliga RR, Neinaber CA, Isselbacher EM, Eagle KA (eds). *Aortic dissection and related syndromes*. Springer, 2007: pp. 364.

Clouse WD, Hallett JW Jr, Schaff HV, *et al*. Acute aortic dissection: population-based incidence compared with degenerative aortic aneurysm rupture. *Mayo Clin Proc* 2004;**79**:176–80.

Coady MA, Davies RR, Roberts M, *et al*. Familial patterns of thoracic aortic aneurysms. *Arch Surg* 1999;**134**:361–7.

Isselbacher EM. Thoracic and abdominal aortic aneurysms. *Circulation* 2005;**111**:816–28.

Nkomo VT, Enriquez-Sarano M, Ammash NM, *et al*. Bicuspid aortic valve associated with aortic dilatation: a community-based study. *Arterioscler Thromb Vasc Biol* 2003;**23**:351–6.

Ramanath VS, Oh JK, Sundt TM 3rd, Eagle KA. Acute aortic syndromes and thoracic aortic aneurysm. *Mayo Clin Proc* 2009;**84**:465–81.

Schlatmann TJ, Becker AE. Histologic changes in the normal aging aorta: implications for dissecting aortic aneurysm. *Am J Cardiol* 1977;**39**:13–20.

Schouten O, van Laanen JH, Boersma E, *et al*. Statins are associated with a reduced infrarenal abdominal aortic aneurysm growth. *Eur J Vasc Endovasc Surg* 2006;**32**:21–6.

Abdominal aortic aneurysm

Abdominal aortic aneurysm (AAA) is usually defined by a diameter of ≥3 cm (1.5× normal diameter). Incidence varies based on age and sex: by 65, 5% of men have an AAA with increasing prevalence thereafter (6% per decade). Women are three to four less likely to develop an AAA.

Many AAA remain asymptomatic until rupture occurs. This is still associated with excessive mortality (85%). Thus, AAAs are thought to range among the 15 commonest causes of mortality in Western countries.

Exact pathogenesis of AAA is still unknown, but expansion is driven by inflammatory and proteolytic processes. AAA is more common in patients with atherosclerosis and presence of AAA was consistently related with these factors in screening studies (odds ratio (OR); 95% CI):

- Smoking (2.8; 2.5–3.1)
- Coronary heart disease (1.8; 1.7–2.0)
- Family history (first-degree relatives) (2.0; 1.6–2.5)
- Dyslipidaemia (1.4; 1.3–1.5)
- Arterial hypertension (1.4; 1.3–1.5)
- Diabetes (0.7; 0.6–0.8).

Genetic predisposition: is polygenic (monogenic traits, e.g. Marfan's or Ehlers–Danlos syndrome rare in AAA). Positive family history in about 5%; 20–30% of brothers (6% of sisters) of affected patients develop an AAA.

Presentation: most AAA are detected incidentally on abdominal imaging/examination or, increasingly, by screening. Symptoms, if present, are unspecific (back or abdominal pain) or extremely rare (distal embolization, erosion, or compression of adjacent structures).

Clinical approach

History: key points
- Three-generation pedigree: enquire specifically for aneurysm ruptures.
- Evidence for active aneurismal disease: symptoms, documented growth (consider earlier abdominal imaging, also for unrelated causes).
- Cardiovascular risk factors and their management.
- Medical history: in particular symptomatic or unstable cardiovascular disease (CHD, cerebrovascular disease, and claudication), chronic obstructive pulmonary disease (COPD), renal insufficiency.
- Ask for symptoms suggestive of neoplastic disease that might need abdominal surgery soon.
- Surgical history: likelihood of intra-abdominal abnormalities (e.g. bowel resection/reconstruction, adhesions) or 'hostile abdomen'. Earlier perioperative complications.
- Allergies (antibiotics, latex, radiological contrast media)
- Medication: in particular, use of and indication for antiplatelet agents, coumarins
- Sexual history: document information on erectile function with regard of later aneurysm repair.

Examination: key points
- Tenderness of AAA on direct palpation?
- Document peripheral aneurysms and distal pulses.
- Complete cardiopulmonary and abdominal examination
- Preoperatively: inspect surgical access sites (infections?)

Special investigations
Three major goals: (1) confirm diagnosis and stratify associated risks; (2) anticipate potential technical difficulties for repair and evaluate anatomical suitability for endovascular repair (EVAR); (3) assess patient fitness.
- Imaging: initial diagnosis usually on ultrasound. CT angiography (or MRI) needed for confirmation/sizing:
  - Maximum diameter of AAA
  - Extension of AAA to juxtarenal position or into iliac/hypogastric arteries?
  - Procedural planning (open repair): suitable for infrarenal clamping (e.g. length/wall quality of infrarenal segment)? Anatomical variants (e.g. additional renal arteries, left renal vein)? Distal anastomoses?
  - EVAR: measure on three-dimensional reconstructions of CT using a central luminal line: landing zones (length, diameter, shape, angulation, wall quality), lengths and tortuosity between landing zones. Size access vessels.
- Cardiac, pulmonary, and renal function tests to determine patient fitness for major vascular surgery; duplex scan of carotid bifurcations to assess risk of stroke.
- Consider coronary angiography/balloon angioplasty; however, never stent without consulting involved surgeon first (need for dual antiplatelet therapy).
- Look for evidence of other aneurysms (duplex scan), establish baseline ankle–brachial index preoperatively.

Emergency (suspected ruptured aneurysm):
- Search for pulsating abdominal mass/widened pulses.
- AAA visible on bedside ultrasound? Quick scan for free intraperitoneal fluid (perihepatic, perisplenic, pelvic). Confined haematoma: most patients can be stabilized for CT (using hypotensive resuscitation, see p. 353).
- Consider Hardman criteria (OR of mortality): age (>76 years; OR 4.7); cardiac ischaemia (ECG) (OR 6.6); creatinin (>0.19 mmol/L; OR 4.1); loss of consciousness (OR 5.4); hb (<9 g%; OR 2.9). Mortality increases with number of criteria present (0, 16%, to ≥3, 80%).

Natural history and management
AAA expand progressively until they rupture. AAA diameter is currently the best predictor of these events.
- AAA <4.0 cm: risk of rupture negligible. Manage by secondary prevention and repeat scan every 1–2 years.
- AAA 4.0–5.4 cm: expansion rate at 10% per year, risk of rupture in randomized controlled trials (RCTs) ≤1% per year (slightly higher in observational studies).
- AAA ≥5.5 cm: markedly increased annual rates of expansion and rupture (e.g. 10–20% for 6.0–7.0 cm).
- Consider: only one in three or fewer patients die of ruptured AAA; most die from other (mostly cardiovascular) causes!

Thus, aim of surgical management is to select patients with exceeding risk of rupture, and to provide surveillance and secondary prevention for all.

Other determinants of AAA expansion and rupture
- Expansion: correlates with continued smoking (positive) and diabetes (negative).

- Risk of rupture: associated independently with smoking, female gender (OR 4), family history of rupture, hypertension, COPD, and eccentric shape of AAA.

Threshold of intervention and surveillance

Many aspects regarding management are based on level 1a/b evidence by well-designed RCTs (see Further reading).
- UK SAT and ADAM: no survival benefit of early repair of small (4.0–5.4 cm) and asymptomatic AAA.
- Surveillance of such AAA is evidence based, even for low operative mortality (2.7% in ADAM). Consider repair at 5.5 cm and/or ≥1 cm growth/year and/or when symptoms arise.
- Most surveillance protocols recommend ultrasound scans every 6 months for AAA of 4.0–4.9 cm and every 3 months for AAA of 5.0–5.4 cm.
- Potentially, patients with risk factors for rupture might benefit from earlier aneurysm repair (e.g. women at 4.5–5.0 cm), but trials were not powered to prove this.

Screening for AAA and its implications

Ultrasound screening of men (65–74 years) almost halved aneurysm-related mortality at acceptable costs (MASS trial, ~68 000). However, overall mortality was similar.
- Note: a single normal scan (<2.6 cm) at age 65 can rule out AAA for life in men (GASP).
- Screening will yield many small AAAs for management.
- Smoking cessation and management of cardiovascular risk factors is a top priority in these patients.
- Dedicated preventive drugs are developed including inhibitors of proteolytic and inflammatory pathways.

Aneurysm repair

At present, aneurysm repair is the only durable solution to the problem of progressive expansion/risk of rupture.

Open repair is the established approach, involving insertion of a synthetic y-shaped/tube-graft into the opened vessel by direct suture. It is very effective, but associated with substantial surgical risks, massive haemodynamic shifts, and ischemia during aortic clamping.
- Operative mortality is often reported in the 3–8% range (recent RCTs ~4.5%; in selected centres 1–2%) and depends on patient fitness and hospital/surgeon volume.
- Complications are mainly in the perioperative period involving cardiac, pulmonary renal and surgical complications. After that, graft-related complications and reinterventions are rare (cumulative 9% and 6% at 4 years (EVAR 1)).
- EVAR was developed in the 1990s to reduce surgical risks for unfit patients. It involves endoluminal insertion of a modular y-shaped stent-graft via femoral axes. It is much less invasive but depends on anatomical requirements/preoperative imaging.
- There is consistent threefold reduction of operative mortality in *fit* patients in EVAR 1/DREAM. However, perioperative survival advantage is not sustained after 1 year.
- Graft-related complications and reinterventions occur more often (cumulative 40% and 20% at 4 years (EVAR 1)) and include endoleaks, device migration, limb occlusion, AAA rupture, and possibly renal failure.

- Surprisingly: there is no benefit of EVAR over best medical treatment in surgically *unfit* patients in RCT (EVAR 2).
- In essence, EVAR and open repair have a similar mid-term outcome. The lower early mortality of EVAR balanced by less certain long-term outcome, higher risk of reintervention, and need for close surveillance. EVAR trials suggest the fittest patients benefit the most from EVAR, whereas unfit patients do not benefit at all from repair.

Emergency repair for ruptured AAA

Because of logistics, most emergency repairs are by open repair.
- Reported operative mortality varies greatly (15–90%); meta-analytic trend from 55% (1960) to 41% (2000).
- Hypotensive resuscitation crucial (= fluid *restriction* to maintain systolic pressures at 50–70 mmHg *until bleeding controlled surgically*): slows haemorrhage, enables tamponade, prevents haemodilution. *Note:* haemodilution but not blood pressure is among Hardman criteria.
- Emergency EVAR may produce lower mortality (15–30%) in selected patients (observational evidence); however, level 1 evidence of advantage is lacking.

Follow-up

After EVAR strict surveillance recommended with regular CT scans depending on presence of endoleaks and shrinkage of AAA sac. However, duplex ultrasound increasingly being used instead and technical improvements likely to reduce the need for surveillance. All patients depend on risk factor control to reduce cardiovascular risk and 'at risk family' members need to be offered screening.

Further reading

ACC/AHA. 2005 Practice Guidelines: executive summary. *J Am Coll Cardiol* 2006;**47**:1239–312.

ADAM: Lederle FA, Wilson SE, Johnson GR, *et al*. Immediate repair compared with surveillance of small abdominal aortic aneurysms. *N Engl J Med* 2002;**346**:1437–44.

DREAM: Blankensteijn JD, de Jong S, Prinssen M, *et al*. Two-year outcomes after conventional or endovascular repair of abdominal aortic aneurysms. *N Engl J Med* 2005;**352**:2398–405.

EVAR trial participants. Endovascular aneurysm repair versus open repair in patients with abdominal aortic aneurysm (EVAR trial 1): randomised controlled trial. *Lancet* 2005;**365**:2179–86.

EVAR trial participants. Endovascular aneurysm repair and outcome in patients unfit for open repair of abdominal aortic aneurysm (EVAR trial 2): randomised controlled trial. *Lancet* 2005;**365**:2187–92.

GASP: Earnshaw JJ, Shaw E, Whyman MR, *et al*. Screening for abdominal aortic aneurysms in men. *BMJ* 2004;**328**:1122–4.

Greenhalgh RM, Powell JT. Endovascular repair of abdominal aortic aneurysm. *N Engl J Med* 2008;**358**:494–501.

MASS: Kim LG, RA PS, Ashton HA, *et al*. A sustained mortality benefit from screening for abdominal aortic aneurysm. *Ann Intern Med* 2007;**146**:699–706.

Powell JT, Greenhalgh RM. Small abdominal aortic aneurysms. *N Engl J Med* 2003;**348**:1895–901.

The United Kingdom Small Aneurysm Trial (UK SAT) participants. Long-term outcomes of immediate repair compared with surveillance of small abdominal aortic aneurysms. *N Engl J Med* 2002;**346**:1445–52.

Aortic dissection

Acute aortic dissection is an emergency condition occurring when a 'false' blood-containing secondary lumen develops within the media of the aortic wall. Classically, entry occurs via a spontaneous tear in the aortic intima raising an intimal flap, which separates the new 'false' and native true lumens. Occasionally, the initiating event is believed to be bleed from the aortic vaso vasorum without an intimal tear. The false lumen commonly re-enters the true lumen via distal re-entry tears. It has an incidence of 3/100 000 patient/years (Golledge and Eagle 2008) with reports of diagnosis only being established in 15% before autopsy (Mészáros et al. 2002). Aortic dissection weakens the aortic wall predisposing to rupture. The pressurized false lumen may compromise blood flow in major aortic branches, particularly the coronary, carotid, renal and visceral arteries, and may also compromise aortic valve function by disrupting the aortic valve commissures. Acute dissection is the commonest of the acute aortic syndromes. Others include acute intramural haematoma and deep penetrating aortic ulceration (DPU). In patients surviving the acute phase, the dissection becomes chronic.

Classification and early natural history

There are two commonly used classifications of aortic dissection: Stanford and DeBakey. A Stanford type A dissection involves the ascending aorta and this encompasses DeBakey types I (dissection involving the ascending aorta and propagating distally) and II (dissection limited to the ascending aorta) whereas a Stanford type B dissection (and DeBakey type III) involves the descending aorta and beyond (Figure 10.5.1). The classifications are pragmatic as involvement of the ascending aorta determines the treatment approach. Acute dissection affecting the ascending aorta is highly lethal, with an untreated 30-day mortality of ≥50%; the majority of risk occurs in the early hours after symptom onset (Nienaber and Eagle 2003). It may cause death by rupture, particularly into the pericardium, by malperfusion of the coronary, carotids, or visceral arteries and by heart failure due to acute aortic regurgitation. Acute dissection involving the descending aorta has an early mortality risk of 10% (Hagan et al. 2000), predominantly due to rupture or malperfusion. After an arbitrary period of 14 days, patients surviving the initial event display chronic dissection and in this circumstance prognosis is primarily determined by whether the weakened false lumen becomes aneurysmal. Intramural haematoma (IMH) is believed to occur as a consequence of medial vasa vasorum rupture and causes crescentic wall thickening of the aortic wall. It is also classified as types A and B on the basis of ascending aortic involvement and is managed in a similar manner to dissection. IMH may regress with medical treatment, but some patients progress to dissection, rupture, or aneurysm formation. DPU is predominantly a disease of the atherosclerotic aorta and may present acutely with pain, IMH, and rupture. In these circumstances urgent treatment is required. Management of DPU recognized in the chronic phase is predominantly managed medically unless new symptoms develop or aneurysmal progression occurs.

Predisposing factors

The age distribution of aortic dissection is bimodal. The majority of older patients have a history of hypertension. Predisposing factors in the younger group include aortopathies associated with Marfan's syndrome, Loeys–Dietz syndrome, Ehlers–Danlos syndrome (type IV) and familial dissection (Nienaber and Eagle 2003). Other factors include Turner's syndrome, aortic coarctation, pseudoxanthoma elasticum, bicuspid aortic valve, annulo-aortic ectasia, peripartum, and a number of vasculitides, including giant cell arteritis, artherosclerosis previous cardiac surgery especially previous repair of aortic aneurysm (Golledge and Eagle 2008). Catheter- or surgically related iatrogenic dissection and blunt trauma are also possible. Only 50% of patients with type A dissection have a ascending aorta ≥5 cm at diagnosis. Patients with Marfan's and Loeys–Dietz syndromes commonly undergo prophylactic prosthetic or valve-sparing aortic root replacement to reduce the risk of future dissection.

Presentation and diagnosis

Although the majority of patients present with sudden-onset severe chest pain (type A 85%; B 63%), back/interscapular pain (type A 46%; B 64%) (Nienaber and Eagle 2003) a significant minority have pain at other sites or present with symptoms related to limb or organ malperfusion or cardiac compromise including syncope, stroke, breathlessness, haemoptysis, haematemesis, upper airway obstruction paraplegia, and paraparesis. This plethora of presentational features leads to a failure or delay in diagnosis in nearly 40% (Nienaber and Eagle 2003) of cases and a high index of suspicion is required to prompt diagnostic investigations. Examination findings are dependent upon the presence of rupture, tamponade, and branch vessel involvement but may reveal hyper- or hypotension, systolic pressure differential (≥20 mmHg) differences in upper limb systolic blood pressure, an early diastolic murmur (40–50% (Nienaber and Eagle 2003)) with or without heart failure, signs of haemorrhagic or cardiogenic shock, or any signs related to central nervous system, limb, or visceral malperfusion. These patients need to undergo diagnostic imaging before any thrombolytic for a suspected acute coronary syndrome is administered.

Despite the very high early risk in acute dissection, the time from initial symptoms to diagnosis and treatment is commonly >12 hours and >24 hours in a substantial minority. Unlike acute coronary syndromes, there is no established biomarker of aortic dissection but such a point-of-care test is urgently required. Normal D-dimer levels make the diagnosis unlikely but attempts to develop a positively discriminant test have been disappointing. Elevated levels of smooth muscle myosin chains (Suzuki et al. 1999), soluble elastin compounds (Shinohara et al. 2004), and calponins have been demonstrated in acute aortic dissection but lack sufficient sensitivity and specificity for routine application. Any patient with suspected acute aortic dissection should be rapidly investigated. The ECG may be normal 30% (Golledge and Eagle 2008), low voltage, display changes of left ventricular hypertrophy, or demonstrate non-specific or specific ST segment changes consistent with acute ischaemia. A posteroanterior chest radiogram demonstrates a blurred contour/widened mediastinum in 60–90% (Nienaber and Eagle 2003) and abnormal aortic contour in 47% (Golledge and Eagle 2008) cases but may also be normal (30%) (Golledge and Eagle 2008). Transthoracic echocardiography (sensitivity 77–80%,

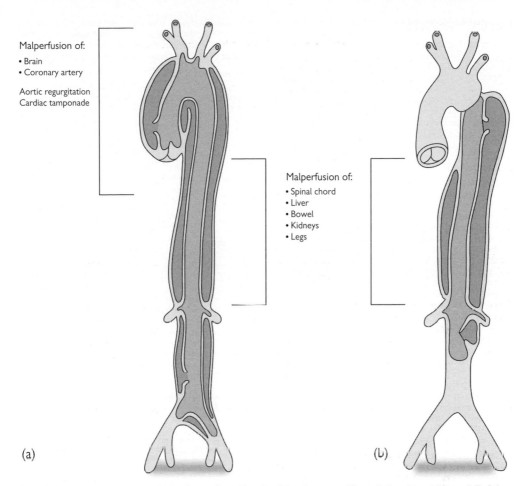

Malperfusion of:
• Brain
• Coronary artery

Aortic regurgitation
Cardiac tamponade

Malperfusion of:
• Spinal chord
• Liver
• Bowel
• Kidneys
• Legs

(a)   (b)

Fig. 10.5.1 Diagram demonstrating aortic dissection and possible malperfusion phenomena. (a) type A dissection and (b) type B (DeBakey type III). A type A dissection involves the ascending aorta and encompasses DeBakey types I and II. A DeBakey type I is depicted; this involves the aorta beyond the ascending section. A DeBakey type II involves the ascending aorta only. The distinction is important: type II dissections have a better prognosis as there is less likelihood of aneurysmal expansion of the distal aorta. Reproduced with permission from Golledge J, Eagle KA, Acute aortic dissection, reprinted from *The Lancet* 372(9632):55–66, copyright 2008, from Elsevier.

specificity 93–96% (Erbel et al. 2001)) may diagnose type A dissection but is insensitive and transoesophageal echocardiography (sensitivity 99%, specificity 89% (Erbel et al. 2001)) or CT scanning (sensitivity 98%, specificity 87%) (Sommer et al. 1996) before and after contrast are the most readily available and useful investigations. Magnetic resonance imaging is also sensitive and specific but has less utility because of the time required and patient instability. The fundamental requirement of imaging is to determine the diagnosis and ascending aortic involvement. Imaging may also reveal the extent and perfusion of the false lumen, pleural or pericardial fluid, aortic side branch involvement, and the presence of co-existing aneurismal aortic disease, and may differentiate other acute aortic syndromes (intramural haematoma/transection). It is also used to locate the intimal tear and flap and detect AR and pericardial tamponade depending on quality of the acoustic windows. Aortic and coronary angiography is rarely required.

Immediately that diagnosis is confirmed, all patients should be discussed with a Cardiothoracic Surgical Centre.

Management
The initial management of all types of suspected acute dissection should include transfer to at least level 2 critical care, resuscitation, pain relief, and antihypertensive therapy. This should include, where possible, intravenous beta-blockade to reduce the force of ventricular contraction and limit the risks of dissection propagation. Therapy should be administered with invasive arterial monitoring. The management of acute type A dissection is nearly always surgical and predominantly comprises emergency graft replacement of the ascending aorta; the segment at most risk of rupture. Some cases suffering independently lethal malperfusion complications may be managed conservatively if surgery is deemed futile. Surgery is conducted utilizing cardiopulmonary bypass and profound cooling is

often used in order to attach a prosthetic graft to or reconstruct the aortic arch. The aims of surgery are to prevent intrapericardial rupture, to re-establish aortic valve competence and to prevent or treat coronary or distal arterial malperfusion. The 30-day mortality of surgery approximates to 25% (Hagan *et al.* 2000; Nienaber and Eagle 2003) with 5-year survival of 60–70% (Hagan *et al.* 2000). Patients of advanced age, rupture, and evidence of branch vessel involvement fare worse. Unfortunately, surgery carries a high risk of neurological complications. There are no randomized trials of medical versus surgical management in acute type A dissection, but multiple observational studies demonstrate that surgery, although high risk, considerably improves survival chances. Medical management on its own in these patients is associated with a mortality rate of 20% within 24 hours of symptoms, 30% by 48 hours 40% by 1 week and >50% by 1 month (Nienaber and Eagle 2003). Late survival is also worse (Tsai *et al.* 2009). There are considerable areas of debate regarding the optimal techniques in the surgery of acute type A dissection including choice of cannulation sites, management of malperfusion, type of repair of the aortic valve, and extent of surgery to effect best short- and long-term outcome. Type B dissections have a lower acute mortality of 10% in the first 30 days (Hagan *et al.* 2000) and if uncomplicated (Nienaber and Eagle 2003) the main initial management remains medical (Tsai *et al.* 2009). Patients should have invasively monitored blood pressure control (systolic <110 mmHg) using analgesics and intravenous beta-blockade if tolerated or in combination with vasodilator drugs, such as sodium nitroprusside or angiotensin-converting enzyme inhibitors (Erbel *et al.* 2001; Nienaber and Eagle 2003). A subgroup of patients with type B dissection present with complications (contained rupture with hypotension, peri-aortic haematoma and branch vessel compromise) and are at much higher risk of early mortality (Nienaber and Eagle 2003). Such complicated patients and should be considered for intervention with the view to relieve life-threatening complications and preventing rupture (Erbel *et al.* 2001). Historically, intervention in complicated type B dissection was by high-risk surgical repair but now endovascular stent placement may be performed at lower risk and is likely to subsume open repair (Erbel *et al.* 2001; Golledge and Eagle 2008; Tsai *et al.* 2009). In certain cases catheter-based fenestration and branch vessel stenting may be needed to treat visceral malperfusion (Nienaber and Eagle 2003). Stenting the aorta after the acute phase does not appear to improve mid-term survival but there are ongoing trials assessing whether stent aortoplasty will accrue long-term benefits.

Late natural history

Residual dissection of untreated aortic segments is very common and predisposes 15–40% of patients to late aneurysm formation and a requirement for further intervention. More extensive surgical repair in acute type A dissection may reduce this risk of aneurysm formation but may increase the risks of the emergency repair. The overall 10-year survival is 40–60%. Marfan's syndrome patients have the highest risk of requiring further aortic procedures. In all patients, long-term aggressive control of blood pressure and imaging surveillance in dedicated aortic clinics is required (Erbel *et al.* 2001; Mészáros *et al.* 2002; Nienaber and Eagle 2003) to assess the need for further surgical or endovascular intervention.

References

Erbel R, Alfonso F, Boileau C, *et al*. Diagnosis and management of aortic dissection. *Eur Heart J* 2001;**22**:1642–81.

Golledge J, Eagle KA. Acute aortic dissection. *Lancet* 2008;**372**:55–66.

Hagan PG, Nienaber CA, Isselbacher EM, *et al*. The International Registry of Acute Aortic Dissection (IRAD): new insights into an old disease. *JAMA* 2000;**283**:897–903.

Mészáros I, Mórocz J, Szlávi J, *et al*. Epidemiology and clinicopathology of aortic dissection. *Chest* 2002;**117**:1271–8.

Nienaber CA, Eagle KA. Aortic dissection: new frontiers in diagnosis and management: Part I: from etiology to diagnostic strategies. *Circulation* 2003;**108**:628–35.

Nienaber CA, Eagle KA. Aortic dissection: new frontiers in diagnosis and management: Part II: therapeutic management and follow-up. *Circulation* 2003;**108**:772–8.

Shinohara T, Suzuki K, Okada M, *et al*. Soluble elastin fragments in serum are elevated in aortic dissection. *J Cardiol* 2004;**43**:96–7.

Sommer T, Fehske W, Holzknecht N, *et al*. Aortic dissection: a comparative study of diagnosis with spiral CT, multiplanar transesophageal echocardiography, and MR imaging. *Radiology* 1996;**199**:347–52.

Suzuki T, Katoh H, Nagai R. Biochemical diagnosis of aortic dissection: from bench to bedside. *Jpn Heart J* 1999;**40**:527–34.

Tsai TT, Trimarchi S, Nienaber CA. Acute aortic dissection: perspectives from the International Registry of Acute Aortic Dissection (IRAD). *Eur J Vasc Endovasc Surg* 2009;**37**:149–59.

Deep vein thrombosis

Deep vein thrombosis (DVT) is a common disorder that can affect apparently healthy as well as hospitalized patients.

Most frequently DVT occurs in the lower limbs, but it can also affect the upper limbs as well as any other district (e.g. splanchnic veins, cerebral veins, retinal veins). Between 40% and 50% of patients presenting with DVT symptoms have concomitant, silent pulmonary embolism.

Overall, DVT occurs for the first time in about 100 people per 100 000 each year (White 2003), and its incidence increases exponentially with age, particularly after age 40 years (Anderson 1991).

Causes

On the whole, DVT is probably best understood as a multicausal disease. The individual risk of DVT varies as a result of a complex interaction between congenital and transient or permanent acquired risk factors. The main processes underlying DVT are summarized in the Virchow's triad: venous stasis, vessel wall injury, and hypercoagulable state (congenital of acquired).

Major risk factors

- Age
- Immobilization longer then 3 days
- Trauma in previous 4 weeks (e.g. major trauma of lower extremity fractures, with bone immobilization)
- Major surgery in previous 4 weeks
- Acute medical illness (e.g. stroke, congestive heart failure, acute myocardial infarction, sepsis, ulcerative colitis, nephrotic syndrome)
- Pregnancy and the postpartum period
- Estro-progestinic drugs
- Cancer
- Congenital thrombophilic disorders (antithrombin deficiency, protein C deficiency, protein S deficiency, prothrombin 20210A mutation, factor V Leiden mutation, elevated factor VIII levels)
- Acquired thrombophilic disorders (e.g. antiphospholipid antibody syndrome, hyperhomocysteinaemia) or hypercoagulable states (e.g. polycythaemia rubra vera, thrombocytosis)
- Intravenous drug abuse
- Previous DVT
- Family history of DVT or pulmonary embolism.

Symptoms and signs

Common symptoms of lower limb DVT are the following:
- Swelling of the lower limb, principally unilateral
- Leg pain, principally unilateral: patients can complain either entirely limb pain or discomfort of the calf
- Tenderness of the limb
- Warmth or erythema of skin.

Many patients with DVT can be asymptomatic or can refer bland symptoms.

Most frequent, but not specific signs are:
- Oedema, principally unilateral
- Tenderness, if present, is usually confined to the calf muscles or along the course of the deep veins in the medial thigh

- Pain exacerbated by dorsiflexion of the foot with the knee straight (Homans's sign)
- Prominence of the subcutaneous veins
- Fever: patients may have a low-grade fever.

Differential diagnoses

Many non-thrombotic conditions produce signs and symptoms suggestive of DVT:
- Arterial insufficiency
- Arthritis
- Asymmetric peripheral oedema secondary to cardiac heart failure, liver disease, renal failure, or nephrotic syndrome
- Cellulitis, lymphangitis
- Extrinsic compression of an iliac vein secondary to cancer
- Lymphoedema
- Muscle or soft tissue injury
- Neurogenic pain
- Post-phlebitic syndrome
- Prolonged immobilization or limb paralysis
- Ruptured Baker's cyst
- Algodystrophic syndrome
- Varicose veins and superficial thrombophlebitis.

Investigations

Neither a single physical finding nor the combination of symptoms and signs are sufficiently accurate to establish the diagnosis of DVT. Ultrasonography is currently the first-line imaging examination for the diagnosis of DVT, because of its relative ease of use, absence of irradiation or contrast material, and high sensitivity and specificity. Ultrasound examination to be performed in a suspected DVT is the so called compression ultrasonography (CUS), either 'complete', exploring in the axial plane with a 5- to 10-MHz transducer both distal and proximal veins, or 'limited', exploring proximal veins (popliteal, superficial femoral, deep femoral, common femoral) only. Compression is intermittently applied to induce complete coaptation of the walls of the patent vein: if the vein does not compress, it is occluded (Heijboer 1993). The two diagnostic strategies, complete CUS and limited CUS have been shown to be equivalent for the management of symptomatic outpatients with suspected DVT (Bernardi 2008).

To reduce the need for imaging tests in all outpatients presenting with suspected DVT, the use of pre-test clinical probability scores (e.g. Wells DVT score) and of D-dimer measurement is currently recommended. This combined approach can safely identify those patients who do not require further objective diagnostic testing.

Outpatients with leg symptoms and signs compatible with DVT should initially have a determination of pre-test probability of DVT using an established prediction score (Table 10.6.1).

If the probability of DVT is 'likely', patients should undergo CUS. If urgent testing is unavailable, imaging can be arranged the following day and patients should receive an injection of low-molecular-weight heparin (LMWH) (treatment dose). In case the pre-test probability is 'unlikely', a D-dimer high sensitivity test should be performed.

D-dimer is a degradation product of fibrin and is elevated in acute DVT. However, D-dimer levels may also be increased

Table 10.6.1 Simplified clinical model for assessment of DVT*

Clinical variable	Score
Active cancer (treatment ongoing or within previous 6 months or palliative)	1
Paralysis, paresis, or recent plaster immobilization of the lower extremities	1
Recently bedridden for 3 days or more, or major surgery within the previous 12 weeks requiring general or regional anesthesia	1
Localized tenderness along the distribution of the deep venous system	1
Entire leg swelling	1
Calf swelling at least 3 cm larger than that on the asymptomatic leg (measured 10 cm below the tibial tuberosity)	1
Pitting oedema confined to the symptomatic leg	1
Collateral superficial veins (non-varicose)	1
Previously documented DVT	1
Alternative diagnosis at least as likely as DVT	−2

≥2, probability of DVT is 'likely'.
≤1, probability for DVT is 'unlikely'.

by non-thrombotic disorders (e.g. recent major surgery, haemorrhage, trauma, malignancy, sepsis, pregnancy, oestrogen therapy). Its potential value is for a negative test result to 'rule out' the diagnosis of DVT. Thus, if the D-dimer test is positive, then CUS needs to be performed, but if the test result is negative, then the diagnosis of DVT can be safely excluded.

When imaging test is indicated and ultrasound is performed, limited CUS is an acceptable strategy. The positivity of the test (lack of complete vein compressibility) will 'rule in' the diagnosis of DVT. In case the test is negative (veins are completely compressible), then a repeat ultrasound no more than 1 week later is generally recommended (Wells 2007).

If the patient has a positive history of DVT, the results of previous ultrasound tests are needed, in particular if ipsilateral recurrence is suspected: an increase in clot diameter by 4 mm or more is suggestive of recurrence.

Treatment

Initial treatment acute DVT
Current guidelines (Kearon *et al.* 2008) recommend initial treatment with LMWH, unfractionated heparin (UFH), or fondaparinux for at least 5 days and until the international normalized ration (INR) is >2.0 for 24 hours. Vitamin K antagonists (VKAs) like warfarin should be initiated together with LMWH, UFH, or fondaparinux on the first treatment day. The dose of VKAs should be adjusted to achieve and maintain a target INR of 2.5 (range 2.0–3.0).

Placement of a vena cava filter has to be considered only if anticoagulant therapy is contraindicated (e.g. in the presence of active bleeding) on if the thrombotic event occurred despite adequate anticoagulant therapy.

Duration of anticoagulant therapy
Optimal duration of secondary prevention of DVT depends on the pathogenesis of the index event. For patients with DVT secondary to a transient (reversible) risk factor, treatment with VKAs for 3 months is recommended. For patients with unprovoked DVT (no major risk factors have been identified), it is currently recommended to administer VKAs for at least 3 months and then to evaluate for all patients the risk-to-benefit ratio of long-term therapy. For patients with a first unprovoked, proximal DVT, in whom risk factors for bleeding are absent and for whom good anticoagulant monitoring is achievable, long-term treatment is suggested with subsequent evaluations over time of the risk to benefit ratio of antithrombotic treatment. A great value is attributed to patients' preferences.

For patients with a second episode of unprovoked VTE and for patients with other permanent risk factors, long-term treatment is recommended.

Elastic stockings with an ankle pressure gradient of 30–40 mmHg should be started as soon as feasible after starting anticoagulant therapy and should be continued for a minimum of 2 years, and longer if patients have symptoms of post-thrombotic syndrome.

Specials situations
* Pregnancy: VKAs should be avoided because of the risk of possible fetal malformation: LMWH can be used safely throughout pregnancy.
* Renal failure: LMWH should not be used in patients with creatine clearance <30 mL/min for the possibility of accumulation with consequent haemorrhagic complication.
* Morbid obesity: as in patients with renal failure, UFH should be preferred.
* Asymptomatic, incidentally detected DVT: current guidelines recommend the same treatment as for proximal DVT, even if the clinical relevance of such events has yet to be established.
* Isolated calf DVT (anterior tibial, posterior tibial, peroneal, or deep muscular veins): current guidelines recommend the same treatment as for proximal DVT (3 months of VKAs). A shorter course of LMWH (i.e. 6 weeks) is largely applied in some European countries, but evidences are lacking.
* Cancer patients: weight-adjusted doses of LMWH are currently recommended for the first 3–6 months after the index event. Subsequently, anticoagulant therapy with VKAs or LMWH should be administered indefinitely or until cancer is resolved given the high risk of recurrence in these patients.

Complications
* Acute pulmonary embolism.
* Phlegmasia cerulea dolens: soft tissue ischaemia associated with massive clot and very high venous pressures. In this case thrombolytic therapy may be considered.
* Post-thrombotic syndrome: pain and oedema in the affected limb without new clot formation. It is a chronic complication of DVT that manifests months to many years after the initial event. Symptoms range from mild erythema and localized induration to massive extremity swelling and ulceration, usually exacerbated by standing and relieved by elevation of the extremity.

- Haemorrhagic complications are the most common adverse effects of anticoagulant therapy. The risk of major haemorrhage while taking VKAs is approximately 1%/year if treatment is managed by expert centres.

Prevention

Every hospital should develop a formal local thromboprophylactic strategy.

Thromboprophylaxis, usually with low-dose LMWH or fondaparinux, is routinely indicated in patients undergoing major general abdominal surgery, major thoracic surgery, major gynaecologic surgery, major open urological procedures, bariatric surgery, major orthopaedic surgery (e.g. elective knee replacement, hip fracture surgery, elective hip replacement), and also in major trauma patients, acutely ill medical patients (e.g. patients with congestive heart failure or severe respiratory disease, or who are confined to bed and have one or more additional risk factors, including active cancer, previous venous thromboembolism, sepsis, acute neurological disease, or inflammatory bowel disease).

Prophylaxis for DVT is generally recommended for all patients with individual additional risk factors (Geerts 2008).

FAQs

- Can a patient with acute DVT ambulate? Early ambulation after initiation of anticoagulant therapy in addition to effective compression is recommended. The fear of dislodging clots thus precipitating a fatal pulmonary embolism is unfounded.
- Is it necessary to hospitalize patients with acute DVT? DVT can be safely treated at home in all patients who do not present contraindications to a home-treatment management. Of course, these should be carefully excluded: suspected or proven concomitant pulmonary embolism, significant cardiovascular or pulmonary co-morbidity, contraindications to anticoagulation, morbid obesity, severe renal failure, unavailability for adequate follow-up visits, possible lack of compliance.

- Is vitamin K intake restriction necessary during treatment with VKAs? During VKAs treatment a normal vitamin K intake is required, thus, diet restrictions are not recommended.
- Is it useful to provide periodic ultrasound follow-up of the thrombus during anticoagulant treatment? Because treatment duration is currently not influenced by the presence of residual thrombosis, regular ultrasound monitoring during treatment is not necessary unless the patient has symptoms or signs of suspected recurrence. CUS with the measurement of residual thrombus dimensions is recommended at the time when anticoagulant suspension is considered.

References

Anderson FA, Wheeler HB, Goldberg RJ, et al. A population based perspective of the hospital incidence and case fatality rates of deep vein thrombosis and pulmonary embolism. The Worcester DVT study. Arch Int Med 1991;**151**:933–8.

Bernardi E, Camporese G, Buller HR, for the ERASMUS study group. Serial 2-point ultrasonography plus D-dimer vs whole-leg color-coded Doppler ultrasonography for diagnosing suspected symptomatic deep vein thrombosis: a randomized controlled trial. JAMA 2008;**300**:1653–9.

Geerts WH, Bergqvist D, Pineo G, et al. Prevention of venous thromboembolism. American College of Chest Physicians Evidence-Based Clinical Practice Guidelines (8th Edition). Chest 2008;**133**:381S–453S.

Heijboer H, Buller HR, Lensing AWA, et al. A comparison of real-time compression ultrasonography with impedance plethysmography for the diagnosis of deep-vein thrombosis in symptomatic outpatients. N Engl J Med 1993;**329**:1365–9.

Kearon C, Kahn SR, Agnelli G, et al. Antithrombotic therapy for venous thromboembolic disease: American College of Chest Physicians evidence-based clinical practice guidelines (8th edition). Chest 2008;**133**:454S–545S.

Wells PS. Integrated strategies for the diagnosis of venous thromboembolism. J Thromb Haemost 2007;**5**:41S–50S.

White RH. The epidemiology of venous thromboembolism. Circulation 2003;**107**:I-4–I-8.

Chapter 11

Cardiac consultations and emergencies

Perioperative evaluation for cardiac surgery

Physiology of bypass

- A systemic inflammatory response created by bloods exposure to the extracorporeal circuits utilized in cardiopulmonary bypass (CPB) alters clotting ability, activates platelets, and can result in lung injury leading to acute respiratory distress syndrome
- The non-pulsatile flow of cardiopulmonary bypass disrupts the normal pulsatile flow of the cardiovascular system altering the feedback loops in the kidneys and brain.

Preoperative risk analysis

The approach to preoperative risk analysis for cardiac surgery encapsulates the same principles for risk analysis for non-cardiac surgery (Eagle et al. 2002).

Non-modifiable risk factors

Age

Patients greater than 80 years of age have twice the risk of death, a markedly higher risk of prolonged ventilation time, more frequent reoperation for bleeding, and longer hospital stays.

Gender

Early mortality has been found to be significantly higher in women undergoing coronary artery bypass graft (CABG) even after adjustment for confounding factors such as low body surface area (Blankstein et al. 2005).

Pregnancy

- Cardiac surgery during pregnancy is associated with increased maternal and fetal mortality rates.
- Poor functional class, age, type of surgery, and reoperation are associated with a higher risk of maternal death.
- Maternal age more than 35 years, functional class, reoperation, emergency surgery, and anoxic time can have adverse effects on fetal survival.

Preoperative medical conditions

Renal dysfunction

- Risk stratification is better using estimated or measured glomerular filtration rate (GFR) rather than serum creatinine.

Mild elevations of preoperative creatinine can significantly increase perioperative mortality, need for haemodialysis, and length of hospital stay (Antunes et al. 2004).

- Dialysis dependence is a major risk with bypass surgery that may be reduced with off-pump CABG (OPCAB).
- Patients who have undergone kidney transplantation show better survival than those on dialysis.

Atrial fibrillation

- Pre-existing atrial fibrillation in patients undergoing CABG is not associated with increased in-hospital mortality or major morbidity. Preoperative atria fibrillation is associated with increased perioperative stroke (Banach et al. 2008).
- If patients in AF require surgical revascularization, it is appropriate to consider performing a concomitant surgical ablation procedure.

Pulmonary disease

Preoperative COPD, defined as those undergoing active therapy or having a FEV_1 <75% of predicted, leads to a higher mortality and higher incidence of postoperative respiratory complications requiring prolonged ICU and hospital stay (Canver et al. 1998).

Stroke

- Preoperative stroke carries a high risk of developing postoperative neurological complications.
- An accepted practice is to wait 2–3 months after a stroke before placing a patient on bypass.
- Patients with remote CVA, even after complete recovery, often exhibit signs of reactivation where some or all of the previous symptoms reappear, albeit in a milder form. Although the prognosis for recovery is good, several weeks are sometimes needed.

Carotid artery disease

- Carotid artery disease may be associated with postoperative stroke.
- Although preoperative screening with bilateral duplex ultrasound of all also left main disease patients is still done in some institutions, limiting this process to patients older than 65, those with a carotid bruit, or those with suspected or established cerebrovascular disease can reduce the screening load with negligible impact on neurological outcomes (Durand et al. 2004).
- In cases where critical, symptomatic carotid artery stenosis exists at the time of CABG, a combined or staged CABG and carotid endarterectomy can be done with excellent results. It is unclear whether a combined or staged technique shows superior outcomes. In staged surgery, carotid endarterectomy is done first.

Hepatic disease

- Liver disease may be associated with complex multifactorial coagulopathies.
- Complication rates can be high for all Pugh Classes, but rates may be lower for OPCAB in such patients (Hayashida et al. 2004).

Haematological/oncological disease

- Whether cardiac surgery is justifiable in patients with malignant tumours is determined by the patients life expectancy based on long-term prognosis of the malignancy.
- Cardiac operations can be performed with acceptable mortality in patients with haematological malignancies but with significant morbidity rates, most often bleeding and infection.

Cardiovascular risk factors

Cigarette smoking

- Smokers are twice as likely to develop postoperative respiratory complications.
- Patients who have stopped smoking for more than 6 months have complication rates similar to those who have never smoked.
- Even smoking cessation for more than 2 months can significantly reduce the rate of respiratory complications.

Obesity

- Long-term survival may be reduced, and higher rates of atrial fibrillation, bleeding, and reoperation may occur in obese patients.
- A BMI >40 leads to significantly more complications, including a higher incidence of postoperative sternal wound infections, prolonged ventilation, and longer hospital stay.

Diabetes

- Diabetics show a significantly higher rate of major post-operative complications including acute renal failure, sternal wound infection, and prolonged postoperative stay (Kubal *et al.* 2005).
- The absence of diabetes-related target organ damage is associated with long-term survival after CABG that is similar to that in patients without diabetes.

Peripheral vascular disease

- Off-pump CABG is safe in PVD patients with a reduced incidence of postoperative stroke, but higher risk for limb ischaemia and leg wound infection.
- When calcification of the ascending aorta is detected on thoracic imaging studies, evaluation with intraoperative epiaortic ultrasound should be considered to map out the location of calcium and to avoid vascular disruption or stroke during cannulation or proximal anastomoses of bypass grafts.
- The presence of the most severe aortic calcification known as 'porcelain aorta' may lead to a decision to pursue OPCAB or an alternative approach to aortic cannulation or proximal grafting.

Preoperative risk calculation

- Two widely used models to estimate perioperative risk are the EuroSCORE additive model and the Society of Thoracic Surgeons (STS) model.
- The EuroSCORE is the most rigorously evaluated scoring system and has been used for estimating perioperative mortality, length of stay, and specific postoperative complications.
- The EuroSCORE is better at predicting 30–day mortality than the STS algorithm for patients undergoing CABG (Nilsson *et al.* 2004).
- The additive EuroSCORE greatly underestimates risk in high-risk patients when compared with the logistic version (Jin and Grunkemeier 2005)
- The additive version generally overestimates mortality at lower scores (EuroSCORE 6) and underestimates mortality at higher values (EuroSCORE >13) (Gogbashian *et al.* 2004).
- A scoring system using blood tests and clinical risk factors to determine thromboembolic risk after heart valve replacement may be used to guide prosthesis choice and antithrombotic management.

Prevention of complications

Case volume

- As a discriminator of quality of care, the use of hospital volumes of cardiac surgery, which may combine the experience of a wide range of individual surgeons, is disputed.
- There is considerable variation in adjusted mortality within low-volume and high-volume groups so that overall, volume criterion alone is a poor discriminator of mortality.
- Volume statistics of individual surgeons seem to be a better quality criterion. Patients treated by low-volume surgeons have significantly higher mortality rates than those treated by medium-volume surgeons (51–100 cases annually), high-volume surgeons (101–150 cases annually), or very-high-volume surgeons (>151 cases annually).

Surgical technique

- Conventional midline sternotomy is the standard.
- Off-pump CABG (OPCAB) may be considered using a median sternotomy or with MIDCAB procedures.
- Among eligible patients OPCAB appears to be as good as, or superior to, on-pump CABG in terms of reduced length of hospital stay, operative morbidity and mortality, and postoperative renal failure, especially in high-risk patients (after acute myocardial infarction (MI)).
- Moderate- or high-risk patients (elderly people with multiple co-morbidities or emergency patients operated within the first 48 hours of acute (MI)) can preferentially be treated using OPCAB when complete revascularization with this technique is possible.
- After risk adjustment, patients with critical left main stem stenosis or those with diffuse coronary disease can undergo OPCAB safely, with results similar to on-pump CABG.
- Anatomical factors against OPCAB include target vessel size less than 1.25 mm, calcification, intramyocardial location of target vessels, and multiple stenoses.
- Experienced OPCAB surgeons have a low risk of acute conversion to CPB.
- Acutely converted patients have a moderately increased risk of in-hospital death and serious complications that are difficult to quantify because conversion is infrequent and unpredictable.
- Minimally invasive direct CABG (MIDCAB), conducted through a left thoracotomy, is limited to patients with amenable coronary anatomy.

Baseline laboratory evaluation

- A high preoperative white blood cell (WBC) count has been associated with more perioperative CVAs, increased neuropsychological morbidity, and higher 1–year mortality (Newall *et al.* 2006)
- Markedly elevated serum troponin levels (e.g. 5–10 times normal) measured within 24 hours before elective CABG identifies patients with higher risk for perioperative MI and higher in-hospital mortality (Thielmann *et al.* 2005)

Preoperative drug therapy

- Preoperative aspirin taken within 5 days preceding CABG is associated with lower in-hospital mortality without an increased risk of reoperation for bleeding or need for blood transfusion.
- The risk versus benefit of preoperative administration of clopidogrel remains unresolved.
- Preoperative clopidogrel is an independent risk factor for increased transfusion requirements and prolonged ICU and hospital length of stay. If administered within 5 days before CABG, early mortality and morbidity are increased, and the risk of death is greatest when the drug is given within 48 hours of surgery (Ascione *et al.* 2005).
- Patients who undergo early CABG after non-ST elevation acute coronary syndromes show significant improvement in cardiovascular outcomes with preoperative clopidogrel therapy, with no significant increase in life-threatening postoperative bleeding.
- It is recommended that surgery in patients on clopidogrel be performed using standard heparinization and antifibrinolytic strategies, platelet transfusion prior to chest closure may have a beneficial effect.

- Preoperative enoxaparin given less than 12 hours before CABG is associated with lower postoperative haemoglobin and higher rates of transfusion when than preoperative unfractionated heparin administration.
- Preoperative statin therapy confers a protective benefit on postoperative outcomes including early mortality, morbidity, MI, and a-fib after surgery.

Neurological

- Prevention of neurological injury by the reduction of atheroembolic episodes related to aortic manipulation can be achieved by the use of aortic imaging.
- The surgeon can carefully select the safest area for cross-clamp application, aortic cannulation, and conduit anastomosis.
- Identifying the presence of atrial fibrillation and initiating appropriate anticoagulation can reduce the risk of perioperative stroke.
- Appropriate screening and identification of carotid artery disease enables planning of a staged or combined procedure when applicable.

Infectious

- Antibiotics should be given to all patients undergoing cardiac surgery 30–60 minutes before skin incision. If the duration of surgery exceeds 3 hours, readministration of antibiotics should occur.
- The cephalosporin class is utilized unless a true penicillin allergy exists, in which case vancomycin is used.
- Unless an infection is present, antibiotics should only be continued for 1 day postoperatively.
- Some centres advocate the use of chlorhexidine gluconate oropharyngeal rinse or nasal ointment for preoperative decontamination of *Staphylococcus aureus*. This type of selective decontamination has reduced rates of nosocomial infection and length of stay.

Atrial arrhythmias

- Postoperative atrial fibrillation is a common complication after cardiac surgery and can potentially be avoided with the preoperative use of beta-blockers or amiodarone.
- Postoperative withdrawal of beta-blockers should be avoided as this increases the risk of postoperative atrial fibrillation considerably.

Early postoperative period

Haemodynamic monitoring

- Invasive haemodynamic monitoring after cardiac surgery is essential as the rapid fluid and electrolyte shifts, transient myocardial depression, and dramatic fluctuations in vascular tone require the use of invasive monitoring to ensure adequate tissue oxygen delivery.

Postoperative haemodynamic changes

- Rewarming near the end of most cardiac procedures, results in systemic vasodilation, decreased systemic blood pressure and the redistribution of blood volume to the periphery.
- Although normally resolved after several hours, maintaining adequate mean arterial pressure with vasoconstricting agents is frequently needed.
- A transient increase in pulmonary vascular resistance, secondary to platelet activation and the administration of protamine and other blood products, may develop.

- When RV function is compromised, the use of pulmonary vasodilators such as milrinone, nitroglycerine, and nitric oxide is needed may be needed.
- Transient RV dysfunction, as a consequence of inadequate myocardial preservation techniques in combination with an increase in pulmonary resistance, can lead to cardiogenic shock secondary to an underfilled left ventricle.

Management of intravascular volume

- A potential consequence of CPB is a generalized, temporary capillary leak syndrome, resulting in intravascular volume depletion with a lowering of ventricular filling pressures, and a decrease in cardiac output and mean arterial pressure.
- The use of homologous blood products is associated with an immunosuppressive, immunomodulary effect, which may increase the risk of viral and bacterial infections.
- The third-spaced fluid should begin to redistribute into the vascular space after 48 hours when the capillary leak ceases.
- Patients may require diuretics if they begin to demonstrate signs or symptoms of a volume-overloaded state.
- Many patients begin to autodiurese between postoperative days 1 and 3.

Postoperative shock and circulatory support

- The hallmark of postcardiotomy cardiogenic shock is low cardiac output/index.
- Correctable aetiologies, such as acidaemia or myocardial ischaemia secondary to arterial spasm or vein graft closure, must be identified and treated.
- If the cardiac index is <2 L/min/m^2 after optimization of heart rate and rhythm, volume status, and haemoglobin levels and factors such as ischaemia and tamponade are ruled out then approaches to improve contractility and cardiac output are needed.
- Some situations present with elevated right ventricular filling pressures and inadequate left ventricular filling pressures consistent with right ventricular failure.
- A variety of inotropes are available to treat low output syndromes including adrenaline (epinephrine), noradrenaline (norepinephrine), dopamine, and dobutamine.
- Milrinone is a phosphodiesterase inhibitor that increases cardiac output and reduces pulmonary and systemic vascular resistance. Milrinone is often used in situations that involve the right ventricle since it reduces pulmonary vascular resistance.
- In some settings, pharmacological intervention remains inadequate requiring the use of mechanical support.
- The most commonly used device is the intra-aortic balloon pump (IABP), which is placed percutaneously and functions by improving coronary blood flow during diastole and reducing afterload during systole.
- Short-term support with temporary ventricular assist devices (VADs) are occasionally necessary. They function by drainage of the ventricle followed by pneumatically driven pulsatile delivery of blood to the aorta, pulmonary artery, or both.
- Weaning from these devices can be attempted when cardiac index is optimized with minimal support and if there is echocardiographic evidence of improving

ventricular function. When unable to be weaned from short-term support, then long-term support can be provided with more durable devices that are best suited for bridging to transplantation.

Tamponade
- The diagnosis of pericardial tamponade should be considered anytime the patient's haemodynamics are impaired.
- The classic presentation of pericardial tamponade is not usually present in the post-cardiac surgery patient.
- Postoperative pericardial constriction may manifest as focal chamber compression by blood or a clot.
- Chest tubes, sternal bandages, or residual mediastinal air compromise the ability to effectively diagnose pericardial tamponade or compression with standard transthoracic imaging. Transoesophageal echocardiography is a much more sensitive tool in this setting.

Postoperative haemostasis
- Management of postoperative bleeding requires an understanding of the patient's history, medication use, and laboratory assessment of the patient's coagulation profile.
- One strategy for decreasing the need for allogeneic blood transfusion is the preoperative donation of autologous blood or the autotransfusion of scavenged mediastinal blood.
- Antifibrinolytics, lysine analogues, and serine protease inhibitors are frequently used to decrease bleeding.
- Lysine analogues are most commonly utilized due to their low cost, especially in first time operations.
- The lysine analogue, aprotinin, is associated with a severe hypersensitivity reaction with re-exposure.
- Cardiopulmonary bypass activates platelets resulting in thrombocytopenia, creates fibrinolysis, and reduces circulating factors.
- Early assessment and correction of underlying aetiologies is imperative. If excessive bleeding continues, re-exploration is indicated while correcting any coagulopathy.
- The phenomenon of heparin rebound refers to the reappearance of a heparin effect after neutralization by protamine. This occurs due to the different elimination of protamine and heparin and because of abnormalities in the rewarming process.

Graft patency
- The use of the left internal mammary artery as a conduit to the left anterior descending artery is now standard of care.
- Revascularization with the internal mammary artery (IMA) yields better long-term outcomes than the use of saphenous vein grafts (SVG) as vein grafts are more prone to intimal proliferation and early atherosclerosis.
- 1-year patency rates are similar, however, at 5 and 10 years, the patency rates for IMA grafts is 88% and 83%, respectively, whereas the rates for SVGs is 74% and 41%.
- SVG patency is enhanced by early use of 325 mg of ASA.
- In patients who are at high risk of mediastinitis, the obese and diabetics, it is best to avoid the use of both internal mammary arteries.

- Radial arteries are prone to vasospasm and patients who receive this type of graft need to receive long-term therapy with a calcium channel blocker or nitrate.
- Postoperative vascular spasm can occur in the native coronary arteries and grafts leading to MI, ventricular arrhythmias, LV dysfunction and death.
- Diagnosis can be made by electrocardiogram or echocardiography with wall motion abnormalities.
- Treatment with nitroglycerine and/or calcium channel blockers can be helpful.

Epicardial pacing
- Epicardial atrial electrodes usually exit from the right side of the chest while ventricular leads exit the left side.
- Placement of two atrial leads allows bipolar pacing and electrogram recording.
- Bipolar pacing requires less energy output which reduces diaphragmatic and chest wall stimulation.
- Ventricular electrograms allow differentiation between ventricular tachycardia and a supraventricular tachycardia with aberrant conduction.

Neurological injury
- Neurological complications including permanent cerebrovascular accidents (type 1 deficit) and cognitive decline (type 2 deficit) occur in 1–4% and 50–80%, respectively, of patients after standard CPB.
- Both injuries are associated with increased mortality, increased length of stay, and increased likelihood of discharge to a nursing home.
- The most predictive risk factor for type 1 deficits is aortic atherosclerosis.
- Strategies aimed at reducing the risk of neurological complications focus on the presence of aortic atherosclerosis, cerebrovascular disease, and cardiac sources of emboli such as in atrial fibrillation.
- Attempts have been made to lessen the amount of aortic manipulation with the single-clamp technique and the use of off-pump procedures.

Infectious complications
- Many patients develop low-grade fevers in the first several days that generally resolve spontaneously, yet an aggressive strategy to identify the pathogen should be undertaken. Most of these are thought to be due to postoperative atalectasis of a lung.
- Deep sternal wound infections and mediastinitis are associated with a two to three times increase in the incidence of death.
- The most important predisposing risk factor for deep sternal wound infections is poorly controlled perioperative blood glucose. Tight glucose control greatly reduces the incidence.
- Other risk factors include re-do procedures and the use of both internal mammary arteries.
- Once a deep sternal wound infection is diagnosed, aggressive antimicrobial therapy, surgical debridement, and early muscle flap coverage are recommended.

References

Antunes PE, Prieto D, Ferrão de Oliveira J, Antunes MJ. Renal dysfunction after myocardial revascularization. *Eur J Cardiothorac Surg* 2004;**25**:597–604.

Ascione R, Ghosh A, Rogers CA, Cohen A, Monk C, Angelini GD. In-hospital patients exposed to clopidogrel before coronary artery bypass graft surgery: a word of caution. *Ann Thorac Surg* 2005;**79**:1210–6.

Banach M, Goch A, Misztal M, *et al*. Relation between postoperative mortality and atrial fibrillation before surgical revascularization—3-year follow-up. *Thorac Cardiovasc Surg* 2008;**56**:20–3.

Blankstein R, Ward RP, Arnsdorf M, Jones B, Lou YB, Pine M. Female gender is an independent predictor of operative mortality after coronary artery bypass graft surgery: contemporary analysis of 31 Midwestern hospitals. *Circulation* 2005;**112** (9 Suppl):I323–7.

Canver CC, Nichols RD, Kroncke GM. Influence of age-specific lung function on survival after coronary bypass. *Ann Thorac Surg* 1998;**66**:144–7.

Durand DJ, Perler B.A, Roseborough GS, *et al*. Mandatory versus selective preoperative carotid screening: a retrospective analysis. *Ann Thorac Surg* 2004;**78**:159–66; Discussion 159–66.

Eagle KA, Berger PB, Calkins H, *et al*. ACC/AHA Guideline Update for Perioperative Cardiovascular Evaluation for Noncardiac Surgery—Executive Summary. A Report of the American College of Cardiology/American Heart Association Task Force on Practice Guidelines (Committee to Update the 1996 Guidelines on Perioperative Cardiovascular Evaluation for Noncardiac Surgery). *J Am Coll Cardiol* 2002;**39**:542–53.

Gogbashian A, Sedrakyan A, Treasure T. EuroSCORE: a systematic review of international performance. *Eur J Cardiothorac Surg* 2004;**25**:695–700.

Hayashida N, Shoujima T, Teshima H, *et al*. Clinical outcome after cardiac operations in patients with cirrhosis. *Ann Thorac Surg* 2004;**77**:500–5.

Jin R, Grunkemeier GL. Additive vs. logistic risk models for cardiac surgery mortality. *Eur J Cardiothorac Surg* 2005;**28**:240–3.

Kubal C, Srinivasan AK, Grayson AD, Fabri BM, Chalmers JA. Effect of risk-adjusted diabetes on mortality and morbidity after coronary artery bypass surgery. *Ann Thorac Surg* 2005;**79**:1570–6.

Lindhout AH, Wouters CW, Noyez L. Influence of obesity on in-hospital and early mortality and morbidity after myocardial revascularization. *Eur J Cardiothorac Surg* 2004;**26**:535–41.

Lindvall G, Sartipy U, Bjessmo S, Svenarud P, Lindvall B, van der Linden J. Aprotinin reduces the antiplatelet effect of clopidogrel. *Interact Cardiovasc Thorac Surg* 2009;**9**:178–81.

Newall N, Grayson AD, Oo AY, *et al*. Preoperative white blood cell count is independently associated with higher perioperative cardiac enzyme release and increased 1–year mortality after coronary artery bypass grafting. *Ann Thorac Surg* 2006;**81**:583–9.

Nilsson J, Algotsson L, Höglund P, Lührs C, Brandt J. Early mortality in coronary bypass surgery: the EuroSCORE versus The Society of Thoracic Surgeons risk algorithm. *Ann Thorac Surg* 2004;**77**:1235–9; Discussion 1239–40.

Thielmann M, Massoudy P, Neuhäuser M, *et al*. Risk stratification with cardiac troponin I in patients undergoing elective coronary artery bypass surgery. *Eur J Cardiothorac Surg* 2005;**27**:861–9.

Perioperative evaluation for non-cardiac surgery

The ageing of society in developed countries has seen increasing ages of people undergoing major surgical procedures and an increasing prevalence of cardiovascular disease in these patients. Improvements in surgical techniques and anaesthetic procedures mean that higher and higher risk patients are being considered, and accepted, for major surgery. A significant related problem is the detection of, and management of, significant cardiovascular disease in patients undergoing major non-cardiac surgery. The reader is also referred to Chapter 11.1, and Chapter 11.4 for further information.

Guidelines

In an increasingly complex medical environment with more and more sophisticated interventions and more powerful drugs available it is increasingly difficult for physicians to keep abreast even in their own subspecialty. It is unrealistic to expect surgeons performing non-cardiac surgery or the anaesthetist for these procedures to be aware of modern cardiovascular disease assessment and treatment, about the issues of anticoagulant and combined antiplatelet therapy for new drug-eluting stents, or the electrophysiological characteristic of complex implantable defibrillator/resynchronization devices. As we enter a dawn of stem cell and gene therapy and new powerful biologics, these issues will become even more problematic. As a result, all doctors are increasingly dependent on guidelines produced by experts and practising physicians and designed to act both as a checklist and informative guide as to what can and should be done in the majority of situations. These guidelines should now be designed with cross-speciality interactions in mind. For this topic the most relevant recent guideline is a report of the ACC/AHA on perioperative cardiovascular evaluation and care for non-cardiac surgery, to which the reader is referred for a more detailed guideline for this area (Lee et al. 2007). Until the recent past perioperative assessment was mainly the preserve of the medical intern on a surgical firm or the anaesthetist doing a preoperative assessment, and on occasion on the surgeon requesting a physician, or in the case of known cardiac disease a cardiologist, for an assessment. This has unfortunately been somewhat ad hoc in many cases with the dual risk of under-investigating and hence not performing necessary precautions in some and performing some unnecessary tests in some other patients unrelated to their initial complaint.

The assessment process

The cost of routine cardiovascular evaluation of all patients undergoing non-cardiac surgery would be prohibitive so this resource needs to be rationed to where it is most needed and has most to offer. Unfortunately, no trials exist that guide evidence-based recommendations of whom to refer for such assessment and no risk calculators have been developed and evaluated in randomized controlled trials to show they truly reduce risk when used. The most widely used, however, is a simple score, the Revised Cardiac Risk Index, which identified six simple independent clinical predictors of risk for major non-cardiac surgery: (1) high-risk type of surgery, (2) history of ischaemic heart disease, (3) history of congestive heart failure, (4) history of cerebrovascular disease, (5) preoperative

treatment with insulin, and (6) preoperative serum creatinine >2.0 mg/dL (Lee et al. 1999). Clinical judgement is needed when using this in practice, taking into account also such other known risks as well age over 50, other diseases and drug therapies.

The assessment

A preoperative cardiovascular assessment should be conducted in the same way as the history and examination described in Chapter 1.1. It should not be an excuse for a quick review of the risk of the proposed surgery and certainly should not be restricted to simply answering the too often quoted request 'assess fitness for surgery' with the answer 'no reason not to proceed'. This does the patient no favour and is a neglect of duty by the assessing physician; if asked to assess a patient the patient should be assessed like any other for whom a consultation is requested. The chance should be taken to do whatever tests and interventions are beneficial to allow the best chances for good outcomes from the proposed surgery in as fast a time as safely possible, combined with the best advice on future management of the patient's cardiovascular condition and that will include advice on long-term investigation and management.

Particular conditions of note

CAD

- Most important is frequency of unstable episodes and functional capacity.
- Special care concerning anticlotting agents.

Hypertension

- Increases risk of stroke if uncontrolled.
- Rapid BP reduction may be harmful.
- Be aware of falsely high BPs (e.g. white coat hypertension in preoperative assessment visit).

Heart failure

- Increases risk of death.
- Functional capacity key to risk, along with arrhythmias.
- Avoid rapidly discontinuing beta-blockade if possible.
- Perioperative fluid management crucial.
- Renal failure common.

Aortic stenosis

- If severe, delay non-urgent surgery until valve treated if correctable.

Mitral stenosis

- If severe, delay non-urgent surgery until valve treated if correctable.
- Take care over anticoagulation.
- Beware of postoperative atrial fibrillation (AF).

Aortic regurgitation

- Treat as for heart failure.
- Intraoperative echo can be useful in very high-risk cases.
- Fluid balance and diuretic doses crucial.

Mitral regurgitation

- Treat as for heart failure.
- Intraoperative echo can be useful in very high-risk cases.
- Fluid balance and diuretic doses are crucial.

Artificial valves (on warfarin) (from Lee et al. 2007)
The Seventh American College of Chest Physicians Consensus Conference on Antithrombotic and Thrombolytic Therapy recommends the following:
- For patients who require minimally invasive procedures (dental work, superficial biopsies), the recommendation is to briefly reduce the international normalized ratio (INR) to the low or subtherapeutic range and resume the normal dose of oral anticoagulation immediately after the procedure.
- Perioperative unfractionated heparin therapy is recommended for patients in whom the risk of bleeding with oral anticoagulation is high and the risk of thromboembolism without anticoagulation is also high (mechanical valve in the mitral position, Bjork–Shiley valve, recent (i.e. less than 1 year) thrombosis or embolus, or three or more of the following risk factors: atrial fibrillation, previous embolus at any time, hypercoagulable condition, mechanical prosthesis, and LVEF less than 30% (Lee *et al.* 2007).

Arrhythmias and ICDs
- Recommend continuation of therapy and perioperative monitoring.

Pulmonary vascular disease and congenital heart disease
- Treat as for heart failure and valve disease.
- Care over oxygenation and clotting risk (if polycythaemic).
- Fluid balance and diuretic doses are crucial.

Renal disease
- Increases risk of death and dialysis.
- May need renal rescue therapy option available.
- Care on drug dosages and avoid nephrotoxic agents.

Diabetes
- Consider insulin management if recently variable control.
- Heightens risk of CV disease.
- Increases infection risk.

Significant COPD
- Increases risk of respiratory complications.
- May worsen cardiac function if become hypoxaemic.
- Functional capacity and response to bronchodilators, should be determined.

Blood disorders and anticoagulants and antiplatelet agents
- Consider options for managing balance of perioperative control of clotting/bleeding risks
- Tranfusions/blood products may be needed at short notice.

Cardiovascular conditions of note in the preoperative assessment (redrawn and summarized from Lee et al. 2007)

Require preop evaluation and treatment

Unstable coronary syndromes.
Class IV, worsening decompensated or recent onset heart failure.
High-grade arrhythmias.
Haemodynamically significant valve disease.
(see also info on antibiotic prophylaxis, Chapter 7.12).

Should be taken into account in planning surgery

Pacemaker or ICD *in situ*.
Orthostatic hypotension.
Peripheral vascular disease.
Diabetes.
Cerebrovascular disease.
COPD.
Renal impairment.
Modifiable CV risk factors.

To be documented and noted

All medication (including OTC).
Allergies.
The patient's functional capacity (thought to be best single guide to operative risk for major surgery) which can be reasonably assessed by questionnaire (Hlatky *et al.* 1989).

References

Hlatky MA, Boineau RE, Higginbotham MB, *et al.* A brief self-administered questionnaire to determine functional capacity (the Duke Activity Status Index). *Am J Cardio* 1989;**64**:651–4.

Lee TH, Marcantonio ER, Mangione CM, *et al.* Derivation and prospective validation of a simple index for prediction of cardiac risk of major noncardiac surgery. *Circulation* 1999,**100**.1013–9.

Lee A, Fleisher JA, Beckman KA, *et al.* ACC/AHA 2007 Guidelines on Perioperative Cardiovascular Evaluation and Care for Noncardiac Surgery: A Report of the American College of Cardiology/American Heart Association Task Force on Practice Guidelines. *Circulation* 2007;**116**:e418–e500.

Perioperative cardiac arrhythmias

Introduction
- Perioperative arrhythmias are common.
- Significant arrhythmias that require treatment are less common.
- Findings from studies conducted in the context of perioperative arrhythmias following cardiac surgery may be carefully applied to patients undergoing non-cardiac surgery.
- The patient's underlying cardiac status is the key to management.

Predisposing factors
Predisposing factors can be divided into preoperative and postoperative conditions. The type of surgery a patient is undergoing can predispose to certain arrhythmias; thoracic, abdominal aortic aneurysm (AAA) repair, infra-abdominal, major vascular, and cardiac surgeries show an increased incidence of supraventricular tachycardias.
- Preoperative conditions can predispose to certain arrhythmias:
  - Older age, hypertension, male sex, prior atrial fibrillation, and pulmonary rales have been shown to predict increased risk of postoperative supraventricular tachycardia and atrial fibrillation
- Postoperative conditions:
  - The increased vagal tone that can be seen after spinal or epidural anaesthesia, laryngoscopy, or surgical intervention predisposes to bradycardia
  - Many forms of decompensation including hypoxia, hypercarbia, myocardial ischaemia, increased catecholamines, electrolyte or acid–base disturbance, pneumonia, and mechanical ventilation have been associated with atrial fibrillation and other arrhythmias
  - Atrial ischaemia due to cardioplegia during bypass surgery, atrial distention, or inflammation may increase incidence of atrial fibrillation.

Perioperative bradyarrhythmias
Bradycardia requiring treatment is rare, occurring in less then 1% of surgeries.

Causes of perioperative bradycardia
Patient-related factors
- Pre-existing sinus node disease predisposes to sinus bradycardia, sinus pauses, and sinus arrest allowing for emergence of junctional or ventricular escape rhythms
- Pre-existing conduction system disease can lead to heart block, although the overall risk of heart block with underlying bifascicular block is low. Heart block can also be precipitated by ischaemia without any underlying conduction system disease.

Extrinsic factors
- Increased vagal tone
  - Due to airway manoeuvres, epidural, or spinal anaesthesia, sedation.
- Medications
  - Beta-blockers, non-dihydropryridine calcium channel blockers, and antiarrhythmics.
- Electrolyte imbalance, acid–base disturbance, hypercarbia.

Treatment
Perioperative bradycardia is most often transient and without haemodynamic consequence, and therefore does not need to be treated. When bradycardia or heart block is symptomatic, initial treatment with antimuscarinics (atropine) or beta-agonists (ephedrine or isoproterenol) can be attempted. Transcutaneous or transvenous pacing may be needed for prolonged bradycardia or heart block that does not respond to the initial treatment.

Perioperative supraventricular arrhythmias
This occurs in about 4% of patients undergoing major non-cardiac surgery and 13% undergoing thoracic surgery.

Multifocal atrial tachycardia
- The irregularly irregular rhythm with three different p-wave morphologies on ECG distinguishes this rhythm from atrial fibrillation.
- It occurs in elderly people, COPD exacerbation, and acutely ill patients.

Management
- Treat underlying condition
- Consider calcium channel blockers or beta-blockers for heart rate control
- Amiodarone may be used as well.

AV nodal re-entry tachycardia (AVNRT)
This is treated similarly to non-surgical patients.

Management
- Carotid sinus massage or adenosine is first line.
- If AV nodal block does not convert the rhythm consider an alternative diagnosis.
- Consider calcium channel blocker or beta-blocker upon return to sinus rhythm.

Accessory pathway re-entry tachycardia
Orthodromic (narrow complex: conducts retrograde through accessory pathway and down AV node).

Management
Similar to AVNRT: carotid massage, adenosine, calcium channel blocker, or beta-blocker.

Antidromic (wide complex, delta wave: conducts retrograde through AV node and down through accessory pathway).

Management
- Avoid medications that block the AV node without blocking the accessory pathway, as this can lead to acceleration of heart rate to dangerous levels.
- Intravenous procainamide or amiodarone is the treatment of choice, as these slow conduction down the accessory pathway.
- Urgent electrical cardioversion for unstable patients.

Atrial fibrillation
This is the most common perioperative arrhythmia requiring treatment in both cardiac (30–50%) and major non-cardiac surgery (4%). Peak occurrence is postoperative days 2 and 3. Perioperative atrial fibrillation often converts to sinus rhythm on its own; 15–30% convert by 2 hours, and 80% convert within 24 hours.

Management
As in non-surgical patients, a decision should be made to attempt to restore and maintain sinus rhythm (rhythm control strategy) or to control ventricular response (rate control).

Rhythm control
- Indicated in haemodynamically unstable patients and those with contraindication for anticoagulation

- Direct electrical cardioversion for unstable patients with hypotension, pulmonary oedema, or myocardial ischaemia
- Pharmacological rhythm control
  - Amiodarone: most frequent first-line antiarrhythmic; safety in ischaemic disease, renal failure; effective
  - Sotalol: less effective; increased beta-blocker activity.

Rate control
- Indicated in most postoperative patients due to high rate of conversion to sinus rhythm
- AV nodal blockers
  - Beta-blockers: frequently in place preoperatively; may be given orally or intravenously
  - Non-dihydropyridine calcium channel blockers: orally or intravenously
  - Digoxin is sometimes added as second or third line.
- Anticoagulation should be considered if atrial fibrillation persists for 48 hours.

Prevention strategies
Recent research has focused on prevention of atrial fibrillation in cardiac surgery patients due to its frequency and evidence for an increased risk of stroke, longer hospital length of stay, and increased 30-day and 6-month mortality.

Beta-blockers
- Continuation of preoperative beta-blockers into the postoperative period can reduce atrial fibrillation by up to 70% in cardiac surgery patients. This provides a rationale for use in high risk non-cardiac surgery patients.
- Class Ia indication in ACC/AHA guidelines for prevention of postoperative atrial fibrillation in cardiac surgery patients.
- Choice of beta-blocker is generally not considered crucial, but a recent trial suggested that carvedilol was more effective than metoprolol in bypass patients.

Amiodarone
- Recent trials show effectiveness when given preoperatively or postoperatively
- The PAPABEAR trial evaluated 600 patients undergoing bypass surgery, valve, or both given amiodarone 10 mg/kg orally 6 days before through 6 days after surgery or placebo. Treatment decreased atrial fibrillation incidence (16% versus 30%, P <0.001). There was no difference in serious complications or 1-year mortality and also ventricular tachycardia (VT) in the treated group; 10% of patients discontinued the study drug because of bradycardia, skin rashes, and QTc prolongation over 650 ms
- The ARCH trial evaluated postoperative intravenous amiodarone 1–2 g daily in cardiac surgery patients and found reduced incidence of postoperative atrial fibrillation (35% versus 47%, P = 0.04)
- Class IIa in the ACC/AHA guidelines for high risk patients undergoing cardiac surgery.

Other preventive strategies
- IV magnesium supplementation is considered safe and has been shown to decrease postoperative atrial fibrillation in cardiac surgery patients.
- Atrial pacing has been shown to be effective but its use is limited due to difficulty in implementation.
- Small studies have shown that omega-3 PUFA supplementation may be effective.

Ventricular arrhythmias
Ventricular arrhythmias are common perioperatively, but they are commonly not sustained, and often do not require treatment.

Non-sustained VT and premature ventricular beats
- Benign in those without structural heart disease.
- May be of significance in those with structural heart disease.
- Perioperative risk is unknown.
- There is some evidence even in patients with structural heart disease, there is no difference in incidence of major complications regardless of the burden of perioperative premature ventricular beats and non-sustained VT.

Sustained VT
When encountered perioperatively a search for correctable causes should be initiated, including ischaemia, infarction, hypoxia, or electrolyte disturbance.

Management
- Unstable VT requires immediate defibrillation.
- Stable monomorphic VT can be considered for antiarrhythmic therapy with agents such as amiodarone.

Torsades de pointes: polymorphic VT in association with prolonged QT interval
Management
- Empiric magnesium should be given.
- Therapy involves decreasing the QT interval by decreasing the RR interval (increasing the heart rate). Thus can be done using isoproterenol, other catecholamines, or atropine. Pacing can also be considered.

Further reading
Asinger RW, Cannom DS, Crijns HJ, et al. ACC/AHA/ESC guidelines for the management of patients with atrial fibrillation: a report of the ACC/AHA/ESC committee for Practice guidelines and Policy Conferences. *J Am Coll Cardiol* 2001;**38**:1266i–lxx.

Calo L, Bianconi L, Coliviccio F, et al. N-3 fatty acids for the prevention of atrial fibrillation after coronary artery bypass surgery: a randomized controlled trial. *J Am Coll Cardiol* 2005;**45**:1723–29.

Fleisher LA Beckman JA, Brown KA, et al. ACC/AHA 2007 Guidelines on Perioperative Cardiovascular Evaluation and Care for Noncardiac Surgery: A Report of the ACC/AHA Task Force on Practice Guidelines (Writing Committee to Revise the 2002 Guidelines on Perioperative Cardiovascular Evaluation for Noncardiac Surgery). *J Am Coll Cardiol* 2007:e159–e242.

Goldman L. Supraventricular tachyarrhythmias in hospitalized adults after surgery. Clinical correlates in patients over 40 years of age after major noncardiac surgery. *Chest* 1978;**73**:450–4.

Haghjou M, Saravi M, Hashemi MJ, et al. Optimal beta blocker for prevention of atrial fibrillation after on pump coronary artery bypass graft surgery: Carvedilol versus metoprolol. *Heart Rhythm* 2007;**4**:1170–4.

Heintz KM, Hollenberg SM. Perioperative cardiac issues: postoperative arrhythmias. *Surg Clin NA* 2005;**85**:1103–14.

Maisel WH, Rawn JD, Stevenson WG. Atrial fibrillation after cardiac surgery. *Ann Intern Med* 2001;**135**:1061–73.

Miller S, Crystal E, Garfinkle M, et al. Effects of magnesium on atrial fibrillation after cardiac surgery: a meta-analysis. *Heart* 2005;**91**:618–23.

Mitchell LB, Exner DV, Wyse DG, et al. Prophylactic oral amiodarone for the prevention of arrhythmias that begin early afterrevascularization, valve surgery, or repair. *JAMA* 2005;**294**:3093–100.

Polancyk CA, Goldman L, Mercantonio ER, Orau EJ. Supraventricular arrhythmia in patients having noncardiac surgery: clinical correlates and effect on length of stay. *Ann Intern Med* 1998;**129**:279–85.

Websites
http://www.acc.org/qualityandscience/clinical/guidelines/arrhythmias/update_index.htm

http://content.onlinejacc.org/cgi/content/full/48/4/e149

http://www.acc.org/qualityandscience/clinical/guidelines/perio/update/periupdate_index.htm

Anaesthesia and the patient with cardiovascular disease

A complete review of this topic can be found in recently published guidelines (Fleisher et al. 2007) There are three classes of anaesthetics: general, regional and local/sedation or monitored anaesthetic care (MAC).

General anaesthesia

- General anaesthesia can best be defined as a state including unconsciousness, amnesia, analgesia, immobility, and attenuation of autonomic responses to noxious stimulation.
- General anaesthesia can be achieved with inhalational agents, intravenous agents, or a combination (frequently termed a balanced technique).
- General anaesthesia can be achieved with or without an endotracheal tube.

The five currently available inhalational anaesthetic agents in addition to nitrous oxide, are enflurane, halothane, isoflurane, sevoflurane, and desflurane, although the first two agents are not used in the United States.

- All inhalational agents can lead to reversible myocardial depressant effects and decreases in myocardial oxygen demand.
- The degree to which they depress cardiac output is a function of concentration.
- Isoflurane, desflurane, and sevoflurane cause negative inotropic effects, potent vascular smooth muscle relaxation, and minimal effects on baroreceptor function.
- Isoflurane has the slowest onset and offset, sevoflurane is intermediate, and desflurane is the fastest.

Outcomes related to inhalational agents

- Several large scale randomized and non-randomized studies of the use of inhalational agents in patients undergoing coronary artery bypass grafting have not demonstrated any increased incidence of myocardial ischaemia or infarction in patients receiving isoflurane compared with other inhalation agents or narcotic-based techniques.
- Desflurane has been shown to be associated with airway irritability and led to tachycardia in volunteer studies.
  - In a large-scale study comparing a narcotic-based anaesthetic to a desflurane-based anaesthetic, the desflurane group had a significantly higher incidence of myocardial ischaemia, although there was no difference in the incidence of myocardial infarction (Helman et al. 1992)
  - Including a narcotic with desflurane can avoid this tachycardia.
- Sevoflurane has been studied in one randomized trial and compared with isoflurane in patients at high risk for cardiovascular disease with no differences in the incidence of myocardial ischaemia observed.
- Overall, at this time, there appears to be no one best inhalation anaesthetic for the patient with coronary artery disease.
- Several investigative groups have demonstrated in vitro and in animal models that these agents possess protective effects on the myocardium similar to ischaemic preconditioning.

Narcotic-based techniques

- High-dose narcotic techniques offer the advantage of haemodynamic stability and lack of myocardial depression.

- Narcotic-based anaesthetics were frequently considered the 'cardiac anaesthesia' and advocated for use in all high-risk patients including those undergoing non-cardiac surgery; however, high-dose narcotics may require postoperative ventilation.
- An ultra-short-acting narcotic (remifentanil) currently available may obviate the need for prolonged ventilation. It has been used in patients undergoing cardiac surgery and shown to facilitate early extubation.
- Several large-scale trials in patients undergoing coronary artery bypass grafting showed no difference in survival or major morbidity compared with the inhalation-based technique (Slogoff and Keats 1989) This led to the abandonment of high-dose narcotics in much of cardiac surgery and an emphasis on early extubation.
- Most anaesthesiologists use a 'balanced' technique, involving the administration of lower doses of narcotics with an inhalational agent, and deriving the benefits of each of these agents while minimizing the side-effects.

Non-narcotic intravenous techniques

- Propofol is an alkyl phenol that can be used for both induction and maintenance of general anaesthesia.
  - It can result in profound hypotension due to reduced arterial tone with no change in heart rate.
  - The major advantage is rapid clearance with few residual effects on awakening.
  - Despite its haemodynamics effects, it has been used extensively to facilitate early extubation after coronary artery bypass surgery.

Spinal, epidural and regional anaesthesia

- Regional anaesthesia includes the techniques of spinal and epidural, as well as peripheral nerve blocks.
- Peripheral techniques, such as brachial plexus or Bier blocks, offer the advantage of causing minimal or no haemodynamic effects.
- Spinal or epidural techniques can produce sympathetic blockade, which can reduce blood pressure and slow heart rate.
- Spinal anaesthesia and lumbar or low thoracic epidural anaesthesia can also evoke reflex sympathetic activation above the blockade, which might lead to myocardial ischaemia.
- Spinal anaesthesia and its associated autonomic effects occur sooner than the same agent administered epidurally.
- Epidural catheters can also be used postoperatively to provide analgesia.
- In one meta-analysis, overall mortality was reduced by about a third in patients allocated to neuraxial blockade, although the findings were controversial since most of the benefit was observed in older studies (Rodgers et al. 2000). There were also reductions in myocardial infarction and renal failure.
- A recent (MASTER) randomized trial demonstrated no difference in outcome between regional and general anaesthesia (Rigg et al. 2002).

Monitored anaesthesia care

- MAC encompasses local anaesthesia administered by the surgeon with or without sedation.
- In a large-scale cohort study, MAC was associated with increased 30-day mortality in a univariate analysis

compared with general anaesthesia, although it did not remain significant in multivariate analysis once patient co-morbidity was taken into account (Cohen et al. 1988).
- The major issue with MAC is the ability to adequately block the stress response, since inadequate analgesia associated with tachycardia may be worse than the potential haemodynamic effects of general or regional anaesthesia.
- Claims data suggest major risk of MAC is airway loss.

Intraoperative haemodynamics and myocardial ischaemia
- Tachycardia is the strongest predictor of perioperative ischaemia in non-cardiac surgery.
- In the absence of tachycardia, hypotension has not been shown to be associated with myocardial ischaemia.
- Although traditionally a heart rate >100 bpm has been defined as the lower limit for tachycardia, slower heart rates may result in myocardial ischaemia.
- Administration of beta-blockers, titrated to effect, reduces the incidence of perioperative ischaemia, although there are recent concerns that acute administration without titration can lead to an increase incidence of stroke and mortality (POISE).
- In coronary artery bypass grafting, the vast majority of episodes of intraoperative ischaemia do not correlate with haemodynamic changes (Leung et al. 1990).

Temperature
- A randomized trial in 300 high-risk patients undergoing a diverse group of intermediate and high-risk procedures and randomized patients to maintenance of normothermia or routine care observed a significantly reduced incidence of peri-operative cardiac morbidity and mortality within 24 hours of surgery in the group which was kept normothermic (Frank et al. 1997).

Monitoring
- Peri-operative ST-segment changes correlate with major cardiac events. the duration, either cumulative or continuous, of perioperative ST changes strongly predict poor outcomes (Fleisher et al. 1995). Patients at low to moderate-risk patients may also develop ST segment changes which may not reflect true myocardial ischaemia.
- There is controversy regarding the value of pulmonary artery catheterization for non-cardiac surgery. Several small randomized trials did not demonstrate significant reduction in major cardiac morbidity and mortality in patients undergoing aortic surgery. A study of patient randomized to goal-directed therapy guided by a pulmonary catheter versus standard care without the use of a pulmonary catheter for patients undergoing urgent or elective major surgery observed no difference in survival, but there was a higher rate of pulmonary embolism in the catheter group than in the standard care group. Current evidence and guidelines do not support the routine use of pulmonary artery catheterization for high-risk patients undergoing major non-cardiac surgery (2003).
- Transoesophageal echocardiography (TEE) is a means of assessing intraoperative cardiac function. It is an extremely sensitive non-invasive tool to monitor intraoperative wall motion abnormalities. TEE monitoring may be valuable to guide treatment in patients with unstable haemodynamics where filling status and/or myocardial function are uncertain.

Transfusion therapy
- No randomized trials have evaluated the optimal transfusion threshold, although there is a study ongoing (FOCUS).
- Several small cohort studies have shown that haematocrits in the 27–29% range represent the point below which there is an increased incidence of myocardial ischaemia and potentially myocardial infarction.
- Data from a large-scale trial of transfusion triggers in the ICU were unable to document increased morbidity and mortality with a transfusion threshold of haemoglobin less than 7 gm/dL, but there were trends for increased morbidity in the subset of patients with ischaemic heart disease (Hebert et al. 1999).
- There is accumulating evidence to suggest that patients with known ischaemic heart disease that has not been revascularized should be maintained perioperatively with a haemoglobin greater than 9 gm/dL.

Further reading

Cohen M, Duncan PG, Tate RB. Does anesthesia contribute to operative mortality? JAMA 1988;**260**:2859–2863.

Fleisher LA, Nelson AH, Rosenbaum SH. Postoperative myocardial ischemia: etiology of cardiac morbidity or manifestation of underlying disease. J Clin Anesth 1995;**7**:97–102.

Fleisher LA, Beckman JA, Brown KA, et al. ACC/AHA 2007 guidelines on perioperative cardiovascular evaluation and care for noncardiac surgery: a report of the American College of Cardiology/American Heart Association Task Force on Practice Guidelines (Writing Committee to Revise the 2002 Guidelines on Perioperative Cardiovascular Evaluation for Noncardiac Surgery): developed in collaboration with the American Society of Echocardiography, American Society of Nuclear Cardiology, Heart Rhythm Society, Society of Cardiovascular Anesthesiologists, Society for Cardiovascular Angiography and Interventions, Society for Vascular Medicine and Biology, and Society for Vascular Surgery. Circulation 2007;**116**:e418–99.

Frank SM, Fleisher LA, Breslow MJ, et al. Perioperative maintenance of normothermia reduces the incidence of morbid cardiac events. A randomized clinical trial. JAMA 1997;**277**:1127–34.

Hébert PC, Wells G, Blajchman MA, et al. A multicenter, randomized, controlled clinical trial of transfusion requirements in critical care. Transfusion Requirements in Critical Care Investigators, Canadian Critical Care Trials Group. N Engl J Med 1999;**340**:409–17.

Helman JD, Leung JM, Bellows WH, et al. The risk of myocardial ischemia in patients receiving desflurane versus sufentanil anesthesia for coronary artery bypass graft surgery. The S.P.I. Research Group. Anesthesiology 1992;**77**:47–62.

Leung JM, O'Kelly BF, Mangano DT. Relationship of regional wall motion abnormalities to hemodynamic indices of myocardial oxygen supply and demand in patients undergoing CABG surgery. Anesthesiology 1990;**73**:802–14.

Practice guidelines for pulmonary artery catheterization: an updated report by the American Society of Anesthesiologists Task Force on Pulmonary Artery Catheterization. Anesthesiology 2003;**99**:988–1014.

Rigg JR, Jamrozik K, Myles PS, et al. Epidural anaesthesia and analgesia and outcome of major surgery: a randomised trial. Lancet 2002;**359**:1276–82.

Rodgers A, Walker N, Schug S, et al. Reduction of postoperative mortality and morbidity with epidural or spinal anaesthesia: results from overview of randomised trials. BMJ 2000;**321**:1493.

Slogoff S, Keats AS. Randomized trial of primary anesthetic agents on outcome of coronary artery bypass operations. Anesthesiology 1989;**70**:179–88.

Cardiogenic shock

Cardiogenic shock (CS) is a life-threatening condition defined as a critical failure of the heart to maintain a sufficient tissue perfusion. As an emergency, it requires immediate workup and therapeutic management. The typical patient with CS suffers from an acute event such as acute myocardial infarction (AMI), a mechanical complication such as papillary muscle or ventricular muscle rupture, pericardial effusion, life-threatening arrhythmia (bradycardiac or tachycardiac), acute myocarditis, or pulmonary embolus. Chronic heart failure may also slowly deteriorate to a stage resembling CS. However, as acute events are the leading causes in patients with CS, immediate management of the underlying disease process is typically the most important therapeutic intervention (Reynolds and Hochman 2008).

AMI is by far the most frequent single cause in patients with CS (80%). In ST segment elevation myocardial infarction (STEMI) patients, CS is an early in-hospital complication (median time = 6 hours post first symptoms), whereas in patients with non-ST segment elevation myocardial infarction (NSTEMI), it occurs at a later stage (hours to days). CS complicates between 6% and 8% of all AMI cases. Although the incidence of patients with AMI admitted with CS has been relatively stable over the last 10 years, the incidence of patients developing CS 24–48 hours after admission for AMI is decreasing because of an increase in early reperfusion rates, especially with PCI. Despite improvements in therapy, the overall in-hospital mortality for patients with CS following AMI is still between 40% and 60%.

Clinical approach

Examination
- History for AMI, CAD, PE, myocarditis
- Vital signs (systemic hypotension, tachycardia, shock index)
- Respiratory status (SOB, tachypnoea, crackles, wheezing, pulmonary oedema)
- Vital organ hypoperfusion (level of consciousness, cool extremities, skin pallor, urine output)
- CVP (elevated JVP)
- Emergency blood tests, especially arterial blood gases, pH, lactate, cardiac enzymes, electrolytes, glucose
- ECG (signs of AMI, LBBB, arrhythmias, signs of pulmonary embolism)
- Echocardiography (left ventricular function, pericardial fluid, right ventricular enlargement, function of aortic and mitral valve, ventricular septal defect (VSD))
- Chest X-ray (signs of acute lung oedema).

Consider monitoring
- ECG
- Arterial pressure (for haemodynamics and continuous blood gases)
- CVP line, pulmonary wedge pressure catheter, or PiCCO system. The benefit of pulmonary wedge pressure catheters has been debated. However, regardless of the system used, some information about filling pressures and CO is needed for initial evaluation and for guiding and aiming therapeutic interventions
- Urine output via catheter.

Haemodynamics and definition of CS

The pathophysiology of CS is determined by tissue hypoxia resulting from severe impairment of ventricular pump function in the presence of adequate intravascular volume. In many cases (as in AMI), this results in further deterioration (vicious cycle or downward spiral), decreased myocardial oxygen supply and final end-stage multi-organ damage. To define patients at risk, the following definition of CS may be used for patients with AMI according to clinical trials (Hochman et al. 1999):

1 Systemic hypotension (systolic blood pressure <90 mmHg) for at least 30 minutes and a heart rate >90 bpm or the need for positive inotropic drugs to maintain a systolic blood pressure >90 mmHg
2 End-organ hypoperfusion (cool extremities, altered mental status or a urine output of <30 mL per hour) or pulmonary oedema
3 Cardiac index <2.2 L/min/m^2 and PCWP >15 mmHg or left ventricular end-diastolic pressure (LVEDP) >20 mmHg.

Caveat: the degree of impairment of left ventricular ejection fraction (LVEF) is only one factor associated with CS. There is no absolute value of contractile dysfunction at which CS occurs. Although the impairment of LVEF remains a prognostic indicator for mortality, the definition of CS is based mainly on clinical and haemodynamic parameters.

Early management

Although initial work-up aims to elucidate the cause of CS, initial management should focus on stabilization of the patients:
- Correct arrhythmias (cardioversion, pacemaker).
- Guarantee oxygen supply (CPAP mask or mechanical ventilation).
- Correct electrolytes and metabolic acidosis, if necessary.
- Give fluids if haemodynamics are the major focus (and oxygen supply is not a problem). With continuous monitoring of MAP and CO, a test bolus of 500 mL of fluid may determine if the patient benefits from further volume.
- Diuretics (40–80 mg of frusemide) and low-dose nitrates may be appropriate for patients with pulmonary oedema to avoid further deterioration.
- Give morphine (5–10 mg IV) to reduce stress and anxiety. Any sedation and/or pain management may result in acute haemodynamic instability because of the adrenergic withdrawal effect (prepare for CPR or inotropes when planning mechanical ventilation!).
- Administer inotropes or vasopressors at as low a dose as possible. In most cases, initial therapy with either dopamine (2–20 µg/kg/min) or dobutamine (2–20 µg/kg/min) is necessary.
- In case of an AMI give ASS (500 mg), heparin (5000 IU), and clopidogrel (600 mg); a GPIIb/IIIa inhibitor may be considered.

Causal therapy

After initial management, steps towards a causal therapy should be initiated. As most patients with CS suffer an AMI, reperfusion therapy is the most important therapeutic measurement (Reynolds and Hochman 2008). Immediate coronary angiography and PCI has been demonstrated in a randomized trial to reduce mortality and should be considered even when not directly available on site. The critical state of patients with CS should not be used as an argument against PCI. Thrombolytic therapy should only be considered for STEMI within 3 hours and no access to a cath lab.

Patients with CS because of a mechanical complication (mitral regurgitation, VSD) should be transferred to cardiac surgery for definite therapy as soon as possible.

Further management with mechanical support

- IABP: intra-aortic balloon counterpulsation has been recommended in guidelines for patients with CS despite the lack of randomized controlled trials (RCTs). Registry data support the use of IABP in patients treated with thrombolytics. As IABP is very easy to use even in the absence of cath lab facilities, it should be considered very early in the management of patients with CS.
- Percutaneous LVAD: all left ventricular assist devices require some interventional or surgical approach. They offer an active support for the failing circulation by either pumping blood from the left ventricle to the aorta (e.g. Impella devices, Abiomed), or from the left atrium to the femoral artery (Tandem Heart, CardiacAssist). They have been investigated in small RCTs and are shown to improve haemodynamic status (Seyfarth et al. 2008; Thiele et al. 2005).
- Surgical implanted cardiac mechanical support: most ventricular assist devices or total artificial hearts require cardiac surgery, which limits the use for the majority of the patients with CS (Baughman and Jarcho 2007). This option should be considered for all patients who received the initial therapeutic steps, recovered to a stable condition, but need further invasive support as a bridge to recover or transplantation.

Pharmacological management

The aim of medical management of patients with CS is to bridge the patient for the first critical hours and days until the failing heart has recovered. MAP >60–70 mmHg may be a target; however, integrative parameters such as serum lactate, oxygenation, urine output, or mental status may be more useful targets for pharmacological management. Table 11.5.1 lists the most important drugs for pharmacological management.

All positive inotropic drugs should be used at as low a dose as possible to avoid increased oxygen demand, myocardial work, and direct toxic effects of these agents. Whenever LVADs are used or MAP is sufficiently high, vasodilators are beneficial to reduce preload and afterload

Table 11.5.1 Drugs for pharmacological management of patients with CS

Indication	Drug	Dose
CO↓ and MAP↓	Dopamine	2–20 µg/kg/min IV
CO↓ and MAP↓	Dobutamine	2–20 µg/kg/min IV
MAP↓ and TPR↓	Norepinephrine	0.05–1.0 µg/kg/min IV
CO↓↓ and MAP↓↓	Epinephrine	0.1–2 µg/kg/min IV
CO↓↓	Levosimendan (Ca-sensitizer)	12 µg/kg over 10 min, then 0.1–0.2 µg/kg/min IV
CO↓↓	Milrinone (PDE-inhibitor)	50 µg/kg over 10 min, then 0.375–0.75 µg/kg/min IV
Congestion and MAP (=)	Vasodilator (nitrates)	

and, thereby, reduce the work of the failing heart. Tilarginine to inhibit excess of nitric oxide has been tested in a large RCT with no observed survival benefit in patients with CS, despite evidence that systemic inflammatory response syndrome (SIRS) is associated with AMI and CS and SIRS might promote the vicious cycle of hypoxia in patients with CS (Alexander et al. 2007).

References

Alexander JH, Reynolds HR, Stebbins AL, et al. Effect of tilarginine acetate in patients with acute myocardial infarction and cardiogenic shock: the TRIUMPH randomized controlled trial. *JAMA* 2007;**297**:1657–66.

Baughman KL, Jarcho JA. Bridge to life—cardiac mechanical support. *N Engl J Med* 2007;**357**:846–9.

Hochman JS, Sleeper LA, Webb JG, et al. Early revascularization in acute myocardial infarction complicated by cardiogenic shock. SHOCK Investigators. Should We Emergently Revascularize Occluded Coronaries for Cardiogenic Shock. *N Engl J Med* 1999;**341**:625–34.

Reynolds HR, Hochman JS. Cardiogenic shock: current concepts and improving outcomes. *Circulation* 2008;**117**:686–97.

Seyfarth M, Sibbing D, Bauer I, et al. A randomized clinical trial to evaluate the safety and efficacy of a percutaneous left ventricular assist device versus intra-aortic balloon pumping for treatment of cardiogenic shock caused by myocardial infarction. *J Am Coll Cardiol* 2008;**52**:1584–1588.

Thiele H, Sick P, Boudriot E, et al. Randomized comparison of intra-aortic balloon support with a percutaneous left ventricular assist device in patients with revascularized acute myocardial infarction complicated by cardiogenic shock. *Eur Heart J* 2005;**26**:1276–83.

Cardiopulmonary resuscitation

Recovery from cardiac arrest depends on an intact 'chain of survival', which comprises:
- Early recognition and call for help
- Early cardiopulmonary resuscitation (CPR)
- Early defibrillation
- Post resuscitation care.

Prevention

In-hospital cardiac arrests are usually not sudden or unpredictable: in about 80% there is deterioration in clinical signs during the preceding few hours. The cardiac arrest rhythm is usually pulseless electrical activity (PEA) or asystole and prognosis is poor. Earlier recognition and treatment can prevent some cardiac arrests, deaths, and unanticipated intensive care unit (ICU) admissions.

Critical care outreach and medical emergency teams (also known as rapid response teams) might reduce the incidence of cardiac arrest. Earlier recognition also enables a do-not-attempt-resuscitation (DNAR) decision to be applied, if this is appropriate.

In-hospital resuscitation

After in-hospital cardiac arrest, the division between basic life support (BLS) and advanced life support (ALS) is arbitrary; in practice, in-hospital resuscitation is a continuum. For all in-hospital cardiac arrests, ensure that cardiorespiratory arrest is recognized immediately; help is summoned using a standard telephone number—it is 2222 in the UK; CPR is started immediately using a compression–ventilation (CV) ratio of 30:2.

Risks to the rescuer

There are few reports of harm to rescuers from carrying out CPR.

Wear gloves: eye protection, aprons and facemasks, may be necessary. Infection risk is lower than perceived. There are reports of infections with tuberculosis (TB), and severe acute respiratory distress syndrome (SARS). HIV transmission has never been reported.

Mechanism for the production of blood flow during chest compressions

Chest compressions generate blood flow by increasing intrathoracic pressure and compressing the heart directly; however, perfusion of the brain and myocardium is, at best, 25% of normal. The coronary perfusion pressure (CPP) achieved during CPR correlates with restoration of spontaneous circulation (ROSC). Frequent interruptions in chest compressions reduce survival from cardiac arrest. Each time chest compressions are stopped the CPP decreases rapidly and takes time to previous levels once chest compressions are resumed. In the presence of ventricular fibrillation (VF), chest compressions increase the amplitude and frequency of the VF waveform and the likelihood that attempted defibrillation will be successful.

The duration of the pre-shock pause (interval between stopping compressions and delivering a shock) influences the shock success. A pre-shock pause of just 10 seconds reduces the chances of successful defibrillation.

Quality of CPR

By incorporating a force transducer in a sternal compression pad and measuring transthoracic impedance with self-adhesive defibrillation pads, some defibrillators can provide real time feedback on compression depth and rate, and ventilation volume and rate. This improves the quality of CPR but has yet to be shown to improve outcome.

Defibrillation

Defibrillation is defined as the termination of VF or, more precisely, the absence of VF/ventricular tachycardia (VF/VT) at 5 seconds after shock delivery; however, the goal of attempted defibrillation is to restore spontaneous circulation. The likelihood of successful defibrillation diminishes rapidly with any delay in shock delivery.

Self-adhesive defibrillation pads

These are preferred to standard 'manual' defibrillation paddles because they are perceived to be safer: they are less likely to cause sparking; they enable the operator to be well away from the patient when the shock is delivered; they are less likely to be influenced by poor technique (frequently, inadequate force is applied to manual paddles). It is also easy to continue chest compressions as self-adhesive pads applied.

CPR versus defibrillation as the initial treatment

After out-of-hospital cardiac arrest (OHCA), if response times exceed 4–5 minutes, a period of 2 minutes of CPR before shock delivery may improve survival compared with immediate defibrillation. After in-hospital cardiac arrest, response times should be much less than 5 minutes: if a shockable rhythm is identified, give a shock immediately.

One-shock versus three-shock sequence

Before 2005, defibrillation was attempted with sequences of up to three shocks. The 2005 CPR guidelines introduced a single-shock protocol followed by immediate resumption of CPR because:
- The delivery of three shocks causes prolonged (up to 1 minute) interruptions to chest compressions.
- Modern, biphasic defibrillators have a first shock efficacy of more than 90%—failure to defibrillate implies that the quality of VF is poor; 2 minutes of high-quality CPR may make the VF 'more shockable'.
- Immediately after a successful shock, despite ROSC, the pulse may not be palpable—at this stage 2 minutes of CPR will maintain some coronary and cerebral blood flow while the myocardial contractility picks up. If the shock has not been successful, there is zero flow while attempting to feel a pulse.

Waveforms and energy levels
- All modern defibrillators deliver a biphasic shock.
- Optimal energy levels for both monophasic and biphasic waveforms are unknown. The recommended energy levels vary between manufacturers, partly because the precise waveform varies between different defibrillators. Although higher energy levels might cause more myocardial injury, the earlier conversion to a perfusing rhythm may outweigh this risk.
- In general, the energy level for the first shock with a biphasic defibrillator should be 150–200 J. If using a monophasic defibrillator, deliver the first and subsequent shocks at 360 J.
- Subsequent shocks can be given at the same energy (fixed) or at higher (escalating) energy level. The strategy

used will depend on the manufacturer's recommendations and the setting available on the defibrillator. Both strategies are acceptable; however, if the first shock is not successful and the defibrillator is capable of delivering shocks of higher energy, it is rational to increase the energy for subsequent shocks.

Advanced life support

The ALS algorithm enables a standardized approach to cardiac arrest management (Figure 11.6.1). Cardiac arrest rhythms are classified simply as shockable (VF/VT) and non-shockable (asystole and PEA).

Treatment of shockable rhythms

- Start CPR and assess the rhythm.
- Without interrupting chest compressions, place self-adhesive pads on the patient's chest—one below the right clavicle and one in the V6 position in the mid-axillary line.
- Select correct energy level: 150–200 J biphasic (360 J monophasic) for first shock and 150–360 J biphasic (360 J monophasic) for subsequent shocks.
- Charge the defibrillator: consider resuming chest compressions while charging the defibrillator (especially if using older equipment that is slow to charge).
- Ensure that oxygen is not flowing across the chest.
- Warn everyone to 'stand clear' and deliver shock.
- Without reassessing the rhythm or feeling for a pulse, start CPR using a ratio of 30:2, starting with chest compressions.
- Continue CPR for 2 minutes, then pause briefly to check the monitor.
- If VF/VT persists:
  - Give a second shock, resume CPR immediately and continue for 2 minutes.
  - Pause briefly to check the monitor; if VF/VT persists give adrenaline 1 mg IV followed immediately by a third shock. Do not delay a shock to wait for adrenaline—if the adrenaline is not ready, give it after delivery of the shock. Resume CPR immediately and continue for 2 minutes.
  - Pause briefly to check the monitor; if VF/VT persists, give amiodarone 300 mg IV followed immediately by a fourth shock; resume CPR immediately and continue for 2 minutes.
  - Give adrenaline 1 mg IV immediately before alternate shocks (i.e. approximately every 3–5 minutes).
  - Give further shocks after each 2 minutes period of CPR and after confirming that VF/VT persists.
- If organized electrical activity compatible with a cardiac output is seen, check for a pulse:
  - If a pulse is present, start post-resuscitation care
  - If no pulse is present, continue CPR and switch to the non-shockable algorithm.
- If asystole is seen, continue CPR and switch to the non-shockable algorithm.

Precordial thump

- If the onset of VF/VT is both witnessed and monitored, consider giving a precordial thump if a defibrillator is not available for immediate delivery of a shock.
- Two recent studies suggest that a precordial thump is only rarely effective.

Treatment of PEA

- Start CPR 30:2.
- Give adrenaline (epinephrine) 1 mg IV as soon as intravascular access is achieved.
- Continue CPR 30:2 until the airway is secured; then continue chest compressions without pausing during ventilation.
- Recheck the rhythm every 2 minutes and check for a pulse if organized electrical activity is seen.
- Give further adrenaline 1 mg IV every 3–5 minutes (alternate loops) until ROSC is achieved.

Treatment of asystole and slow PEA (rate <60 per minute)

- Treat as for PEA but inject atropine 3 mg after the first dose of adrenaline is given. Although recommended in CPR guidelines, there is very little evidence that atropine is beneficial.

Airway and ventilation

- Tracheal intubation provides the most reliable airway during CPR but if a tracheal tube is not already in place, attempts at intubation should be made only by trained personnel.
- A supraglottic airway device (e.g. laryngeal mask airway (LMA) or I-gel) is an alternative to tracheal intubation.
- If a supraglottic airway device has been inserted, attempt continuous chest compressions without stopping for ventilations. If gas leakage is excessive, interrupt the chest compressions to enable adequate ventilation.

Drug delivery

There is very little clinical evidence that any drug improves long term outcome in cardiac arrest—the priority is to provide high quality chest compressions with minimal interruptions, and rapid defibrillation when indicated. Peak drug concentrations are higher and circulation times are shorter when drugs are injected into a central vein compared with a peripheral vein; however, insertion of a central venous catheter is not an immediate priority—it requires interruption of CPR and is associated with several potential complications. Peripheral venous cannulation is quicker, easier, and safer. Flush drugs injected peripherally with at least 20 mL of fluid and elevate the extremity for 10–20 seconds to facilitate drug delivery to the central circulation. Consider the intraosseous route if the intravenous route is impossible. Giving a drug through the tracheal tube results in highly variable, and usually ineffective, plasma drug concentrations.

Reversible causes

Identify and treat reversible causes during CPR for all cardiac arrests. This is particularly important in the ICU where potentially reversible causes are more common:

- Hypoxia
- Hypovolaemia
- Hyperkalaemia, hypokalaemia, hypocalcaemia, acidaemia, and other metabolic disorders
- Hypothermia
- Tension pneumothorax
- Tamponade
- Toxic substances
- Thromboembolism (pulmonary embolism or coronary thrombosis).

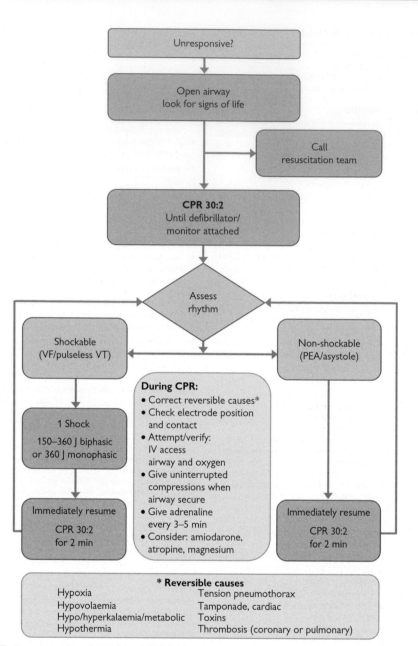

Fig. 11.6.1 The Resuscitation Council (UK) Advanced Life Support algorithm. With permission from The Resuscitation Council UK.

Focused echo entry level (FEEL)

The widespread availability of small, high-quality portable echocardiography devices is impacting significantly on practice in acute medicine. During cardiac arrest, as chest compressions are paused to assess the rhythm, a rapid sub-xiphoid echocardiographic examination can be attempted. This may enable reversible causes to be identified and treated (e.g. hypovolaemia, pericardial tamponade). In many of these cases, echocardiography will show pseudo-PEA,

i.e. cardiac wall motion detected but no palpable pulses. The use of echocardiography during ALS must not be allowed to cause prolonged interruptions to chest compressions: the aim is to obtain a subxiphoid view within 10 seconds.

Post-cardiac arrest syndrome

With the exception of patients resuscitated from a very brief period of cardiac arrest, most of those who achieve

ROSC will initially be comatose and many of these will require admission to an intensive care unit (ICU). Unconscious, mechanically ventilated survivors of cardiac arrest account for 6% of all admissions to ICUs in the UK.

Organ injury caused by ischaemia and hypoxia during prolonged cardiac arrest is compounded by reperfusion injury that occurs when a spontaneous circulation is restored. These insults trigger a systemic inflammatory response, similar to that associated with sepsis. The four key components of post-cardiac arrest syndrome are:

1 post-cardiac arrest brain injury
2 post-cardiac arrest myocardial dysfunction
3 systemic ischaemia/reperfusion response
4 unresolved pathology that caused of the arrest.

Post-cardiac arrest brain injury

Post-cardiac arrest brain injury is a common cause of morbidity and mortality: two-thirds of patients dying after admission to ICU following OHCA die from neurological injury and 25% of patients dying after admission to ICU following in-hospital cardiac arrest die from neurological injury. The following therapeutic strategies may improve neurological outcome.

Optimizing cerebral perfusion

After resuscitation from cardiac arrest, normal cerebral autoregulation is lost, leaving cerebral perfusion dependent on mean arterial pressure. Hypotension will compromise cerebral blood flow severely and will compound any neurological injury; therefore, maintain mean arterial pressure at the patient's normal level.

Prevention and control of seizures

Seizures and/or myoclonus occur in 5–15% of those achieving ROSC, and in 10–40% of those who remain comatose. Seizures increase cerebral metabolism by up to threefold. Status epilepticus and, in particular, status myoclonus are associated with a poor outcome, but transient seizures do not necessarily predict a poor outcome. Prolonged seizure activity may cause cerebral injury, and should be treated promptly and effectively with benzodiazepines, phenytoin, sodium valproate, propofol, or a barbiturate. Clonazepam is the drug of choice for the treatment of myoclonus, but sodium valproate and levetiracetam may also be effective.

Blood glucose control

There is a strong association between high blood glucose after resuscitation from cardiac arrest and poor neurological outcome. Tight control of blood glucose (4.4–6.1 mmol/L) has been shown to reduce mortality in critically ill surgical patients and medical patients in ICU for more than 3 days. But, comatose patients are at particular risk from unrecognized hypoglycaemia, and the risk of this complication occurring increases as the target blood glucose concentration is lowered. More recent evidence suggests that strict glucose control may be harmful if applied generally to all ITU patients, and is associated with increased markers of cellular stress in those with brain injury. A more moderate blood glucose target range of below 8–10 mmol/L may be optimal.

Temperature control and therapeutic hypothermia

A period of hyperthermia is common in the first 48 hours after cardiac arrest. The risk of a poor neurological outcome increases for each degree of body temperature >37°C. Treat any hyperthermia occurring in the first 72 h after cardiac arrest with antipyretics or active cooling.

Mild hypothermia started after ROSC reduces the neurological injury caused by reperfusion and the post cardiac arrest syndrome. Assuming active treatment is appropriate, unconscious adult patients with ROSC after out-of-hospital VF cardiac arrest should be cooled to 32–34°C. Start cooling as soon as possible and continue for at least 24 hours. Although supported only by lower level evidence, induced hypothermia might also benefit unconscious adult patients after OHCA from a non-shockable rhythm, or after in-hospital cardiac arrest. Rapid infusion of ice-cold fluid 30 mL/kg is a very effective, simple method for initiating cooling. Treatment is continued using either intravascular cooling or external techniques (e.g. circulating water blankets). Treat shivering by ensuring adequate sedation and giving neuromuscular blocking drugs. Rewarm slowly (0.25–0.5°C/hour) and avoid hyperthermia. Complications of mild therapeutic hypothermia include increased infection, cardiovascular instability, hypovolaemia, coagulopathy, hyperglycaemia, and electrolyte abnormalities such as hypophosphataemia and hypomagnesaemia.

Post-cardiac arrest myocardial dysfunction

Haemodynamic instability is common after cardiac arrest and manifests as hypotension, low cardiac index, arrhythmias, and impaired contractility. This post-resuscitation myocardial dysfunction is usually transient and often reverses within 48–72 hours. Infusion of fluids may be required to increase right heart filling pressures or, conversely, diuretics, vasodilators and inotropes/balloon pump may be needed to treat myocardial dysfunction.

In the presence of the significant inflammatory response that is part of the post-cardiac arrest syndrome, noradrenaline (norepinephrine) may be required to maintain an adequate blood pressure. Early echocardiography will enable the extent of myocardial dysfunction to be quantified and may guide therapy.

Coronary revascularization

The majority of OHCA patients have coronary artery disease, and acute myocardial infarction is the commonest cause of sudden cardiac death. Acute changes in coronary plaque morphology occur in 40–86% of cardiac arrest survivors and in 15–64% of autopsy studies. Thus, early post-cardiac arrest coronary angiography with subsequent percutaneous coronary intervention (PCI) is appropriate not just for those patients with ST elevation myocardial infarction (STEMI) but also for those who are suspected of having an acute coronary syndrome (ACS). Several studies have evaluated the use of primary PCI for patients with STEMI following resuscitation from cardiac arrest and have reported survival to discharge rates in the range 55–80%. When appropriate, the combination of mild hypothermia and primary PCI results in better outcomes than PCI alone. Chest pain and/or ST elevation may be poor predictors of acute coronary occlusion in post-cardiac arrest patients, and prospective studies are needed to determine if immediate coronary angiography should be performed on all patients that regain ROSC after OHCA. If there are no facilities for immediate PCI, patients with STEMI should be thrombolysed. The safety of thrombolysis after CPR is well established: prior CPR is not a contraindication to thrombolysis; restoration of coronary perfusion is a priority.

Systemic ischaemia/reperfusion response
The whole body ischaemia/reperfusion of cardiac arrest activates immunological and coagulation pathways increasing the risk of multiple organ failure and infection. As occurs in sepsis, activation of blood coagulation without adequate activation of endogenous fibrinolysis may also contribute to microcirculatory reperfusion disorders after cardiac arrest. Clinical manifestations of systemic ischaemic–reperfusion response include intravascular volume depletion, impaired vasoregulation, impaired oxygen delivery and utilization, and increased susceptibility to infection.

Persisting precipitating pathology
Post-cardiac arrest syndrome is commonly associated with persisting acute pathology that caused the cardiac arrest. The diagnosis and treatment of ACS, pulmonary diseases, haemorrhage, and sepsis, is often complicated in the setting of post-cardiac arrest syndrome.

Prediction of outcome in comatose survivors after cardiopulmonary resuscitation
Predicting the final outcome of individual patients remaining comatose after resuscitation from cardiac arrest is problematic. Prognosis cannot be based reliably on the circumstances surrounding cardiac arrest and cardiopulmonary resuscitation. Absent pupil or corneal reflexes within days 1–3 after CPR, or absent or extensor motor responses 3 days after cardiac arrest reliably predict a poor outcome in the normothermic patient. The use of therapeutic hypothermia probably invalidates these criteria because they were derived before this treatment was introduced into clinical practice.

Outcome
The outcome from OHCA remains relatively poor, with a survival rate to hospital discharge of approximately 5–10%. After in hospital cardiac arrest, the survival rate to hospital discharge is 15–20% (40% after VF and 6% after PEA or asystole). Of those patients admitted to ICU after cardiac arrest, about 40% survive to leave the ICU and about 30% survive to hospital discharge. Of the patients that survive to hospital discharge, approximately 60–80% have a good neurological outcome.

Cardiac arrest centres
It has been suggested that post-cardiac arrest patients should be admitted directly to cardiac arrest centres (similar in concept to level one trauma centres), which would provide a 24/7 PCI facility along with experience in therapeutic hypothermia and a neurological rehabilitation service. Whether this improves outcome is unknown.

Further reading
Deakin CD, Nolan JP. European Resuscitation Council guidelines for resuscitation 2005. Section 3. Electrical therapies: automated external defibrillators, defibrillation, cardioversion and pacing. *Resuscitation* 2005;**67**(Suppl 1):S25–37.

Hypothermia After Cardiac Arrest Study Group. Mild therapeutic hypothermia to improve the neurologic outcome after cardiac arrest. *N Engl J Med* 2002;**346**:549–56.

Nolan JP, Deakin CD, Soar J, et al. European Resuscitation Council guidelines for resuscitation 2005. *Section 4. Adult advanced life support. Resuscitation* 2005;**67**(Suppl 1):S39–86.

Nolan J, Soar J, Lockey A, et al. *Advanced life support*, 5th edn. London: Resuscitation Council (UK) 2006.

Nolan JP, Neumar RW, Adrie C, et al. Post-cardiac arrest syndrome. Epidemiology, pathophysiology, treatment, and prognostication. *Resuscitation* 2008;**79**:350–79.

Sandroni C, Nolan J, Cavallaro F, Antonelli M. In-hospital cardiac arrest: incidence, prognosis and possible measures to improve survival. *Intensive Care Med* 2007;**33**:237–45.

Others

Genetic abnormalities and structural heart diseases

Genetic abnormalities leading to structural heart diseases can be broadly categorized into cardiomyopathies, congenital heart diseases (CHD), and cardiac tumours. In this chapter, the general approach to diagnosing and treating patients with suspected genetic heart disease is discussed, followed by descriptions of diagnoses to consider. Inherited cardiac arrhythmia syndromes are discussed separately in Chapter 12.2.

Clinical approach

The approach is primarily to identify and distinguish between familial forms of structural heart diseases.

History: key points
- Family history of genetic heart diseases.
- Cardiac: syncope, palpitations, signs of congestive heart failure (CHF) such as dyspnoea, fatigue, exercise intolerance, angina, or oedema.
- Associated malformations: renal, intestinal malrotation, biliary atresia, and craniofacial anomalies.
- Neurodevelopmental delay.

Examination: key points
- General: cyanosis.
- Cardiac: check for tachycardia, congestion, murmurs, S_3, S_4, abnormal location of apex beat (e.g. valvular or septal defects, cardiomyopathy).
- Facial dysmorphisms: simplified ears, cleft palate (DiGeorge syndrome), hypertelorism (Noonan syndrome), facial asymmetry (CHARGE syndrome).
- Skeletal abnormalities: short stature (Noonan syndrome, Turner syndrome).
- Also examine first-degree relatives.

Special investigations
- Lab: Ca^{2+} level (hypocalcaemia in DiGeorge syndrome, hypercalcaemia in Williams syndrome).
- Electrocardiogram (ECG), transthoracic echocardiography (TTE).

Some diagnoses to consider

Cardiomyopathies
Cardiomyopathies with a known genetic cause include hypertrophic cardiomyopathy (HCM), dilated cardiomyopathy (DCM), restrictive cardiomyopathy (RCM), arrhythmogenic right ventricular cardiomyopathy/dysplasia (ARVC/D), and left ventricular non-compaction (LVNC) (Hershberger et al. 2009).

General diagnostic approach to cardiomyopathies
- Family history: inheritance pattern, age of onset, penetrance, lethality, and response to treatment.
- Clinical screening: history and physical exam, ECG, TTE, CK-MM at initial evaluation, signal averaged ECG and magnetic resonance imaging (MRI) (ARVC/D), Holter monitoring (HCM, ARVC/D), exercise-stress test (HCM).
- Genetic testing should be considered for probands and affected family members. Family counselling is also recommended. If a mutation is present, screening needs to be performed yearly in childhood (DCM, LVNC, RCM), or from age 10 (ARVC/D), or every 3 years until 30 years (HCM). Also recommended for asymptomatic first-degree relatives.

- Medical and/or device therapy is recommended based on cardiac phenotype. Patients with a positive family history of sudden cardiac arrest/death (SCA/D) or DCM due to a *LMNA* mutation should be considered for an implantable cardioverter-defibrillator (ICD), even if left ventricular ejection fraction (LVEF) is between 30% and 35%.

Hypertrophic cardiomyopathy (HCM)
Familial HCM is the most common genetic heart disease, affecting nearly 1 in 500 people. Inherited HCM is predominantly caused by autosomal-dominant (AD) mutations in genes encoding sarcomeric proteins.

Clinical presentation and examination
HCM is the most common cause of SCD during vigorous exercise, particularly in athletes <40 years of age. Since most patients are asymptomatic, the diagnosis is often incidental during investigation of asymptomatic murmurs or with family screening. Symptoms may include palpitations or signs of CHF. TTE is used to establish left ventricular hypertrophy (LVH), which is typically asymmetric. A maximal left ventricular (LV) wall thickness ≥15 mm is diagnostic. Doppler tissue imaging may reveal early signs of diastolic abnormalities. ECG often reveals signs of cardiac hypertrophy (S wave in lead V1 plus R wave in lead V5 or V6 >35 mm).

Genetic testing
- AD mutations in β-myosin heavy chain (*MYH7*), which cause 30–40% of HCM, manifest as severe LVH, CHF, and SCD.
- Myosin-binding protein C (*MYBPC3*) mutations (AD; 30–40%) cause mild disease with a late onset.
- Cardiac troponin T (*TNNT2*) mutations (AD; 10–20%) cause mild LVH, and SCD is more common.
- Myosin regulatory light chain (*MYL2*) and myosin essential light chain (*MYL3*) each cause 2–5%.
- Rare (<1%) AD mutations in cardiac actin (*ACTC*), titin (*TTN*), α-myosin heavy chain (*MYH6*), or telethonin (*TCAP*) also cause HCM.
- X-linked HCM associated with Fabry disease is caused by α-galactosidase (*GLA*) mutations.
- X-linked HCM associated with Danon disease is caused by lysosome-associated membrane protein 2 (*LAMP2*) mutations.
- Familial HCM can also be associated with infiltrative or metabolic diseases, such as Pompe disease, glycogen storage disease type III, LEOPARD syndrome, or Friedreich's ataxia.

Prevention and treatment
- Symptoms of CHF are treated conventionally. There is no evidence that pharmacological therapy may alter the clinical course.
- Verapamil may be used in case of severe outflow tract obstruction.
- Myectomy in drug-refractory patients with obstruction can promote survival and improve symptoms.
- Cardiac arrest survivors and patients with multiple episodes of sustained ventricular tachycardia (VT) are high risk and candidates for ICD implantation.
- Patients with severe HCM are candidates for heart transplantation; an ICD should be considered too.

Dilated cardiomyopathy

Familial DCM is defined as DCM of unknown cause in two or more closely related family members. DCM is characterized by an increase in both myocardial mass and volume.

Clinical presentation and examination

Symptoms may vary widely due to incomplete penetrance, and are related to CHF or complications (e.g. arrhythmias, thromboembolic events, stroke). Screening involves ECG and TTE for probands and first-degree relatives. Rule out myocarditis.

Diagnostic criteria

The presence of two or more affected first-degree relatives, and
- Established diagnosis of DCM, or
- Unexplained SCD <30 years of age, or
- Two major echocardiographic criteria:
  - Left ventricular end-diastolic dimension >117% of predicted value
  - Fractional shortening (FS) <25%, or
- Three minor echo and/or ECG criteria:
  - LVEDD >112% of predicted value
  - FS <28%
  - Unexplained conduction defects
- Or a first-degree relative of DCM patient with a well-documented unexplained SCD <35 years.

Genetic testing

Mode of inheritance is predominantly AD with a reduced penetrance due to modifier genes. Autosomal-recessive (AR) and X-linked inheritance is also seen.
- AD mutations in lamin A/C (*LMNA*) (~7%) are often associated with conduction disease. Mutations in *MYH7* cause 6%, *TNNT2* mutations cause 3%.
- Mutations in β- or δ-sarcoglycan (*SGCB*, *SGCD*) are associated with muscular dystrophy, desmin (*DES*) mutations also cause skeletal myopathy.
- Rare (<1%) AD mutations may be identified in: α-tropomyosin (*TPM1*), metavinculin (*VCL*), muscle LIM protein (*CSRP3*), α-actinin-2 (*ACTN2*), phospholamban (*PLN*), cipher/LIM binding protein 3 (*ZASP/LDB3*), SUR2A (*ABCC9*), presenilin 1/2 (*PSEN1/2*), troponin C (*TNNC1*), Na⁺ channel (*SCN5A*), thymopoietin (*TMPO*), eyes-absent 4 (*EYA4*), *MYBP3*, *ACTC*, *TTN*, *TCAP*, and *MYH6*.
- AR inherited DCM can be caused by mutations in cardiac troponin I (*TNNI3*).
- X-linked DCM can be caused by mutations in dystrophin (*DMD*; associated with skeletal myopathy) or tafazzin (*TAZ/G4.5*; associated with neutropenia and short stature).

Prevention and treatment

- Pharmacological treatment may include angiotensin-converting enzyme (ACE) inhibition for CHF symptoms, diuretics for oedema, and β-blockers for reduced LV ejection fraction.
- Cardiac resynchronization therapy (CRT) is used to treat conduction disturbances in CHF.
- Heart transplantation or LV assist device (LVAD) are considered in case of end-stage CHF.

Restrictive cardiomyopathy

RCM is the least common of cardiomyopathies, but has the highest mortality. Patients with RCM often present with SCD or symptoms of CHF. Up to a third of patients may present with embolic complications.

Genetic testing

- RCM can be idiopathic or secondary to rare metabolic disorders (i.e. Gaucher's disease, mucopolysaccharidoses, Fabry's disease).
- AD mutations in *MYH7* and *TNNI3* have been linked to RCM.

Arrhythmogenic right ventricular cardiomyopathy/dysplasia

In ARVC/D, there is progressive replacement of normal cardiac tissue with fat and fibrous tissue, predominantly in the right ventricle (RV). ARVC/D affects 1:1000–5000 individuals.

Clinical presentation and examination

Symptoms start around 30 years of age, and are due to arrhythmias (palpitations, syncope). SCA/D may be the presenting symptom. ECG may reveal RV tachycardia. MRI may reveal right and/or LV dysplasia.

Diagnostic criteria

Diagnosis is positive in the presence of two major and two minor, or four minor criteria:
- Family history: confirmed (major) or suspected (minor) history of SCA <35 years due to ARVC/D.
- ECG: epsilon waves or QRS ≥110 ms in V1–V3 (major), late potentials (minor), or inverted T-waves in V1–V3 in absence right bundle branch block (RBBB) (minor).
- Holter: LBBB-type VT or >1000/24 hours ventricular extrasystoles (both minor).
- Biopsy: fibrofatty tissue replacement (major).
- Imaging: severe dilation and reduced ejection fraction, RV aneurysms, severe segmental RV dilation (all major), mild global or segmental RV dilation, or regional RV hypokinesia (all minor).

Genetic testing

- AD mutations in desmoglein-2 (*DSG2*) and plakophilin-2 (*PKP2*) each cause 10–40% of ARVC/D.
- AD mutations in desmoplakin (*DSP*) are causative in 6–16% of cases.
- Rare (<1%) forms of ARVC/D are caused by mutations in transforming growth factor-β3 (*TGFβ3*), desmocolin-2 (*DSC2*), transmembrane protein 43 (*TMEM43*), and plakoglobin (*JUP*).
- Rare AR mutations in *JUP* and *DSP* are linked to Naxos syndrome, which is associated with woolly hair and ketaroderma.

Prevention and treatment

Therapy goal is prevention of SCD. An ICD is often effective. Milder forms are treated with β-blockers.

Left ventricular non-compaction

LVNC is characterized by non-compacted or spongy myocardium, and often associated with other cardiac diseases. Half of all cases are familial.

Clinical presentation and examination

LVNC is most easily detected using TTE, although other imaging modalities including MRI are also used.

Diagnostic criteria

- More than three coarse prominent trabeculations apical to papillary muscle not connected to papillary muscle.
- Ratio of non-compacted–compacted myocardium >2.

Genetic testing

Most common causes are:

- AD mutations in *MYH7*, *ACTC*, *TNNT2*, or *MYBPC3* are also associated with HCM
- Mitochondrial disorders (mtDNA genes)
- Barth syndrome (*G4.5*, *TAZ*)
- 1p36 deletion syndrome.

Prevention and treatment

Mostly symptomatic for CHF manifestations.

Congenital heart diseases

CHD occur in 5–8:1000 live births with apparently complex inheritance pattern. Numerous environmental and genetic factors have been implicated in the pathogenesis of CHD (Bruneau 2008). Congenital rubella infection, *in utero* exposure to retinoids, and maternal diabetes are implicated. Cytogenetic abnormalities such as trisomy 21 and Turner syndrome (45, X) often cause CHD.

Clinical presentation and examination

Signs and symptoms depend on the type and severity of disease. Some patients exhibit no symptoms, while others present with respiratory distress, cardiac murmurs, and failure to thrive. CHD can be detected by auscultation, chest X-ray, and TTE.

Genetic testing

Genetic testing for some of the inherited CHD syndromes may be available. Prenatal ultrasound scans can often detect the CHD and extracardiac defects. Counsel as appropriate for the underlying syndrome.

Prevention and treatment

Some forms of CHD improve spontaneously without treatment. However, most forms of CHD require surgery and/or medications such as diuretics, digoxin, and inotropes.

DiGeorge syndrome/velocardiofacial syndrome

The prevalence is estimated to be 1 in 6000. Microdeletions within chromosome 22q11.2 encompassing T-box 1 (*TBX1*) gene can cause conotruncal malformations such as tetralogy of Fallot, interrupted aortic arch and truncus arteriosus, velopharyngeal incompetence, cleft palate, immune deficiency, hypocalcaemia, and learning problems.

Genetic testing

The diagnosis is made by fluorescence *in situ* hybridization (FISH) for the 22q11.2 deletion.

Noonan syndrome

The prevalence of Noonan syndrome (NS) is 1 in 1000 to 1 in 2500, and is characterized by short stature, CHD (pulmonic stenosis, HCM), webbed neck, pectus deformity, cryptorchidism, coagulation defects, and lymphatic dysplasias.

Genetic testing

NS is caused by mutations in protein tyrosine phosphatase, non-receptor type 11 (*PTPN11*) in 50% of the cases. Mutations in v-raf-1 murine leukaemia viral oncogene homologue 1 (*RAF1*), son of sevenless homologue 1 (*SOS1*) and v-Ki-ras2 Kirsten rat sarcoma viral oncogene homologue (*KRAS*) can also cause NS.

Alagille syndrome

Alagille syndrome (prevalence 1 in 70 000) is characterized by cholestasis due to bile duct paucity, CHD (primarily involving the pulmonary arteries), posterior embryotoxon in the eye, and butterfly vertebrae.

Genetic testing

Alagille syndrome is predominantly caused by mutations in jagged 1 (*JAG1*) gene. Rare individuals have mutations in Notch homologue 2 (*NOTCH2*).

CHARGE syndrome

CHARGE syndrome (prevalence 1 in 8500) is characterized by coloboma of the iris or retina, choanal atresia, cranial nerve dysfunction, hearing loss, absent or hypoplastic semicircular canals, CHD (conotruncal anomalies, AV canal defects, aortic arch anomalies and septal defects), and growth deficiency.

Genetic testing

Mutations in chromodomain helicase DNA binding protein 7 (*CHD7*) are detected in 60–65% of cases.

Williams syndrome

Williams syndrome (WS) (prevalence 1:7500) is characterized by distinctive facies, CHD (peripheral pulmonary stenosis, supravalvular aortic stenosis), mental retardation, and endocrine abnormalities (hypercalcaemia, hypercalciuria, hypothyroidism).

Genetic testing

Most individuals have contiguous gene deletion encompassing the elastin (*ELN*) gene on chromosome 7q11.23, detected by FISH.

Syndromic and non-syndromic septal defects

Septal defects commonly occur in the interatrial (ASD) or interventricular septum (VSD). Non-syndromic and syndromic forms of septal defects are distinguished clinically.

Genetic testing

- Familial ASD can be caused by mutations in transcription factors such as GATA binding protein 4 (*GATA4*), NK2 transcription factor related, locus 5 (*NKX2-5*), and *MYH6*.
- *TBX20* mutations are associated with a wide spectrum of defects including ASD and VSD.
- Actin alpha cardiac muscle 1 (*ACTC1*) mutations can cause ASD without cardiomyopathy.
- More than 70% of individuals with Holt–Oram syndrome (characterized by ostium secundum ASD, VSD, conduction disease, and upper limb malformations) have mutations in the *TBX5* gene.

Heterotaxy

CHD in heterotaxy (abnormal placement of organs due to failure to establish the normal left–right patterning) is related to incomplete or impaired rotation of the heart. Defects include endocardial cushion defects, persistence of a left-sided superior vena cava, anomalous pulmonary venous return, and double outlet RV.

Genetic testing

Mutations in *ZIC3* (X-linked), *CFC1*, *LEFTY2*, *CRELD1*, and *GDF1* are known to cause heterotaxy.

Bicuspid aortic valve

The population frequency of bicuspid aortic valve (BAV) is 0.9–1.36%, with a male–female ratio of 2:1.

Genetic testing

Mutations in *NOTCH1* have been described in non-syndromic AD families with BAV.

References

Bruneau BG. The developmental genetics of congenital heart diseases. *Nature* 2008;**451**:943–8.

Hershberger RE, Lindenfeld J, Mestroni L, *et al.* Genetic evaluation of cardiomyopathy—a Heart Failure Society of America Practice Guideline. *J Card Fail* 2009;**15**:83–97.

Inherited cardiac arrhythmia syndromes

Inherited cardiac arrhythmia syndromes are an important cause of morbidity and mortality. These syndromes typically manifest during childhood or adolescence with a clinical presentation ranging from sudden cardiac arrest or death (SCA/D) to an incidental finding on ECG. This chapter will provide an overview of genetic arrhythmia syndromes that may cause life-threatening arrhythmias in the absence of structural heart disease, including congenital long QT syndrome (LQTS), Brugada syndrome (BrS), catecholaminergic polymorphic ventricular tachycardia (CPVT), and short QT syndrome (SQTS). Other inherited arrhythmia syndromes will be covered briefly, such as familial sick sinus syndrome (SSS), inherited Wolff–Parkinson–White (WPW) syndrome, progressive familial heart block (PFHB), and familial atrial fibrillation (AF). Inherited forms of cardiomyopathies associated with ventricular arrhythmias are discussed in Chapter 12.1.

Clinical approach

The approach is primarily to identify and distinguish between inherited arrhythmia syndromes.

History: key points
- Syncope: frequency, duration, time of the day, mode of onset (typical triggers include exercise, stress, loud noise, and swimming).
- Epilepsy may be a primary consequence of inherited defect, or secondary due to brain ischemia.
- Family history: syncope or SCA/D in pedigree. Consanguinity in parents may indicate an autosomal recessive (AR) syndrome.
- Associated hearing loss.
- Associated malformations (e.g. syndactyly).

Examination: key points
- General: usually normal although fever may be a trigger for some forms of arrhythmias.
- Cardiac: rule out signs of structural heart disease such as murmurs, S3, S4, and abnormal location of apex beat (e.g. valvular or septal defects, or hypertrophic cardiomyopathy).
- Ears: signs of sensorineural deafness (Jervell and Lange–Nielsen syndrome (JLNS)).

Special investigations
- Lab: rule out conditions that may exacerbate arrhythmias, such as metabolic abnormalities and ischaemia.
- Electrocardiogram (ECG): look for abnormal QTc intervals, T-wave notch, T-wave alternans, bradycardia. AF, or signs of conduction disease.
- Non-invasive tests: 24-hour Holter recording, echocardiogram, and exercise stress test.
- Invasive tests: programmed electrophysiological study (PES), coronary angiography, right and left ventricular cine-angiography, and/or MRI (in case of suspected arrhythmogenic right ventricular dysplasia/cardiomyopathy).
- EEG: in case of suspected or witnessed epilepsy.
- DNA analysis: recommended if clinical diagnosis is strongly suspected. Screening for mutations in arrhythmia syndrome-associated genes.
- Consider clinical and genetic evaluation of first- and second-degree relatives.

Some diagnoses to consider

Long QT syndrome
Congenital long QT syndrome (LQTS) is characterized by delayed repolarization, syncope due to Torsade de Pointes (tdp) tachycardia, and SCA/D due to ventricular fibrillation (VF). JLNS is associated with congenital deafness.

Epidemiology
Prevalence is estimated to be approximately 1:2500 to 1:5000. Congenital LQTS may be responsible for approximately 5000 deaths in the United States each year.

Diagnostic criteria
The Schwartz–Moss score is used for the clinical diagnosis, and a positive score has a considerable relevance for prognosis and clinical management (Morita et al 2008). Probability of LQTS is high with ≥4 points, low with ≤1, and intermediate with 2–3. Scoring criteria are:
- QTc (QT/√RR): ≥480 ms, 3 points (pts); 460–470 ms, 2 pts; 450 ms and male gender, 1 pt
- tdp: 2 pts
- T-wave alternans, 1 pt
- Notched T wave in at least three leads, 1 pt
- Low heart rate for age, 0.5 pt
- Syncope (with stress, 2 pt; without stress, 1 pt)
- Congenital deafness, 0.5 pt
- Family history: definite LQTS, 1 pt; SCD in immediate family age <30, 0.5 pt.

Clinical presentation
Mean age of onset of LQTS is usually during teenage years, and earlier onset is associated with more severe form of the disease. Death is the first symptom in 10–15% of LQTS patients. Triggers of arrhythmia and syncope vary by genotype: 99% of cardiac events during swimming are due to LQT1, and 80% of events precipitated by acoustic stimuli are due to LQT2.

Electrophysiological examination
Prolonged QTc intervals are found in 70–80% of LQTS patients. Some patients show atypical T-wave abnormalities. Exercise or epinephrine injection may show failure of normal QTc shortening, or even paradoxical prolongation of QTc.

Genetic testing
Genetic testing is recommended for all patients with a firm clinical diagnosis of LQTS irrespective of the presence of symptoms and/or affected family members. At-risk family members need to be evaluated too. The expected yield of genetic testing is about 50–60% in correctly diagnosed probands. About 90% of genotyped LQTS cases are caused by mutations in *KCNQ1* (LQT1), *KCNH2* (LQT2), or *SCN5A* (LQT3). Compound heterozygosity is present in 4% of LQTS patients. Genetic testing is strongly recommended for patients with a clinical diagnosis of JLNS, or Timothy or Andersen syndromes.
- LQT1 is caused by autosomal-dominant (AD) loss-of-function mutations in *KCNQ1*, which encodes the α-subunit of the slow delayed rectifier K^+ current I_{Ks}. It is the most common type of LQTS. Rare AR mutations in *KCNQ1* result in JLNS.
- LQT2 is caused by loss-of-function mutations in *KCNH2*, the α-subunit of the rapid delayed rectifier K^+ current I_{Kr}.

- LQT3 is caused by gain-of-function mutations in *SCN5A*, the α-subunit of the Na$^+$ current I$_{Na}$.
- LQTS may be caused by rare mutations in other ion channel genes, including *KCNE1* (LQT5), *KCNE2* (LQT6), *KCNJ2* (LQT7, or Andersen–Tawil syndrome), *CACNA1c* (LQT8, or Timothy syndrome), and *SCN4B* (LQT10). Mutations also occur in genes encoding channel-associated proteins, including *ANK2* (LQT4), *Cav3* (LQT9), *AKAP9* (LQT11), and *SNTA1* (LQT12).
  - LQT4 patients may also exhibit AF and conduction disorders.
  - LQT7, or Anderson–Tawil syndrome, also manifests with periodic paralysis, and skeletal developmental abnormalities (syndactyly, short stature, scoliosis, small mandible, hypertelorism).
  - LQT8, or Timothy syndrome, may also exhibit congenital heart diseases, syndactyly, dysmorphic facial features, cognitive deficits, and autism. Average age of death is 2.5 years.

Prevention and treatment
Avoidance of competitive sports, swimming (LQT1), acoustic stimuli (LQT2), and drugs that further prolong QT intervals.
- Beta-blocking agents decrease the risk of stress-induced arrhythmias in patients with clinically diagnosed LQTS, or a LQTS-associated mutation with normal QTc intervals. Beta-blockers may be ineffective in patients with LQT3.
- Pacemakers may be needed in patients with symptomatic bradycardia with use of beta blockers.
- An implantable cardioverter-defibrillator (ICD) is advised in patients with LQT3 or LQT8; with poor prognostic factors, such as QTc >500 ms; repetitive syncope; or previous SCA.
- Potassium supplementation may shorten QTc intervals in patients with LQT2.
- Mexilitine blocks pathogenic sustained Na$^+$ current in patients with LQT3.
- Left cardiac sympathetic neural denervation (stellectomy) might be considered in case of refractory syncope and SCA, but an ICD is usually preferred.

Brugada syndrome
BrS, or idiopathic ventricular fibrillation, is an AD inherited arrhythmia syndrome characterized by ST segment elevation in the right precordial leads, right bundle branch block (RBBB), and susceptibility to ventricular tachycardia (VT) at rest.

Epidemiology
The prevalence of BrS is estimated to be around 1:200 to 1:1000. The male-to-female ratio is 8:1. In Southeast Asia, BrS is the most common cause of natural death in men <50 years.

Diagnostic criteria
Three ECG repolarization patterns in the right precordial leads are used to diagnose BrS (Wilde *et al* 2002):
- Type 1: coved ST segment elevation ≥2 mm followed by a negative T wave in >1 right precordial lead (V1–V3) is diagnostic of BrS. Concealed ECG signs might be unmasked by Na$^+$ channel blockers (e.g. ajmaline, flecainide).
- Type 2: saddleback ST segment elevation with high take-off ≥2 mm, a through >1 mm ST elevation, and positive or biphasic T-wave.

- Type 3: saddleback or coved ST elevation of <1 mm.
- Type 2 and 3 ECG patterns are not diagnostic of BrS. The diagnosis is considered positive when a type 2/3 ST-segment elevation is observed in >1 lead (V1–V3) under basal conditions, and conversion to type 1 occurs after Na$^+$ channel blockade.
- A definitive diagnosis of BrS is made when one of the following is also present: documented VF, polymorphic VT, family history of SCD <45 years, coved-type ECGs in relatives, VT inducibility with PES, syncope, or nocturnal agonal respiration.

Clinical presentation
BrS typically first manifests in the third decade of life. Syncope and SCA are the most common clinical manifestations leading to the diagnosis. In many cases, SCD occurs during rest or sleep. Sometimes the diagnosis is made on the basis of typical findings on a routine ECG. Occasionally, fever has been reported to exacerbate the disease phenotype. Physical examination is required to rule out cardiac causes associated with syncope. Up to 20% of BrS patients develop supraventricular arrhythmias such as AF.

Electrophysiological examination
ECG findings include the presence of typical ST-segment elevation patterns and pseudo-RBBB (elevation of J point) in V1 to V3. Some patients exhibit prolongation of P wave, PR and QTc intervals. EPS can identify high-risk patients in need of treatment.

Genetic screening
Genetic screening is recommended to support the clinical diagnosis and for early detection of relatives at risk. Tests for mutations in *SCN5A* are commercially available, but the prevalence of this defect is only 18–30%, and average penetrance is just 16%.
- BrS1 is caused by loss-of-function mutations in *SCN5A*, the α-subunit of the Na$^+$ current I$_{Na}$, which accounts for 15–30% of all BrS cases.
- BrS2 is rare (1%), caused by mutations in glycerol-3 phosphate dehydrogenase 1-like gene (*GPD1L*). Mutant GPD1L reduces the I$_{Na}$ current.
- BrS3 and BrS4 are caused by mutations in the α1-subunit (*CACNA1C*) and β-subunit (*CACNB2b*) of the L-type Ca^{2+} channel, respectively. Accounts for 8–10% of all BrS, and is often associated with short QT syndrome.
- BrS5 is caused by mutations in *KCNE3*, the β-subunit of the I$_{TO}$ outward K$^+$ channel.
- BrS6 is caused by mutations in *SCN1B*, the β1-subunit of the cardiac Na$^+$ channel.

Prevention and treatment
BrS patients who present with a first episode of SCA are at a high risk of recurrence (70% in next 5 years). Patients with type 1 ST-segment elevation are at the highest risk for syncope. Male gender is another risk factor for SCA/D. Sustained VT induced by PES is the strongest marker of risk. ICD implantation is the only proven effective treatment for BrS, and is indicated in patients with a history of SCA; symptomatic patients with type 1 ST-segment elevation and positive PES study; or asymptomatic patients with type 1 ST-segment elevation, a family history of SCD, and a positive PES study. Certain class 1A agents (e.g. quinidine, tedisamil) might reduce the number of ICD discharges.

Catecholaminergic polymorphic ventricular tachycardia

CPVT is a familial arrhythmogenic disorder characterized by exercise- and stress-related VT manifesting as syncope or SCA/D in patients with structurally normal hearts. CPVT1 has an AD inheritance, whereas the rare CPVT2 subtype has AR inheritance.

Epidemiology

CPVT prevalence is estimated to be 1:10 000.

Diagnosis

No specific diagnostic criteria have been established for CPVT. Exercise- or stress-induced bidirectional or polymorphic VT is a fairly specific finding.

Clinical presentation

About 30% of patients present with a family history of stress-induced syncope, seizures, or SCA/D. Syncope or SCA triggered by physical or emotional stress typically manifests during childhood and adolescence with a mean age of onset being 8 ± 4 years. In ~60% of all cases, SCA/D is the first clinical manifestation. About 20% may have no phenotype.

Electrophysiological examination

Baseline ECG is usually normal, although some patients exhibit prominent U waves or U wave alternans. Sinus bradycardia or AF is observed in some patients. Ventricular extrasystoles can be elicited in most patients during exercise when heart rates exceed 120–130 bpm. Exercise stress testing is recommended in family members to identify exercise-induced VT, but the sensitivity of this test is currently unknown.

Genetic testing

Genetic testing is recommended for individuals with clinical features consistent with CPVT. The diagnostic yield is less than that for LQTS (<50%), but mutation identification has an important prognostic value for both the proband and family members. First-degree relatives should be screened genetically if the mutation is known, or using exercise-stress testing if the genetic defect is unknown. Because of the massive size of the *RyR2* gene, a targeted approach is usually undertaken in which only exons that have been previously implicated are screened.

- CPVT1 is caused by gain-of-function mutations in *RyR2*, the cardiac ryanodine receptor, resulting in diastolic Ca^{2+} release from the sarcoplasmic reticulum (SR) and delayed afterdepolarizations. *RyR2* mutations account for 50% of all CPVT cases.
- CPVT2 is caused by less common *CASQ2* defects. Loss-of-function mutations cause reduced Ca^{2+} buffering within the SR, which is associated with defective Ca^{2+} release and arrhythmias.

Prevention and treatment

- Untreated mortality rate of CPVT is 30–50% by the age of 40.
- Affected people should avoid competitive sports and strenuous exercise.
- Prophylactic β-blocker treatment, with the dose titrated by treadmill testing, is recommended for patients with confirmed spontaneous or stress-induced VT/VF, or genetically diagnosed CPVT in childhood. In up to 40% of patients, in particular males, β-blockade is ineffective.
- ICD implantation, in addition to β-blockers, is recommended in CPVT survivors of SCA.

- Flecainide might have therapeutic effects in patients with CPVT2.

Short QT syndrome

SQTS is an AD inherited disorder characterized by a persistently short QT interval, paroxysmal AF, and increased risk of SCD in the absence of structural heart disease.

Epidemiology

Prevalence is rare and estimated to be <1:1000.

Diagnosis and clinical presentation

- Often diagnosed in childhood, when patients present with syncope or palpitations.
- Most patients have a family history of SCA/D.
- QTc of ≤360 ms is suggestive (≤320 ms is typical).
- Tall and peaked T-wave pattern (as seen in hyperkalaemia) is often observed.
- Bradycardia and/or AF (24% of cases) are sometimes associated.
- PES studies reveal shortening of effective refractory periods and a high percentage of inducibility of ventricular tachyarrhythmias (60%).

Genetic testing

Genetic testing is recommended for individuals with short QT intervals (<320 ms).

- SQT1: gain-of-function mutations in *KCNH2* increase I_{Kr} current, thus shortening action potentials.
- SQT2: gain-of-function mutations in *KCNQ1* increase I_{Ks} current.
- SQT3: gain-of-function mutations in KCNJ2 increase I_{K1} outward K^+ current; typical asymmetric T waves (normal ascending/rapid terminal phase).
- SQT4/SQT5: loss-of-function mutations in *CACNA1C* and *CACNB2b* affect the I_{Ca} current.

Prevention and treatment

- Quinidine can be efficacious by prolonging QT intervals and preventing SCA in some patients.
- Implantation of an ICD is needed for prevention.

Familial sick sinus syndrome

Familial SSS is characterized by sinus bradycardia and sinus arrest in absence of structural heart disease.

Epidemiology

The prevalence of SSS is 1:600 of all cardiac patients >65 years of age, a fraction of which is due to familial SSS.

Diagnosis and clinical presentation

SSS can either be asymptomatic or present with syncope, fatigue, dyspnoea, angina, disturbed sleep, confusion, or palpitations.

Electrophysiological examination

SSS may present as sinus bradycardia, sinus arrest or exit block, combinations of SA and AV node defects, or atrial tachycardia ('tachy-brady syndrome').

Genetic testing

- SSS1: AR mutations in *SCN5A* lead to loss of I_{Na}.
- SSS2: AD mutations in *HCN4* lead to loss of I_f channel function, due to faster I_f deactivation.
- SSS is also a common finding in LQT4 patients with loss-of-function mutations in *ANK2*.

Prevention and treatment

Pacemaker is indicated in case of symptomatic bradycardia.

Wolff–Parkinson–White syndrome

WPW syndrome is a pre-excitation syndrome characterized by premature depolarization of ventricles via an accessory pathway. Whereas WPW might occur as syndromic pre-excitation (e.g. Ebstein's anomaly; not covered in this chapter), WPW can also occur as a single gene disorder.

Epidemiology
Prevalence of WPW is 1:300 to 1:700, of which <5% might be inherited forms of WPW.

Diagnosis and clinical presentation
Patients with WPW syndrome present clinically with palpitations, presyncope, or SCD.

Electrophysiological examination
- Shortened PR interval (<120 ms)
- Widened QRS (>100 ms) with delta wave (slurring of the QRS onset)
- ST changes that are opposite to the direction of QRS complex
- Supraventricular tachycardia
- Diagnosis is typically confirmed using PES
- Familial WPW syndrome differs from other forms in that affected patients may also develop conduction abnormalities (usually in the fourth decade of life).

Genetic testing
Familial WPW syndrome is caused by AD missense mutations in PRKAG2, which encodes an AMP-activated protein kinase. It accounts for approximately 3.4% of all patients with WPW syndrome, and is clinically associated with conduction disease and HCM. Since PRKAG2 mutations are rare, genetic screening is not recommended at this stage.

Treatment
- Ablation of the accessory pathway.
- In familial WPW: permanent pacemaker.

Progressive familial heart block

PFHB is an AD bundle branch disorder that may progress to complete heart block. The adult form is also known as hereditary Lenegre–Lev disease.

Epidemiology
Incidence of PFHB is very rare.

Diagnosis and clinical presentation
- Age of presentation is variable.
- Symptoms may include dyspnoea, syncope or SCA.

Electrophysiological examination
- PFHB1 is a progressive disorder manifesting as RBBB, left anterior or posterior hemiblock, and/or complete heart block with broad QRS complexes.
- PFHB2 manifests as sinus bradycardia, atrioventricular block, idionodal escape rhythm, and/or complete heart block with narrow QRS complexes.

Genetic testing
- PFHB1A: AD loss-of-function defects in SCN5A resulting in reduced I_{Na} current.
- PFHB1B: AD inheritance, mapped to locus 19q13.2-q13.3.
- PFHB2: AD inheritance, mapped to locus 1q32.

Prevention and treatment
Regular follow-up with ECG and timely implantation of a pacemaker is recommended.

Familial atrial fibrillation (FAF or ATFB)

FAF is a monogenetic disorder typically identified when several members of the same family exhibit AF.

Epidemiology
Familial forms are a rare cause of AF.

Diagnosis and clinical examination
Clinical presentation is similar to patients with non-familial AF, which includes palpitations, syncope, dyspnoea and/or angina.

Electrophysiological examination
ECG is similar to that in lone AF: absence of P waves, and irregular RR intervals.

Genetic testing
- ATFB1: AD inheritance, locus on 10q22-q24.
- ATFB2: AD inheritance, locus on 6q14-q16.
- ATFB3: AD gain-of-function mutations in KCNQ1 lead to more I_{Ks} current.
- ATFB4: AD gain-of-function mutations in KCNE2, the β-subunit of the I_{Kr} channel.
- ATFB5: locus identified on 4q25.
- ATFB6: AD inheritance, mutations in NPPA gene (natriuretic peptide precursor A).
- ATFB7: AD mutations in KCNA5, which encodes the Kv1.5 K⁺ channel.
- Additional mutations have been identified in:
  - KCNJ2, causing gain-of-function of I_{K1} current.
  - SCN5A, causing gain-of-function of I_{Na} current.
  - NUP155, leading to loss-of-function.

Treatment and prognosis
The guidelines for lone atrial fibrillation apply (see Chapters 3.3 and 3.8).

Online support

Additional information about specific genes is available at the Online Mendelian Inheritance in Man website (http://www.ncbi.nlm.nih.gov/sites/entrez?db=omim). Available gene tests can be accessed at www.genetests.org, a NIH funded resource. The website of the Sudden Arrhythmia Death Syndrome Foundation (www.sads.org) contains clinically relevant information about the management of patients with inherited arrhythmia syndromes.

References
Katz G, Arad M, Eldar M. Catecholaminergic polymorphic ventricular tachycardia from bedside to bench and beyond. *Curr Probl Cardiol* 2009;**34**:9–43.

Morita H, Wu J, Zipes DP. The QT syndromes: long and short. *Lancet* 2008;**372**:750–63.

Wilde AA, Antzelevitch C, Borggrefe M, et al. Proposed diagnostic criteria for the Brugada syndrome. *Eur Heart J* 2002;**23**:1648–54.

Grown-up congenital heart disease

General principles

Continuous improvement of medical and surgical therapy over the past five decades has led to more than 85% of children with congenital heart lesions surviving into adulthood.

There are in fact more than 250 000 adults with congenital heart disease currently living in the UK and this number continues to grow. However, treatment of congenital heart disease can rarely be considered as being curative and about half of adults with congenital heart disease face the prospect of further surgery or non-surgical intervention, arrhythmia, heart failure, and—if managed inappropriately—premature death.

As patients with congenital heart disease grow older acquired heart or general health problems impose on the underlying cardiac anomaly. This becomes an increasing problem as the patient population ages.

Patients with congenital heart disease may present in adulthood with mild unrepaired lesions, undetected defects (often during pregnancy) or residua or sequelae from surgical repair. Attendance of a specialized centre is required for:

- The assessment of patients if congenital heart disease is suspected
- Follow-up and continuous care for patients with congenital heart disease
- Further surgery or non-surgical interventions
- Risk assessment and counselling on non-cardiac surgery
- Risk assessment and counselling on pregnancy
- Counselling on contraception.

The care for patients with congenital heart disease should ideally be provided by tertiary adult congenital heart disease centres to provide optimal care for these patients reducing errors and avoiding crisis management, sufficient training for medical and non-medical stuff, and to facilitate research. But tertiary care is not possible for any patient at any time for many reasons including geography, lack of capacity, and need for local emergency care. It is therefore essential that tertiary centres offer educational resources to patients and a broader professional audience including not only paediatric an adult cardiologists but also family physicians, obstetricians, surgeons and anaesthetists. Education is in fact the key to improve the care for adults with congenital heart disease.

Transition of care from paediatric cardiology to adult congenital heart disease

Paediatric cardiology centres play a key role in securing appropriate lifelong care for patients with congenital heart disease. Not only do these centres often form the nucleus for adult congenital heart units but also do they have to transfer care to the adult unit when patients reach adulthood. Transition of care has to be secured, transition pathways need to be identified, and transition should take place in a structured way. A transition clinic run jointly with the paediatric cardiologist and the specialist in adult congenital heart would be an ideal model. Patients need to be prepared and educated regarding their diagnosis and specific health behaviours prior to transition, and this needs to be reinforced during transition. Comprehensive information including diagnosis, previous surgical and/or catheter interventions, medical therapy, investigations, current outpatient clinic reports, and medication should be copied to the patients and be provided to the adult congenital heart disease facility. Furthermore, to facilitate care in site it is essential to share this information with local general cardiologists and family physicians.

Specific congenital heart lesions

Patients with congenital heart disease require lifelong follow-up. The most common congenital heart lesions will briefly be reviewed to support this thesis.

Left to right shunt lesions

Ventricular septal defect

Most patients with a ventricular septal defect (VSD) will have been repaired by adulthood but adult patients can present with a native or residual shunt. The haemodynamic consequences of this are dependent on the shunt size. Small restrictive VSDs are often found incidentally and may result in mild left atrium (LA) and left ventricular (LV) dilatation whereas a large (non-restrictive) VSD results in significant LA and LV dilatation and can lead to pulmonary hypertension and Eisenmenger's syndrome.

Clinical issues and outcome in adulthood

- Atrial or ventricular arrhythmia from atrial and ventricular enlargement
- Complete heart block from previous surgery with damage to the atrioventricular (AV) node
- Pulmonary hypertension can progress in patients even after successful closure of the defect late in childhood (>6 months of age)
- Aortic regurgitation (5%) from prolapse of the aortic valve (if the defect is perimembranous)
- Heart failure resulting from left to right shunting or aortic regurgitation
- Pulmonary artery stenosis (from previous pulmonary artery banding)
- Endocarditis.

Patients with a restrictive VSD and patients after successful closure have an excellent long-term outcome. Their life expectancy is close to normal.

Indications for intervention

- LA and LV enlargement with or without early LV dysfunction.
- Reversible pulmonary hypertension (mild)—only consider if the patient is pink and remains pink during exercise, has a significant left to right shunt and, when tested, there is a positive acute vasoreactive response in the catheter laboratory.
- Significant aortic regurgitation in a perimembranous or doubly committed VSD.
- Significant right ventricular (RV) outflow tract obstruction (RV pressure more than two-thirds systemic).

Interventional options are either surgical patch repair or device closure if it is an isolated muscular VSD.

Atrial septal defect

There are three main types of atrial septal defect (ASD):
- Sinus venosus defects are found in the upper part of atrial septum—may be associated with partial anomalous drainage of pulmonary veins to superior vena cava or right atrium (RA).

- Ostium secundum defects (75%) are found in the area of fossa ovalis.
- Ostium primum (atrioventricular septal) defects are found in the lower part of atrial septum—are associated with a trileaflet left AV valve, which is often regurgitant.

Clinical issues and outcome in adulthood

Haemodynamic consequences of the ASD are dependant on the size of the defect, the compliance of the ventricles and the resultant size of the shunt.

Adult patients with an unrepaired ASD with significant LR shunt can present with:
- Dyspnoea and exercise intolerance
- Atrial arrythmias from RA dilatation
- Cerebrovascular events from paradoxical embolisms
- Right heart failure from RV dilatation
- Reduced LV compliance
- Occasionally with pulmonary arterial hypertension.

Patients who had ASD closure before the age of 25 years have a normal long-term survival. Conditions that decrease LV compliance will increase the LR shunt and worsen symptoms. Patients who underwent closure at an older age and those with elevated pulmonary artery pressure before closure have lower long-term survival rates. But even patients who present at an age >40 years benefit from ASD closure in that it improves survival, functional class, exercise tolerance, and reduces the risk of heart failure and pulmonary hypertension. The risk for arrhythmia is not abolished in these patients after late closure.

Indications for intervention
- An ASD with significant LR shunting, resulting in RA/RV enlargement with a mean pulmonary artery pressure of approximately half of the patients age should be closed irrespective of symptoms.
- Cryptogenic thromboembolic event.
- Interventional options—device closure for most secundum ASDs or surgical for all other ASD types.

Atrioventricular septal defect

This term covers a spectrum of defects, all sharing a common AV junction. Abnormalities of the AV valves are universal (single valve in patients with complete atrioventricular septal defect (AVSD), two separate valves in partial AVSD or ostium primum ASD). These defects are found in a third of patients with Down's syndrome.

Clinical issues and outcome in adulthood

The physiological consequences of an AVSD are similar to a VSD and ASD. Adult patients with repaired AVSDs can present with
- Complete AV block
- AV regurgitation or stenosis
- Pulmonary hypertension or heart failure
- Subaortic stenosis.

Patent ductus arteriosus

Patent ductus arteriosus (PDA) is a persistent communication between the proximal left pulmonary artery and the descending aorta resulting in a left to right shunt.

Clinical issues and outcome in adulthood

Usually none, unless there is a moderate or large PDA that can lead to LV dilatation and pulmonary arterial hypertension.

Indications for intervention
- Controversial for small PDAs—there is an associated risk of endarteritis with all except small silent PDAs, albeit small, which is the reason some advocate closing all except silent PDAs
- LV dilatation
- Pulmonary arterial hypertension
- Interventional options—most PDAs are suitable for device closure. Surgical closure should be re-served for those with large PDAs.

Cyanotic congenital heart defects

Tetralogy of Fallot

Tetralogy of Fallot (TOF) comprises a large VSD, RV outflow tract obstruction, consequent RV hypertrophy, and an aorta overriding the septum. The overall survival of those who have had operative repair is excellent. DiGeorge syndrome is found in 15% of those with TOF genetic testing should be offered to any TOF patient of reproductive age—following counselling—as the recurrence risk of DiGeorge syndrome is 50%.

Clinical issues and outcome in adulthood

The majority of adults with TOF will have undergone complete repair, which involves relief of the RV outflow tract obstruction and closure of the VSD. Many patients will also have had a prior systemic-to-pulmonary artery shunt (i.e. Blalock–Taussig, Waterston, Potts) (Table 12.4.1) to increase pulmonary blood flow in severe cases of pulmonary stenosis or pulmonary atresia, and a small number will only have had these palliative shunts and no repair attempted.

The issues which may arise in this group in adulthood are:
- Branch pulmonary artery stenosis from previous shunt procedure (especially Waterston and Potts shunts).
- RV outflow tract obstruction (subvalvar, valvar, or supravalvar pulmonary stenosis).
- Pulmonary regurgitation is almost always present when transannular patch enlargement of the RV outflow tract was performed at repair, when mild or moderate, usually well tolerated long term.
- Aortic regurgitation can result from damage to the valve during VSD closure or secondary to intrinsic abnormalities of a dilated ascending aorta ('cystic medial necrosis').
- LV dysfunction can be associated with severe RV enlargement and dysfunction, the latter may result from long standing pulmonary regurgitation. Long standing cyanosis, repeated cardiac surgery or chronic volume overload of the left ventricle (residual VSD, longstanding palliative shunt before repair, aortic regurgitation) can cause LV dysfunction as well.
- Atrial arrhythmia is common late after repair of TOF (atrial flutter or atrial fibrillation). It occurs in about 30% of adult patients after repair.
- Ventricular tachycardia is less common than atrial tachycardia. It is associated with RV dilatation and dysfunction. The QRS duration of the surface ECG has been shown to correlate with right ventricular size; a QRS duration >180 ms is a highly sensitive marker for sustained VT and sudden death.
- Sudden death is reported to occur with an incidence between 0.5–6% over a period of 30 years after repair.

Table 12.3.1 Common surgical procedures in patients with adult congenital heart disease

Operation	Condition in which it may be used	First performed	Details of operation
Arterial switch (Jantene)	Transposition of the great arteries	1976	Switching the great vessels to their correct position and reimplantation of the coronary arteries on the neoaorta
Atrial switch Mustard Senning	Transposition of the great arteries	1963 1959	Redirection of venous blood to contralateral ventricle Using pericardium or synthetic patch Using atrial wall and septum
Bentall procedure	Aortic valve and root pathology	1968	Replacement of aortic valve and ascending aorta with a conduit and valve and reimplantation of the coronary arteries
BT shunt	Pulmonary stenosis (TOF) or pulmonary atresia	1944	Subclavian artery to ipsilateral pulmonary artery (end to side) anastomosis (Modified BT shunt uses a interposition graft (side to side) anastomosis)
Fontan Classic Fontan Total cavopulmonary connection (TCPC) Extracardiac	Tricuspid atresia	1971	Diversion of systemic venous return to pulmonary artery Right atrium connected to pulmonary artery Glenn plus IVC connected to pulmonary artery with an intra-atrial tunnel Glenn plus IVC connected to pulmonary artery with an extracardiac conduit
Glenn shunt	Pulmonary stenosis or pulmonary atresia		Superior vena cava to ipsilateral pulmonary artery anastomosis
Konno procedure	LV outflow tract obstruction	1974	Repair and reconstruction of the LVOT which is enlarged by inserting a patch in the interventricular septum
Potts shunt	Pulmonary stenosis or pulmonary atresia	1946	Descending aorta to left pulmonary artery anastomosis
Rastelli	Transposition of the great arteries with VSD and PS	1968	Closure of VSD so that the patch connects the aorta to the LV. A conduit is placed to connect the RV to the pulmonary trunk
Ross procedure	Aortic valve stenosis or regurgitation	1967	Transplantation of patient's pulmonary valve to the aortic position and placement of a homograft in the pulmonary position
Tetralogy of Fallot repair	Tetralogy of Fallot	1954	Transannular patch enlargement of right ventricular outflow tract or implantation of conduit from RV to pulmonary artery (for pulmonary atresia)
Waterston Shunt	Pulmonary stenosis or pulmonary atresia	1962	Ascending aorta to right pulmonary artery anastomosis

Indications for further intervention

All patients who have had only palliative procedures should be offered reparative surgery if possible.

- Pulmonary valve replacement should be offered to patients with severe pulmonary regurgitation and progressive moderate to severe RV dilatation and or symptoms, or documented decline of exercise capacity.
- In the long term, the development of clinical arrhythmias like ventricular tachycardia and atrial flutter/fibrillation warrants both full electrophysiological assessment and thorough review of the haemodynamics.
- Target lesions should be repaired (e.g. VSD with large left to right shunt and significant pulmonary stenosis).

Complete transposition of the great arteries (TGA)

In complete transposition of the great arteries the right atrium connects to the morphological right ventricle which gives rise to the aorta and the left atrium connects to the morphological left ventricle which gives rise to the

pulmonary artery. This is incompatible with life, so adults with transposition of the great arteries (TGA) have had operations in childhood.

The patient after 'atrial switch operation'

Currently the majority of adult patients with transposition of the great arteries will have had an 'atrial switch' (Mustard or Senning) operation (Table 12.4.1). The right ventricle remains the systemic ventricle in this situation.

Clinical issues and outcome in adulthood

- By 16 years post-atrial switch only 18% of patients remain in permanent sinus rhythm. Sinus node dysfunction with junctional escape rhythm are common; patients may need permanent pacing.
- Atrial arrhythmia (atrial flutter/fibrillation) occurs in 20% of patients by the age of 20; extensive atrial surgery and systemic RV dysfunction are both contributory.
- Right (systemic) ventricular dysfunction is common, as the RV is not built to support the systemic circulation.
- Tricuspid regurgitation can accompany right heart failure.

- Obstruction of the atrial pathways ('baffle obstruction') can lead to systemic or pulmonary venous congestion.

Although most of these patients do well for many years, life expectancy is clearly limited by eventual failure of the systemic RV.

Indications for intervention

Thorough assessment of RV and tricuspid valve function, heart rhythm, and the integrity of intra-atrial venous pathways is paramount. Therapeutic options include catheterization techniques such as balloon dilatation and stenting for pathway obstruction. Procedures like tricuspid valve replacement or even conversion to the arterial switch operation (for highly selected patients—banding of the pulmonary artery is needed to retrain the left (subpulmonary) ventricle) may be considered. The end of the therapeutic spectrum is heart transplantation. Experts must perform transvenous pacing for bradyarrhythmias, as placement of the leads within the atria and into the left ventricle can be troublesome.

The patient after arterial switch operation

In this present decade the number of adults who survived the arterial switch procedure ('Jatene operation') will increase. Arrhythmias are less common in these patients and ventricular function is usually well preserved.

Clinical issues and outcome

- The arterial switch procedure carries the need for suture lines in the pulmonary trunk, which can cause pulmonary trunk stenosis.
- The procedure brings the pulmonary bifurcation in a position anterior to the ascending aorta, which can cause peripheral pulmonary artery stenosis.
- Progressive dilatation of the aortic root (former pulmonary root) can cause aortic regurgitation.
- As the arterial switch operation includes coronary artery reimplantation there is the potential for coronary stenosis and ischaemia.

Indications for intervention

- Significant RV outflow tract obstruction at any level.
- Myocardial ischaemia from coronary artery obstruction.
- Neo-aortic valve regurgitation.
- Ejection systolic heart murmur from pulmonary artery stenosis.
- Diastolic heart murmur from aortic regurgitation.

Congenitally corrected transposition of the great arteries

Systemic venous return to the RA enters a morphological LV, which pumps into the pulmonary artery. Pulmonary venous blood returns to the LA and then via the morphological right ventricle to the aorta. The circulation is physiologically corrected but the systemic circulation is supported by a morphological RV. Congenitally corrected TGA (ccTGA) is often associated with other heart lesions such as systemic (tricuspid) AV valve abnormalities with valve insufficiency, VSD, subpulmonary stenosis, complete heart block and Wolff–Parkinson–White syndrome. ccTGA can occur with dextrocardia.

Clinical issues and outcome

Patients with no associated abnormalities may survive until the sixth or seventh decade and may go unrecognized until problems arise. Patients may have been operated for their associated lesions.

- Progressive RV (systemic) dysfunction is common as the RV is not built to support the systemic circulation.
- Progressive systemic (tricuspid) AV valve regurgitation can manifest and aggravate heart failure.
- ccTGA patients are at risk of developing both bradyarrhythmia (complete AV block develops in 2% of the patients per year) and tachyarrhythmia (atrial tachycardia or SVT due to WPW syndrome).

Indication for intervention

Preservation of systemic (RV) ventricular function is crucial. Tricuspid (systemic) valve regurgitation has to be treated surgically before ventricular dysfunction becomes irreversible. Valve replacement and not repair is required because of the abnormal, often 'Ebstein-like' anatomy of the tricuspid valve. Complete AV block may require pacemaker implantation.

The single ventricle

Hearts with an 'anatomically' or 'functionally' single ventricle receive the systemic and pulmonary venous blood in 'one' ventricle and are therefore cyanotic. The single ventricle pumps blood into the pulmonary artery (when not atretic) and the aorta. The single ventricle can be predominantly of left or right ventricular morphology.

In case of an 'ideal' anatomy, blood flow into the single ventricle is unrestricted, and if ventricular function is good an adequate and equivalent amount of blood should be delivered to the lungs and into the body. In this 'well-balanced' situation, almost universally excessive pulmonary blood flow is avoided by an obstruction of the pulmonary outflow tract. If pulmonary outflow tract obstruction is not present, excessive blood flow into the lungs will lead to pulmonary arterial hypertension and the Eisenmenger's syndrome. Severe pulmonary outflow tract obstruction with reduced pulmonary blood flow causes severe cyanosis.

Indication for intervention

Surgery in patients with single ventricles is always palliative and aims to secure adequate pulmonary and systemic blood flow and maintain systemic ventricular function:

- Systemicopulmonary shunts (e.g. Blalock–Taussig) are commonly performed in early infancy to improve pulmonary blood flow
- Pulmonary artery banding will be performed to protect patients from pulmonary hypertension when pulmonary blood flow is unobstructed
- Systemic venous to pulmonary artery connections like the Glenn shunt or the Fontan operation (Table 12.4.1) are performed as definitive palliations to improve pulmonary blood flow and separate the pulmonary from the systemic circulation while unloading the systemic ventricle.

The patient after Fontan operation

Many adult patients with a single ventricle have undergone Fontan operations as definitive palliation. Following this operation, all systemic venous return is diverted to the pulmonary circulation without employing a subpulmonary ventricle. Blood flow to the lungs is only driven by systemic venous pressure. Therefore vasodilation or intravascular depletion can have significant impact on haemodynamic stability.

Clinical issues and outcome

A good 'Fontan patient' has no murmurs with a single second heart sound (systolic murmurs can indicate AV valve incompetence). Peripheral oedema can result from heart failure or protein losing enteropathy (PLE) or a combination of both.

- Atrial flutter/fibrillation related to scarring from surgery or to atrial distension from high venous pressure. Atrial arrhythmias in Fontan patients need prompt treatment as they can cause profound haemodynamic deterioration.
- Sinus node dysfunction may warrant pacemaker implantation.
- Thromboembolism can be associated with sluggish venous blood flow in dilated systemic venous pathways.
- PLE occurs in 10% of 'Fontan patients' and is characterized by intestinal protein loss leading to low serum protein levels and subsequently to peripheral oedema and ascites. The condition is associated with a poor prognosis.
- Deterioration of ventricular function is part of the 'natural' history especially if the ventricle is of right ventricular morphology.
- Hepatic dysfunction resulting from high hepatic venous pressure has to be excluded.
- Cyanosis often results from persistent systemic to pulmonary venous connections or intrapulmonary arteriovenous malformations leading to RL shunting.
- Long-term survival is clearly impaired in these patients. The 10-year survival rate is ~70%. If PLE develops, the 5-year survival is approximately 50%. Reoperation following the Fontan procedure carries a high mortality.

Management

'Fontan patients' are one of the most challenging groups of patients in cardiology and require close follow up (every 6–12 months). Treatment aims to maintain optimal pulmonary and systemic circulation and to preserve ventricular function. Therefore the above named complications need to be treated promptly.

Fontan conversion to a total cavopulmonary connection (TCPC) with concomitant arrhythmia surgery is an option for patients with a 'failing Fontan circulation' (arrhythmia, ventricular dysfunction, PLE, thrombus formation) and can improve clinical status and exercise tolerance and reduce arrhythmia propensity. Highly selected patients should only be considered, and the procedure nevertheless carries a high mortality/morbidity risk. Transplantation may be an alternative.

The cyanosed patient

Cyanosis secondary to RL shunting or decreased pulmonary blood flow results in hypoxaemia; multiple adaptive mechanisms ensue to increase oxygen delivery to the tissue. These include a rightward shift in the oxyhaemoglobin binding curve and a haemoglobin rise (secondary erythrocytosis and not polycythaemia).

Clinical issues and outcome

- Haematological: iron deficiency often results from an excessive demand for and inadequate iron uptake or due to repeated, inappropriate venesections. Coagulopathy with bleeding diathesis results from thrombocytopenia and impaired clotting function
- Neurology: brain injury from paradoxical embolism, haemorrhage, abscesses
- Renal: hypoxaemia induced glomerulopathy (haematuria, proteinuria) and nephrolithiasis (uric acid)
- Rheumatology: gout and osteoarthropathy.

Management

- Very few indications for venesection; it may be considered for patients with severe 'hyperviscosity symptoms'

(intense headache, dizziness, fatigue, visual disturbances, tinnitus, and myalgia (not common in patients with stable, compensated secondary erythrocytosis)) which persist following rehydration and with a haematocrit >65%. Noteworthy that many of these symptoms are also symptoms of iron deficiency, which is very common amongst cyanotic patients. There is no justification for routine venesection to keep the haemoglobin below a certain level because it increases the risk of stroke and compromises the oxygen-carrying capacity and, thus, tissue delivery. When venesection is performed, no more than 250–500 mL of blood should be to be removed over a period of 45 minutes and replaced with dextrose. IV 'air filters' must be used.
- Iron deficiency needs to be treated by oral or IV iron supplements.
- Anticoagulation: no general consensus on routine anticoagulation exists.

Eisenmenger's syndrome

Uncorrected left to right shunting in the lesions mentioned above may eventually lead morphological changes to the pulmonary vascular bed in response to the increased pulmonary blood flow result in an obliterative arteritis and progressive pulmonary arterial hypertension and eventually reversal of the shunt and cyanosis.

Clinical issues and outcome

Key clinical findings in these patients are cyanosis (not all are cyanosed at rest), clubbing, loud second heart sound, no murmur from original lesion.

ECG: RV hypertrophy.

CXR: oligaemic lung fields, enlarged proximal pulmonary arteries.

Most patients will have impaired exercise tolerance but their symptoms may be well compensated for years. They may present with the following:

- Atrial arrythmias
- Chest pain
- Syncope and sudden cardiac death
- Haemoptysis and intrapulmonary bleeding
- Pulmonary thromboembolic disease
- Brain abscesses.

The rate of survival at 30, 40, and 55 years has been noted to be 75%, 70%, and 55% respectively.

Management

- Anticoagulation: intrapulmonary thrombi complicate up to a third of patients with Eisenmenger's physiology; however, due to the risk of haemoptysis there are differing opinions on whether these patients should be routinely anticoagulated. Involvement of a haematologist for titrating anticoagulants is paramount.
- Advanced therapy for Eisenmenger patients (bosentan, an endothelin antagonist, and sildenafil, a phospodiesterase inhibitor) are safe and improve functional and pulmonary haemodynamics. Class III patients are currently considered for advance therapy.

Left-sided obstructive lesions

Aortic stenosis and regurgitation are discussed in Chapters 7.6 and 7.7 respectively.

LV outflow tract obstruction can occur at different levels:

- Supravalvar
- Valvar (see AS): in the adult patient with CHD is usually due to bicuspid aortic valve and is associated with other abnormalities, the most common being coarctation of

the aorta (which should be sought), PDA, or ascending aortopathy
- Subvalvar patients with a discrete fibromuscular subaortic stenosis have usually undergone surgery in childhood. But this lesion has a tendency for regrowth (~30% at 10 years after repair). Predictors for recurrence are a preoperative gradient >40 mmHg, a postoperative gradient >10 mmHg and young age at repair. Aortic regurgitation resulting from longstanding turbulent blood flow in the left ventricular outflow tract may develop with this lesion. Surgical therapy (resection of fibrous tissue plus myomectomy) is indicated in a symptomatic patient, if the peak pressure gradient is >60 mmHg or if aortic regurgitation occurs.

Coarctation

Most adults with coarctation of the aorta will have had a corrective procedure. Significant aortic coarctation is usually one with right arm hypertension and a peak pull back gradient of more than 20 mmHg across the coarctation site at angiography. Clinically this may be picked up by a continuous murmur in the back, upper limb hypertension and differential arm–leg pulses (20 mmHg higher pressure in the right arm than left pressure would suggest significant coarctation).

If there is extensive collateral circulation, a significant aortic coarctation may have minimal or no pressure gradient between upper and lower limbs.

Clinical issues and outcome in adulthood
- Systemic hypertension
- Recoarctation of residual coarctation
- Aneurysm formation at the site of repair and aortic dissection
- Progressive aortic valve disease (75% of patients with coarctation have an associated bicuspid valve)
- Cerebral stroke from a ruptured Berry aneurysm
- Heart failure from longstanding LV pressure load
- Life expectancy is reduced in coarctation patients, because of systemic hypertension and propensity to early atherosclerosis. It is therefore, paramount to avoid other risk factors for ischaemic heart disease.

Management and intervention
- Meticulous control of systemic hypertension
- In case of a pressure peak-to-peak gradient across the coarctation of >20 mmHg and/or proximal hypertension catheter stenting or surgical relief of coarctation should be offered
- Interventional implantation of an endovascular stent graft can be offered in specialized centres to seal aneurysms at the site of coarctation.

Cardiac assessment in pregnancy

Introduction

The ability of women to bear children and to survive to bring them up is fundamental to the health of any society. In the developed world, pregnancy is remarkably safe with a maternal mortality rate (MMR) of 9 per 100 000 maternities. In contrast, pregnancy causes many deaths in developing countries; the MMR is 450 in the developing world, ranging from 130 in Latin America to 900 in sub-Saharan Africa (WHO 2007). Maternal deaths in the developing world reflect poor socioeconomic conditions, a lack of education, transport, and organization of basic obstetric services, and are largely due to direct obstetric causes such as obstructed labour, haemorrhage, and infection. Not until these issues are addressed are maternal deaths due to medical disorders like heart disease revealed.

Heart disease is a major cause of maternal death in the developed world; in the UK it is the commonest cause of pregnancy-related death (Table 12.4.1) (Lewis 2007). Furthermore, in developing countries that have sufficient infrastructure to investigate maternal deaths, cardiac disease is also emerging as a major cause of death in pregnant women (Hahthotuwa et al. 2009). In the developed and developing world, substandard care has been consistently identified as an important contributory factor to maternal death. However, the types of heart disease resulting in maternal death differ between societies. In the developing world, rheumatic mitral stenosis is the major cause (James et al. 2006; Nqayana et al. 2008), whereas in the UK coronary artery disease, ventricular dysfunction, and puerperal cardiomyopathy account for more than half of cardiac maternal deaths.

Since maternal death is a rarity in the developed world, morbidity and 'near miss' data are of particular interest. Small series of pregnancy outcome for specific conditions are available, but there are little population based data. A nationwide study in the USA estimated the incidence of

Table 12.4.1 Major cardiac causes of maternal death in the UK 2003–5 (Lewis 2007)

Cause of death	Number of deaths during pregnancy and up to 1 year post delivery
Ischaemic heart disease	20
Ventricular dysfunction	10
Peripartum cardiomyopathy	12
Sudden*	12
Aortic dissection	9
Congenital heart disease	5
Endocarditis	4
Pulmonary hypertension	3
Rheumatic heart disease	3

Maternal mortality is defined as death during pregnancy or up to 42 days after delivery. The Confidential Enquiry also collects data on late deaths, up to a year post delivery.
There were a total of 149 maternal deaths in this period.
*Sudden: no underlying heart disease found; presumed arrhythmic.

pregnancy related acute myocardial infarction to be 6.2 per 10 000 deliveries, with a case fatality rate of 5.1%. UKOSS (UK Obstetric Surveillance System) collects information on the outcome of rare conditions in pregnancy, and pulmonary vascular disease and acute myocardial infarction are currently under surveillance. UKOSS publications to date include data on pulmonary embolism, including incidence (1.3 per 10 000 maternities), case fatality (3.5%), and identification of substandard care (Knight 2008).

Pregnancy has no long-term deleterious effects on the normal heart. The long-term effects of pregnancy on the abnormal heart are ill understood, but in some conditions changes that occurred in pregnancy may not recover.

Women with pre-existing abnormal ventricular function may be at particular risk; but again data are limited. A reduction in systemic right ventricular function and functional class that occurred during pregnancy did not recover in a small study of women who had undergone a Mustard procedure for transposition of the great arteries (Guedes et al. 2004).

This section will consider pre-pregnancy assessment and counselling, antenatal, intrapartum, and postpartum care.

Assessing risk

Pre-pregnancy assessment

Pre-pregnancy assessment includes assessing the risk to the mother and fetus, optimizing the maternal condition to minimize the risks, planning antenatal care and counselling the woman and her partner so they may make an informed decision whether to embark on a pregnancy.

All women with heart disease should receive pre-pregnancy counselling by a cardiologist and obstetrician with particular expertise of heart disease in pregnancy. Counselling should begin, in general terms, as soon as heart disease is diagnosed, and from adolescence in patients with congenital heart disease, so that they are aware of their likely childbearing potential.

However, the majority of women who die of heart disease in pregnancy are undiagnosed until pregnancy reveals or precipitates their condition; these women do not have access to pre-pregnancy counselling (Malhotra and Yentis 2006). It is therefore very important that providers of routine antenatal care are able to distinguish cardiac symptoms such as chest pain, breathlessness, and palpitations from the symptoms of normal pregnancy—and to act quickly and appropriately.

Maternal risk

Risk assessment should take into account both the effects of the pregnancy on the mother's heart, and the effects of the heart and any maternal medication on the pregnancy (Fig. 12.4.1).

In estimating maternal risk, the following should be considered:

1 physiological changes of pregnancy
2 maternal functional status (NYHA)
3 risk-scoring systems
4 any published lesion-specific data.

Physiological changes of pregnancy

The risk of pregnancy in a woman with heart disease depends on the ability of the heart to sustain the marked changes in cardiovascular physiology demanded by pregnancy and delivery (Fig. 12.4.2).

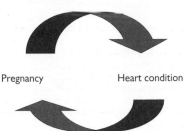

Pregnancy   Heart condition

Fig. 12.4.1 Interaction between pregnancy and maternal heart condition.

Both systemic and pulmonary vascular resistance fall, so that the total peripheral vascular resistance drops to 40–70% of pre-pregnancy levels. Blood volume rises by 30–50%, causing a dilutional anaemia, and heart rate rises by 10–20 bpm. Cardiac output therefore increases rapidly, by around 35% during the first trimester, and then rises more gradually to ~50% of the pre-pregnancy state by the end of the second trimester. During labour, cardiac output increases by a further 30% during each contraction because of an increase in stroke volume, and peaks still higher during the second (pushing) stage of labour. Post delivery,

cardiac output falls rapidly to around half pre-pregnancy levels by 6 weeks postpartum, and then declines to pre-pregnancy levels by ~24 weeks post delivery. As a result of these changes, pregnancy increases preload because of increased blood volume, and decreases afterload because of a fall in vascular resistance. Changes in blood pressure are relatively small; it may fall in early pregnancy due to a fall in vascular resistance and then rise to back to normal as blood volume and cardiac output.

Maternal functional status
Poor functional status (NYHA II or worse) is an independent risk factor for poor maternal and fetal outcome (Siu *et al.* 2001). Pre-pregnancy cardiopulmonary exercise testing is a useful tool in assessing maternal functional status.

Risk scoring systems
The risk of cardiovascular morbidity during a pregnancy in a woman with pre-existing heart disease can be estimated. A prospective study identified 4 predictors of an adverse cardiovascular event during pregnancy (Siu *et al.* 2001):
- Prior cardiovascular event (heart failure, cerebrovascular event, arrhythmia)
- Baseline NYHA >II or maternal cyanosis
- Left heart obstruction (mitral valve, aortic valve, left ventricular outflow tract obstruction)

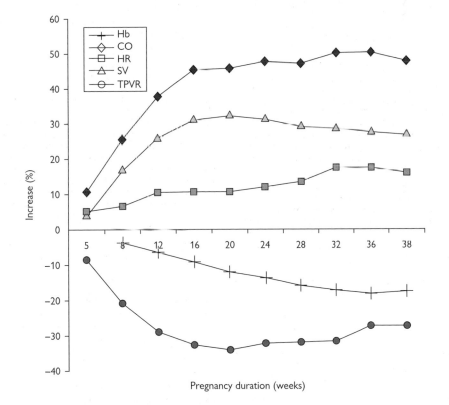

Changes in cardiac output (CO), stroke volume (SV), plasma volume (PV), total peripheral vascular resistance (TPVR), heart rate (HR), haemoglobin concentration (Hb) during pregnancy

Fig. 12.4.2 Cardiovascular changes in pregnancy. Reproduced from *Expert Rev Cardiovasc Ther* 2007;5(5):859–69 with permission of Expert Reviews Ltd.

• Left ventricular dysfunction (ejection fraction <40%)

If one point is assigned to each risk factor, a score of 0 correlated with a 5% maternal cardiovascular event risk, a score of 1 with a 27% risk and a score of >1 with a 75% risk.

Lesion specific risk

Data from small studies on specific cardiac conditions are helpful in assessing risk. However, there is little information for many conditions, so risk must be estimated on an individual basis for most women. Table 12.4.2 summarizes some low, moderate, and high-risk conditions. Risks are additive and may shift a condition from low to moderate or high risk. Non-cardiac risk factors such as obesity, hypertension, and diabetes should also be taken into account, as they too increase the risk of pregnancy.

Fetal risk

The risks to the fetus are of death, prematurity and malformation.

The fetus may be at risk from:
• Maternal drugs
• Maternal cardiovascular state:
  • Hypotension, low cardiac output
  • Cyanosis
• Recurrence of maternal congenital heart disease.

Maternal drugs

Many cardiac drugs cross the placenta and may cause fetal effects, but there are frequently little data. Table 12.4.3 summarizes the risk of some commonly used cardiac drugs. For drugs that have known or possible fetal effects, the

Table 12.4.2 Risk of pregnancy for different maternal cardiac conditions

Risk of maternal death or major morbidity	Maternal condition	Specific high-risk features	General high-risk features
Low (≤1%)	Unoperated, small, or mild Most mild stenotic valvar lesions	AS: non-pregnant PG >30 mmHg, MG >15 mmHg, AVA <1.5 cm^2 MS: MVA <1.5 cm^2	Features that shift the maternal risk to a higher risk group: Ventricular dysfunction NYHA class III or IV
	Most regurgitant valvar lesions		Raised pulmonary vascular resistance
	Septal defects		Obesity
	Patent arterial duct		Diabetes
	Repaired coarctation with no adverse features	Hypertension, aneurysm, recoarctation	Smoking
Significant (1–10%)	Mechanical valve	Mitral position, small valve, valve thrombosis, arrhythmia	
	Moderate stenotic lesions	AS: non-pregnant PG >80 mmHg, MG >50 mmHg, AVA <0.7 cm^2 MS: MVA <1.0 cm^2	
	Ischaemic heart disease	Ongoing ischaemia. Drug eluting stent or other need to continue clopidogrel at delivery	
	Mild systemic ventricular dysfunction (EF 45–50%)		
	Aortic coarctation	Unrepaired coarctation, aortic aneurysm, recoarctation, hypertension, Turner's syndrome	
	Cyanotic heart disease	Pulmonary hypertension	
	Systemic right ventricle	Impaired RV function, co-existent TR	
	Fontan circulation	Previous arrhythmia, dilated RA	
Who 4	Pulmonary arterial hypertension	Severity of PAH RV dysfunction	
	Severe systemic ventricular dysfunction	EF <30%, NYHA III or IV	
	Aortopathy with aortic aneurysm	Dilated aortic root - >4cm for Marfan (no data for other aortopathies). Loeys– Dietz and Ehlers–Danlos type 4	
	Severe stenotic valvar lesions		

Table 12.4.3 Cardiovascular drugs used in pregnancy

Drug	Fetal risk	Comments	Breast feeding
Amiodarone	C	Possible risk of neonatal goitre and hypothyroidism abnormality. However, (i) if life-threatening arrhythmia not controlled by other drugs, risk of stopping is unlikely to outweigh benefit, (ii) if chose to stop amiodarone, must do so 3–6 months before conception, since half-life so long. There may be little point in stopping amiodarone once pregnancy is confirmed: the fetus will be exposed to amiodarone anyway	Contraindicated: Amiodarone (iodine) concentrated in breast milk
Angiotensin converting enzyme inhibitors (ACEI)	D	Teratogenic/adverse effects throughout pregnancy. Cause decreased fetal renal blood flow leading to renal hypoplasia, oligohydramnios, which in turn causes pulmonary hypoplasia, limb and facial deformities. Risk of major abnormality ~17%	Varying passage into breast milk. Enalapril not present in significant amounts
Angiotensin-receptor antagonists	D	Little data, consider as for ACEI	Present in significant amounts in rat milk, suggest avoid
Aspirin: low dose	B	Consider safe	Safe
Beta-blockers	B/C	Most data available on atenolol (C): possible growth retardation (GR) if high dose throughout pregnancy. GR may relate instead to underlying maternal disease. If truly related to atenolol, likely to be a class effect, so regular fetal growth scans recommended for all women on beta-blockers. Transient neonatal bradycardia, hypoglycaemia, hypotension possible, so paediatrician present at delivery	Present in breast milk, but adverse effects not reported. Breastfeeding should not be discouraged
Bosentan	X	Avoid (teratogenic in *animal* studies); effective contraception required during and for at least 3 months after administration (hormonal contraception not considered effective); monthly pregnancy tests advised	Manufacturer advises avoid—no information available
Calcium channel blockers	B/C/D	May inhibit labour. Nifedipine likely to be safe (B). Diltiazem may be teratogenic (D), limited data on verapamil, but may reduce placental blood flow and cause fetal hypoxia (C)	Present in breast milk, but adverse effects not reported. Breast feeding should not be discouraged
Clopidogrel	C	Very limited data, but no adverse reports. Risk of obstetric bleeding and bleeding related to regional analgesia: stop 1 week pre delivery	No data: avoid
Digoxin	B	No studies, but adverse fetal effects not reported	Safe
Disopyramide	C	Third trimester: may induce labour	Present in milk—use only if essential and monitor infant for antimuscarinic effects
Fleccainide	C	Used in pregnancy to treat maternal and fetal arrhythmias in specialist centres; toxicity reported in animal studies; infant hyperbilirubinaemia also reported	Significant amount present in milk but not known to be harmful
Glycoprotein IIb/IIIa inhibitors	C	Isolated case reports only	No data
Heparin (unfractionated and low molecular weight)	B	Does not cross placenta so no adverse fetal effect. May cause maternal or placental bleeding and pregnancy loss. Discontinue 12 hours before delivery	Safe
Morphine	C	Crosses placenta and causes transient neonatal respiratory depression	Present in insignificant amounts
Nitrates	B	Care to avoid maternal hypotension resulting in placental hypoperfusion. Tocolytic so may slow labour	No data
Propafenone	C	Manufacturer advises avoid—no information available	Manufacturer advises avoid—no information available
Spironolactone	C	Not teratogenic but may have fetal anti-androgenic effects	Little data

(Contd.)

Table 12.4.3 *(Contd.)*

Drug	Fetal risk	Comments	Breast feeding
Statins	X	Teratogenic and may interfere with synthesis of fetal steroids and cell membranes	No data
Warfarin	D	Crosses placenta. Embryopathy in first trimester. Risk of fetal bleeding and fetal loss throughout. Risk less if mother adequately anticoagulated on <5 mg. For those at high risk of thrombosis, e.g. mechanical valve, weigh risk to fetus of warfarin against increased risk of thrombosis if mother takes heparin	Safe. In breast milk in insignificant amounts

The categories of fetal risk are:
A: Safe. Controlled studies do not show fetal harm: possibility of harm remote.
B: Likely to be safe. No fetal harm shown in animal studies, or harm shown in animal studies but not in controlled human studies.
C: Fetal harm possible: only use if potential benefit outweighs the risk. No data, or fetal harm in animal studies, but no studies in humans.
D: Proven fetal risk, use may be justified if maternal benefit outweighs risk.
X: Proven fetal risk that outweighs any possible maternal benefit.

fetal risk of using the drug should be individualized and weighed against the maternal (and therefore fetal) risk of not using it. The woman should understand the risks and benefits so she can take an informed decision about whether to use a drug. In general, the fewest possible drugs at the lowest effective doses should be used in pregnancy.

Maternal cardiovascular state
Anything that causes maternal haemodynamic compromise also places the fetus at risk. A low cardiac output state in a woman with heart failure or a Fontan circulation is likely to result in poor fetal and placental perfusion, with restricted fetal growth. Acute maternal haemodynamic compromise during, for example, tachyarrhythmia or an acute coronary syndrome, will also affect the fetus.

Women with cyanotic heart disease usually tolerate the increased cyanosis associated with pregnancy. However, cyanosis has a profound effect on fetal wellbeing, causing miscarriage, low birth weight and prematurity. If pre-pregnancy maternal SaO$_2$ is ≥90%, the chances of a live birth are good, around 92%. If pre-pregnancy maternal SaO$_2$ is <85%, there is only a 12% chance of a live birth (Presbitero *et al.* 1994).

Recurrence
In general terms the risk of recurrence of congenital heart disease in the fetus is around 5%. However, for those with chromosomal disorders, the risk is higher: 50% for single gene disorders like Holt Oram syndrome and Marfan syndrome, and for deletions like the chromosome 22q11 microdeletion (di George syndrome). Although many syndromes associated with chromosomal abnormalities are easily recognized, some, such as the 22q11 microdeletion, which is associated with tetralogy of Fallot, may be easily missed. Clinicians should therefore have a low threshold for referring these conditions to a geneticist, especially is there is a family history of congenital heart disease.

The pre-pregnancy assessment clinic
Pre-pregnancy counselling is important, not only for women at high risk from pregnancy, but also for those with minor disease for whom counselling is likely to be permissive.

The clinic should be run jointly by a cardiologist and obstetrician, both of whom have specialist knowledge of pregnancy in heart disease, with input from the specialist midwife, cardiac nurse specialist, haematologist, and obstetric anaesthetist and geneticist.

Information should be available from echocardiography, exercise testing and if necessary MRI and catheter data to allow an estimate of maternal risk in pregnancy. Any options to reduce maternal and fetal risks should be discussed, to allow the patient and her partner to choose to delay pregnancy until her condition is optimized. Risks should be explained clearly and simply and the consultation followed up with a letter detailing the discussion. An outline antenatal care plan should be discussed. Counselling should be non-directive, allowing the woman to make her own informed decision about whether to embark on a pregnancy.

Alternatives to pregnancy should be discussed, especially for women in whom it carries high risk:
1 no pregnancy—contraceptive counselling needed
2 adoption—those with severe cardiac disease may not be accepted by adoption agencies
3 surrogacy—risk of ovarian hyperstimulation syndrome if ovary-stimulating drugs used.

Women with heart disease and fertility problems may be at particular risk. Those undergoing fertility treatment that involves ovarian stimulation are at risk of developing ovarian hyperstimulation syndrome resulting in life-threatening massive fluid retention. They are also at increased risk if they have a multiple pregnancy. Close liaison is needed with the fertility team to minimize the risks for each individual who wishes to explore fertility treatment.

Contraception
For each contraceptive method, both its cardiovascular safety and contraceptive efficacy should be considered.

Barrier methods
There are no cardiac contraindications to barrier methods, and they are effective at preventing sexually transmitted diseases; however, their efficacy is user-dependent, so additional methods should be used for women at high risk.

Oestrogen-containing methods
The commonest and most popular contraceptive method is the combined oral contraceptive pill (COC). All oestrogen-containing preparations carry a risk of venous and arterial thrombosis, so alternative methods should be considered for women at particular risk for thromboembolism, for example those with atrial fibrillation or dilated cardiomyopathy. In addition, those with a potential right to left shunt should

Table 12.4.4 Describes the indications and contraindications to using the combined oral contraceptive pill

WHO 1 Always useable	WHO 2 Broadly useable	WHO 3 Caution in use		WHO 4 Do not use	
Minor valve lesions; mitral valve prolapse with trivial mitral regurgitation; bicuspid aortic valve with normal function Mild pulmonary stenosis	Tissue prosthetic valve lacking any WHOs 3 or 4 feature	Thrombotic risk, even on warfarin	Mechanical valves: bileflet valve	Thrombotic risk, even on warfarin	Mechanical valves: Starr Edwards; Bjork Shiley; any tricuspid valve
Repaired coarctation with no hypertension or aneurysm	Uncomplicated mild native mitral and aortic valve disease		Previous thromboembolism		Ischaemic heart disease
Simple congenital lesions successfully repaired in childhood and with no sequelae	Most arrhythmias other than atrial fibrillation or flutter		Atrial arrhythmia		Pulmonary hypertension any cause
	Hypertrophic cardiamyopathy locking any WHO 3 or 4 features		Dilated left atrium (>4 cm)		Dilated cardiomyopathy and LV dysfunction any cause LVEF <30%
	Post cardiomyopathy, fully recovered, Including peripartum cardiomyopathy				Fontan circulation
	Uncomplicated Marfan syndrome				Previous arteritis involving coronary arteries, e.g. Kawasaki disease
	Congenital heart disease lacking any WHO 3 or 4 features; small left to right shunt not reversible with physiological manoeuvres, e.g. small VSD	Risk paradoxical embolism	Potential reversal of left to right shunt: unoperated ASD	Risk paradoxical embolism	Cyanotic heart disease; pulmonary AVM

ASD, atrial septal defect; AVM, arteriovenous malformation; LV, left ventricular; LVEF, left ventricular ejection fraction; VSD, ventricular septal defect.
WHO, World Health Organization
WHO 1: Risk no higher than the general population
WHO 2: Small increased risk; advantages of method generally outweigh risk
WHO 3: Risks usually outweigh advantages. Other methods preferable. Exceptions if: patient accepts risks and rejects alternatives, or risk of pregnancy very high and other methods less effective
WHO 4: Method contraindicated: unacceptable risk.

avoid the COC, because of the risk of paradoxical emboli. COCs with the lowest dose of oestrogen, and those combined with progestogen levonorgestrel are thought to carry the lowest thromboembolic risk (Lidegaard et al. 2009). However, in general, progestogen-only alternatives are a better option for women with risk factors for thromboembolism.

An oestrogen-releasing patch is also available in the UK; the risks and side-effects are the same as the COC.

Progestogen-only preparations
There is no increased risk of thrombosis with progestogen-only preparations, so, in general, they may be used in women with heart disease. Their suitability is influenced by their mode of delivery, contraceptive efficacy and menstrual effects. Irregular menstrual bleeding can be a problem in the initial months of use for all progestogen-only methods; it usually subsides after the first few months and (reversible) amenorrhoea may follow.

The progestogen-only pill (POP, minipill) is safe for all women with heart disease, but its poor contraceptive efficacy contraindicates its use in patients in whom pregnancy is high risk.

The newer desogestrel-containing progestogen-only pill, Cerazette, is safe for all women with heart disease and has a contraceptive efficacy similar to that of the COC. Used on its own, it is not associated with any increased thrombotic risk. It is therefore a good choice for women in whom oestrogen-containing methods are contraindicated.

Emergency contraception with the progestogen-only pill Levonelle is safe for all women with heart disease who have had unprotected sex. It potentiates the effects of warfarin, so the international normalized ratio (INR) should be checked within 48 hours.

Long-acting progestogen-only preparations include:

- Depot injections (Depo Provera)
- Progestogen-eluting intrauterine device (Mirena Intra-uterine System)
- Progestogen-eluting subdermal implant (Implanon)

All provide highly effective contraception; the Mirena IUS and Implanon are more effective than sterilization. The only significant precaution is in inserting the Mirena IUS; cervical instrumentation may be associated with a vagal response that may cause cardiovascular collapse in some conditions such as pulmonary hypertension or a Fontan circulation.

With such effective long-acting contraceptive methods, sterilization is not necessarily the best option for women with severe heart disease. Female sterilization is highly effective, but the laparoscopic procedure carries a risk to women with severe heart disease. Male sterilization assumes mutual monogamy, and leaves the male partner unable to have children with any new partner.

Antenatal care

A multidisciplinary team including obstetrician, cardiologist, anaesthetist, midwife, and haematologist should provide antenatal care for women with heart disease. The level of care depends on the risk of pregnancy; many women with heart disease can have much of their care delivered by midwives, but those at the highest risk should be seen in a joint cardiac obstetric clinic. The woman's handheld notes should contain a description of her cardiac condition, and a clear delivery plan.

It is important to distinguish between the signs and symptoms of normal pregnancy and those of cardiac decompensation. The following signs and symptoms may occur in normal pregnancy:

- Breathlessness on exertion
- Palpitation due to atrial and ventricular ectopics
- Mild peripheral oedema
- Heart rate 10–20 bpm higher than pre-pregnancy
- Jugular venous pulse visible +2 cm
- Third heart sound
- Soft ejection systolic murmur.

The following signs and symptoms during pregnancy are not normal and require investigation:

- Extreme breathlessness, e.g. when talking and eating
- Marked peripheral oedema
- Sinus tachycardia persistently >100 bpm
- Jugular venous pulse >2 cm
- Fourth heart sound
- Diastolic murmur
- Pleural effusion
- Sustained tachyarrhythmia.

If the pregnant patient with heart disease decompensates during pregnancy despite medical management, consideration should be given either to early delivery followed by cardiac intervention, or, if gestational stage does not allow safe delivery, cardiac intervention—with or without interrupting the pregnancy.

Appropriate investigation and treatment should not be withheld from pregnant women who present with acute cardiac symptoms: the fetal risks of chest X-ray, chest CT, angiography, cardioversion or the use of emergency cardiac drugs are likely to be outweighed by the maternal and fetal benefits.

Delivery

The safest mode of delivery for the majority of women with heart disease is a spontaneous normal vaginal delivery at term, with regional analgesia and a low threshold for forceps assistance. There is less blood loss, and fluid shifts are less rapid than with delivery by caesarean section; recovery time is also shorter.

There are few cardiac indications for delivery by section; aortic aneurysm is the main reason for a planned section. However, if the mother's cardiac condition deteriorates during pregnancy, or there is fetal compromise necessitating an early delivery, caesarean section is likely. Induction of labour to achieve a vaginal delivery may fail, especially if attempted before 38 weeks' gestation, risking both fetal and maternal compromise.

Postnatal care

Most of the circulatory changes of pregnancy return to normal within the first 48 hours of delivery, so patients with significant heart disease should be cared for in a high dependency setting for this time. Drugs that had to be withheld during pregnancy can be introduced post delivery, with consideration given to the patient's desire to breast feed. Appropriate contraceptive counselling should be offered. Early outpatient review should be planned with repeat echocardiography at around 6 weeks, to ensure that cardiac dimensions and function have returned to their pre-pregnancy state.

Heart diseases and pregnancy

This section will consider specific cardiac conditions in pregnancy.

Acute coronary syndrome

Acute myocardial infarction in pregnancy carries a maternal mortality of around 5% and is now the leading cause of pregnancy-related cardiac death in the UK. The majority have risk factors such as hypertension, diabetes, obesity, smoking, or age >35 years. In those who die, failure to recognize symptoms and act quickly has been identified in around one-third of cases.

Presentation is often with typical chest pain and nausea and clear ECG changes of ischaemia or infarction. Troponin levels are unaffected by pregnancy and should be interpreted as for the non-pregnant state.

Whatever the gestational stage, an acute coronary syndrome should be treated before delivering the fetus. Primary percutaneous intervention is the treatment of choice since thrombolysis carries a risk of obstetric haemorrhage. In addition, if the cause of the acute coronary syndrome is coronary artery dissection (more common in pregnancy), thrombolysis is ineffective.

In general, bare metal stents should be used in preference to drug-eluting stents since the risk of acute stent thrombosis is less when clopidogrel has to be stopped for delivery. Ideally clopidogrel should be given for at least 6 weeks after stent implantation, discontinued for a week prior to delivery and then restarted as soon as possible. Aspirin should always be continued. Inevitably there are occasions when this practice cannot be followed; the cardiologist and obstetrician should make an individualized lowest risk plan.

Aortic dissection

Pregnancy itself is a risk factor for aortic dissection. As well as the haemodynamic stresses of pregnancy, hormonal changes promote aortic dilation, with fragmentation of the reticulum fibres, reduced mucopolysaccharides and loss of the normal configuration of elastic fibres seen in the aortas of pregnant women (Manalo-Estrella and Barker 1967).

Those with the autosomal dominant inherited Marfan, Loeys Dietz and Ehlers–Danlos type IV syndromes are at particular risk. Although aortic dissection can occur in normal women, a retrospective diagnosis of a high-risk syndrome may be made. This is not only important to the woman if she survives, but allows genetic counselling to be offered to her family. Women with bicuspid aortic valve and a dilated aortic root may also be at some increased risk of dissection in pregnancy, but data are lacking.

Women known to have a dilated aorta should be counselled prior to conception. Those with Marfan syndrome and a normal-sized aortic root are at ~1% risk of dissection during pregnancy; this risk rises to 10% for those with an aortic root diameter >4 cm. Aortic root replacement should be offered before pregnancy in women with Marfan syndrome and a dilated root >4.5 cm.

There are no data to aid pre-pregnancy counselling for women with bicuspid aortic valve and dilated root. The decision of whether to replace the root prior to pregnancy may be influenced by the absolute size of the aortic root and the rate of progression of dilatation.

Women with a dilated aortic root who are pregnant should be monitored closely with echo and MRI throughout pregnancy and the first 6 months after delivery. β-blockade is considered standard care and is thought to reduce aortic wall stress. Fetal growth should be monitored when the mother is taking α-blockers. If the aorta dilates further during pregnancy and the fetus can be safely delivered, delivery by caesarean section should be performed before aortic root replacement. If the fetus cannot be delivered safely, aortic root replacement should be performed during the pregnancy.

Cardiac surgery during pregnancy carries a risk to the mother of obstetric bleeding, and a risk of fetal loss of up to 25%. Fetal risk may be reduced by using high-flow, high-pressure normothermic perfusion, but normothermia precludes an open distal aortic repair.

If aortic dissection is suspected, urgent CT or MRI imaging should be performed to confirm the diagnosis. Senior cardiothoracic and obstetric staff should be involved immediately, and depending on gestational age, the fetus delivered and aorta repaired immediately afterwards, or the aorta repaired with the fetus *in situ*.

Heart failure

Women with known impairment of left ventricular function should be carefully assessed and counselled before embarking on a pregnancy.

Those with NYHA III functional capacity or worse, left ventricular ejection fraction ≤30%, atrial fibrillation or significant mitral regurgitation are at high risk of decompensation and permanent reduction in cardiac function. The risk of death may approach 10%. These women should be counselled against pregnancy.

Counselling women with less severe ventricular dysfunction who are less symptomatic is more difficult; their risk of major morbidity and death is likely to be lower, but they may still suffer a permanent deterioration in cardiac function.

Antenatal care should include frequent joint obstetric and cardiology assessment and echo monitoring. Timing and mode of delivery depends on the maternal and fetal condition.

If overt heart failure develops during pregnancy, the choice of heart failure drugs is limited (see Table 12.4.3). Bed rest, prophylactic anticoagulation, and furosemide can all be used. β-blockers can be used with fetal growth monitoring. Angiotensin-converting enzyme inhibitors (ACEIs) carry a known significant risk of fetal renal agenesis, cardiac malformation and fetal loss. Angiotensin II receptor blockers are likely to have similar effects. Spironolactone may cause fetal feminizing effects. The potential fetal risks of using a drug must be weighed against the risk to the mother (and therefore fetus) of withholding effective heart failure treatment; thus in some situations the benefits of using ACEIs may outweigh the risks.

If medical therapy fails, the fetus should be delivered if gestation allows, or termination of pregnancy should be considered, if necessary with ionotropic or and mechanical support.

After delivery, early assessment for transplantation should be made if cardiac function remains poor.

Peripartum cardiomyopathy

This condition is uncommon, occurring in one in every 3000–15 000 pregnancies. It is defined as left ventricular dysfunction (ejection fraction <45%) with no other identifiable cause, occurring during the last month of pregnancy or first 5 months after delivery. The aetiology is unknown, but histology usually shows a myocarditic process.

Mortality is reported to be around 20%, most deaths occurring close to presentation. Around 50% make a complete recovery; long-term prognosis is reduced in those with persistent ventricular dysfunction (Elkayam et al. 2001).

There is a high recurrence rate in subsequent pregnancies. Those in whom ventricular function has not returned to normal face a 50% risk of recurrence or deterioration and a 20% risk of death. For those in whom ventricular function does return to normal prior to a subsequent pregnancy, the risk of death is probably low, but the risk of recurrence and long-term deterioration is around 20%.

Arrhythmias in pregnancy

The increased sympathetic drive, haemodynamic and hormonal changes of pregnancy may cause worsening of any tachyarrhythmia, and palpitation occurs in around 50% of all pregnant women.

The majority of symptoms are due to atrial and ventricular ectopy and require simple reassurance. However, ECG diagnosis of sustained palpitation is important, since palpitation may be symptomatic of underlying heart disease.

Pregnant women who present with acute-onset tachyarrhythmia or who are haemodynamically compromised should not be denied appropriate treatment because of concerns for the fetus; fetal wellbeing is more likely to be adversely affected by persistent maternal tachyarrhythmia. Adenosine is safe in pregnancy, as is electrical cardioversion, performed with a pelvic wedge placed under the right hip. As a general rule, antiarrhythmic drugs should be used in the smallest effective dose, avoiding drug combinations (see Table 12.4.3).

Supraventricular tachycardias

Re-entry tachycardias occur most often in women with structurally normal hearts. They occur more commonly in pregnancy and indeed some women only experience them during pregnancy. If self-limiting and infrequent, no treatment is required, but if recurrent, regular antiarrhythmic medication may be required.

Atrial flutter and atrial fibrillation

Both these arrhythmias should trigger a search for underlying heart disease or conditions such as thyrotoxicosis. If presenting acutely, electrical cardioversion is indicated and consideration should be given to anticoagulation with low-molecular-weight heparin. β-blockers and digoxin are useful for rate control, and beta-blockers and flecainide may be helpful in maintaining sinus rhythm.

Ventricular tachycardia

Ventricular tachycardia signifies underlying heart disease. It should be terminated with electrical cardioversion, and recurrence treated with beta-blockers or amiodarone, despite the latter's possible fetal effects. Pregnancy is possible with an implantable automatic defibrillator.

Bradyarrhythmias

Congenital complete heart block should usually be treated with a permanent pacemaker prior to pregnancy, since the increased cardiac output can only otherwise be achieved by an increase in the diastolic volume of the heart and may cause long-term ventricular dysfunction. If needed, a permanent pacemaker may be placed during pregnancy with minimal X-ray screening.

Valvular heart diseases

Valvar regurgitation

Regurgitant lesions are generally well tolerated in pregnancy, provided ventricular function is maintained. However, the volume load of pregnancy may result in ventricular dilation and worsening of valvar regurgitation, as well as a deterioration in ventricular function. Women may become symptomatic for the first time in pregnancy and require treatment with diuretics. Early delivery may be necessary if ventricular function deteriorates.

The decision to replace a regurgitant valve before pregnancy is influenced by balancing the risk of pregnancy with the regurgitant valve against the additive risks of cardiac surgery and the risk of a pregnancy with a valve prosthesis. Thus the risk of pregnancy with severe mitral regurgitation and a normal-sized, normally functioning left ventricle may be lower than the combined risk of cardiac surgery to replace the mitral valve and a subsequent pregnancy with a mechanical mitral valve.

Mitral stenosis

Mitral stenosis is usually due to rheumatic heart disease and in the UK is almost entirely confined to the immigrant population. It is particularly dangerous in pregnancy, and is the commonest cardiac cause of death in the developing world (Thorne et al. 2006); it has also re-emerged as a cause of cardiac death in the UK. Most women with mitral stenosis are asymptomatic and unaware that they have

heart disease until pregnancy precipitates symptoms for the first time. They therefore rarely have access to pre-pregnancy counselling and treatment. If mitral stenosis is diagnosed before pregnancy, all but the mildest lesions should be treated first.

Presentation is usually with breathlessness and orthopnoea in the second trimester. The mainstay of medical treatment is to reduce left atrial pressure, with diuretics and beta-blockers, the latter to reduce heart rate to allow time for ventricular filling. If medical therapy fails, and the fetus cannot be safely delivered, balloon mitral valvuloplasty should be considered. In the majority of women of childbearing age with mitral stenosis, the valve is pliable and not calcified, so as long as there is no significant mitral regurgitation, the valve is likely to be suitable for balloon valvuloplasty. In order to reduce X-ray screening time and reduce the risk of causing significant regurgitation that requires emergency valve replacement, this procedure should only be performed by a high-volume operator. Following successful valvuloplasty, the majority of women should be able to continue their pregnancy uneventfully.

Aortic stenosis

In contrast to mitral stenosis, aortic stenosis in women of childbearing age is usually due to congenital bicuspid valve disease. Most women are already aware of their condition and should have had access to pre-pregnancy counselling. As a rule, pregnancy is likely to be well tolerated if, before pregnancy the patient has or is:

- Asymptomatic
- Normal resting ECG
- Normal exercise capacity, with no ECG changes and a normal blood pressure rise to exercise
- Good left ventricular function on echo
- Peak aortic valve gradient <80 mmHg, mean <50 mmHg
- Valve area >1.0 cm^2.

Careful antenatal follow up is required, with attention to new symptoms or ECG changes. Regular echo should show a rise in transvalvar velocities during pregnancy, reaching an increase of up to 20% of pre-pregnancy levels at term, giving a significant rise in the estimated transvalvar gradient. The rise in estimated aortic valve gradient reflects the ability of the normally functioning ventricle to increase stroke volume and cardiac output.

Indicators of the onset of deterioration are:

- Severe breathlessness
- Onset of angina
- Syncope
- New ischaemic ECG changes
- A fall or failure to increase, of the transvalvar velocity (suggesting ventricular failure)
- Left ventricular dysfunction.

A patient who starts to deteriorate should be admitted for rest. Pulmonary oedema should be treated with diuretics. Vasodilators should be avoided. Cautious β blockade may be considered. If there is no improvement and gestational stage allows, the fetus should be delivered: delivery should result in an improvement in the maternal condition, and allow a measured approach to surgical intervention.

If the fetus cannot be safely delivered, aortic valve intervention should be performed without interrupting the pregnancy, or termination of pregnancy may be considered. Although not usually calcified, the morphology of the bicuspid aortic valve in women of child bearing age is frequently not ideal for balloon valvuloplasty. It may be difficult to predict how the valve commissures will split on ballooning: sudden onset severe aortic regurgitation may occur leading to serious decompensation and the need for emergency cardiac surgery. Any percutaneous intervention should be carried out by an operator experienced in treating bicuspid aortic stenosis in children and young adults.

In some cases surgical aortic valve replacement will need to be carried out during pregnancy. The maternal and fetal risks of cardiac surgery in pregnancy are discussed above.

Mechanical valves

The major risks associated with mechanical heart valves in pregnancy are thromboembolism and haemorrhage. The risk of maternal death is up to 4%, mostly due to mechanical valve thrombosis. The interests of the mother and fetus are in conflict; warfarin is the most effective maternal anticoagulation regime but risks fetal ill effects and pregnancy loss, whereas heparin is the safest regime for the fetus, but puts the mother at risk of life-threatening thromboembolic events.

Pregnancy is a pro-thrombotic condition, so the risks of thrombotic complications are higher than in the non-pregnant state. The levels of certain clotting factors (VIII, IX, X, fibrinogen) are increased and fibrinolytic activity, protein S and antithrombin III all decrease.

Warfarin crosses the placenta and is associated with a first trimester embryopathy. The embryopathy occurs between 6 and 12 weeks of gestation, so it is safe to conceive on warfarin, as long as it is stopped within 2 weeks of a missed period. It anticoagulates the fetus and may cause cerebrovascular bleeding and neurodevelopmental delay as well as miscarriage and stillbirth. In addition, if warfarin is used after 36 weeks, there is a risk of retroplacental bleeding as well as neonatal bleeding, since the immature neonatal liver takes time to metabolize the warfarin. The adverse fetal effects of warfarin are dose related and are uncommon if the mother is adequately anticoagulated on ≤5 mg warfarin (note the dose of warfarin should NOT be reduced to <5 mg at the expense of a suboptimal INR).

In contrast, heparin does not cross the placenta and is not associated with adverse fetal effects. However, it does reach the placenta, so placental bleeding may occur. The main risk with heparin is of valve thrombosis, and even with meticulous control of heparin therapy, fatal thromboses are reported. The safest heparin regime is probably twice daily low molecular weight heparin (e.g. enoxaparin 1 mg/kg bd) maintaining anti-Xa levels >1.0, with adjunctive aspirin 75 mg daily. The long half-life of low-molecular-weight heparin means that fairly stable levels of anticoagulation are maintained. By comparison, unfractionated heparin has a short half-life, and even if given 8 hourly subcutaneously, is likely to be associated with periods of inadequate anticoagulation.

The highest risk situations for mechanical valve thrombosis are:
- Valve in mitral position
- Single leaflet tilting disc and ball in cage valves
- More than one mechanical valve
- Small mechanical valve (e.g. one placed in childhood)
- Heparin anticoagulation.

Possible anticoagulation regimes are:
1 Warfarin throughout the pregnancy, converting to monitored twice daily low-molecular-weight heparin and aspirin 75 mg od at 36 weeks.

2 Monitored twice daily low molecular weight heparin and aspirin 75 mg od throughout pregnancy.
3 Monitored twice daily low-molecular-weight heparin and aspirin 75 mg od for the 1st trimester, then warfarin until 36 weeks, then heparin and aspirin.

There is no risk-free regime. The choice of anticoagulation should be individualized to the mother's particular risk, and she should be given enough information to be able to make an informed decision.

If delivery by caesarean section is planned, a prophylactic dose of low molecular weight heparin should be given on the evening before. Delivery should take place the following morning, with regional analgesia. For vaginal delivery, heparin should be withheld once the woman starts labour. Regional analgesia can only be used 12 hours after a prophylactic dose, and 24 hours after a treatment dose of low-molecular-weight heparin. After delivery, a prophylactic dose of heparin should be given 3–4 hours later if there is no bleeding, and full dose heparin restarted that evening.

Warfarin should not be reintroduced for 48 hours post delivery because of the risk of major obstetric or genital tract haemorrhage.

Congenital heart disease in pregnancy

All women with congenital heart disease should have access to specialist congenital cardiac pre-pregnancy assessment and if necessary, antenatal care. For many, counselling can be permissive, e.g. those with isolated mild pulmonary stenosis, but for others pregnancy may carry a considerable risk and requires specialist management (Thorne et al. 2006).

It is beyond the scope of this section to examine all forms of congenital heart disease, so pregnancy in the following situations will be considered.
- Coarctation of the aorta
- Pulmonary regurgitation: the volume-loaded right ventricle
- Systemic right ventricle: the pressure-loaded right ventricle
- The Fontan circulation
- Cyanosis with normal pulmonary vascular resistance
- Pulmonary arterial hypertension.

Coarctation of the aorta

Unoperated coarctation: coarctation of the aorta should be relieved prior to any pregnancy. It is rarely diagnosed during pregnancy, and although it carries a risk of hypertension and dissection, death is uncommon (Beauchesne et al. 2001). Intervention to relieve coarctation is rarely justified during pregnancy—balloon dilatation and stenting during pregnancy may carry a significant risk of aneurysm formation or aortic rupture. The coarctation site should be monitored with MRI during pregnancy and hypertension treated with beta-blockade with the addition of methyl dopa if necessary. Fetal growth should be carefully monitored. Delivery should be by elective section at around 35 weeks' gestation.

Repaired coarctation: the risk of pregnancy following repair of coarctation depends on the repair site and blood pressure. The aorta should be assessed by MRI prior to pregnancy, or early in the second trimester. If the woman is normotensive and there is no recoarctation or aneurysm, then vaginal delivery at term, with regional analgesia and avoidance of a prolonged second stage should be considered. If there is an aneurysm at the site of repair, then planned caesarean section is preferable.

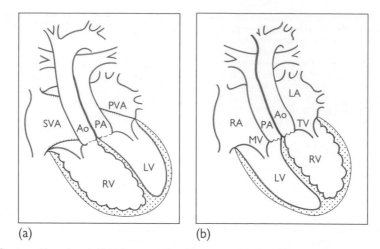

(a)   (b)

Fig. 12.4.3 (a) Senning or Mustard repair of simple transposition of the great arteries. From Thorne and Clift, *Adult Congenital Heart Disease* (2009), plate 6a with permission from Oxford University Press. (b) Congenitally corrected transposition of the great arteries. From Thorne and Clift, *Adult Congenital Heart Disease* (2009), plate 5b with permission from Oxford University Press.

Pulmonary regurgitation—volume-loaded right ventricle

Severe pulmonary regurgitation is common following repair of tetralogy of Fallot or pulmonary stenosis. Consideration should be given to pulmonary valve replacement prior to pregnancy if the woman is symptomatic or there is any dysfunction of a dilated right ventricle. However, as long as right ventricular function is good, pregnancy in the presence of severe pulmonary regurgitation is likely to be well tolerated. Nonetheless, the additional volume loading effects of pregnancy may have a long-term deleterious effect on right ventricular function (Khairy *et al.* 2006; Pedersen *et al.* 2008).

Systemic right ventricle—pressure-loaded right ventricle

Patients with congenitally corrected transposition of the great arteries or Senning or Mustard repair of simple transposition have a systemic right ventricle (see Fig. 12.4.3). The right ventricle is pressure loaded, supporting the systemic circulation, and is at least mildly impaired in the majority of patients of childbearing age. The tricuspid valve is also in the systemic circulation and is usually regurgitant. Pregnancy may precipitate ventricular failure and a worsening of tricuspid regurgitation (Bédard *et al.* 2009).

Those with congenitally corrected transposition may also have heart block. A pacemaker should be inserted pre-pregnancy, or during pregnancy.

Those with previous Mustard or Senning repair of transposition may also have:

- Atrial tachyarrhythmias—if presenting acutely, electrical cardioversion should be performed, and sinus rhythm maintained with beta-blockers
- Sinus node disease and sinus bradycardia—should be treated pre pregnancy with an atrial pacemaker. The atrioventricular node usually functions normally
- Pulmonary venous pathway obstruction—this should be sought and relieved pre-pregnancy. It is not usually amenable to catheter intervention and requires with a surgical approach. If not detected until pregnancy, it behaves like mitral stenosis and the pregnancy may need to be terminated.

Fontan circulation

The chronic low cardiac output state of the Fontan circulation means that pregnancy may be poorly tolerated. Pregnancy may precipitate atrial arrhythmia as well as heart failure. There is a high (up to 30%) risk of miscarriage. Low-molecular-weight heparin should be used throughout the pregnancy. If the woman remains well, delivery may be vaginal at term; however, early delivery by section is often necessary because of maternal and/or fetal compromise.

Cyanotic heart disease with normal pulmonary vascular resistance

The main risk to the mother is of heart failure due to the increased volume load of pregnancy. In addition, the right to left shunt puts her at risk of paradoxical embolism. Obstetric haemorrhage is also a significant risk.

The fetal effects of maternal cyanosis are addressed under the section on Fetal risk, p. 398.

Pulmonary arterial hypertension

The risk of maternal death in the presence of pulmonary artery hypertension is at least 25%, whether secondary to congenital heart disease, connective tissue disease or idiopathic pulmonary hypertension. These women should be advised against pregnancy and given access to safe and effective contraception. Women who wish to pursue a pregnancy should be treated in specialist pulmonary hypertension centres. Anticoagulation, inhaled prostacyclin and sildenafil, close monitoring, and elective delivery by section at around 24 weeks gestation may be have reduced mortality from the 40% seen for many decades to around the 25% more recently cited.

Summary

The majority of women with heart disease can tolerate pregnancy. However, for a sizeable minority, it carries a significant risk of death or major morbidity.

Increasing numbers of women of childbearing age have survived complex congenital heart disease or are at risk of ischaemic heart disease. Their risks can be minimized by careful pre-conception assessment, and antenatal and peripartum care.

References

Beauchesne LM, Connolly HM, Ammash NM, Warnes CA Coarctation of the aorta: outcome of pregnancy. *J Am Coll Cardiol.* 2001;**38**:1728–33.

Bédard E, Dimopoulos K, Gatzoulis MA. Has there been any progress made on pregnancy outcomes among women with pulmonary arterial hypertension? *Eur Heart J.* 2009;**30**:256–65.

Elkayam U, Tummala PP, Rao K, *et al.* Maternal and fetal outcomes of subsequent pregnancies in women with peripartum cardiomyopathy. *N Engl J Med.* 2001;**344**:1567–71.

Guedes A, Nercier LA, Leduc L, *et al.* Impact of pregnancy on the systemic right ventricle after a Mustard operation for transposition of the great arteries. *J Am Coll Cardiol* 2004;**44**:433.

Hahthotuwa HR, Attygalle D, Jayatilleka AC, *et al.* Maternal mortality due to cardiac disease in Sri Lanka. *Int J Obstet Gynecol* 2009;**104**:194–8.

James AH, Jamison MG, Biswas MS, *et al.* Acute myocardial infarction in pregnancy: a United States population-based study. *Circulation.* 2006;**113**:1564–71.

Khairy P, Ouyang DW, Fernandes SM, *et al.* Pregnancy outcomes in women with congenital heart disease. *Circulation.* 2006;**113**:517–24.

Knight M on behalf of UKOSS. Antenatal pulmonary embolism: risk factors, management and outcomes. *BJOG* 2008;**115**:453–61.

Lewis GE. The confidential enquiry into maternal and childhealth (CEMACH). Saving others lives: reviewing maternal deaths to make motherhood safer: 2003–2005. http://www.cemach.org.uk; 2007.

Lidegaard Ø, Løkkegaard E, Svendsen AL, Agger C. Hormonal contraception and risk of venous thromboembolism: national follow-up study. *BMJ* 2009;**338**:557–60.

Malhotra S, Yentis SM. Reports on confidential enquiries into maternal deaths: management strategies based on trends in maternal cardiac deaths over 30 years. *Int J Obstet Anaesth* 2006;**15**:223–6.

Manalo-Estrella P, Barker AE. Histopathologic findings in human aortic media associated with pregnancy. *Arch Pathol* 1967;**83**:336–41.

Nqayana T, Moodley J, Naidoo DP. Cardiac disease in pregnancy. *Cardiovasc J Africa* 2008;**19**:145–51.

Pedersen LM, Pedersen TA, Ravn HB, Hjortdal VE. Outcomes of pregnancy in women with tetralogy of Fallot. *Cardiol Young.* 2008;**18**:423–9.

Presbitero P, Somerville J, Stone S, *et al.* Pregnancy in cyanotic congenital heart disease. *Circulation* 1994;**89**:2673–6.

Siu SC, Sermer M, Colman JM, *et al.* Prospective multicenter study of pregnancy outcomes in women with heart disease. *Circulation* 2001;**104**:515–21.

Thorne SA, MacGregor AE, Nelson Piercy C. Risk of contraception and pregnancy in heart disease. *Heart* 2006;**92**:1520–5.

WHO. *Maternal Mortality in 2005.* World Health Organization 2007, Geneva.

Heart disease and obesity

Definition

Obesity is a condition of excess body fat. Although this is a simple concept, the clinical definition has been problematic. The most widely used metric is the body mass index (BMI) (weight/height^2 in SI units). A BMI <25 is the upper limit of normal, with 25–30 being considered overweight and >30 obese. However, there are obvious shortcomings in relation to racial differences (the upper limit of normal is 23 in Asian subjects) and the failure of this parameter to reflect body composition (e.g. many athletes would be considered as obese using this simple marker). Fat location is important, with central adiposity most associated with metabolic complications. Two simple but under-used clinical parameters that take account of the distribution of adiposity are waist circumference (normal <102 cm in men and 88 cm in women) and waist–hip ratio (normal <1 in men and 0.8 in women).

Sophisticated investigations such as hydrostatic weighing are not feasible in clinical practice. Skinfold estimations are complicated and have limited reproducibility. Two relatively simple tests are dual energy X-ray absorbtiometry (DEXA) and bioimpedance. Imaging of visceral adipose tissue using computed tomography and magnetic resonance has proven valuable in trials.

Epidemiology

The prevalence of obesity increased by >100% over the 20 years between 1980 and 2000. In the USA, the majority of the population (approximately 65%) are overweight and 30% are obese (Flegal et al. 2002).

The health burden of obesity is huge, both with respect to morbidity and mortality. Excess weight accounts for about 300 000 excess deaths/year in the USA (Allison et al. 1999) and medical spending on weight-related conditions is similar to that associated with smoking.

Aetiology

The most common cause of obesity is environmental (nutrition and inactivity). There are important but complex genetic contributors to obesity. A number of endocrine disorders (polycystic ovarian disease, Cushing's syndrome, hypothyroidism, and disorders of the hypothalamus/pituitary) should be considered, although they are quite uncommon.

Obesity as a cardiovascular risk factor

The relatively recent onset of this epidemic has implications for the understanding of obesity as a risk factor. For example, it is not represented in the Framingham risk profile. The degree of obesity has been shown to be proportionate to life expectancy.

Obesity has a number of links with atherosclerotic vascular disease. First, the effect of obesity may be mediated through other cardiovascular risk factors such as diabetes, hypertension, hyperlipidaemia, dysglycaemia, etc., which are associated with obesity. Second, obesity is linked with inflammation and prothrombotic states, which are themselves risk factors. Third, obesity is linked with inactivity, which itself is associated with poor health. From a risk standpoint, it appears that fit overweight individuals are at substantially lower risk than their unfit counterparts. Finally, obesity itself is an independent risk factor (Poirier et al. 2006).

Pathogenesis of complications

The fundamental problems arise from

1 metabolic disturbance: insulin resistance, impaired glucose tolerance, type 2 diabetes mellitus (T2DM), and dyslipidaemia (low high-density lipoprotein (HDL), high triglyceride, increased small dense low-density lipoprotein (LDL), and apoB). The association between obesity and dyslipidaemia appears stronger in younger subjects.

2 Neuroendocrine changes: including disturbances of the renin–angiotensin–aldosterone and sympatho-adrenal axes that relate to fat mass and circulating fatty acids.

3 Inflammation: attributed to production of cytokines and chemokines in fat.

4 Thrombosis: due to procoagulant factors (including increased fibrinogen and factor VII) and reduced fibronolysis (e.g. due to increased PAI-1).

5 Endothelial dysfunction: the mechanisms of which are speculative, but may include any of the above.

Cardiovascular complications

The evidence linking obesity and cardiovascular disease originated in the Framingham study, which showed a 40% increment of CVD risk in obese men and women, a 24% increment of risk in overweight (Wilson et al. 2002). Although these data showed no significant increment of risk in overweight women, the Nurses' Health Study showed the risk of death in women with a BMI >27 significantly exceeded that in women with a BMI of 19.

1 Atherosclerotic vascular disease, especially in men, causing myocardial infarction and stroke. The link between obesity and atherosclerosis has been particularly well defined in the carotid arteries. Stroke risk is increased in both overweight (by 30%) and obese (by 90%); with each unit increment of BMI, the risk of thrombotic and haemorrhagic stroke increases by 4% and 6%, respectively. This effect of obesity (independent of confounders such as hypertension and T2DM) is attributed to the thrombotic and inflammatory consequences of obesity.

2 Hypertension, leading to heart failure and contributing to atherogenesis. This is related to hormonal disturbances, increased arterial stiffness, sleep apnoea and hyperaldosterism. Every 10 kg of weight gain is associated with an increment of 2–3 mmHg of diastolic and systolic BP and parallels a 12–24% increase in coronary heart disease and cerebrovascular disease risk. There is an 'obesity paradox' whereby obese hypertensive subjects appear to have a more favourable outcome than lean hypertensive subjects—but still worse than normotensive subjects!

3 Left ventricular (LV) dysfunction, which occurs independent of the 'usual culprits'—hypertension, left ventricular hypertrophy and coronary disease. Factors that are related to this problem include disturbances of myocardial metabolism (related to disturbances of substrate metabolism including increased circulating free fatty acids, adipokines and insulin resistance), fibrosis related to renin–angiotensin system activation and sympathetic system activation (Wong and Marwick 2007). The LV remodelling that occurs in response to these stimuli includes LV hypertrophy and enlargement, and histological changes include myocyte hypertrophy and fibrosis. Even before heart failure becomes apparent, diastolic

dysfunction, changes of cardiac performance with exercise and subtle alterations of systolic function (e.g. tissue velocity and deformation) may be identified.

4 Heart failure has a strong association with obesity: with each unit increment of BMI, the risk of congestive heart failure (CHF) increases 5% in men and 7% in women. This feature seems eclipsed in the minds of patients and their physicians by concerns about the association of obesity with atherogenesis. Heart failure occurs because of the high output state (attributable to the vascularity of adipose tissue) causing increased preload, together with increased afterload from hypertension and primary myocardial disease. The duration of obesity appears to be an important contributor to the development of heart failure (although older subjects are in any case more likely to develop heart failure). Curiously, in overt heart failure, there is an 'obesity paradox' of lower death and hospitalization risk in overweight subjects, even when the comparison is made to those with a normal BMI (i.e. it does not simply reflect the mortality associated with cardiac cachexia).

5 Arrhythmias and sudden death are more common in obese than lean individuals—an association that has been recognized since antiquity. This is true even in the absence of cardiac dysfunction—the Framingham data show a 40-fold higher sudden death rate than in a matched non-obese group. The causes of this are less clear, but include sleep apnoea, overt, and subclinical cardiomyopathy and prolonged QT (itself due to disturbed sympathovagal balance, increased circulating catecholamines, or increased circulating free fatty acids). Heart rate variability and late potentials may be markers of this risk, but the appropriate management steps (other than weight reduction) are less clear.

6 Venous insufficiency and pulmonary embolism: venous insufficiency is a major contributor to oedema, in addition to increased intravascular volume, inactivity, and right heart failure. The rates of venous thrombosis and pulmonary embolism are increased—especially in women—probably related to stasis and the prothrombotic state.

Non-cardiovascular sequelae

In the obese patient with cardiovascular disease it is prudent to consider the presence of other associated features.

1 Obstructive sleep apnoea: pulmonary pressures are increased in >50% of obese subjects, with increases in pulmonary artery systolic pressure of up to 0.5 mmHg for each 1 unit increment of BMI.

2 T2DM: associated with a doubling or tripling of coronary disease risk and is sometimes considered a risk equivalent to coronary disease. Investigations have demonstrated that the risk of developing diabetes can be reduced by 25–50% by lifestyle and medical therapy.

3 Insulin resistance: an important association of obesity. It is important to realize that not all overweight patients have insulin resistance and not all patients with insulin resistance are overweight. Insulin resistance is a difficult parameter to measure, not the least because of variations between insulin assays. The HOMA score is the simplest clinical parameter but it only expresses insulin resistance in the basal state rather than in response to a meal. The insulin response to a glucose tolerance test may be a relatively simple way of demonstrating insulin resistance although the results require careful processing.

Hyperinsulinaemic, euglycaemic clamps are of value for research but impractical for clinical purposes.

4 Metabolic syndrome—the incremental predictive benefit of combining the constituents of the metabolic syndrome remains controversial. There are two sets of diagnostic criteria—ATP III (abdominal obesity, hypertension, high fasting glucose and triglycerides, low HDL) and WHO (hypertension, central obesity, hyperlipidaemia, microalbuminuria).

5 Non-alcoholic fatty liver disease (NAFLD) is present in at least 15% of the adult population and is responsible for liver enzyme abnormalities in many obese subjects. Although generally benign, some patients develop non-alcoholic steatohepatitis, of whom a few proceed to cirrhosis. Observational data from the West of Scotland (WOSCOPS) study suggests that the presence of fatty liver may be an important predictor of T2DM (Sattar et al. 2007).

Clinical features: the CVD patient with obesity

Obesity may be a substantial challenge in the clinical evaluation of patients presenting with cardiovascular symptoms.

In obese patients with suspected heart failure, jugular venous pressure estimation is almost impossible and examination of hand vein distension is an imperfect but useful alternative. The dorsal veins of the hand are normally filled when the hand is positioned below the heart. Elevation of the arm above this level should lead them to empty and the height where emptying occurs above the sternal angle is a reflection of the venous pressure. Pulmonary hypertension related to obstructive sleep apnoea may be an alternative cause for dyspnoea, and the pulmonary component of the second heart sound may be apparent in the first (rather than the second) left intercostal space.

In obese patients with known cardiac disease, seeking other complications of obesity is prudent and may impact on management—for example the co-existence of obstructive sleep apnoea in the subject with heart failure.

Clinical features: the obese patient and CV concerns

Most obese subjects are aware of the CV risks of their weight problem and may seek reassurance regarding the absence of CVD. The initial step should be to define the overall risk factor profile of the patient with blood biochemistry, lipid profile, glucose tolerance (if appropriate), and assessment of albuminuria. Blood pressure should be assessed with a large cuff—the bladder should cover 75% of the length of the arm and the cuff length (which should be about twice the bladder width) should almost encircle the arm. Ambulatory blood pressure monitoring may be considered (see Chapter 4.2).

• Screening for CAD remains a contentious topic, with the recent DIAD study reporting no change in outcome after the use of perfusion scintigraphy to seek CAD in low-risk subjects with T2DM. Although many of these patients have multiple risk factors, testing with the intent of identifying occult CAD is difficult to justify. However, the use of testing to identify subclinical atherosclerosis (evaluation of coronary calcium or carotid intima-medial thickness) may help to guide the intensity of preventive strategies and improve treatment adherence in some circumstances.

Clinical evaluation of the obese patient

Body mass index.
Fat distribution (waist circumference, waist-hip ratio).
Consider secondary causes.
History suggesting obstructive sleep apnoea, heart failure.
Blood pressure (large cuff), complications of hypertension.
Evidence of atherosclerotic vascular disease.
Clinical clues of pulmonary hypertension.
Venous insufficiency.
ECG (QTc).
Biochemistry—liver function tests, glucose (or oral glucose tolerance), lipid profile.
Albuminuria.
Consider echocardiography (systolic and diastolic function).

- Difficulties are often posed by attribution of symptoms to overweight—especially dyspnoea and fatigue. Increasing emphasis is being placed on early detection of heart failure, and the detection of abnormal cardiac structure would place the subject in ACC/AHA Stage B. Therefore the use of echocardiography to identify LV hypertrophy or LV systolic or diastolic dysfunction is appropriate. The use of B-type natriuretic peptide (BNP) may be problematic (see below).

Impact on investigations

The cardiovascular investigation of obese subjects may be significantly influenced by their obesity.

1 Biochemistry—abnormal liver function tests, abnormal lipid profile and inflammatory markers (e.g. C-reactive protein).

2 Brain natriuretic peptide (BNP) levels are lower in obese than non-obese subjects and this may produce misleading results in obese subjects. The mechanism of this is unclear—there is some suggestion of increased BNP clearance via clearance receptors on adipocyte cells. The prognostic implications of raised BNP still apply, although lower thresholds need to be applied.

3 12-lead ECG—changes relate to cardiac position, workload, distance from the surface, and chronic lung disease. Horizontal cardiac position (due to raised hemidiaphragms in the supine position) may lead to mistaken diagnoses of inferior myocardial infarction. Increased workload may cause strain patterns, but LV hypertrophy is under-diagnosed by voltage criteria in obesity and Cornell criteria appear to be most reliable. PR, QRS, and QT intervals may be prolonged despite an increase in heart rate. Voltages are often reduced due to overlying soft tissue.

4 Chest X-ray—elevated hemidiaphragm, related to increase in liver size, and omental fat, as well as an apparent increase in cardiothoracic ratio related to an epicardial fat-pad.

5 Ultrasound studies may be compromised by obesity although its location in relation to the ultrasound window is critical. Epicardial fat is sometimes mistaken for pericardial fluid or tumour, but if an effusion is present, adjacent fat may lead to underestimation of its size. However, as epicardial fat is visceral fat, and its presence may relate to some of the adverse metabolic effects of overweight on the heart, the measurement of this structure may be of value.

- Lipomatous hypertrophy of the interatrial septum is usually linked with septal fat deposits of >2 cm, but may not be linked with obesity.

- Echo contrast agents may salvage technically difficult studies, and transoesophageal echo is an alternative for imaging structures. It should be remembered that the signal–noise relationship of Doppler is more favourable than grey-scale imaging and diagnostic Doppler studies are obtainable even in the presence of poor quality images. Diastolic dysfunction (see Chapter 1.4) is commonly identified and LV filling pressure may be assessed from the ratio of transmitral flow and annular tissue velocity.

6 Sleep studies and oxygen desaturation may arise from obstructive sleep apnoea.

7 Computed tomography and coronary angiography might be compromised by attenuation of X-rays. Many equipment tables may have upper load limits of 150–200 kg. It is important to consider the potential load if resuscitation might be required during an intervention.

8 Scintigraphic procedures (e.g. SPECT)—weight is a potentially significant problem during which may be reduced with attenuation correction.

Management

The management of overweight includes dietary and lifestyle change, medical therapy and surgery. Weight loss has been associated with improvements of left ventricular function, obstructive sleep apnoea, hypertension, the inflammatory process and the metabolic profile (including lipids, insulin resistance and diabetes).

Dietary-lifestyle change

Patients presenting with cardiovascular disease and overweight have usually made multiple attempts to lose weight without success. This is best managed as a chronic disease with education, goal setting and self monitoring. Clinical guidelines for obese subjects (BMI >30) and overweight subjects (BMI 25–30) with coronary heart disease or multiple risk factors have proposed a three-part strategy comprising caloric restriction, behaviour therapy and structured physical activity (http://www.nhlbi.nih.gov/guidelines/obesity/). Simple dietary interventions include reduction of portion size, reduced carbohydrate and fat intake and avoidance of alcohol and simple sugars. Group therapy is often more effective than individual effort.

Physical activity has an important role. Population studies demonstrate overweight to be associated with lower levels of activity. Despite the high energy efficiency of humans, which requires long periods of activity in order to burn up relatively few calories, activity seems to have an important role in weight reduction.

Medical therapy of obesity

A number of medical therapies have been attempted:

- Appetite suppressants have been withdrawn from the market, because of cardiac side-effects.
- Orlistat reduces the absorption of dietary fat.
- Sibutramine reduces intake of dopamine and noradrenaline, and is an effective appetite suppressant.

- Peroxisome proliferator-activated receptors (PPARs) agents provoke improvements of metabolic profile, but this may be at the cost of a small increment of weight.
- Ribonabant therapy seeks to influence appetite and energy expenditure through the endocannabinoid system.

Adjunctive therapy unrelated to weight control

Established heart failure and coronary artery disease should be treated along standard lines, and blood pressure control is crucial, as usual. Theoretical considerations relating to both cardiac and metabolic effects favour the use of renin–angiotensin–aldosterone system antagonists, as well as beta-adrenosceptor blockers. There are potential metabolic benefits of treatment with metformin or thiazolidinediones, but the clinical evidence in support of this is limited.

Surgery

Weight loss surgery was previously associated with significant risk, but recent laparoscopic procedures such as gastric banding appear to be safer. Weight loss with bariatric surgery is substantial (20–40% being not unusual), and is associated with regression of cardiac changes as well as improved survival and reduced morbidity and metabolic sequelae.

Myocardial revascularization

Revascularization may be considered in obese patients with angina uncontrolled with medical therapy. These patients are often younger than their non-obese counterparts and have insulin resistance and other co-morbidities. Obesity offers technical challenges to both percutaneous intervention and bypass surgery, and is associated with sternal and vein harvest site infections and atrial fibrillation. Surprisingly, pulmonary complications are not increased (although very obese subjects, BMI >35, are at risk of requiring longer postoperative ventilation), and perioperative mortality or stroke are not increased.

Obesity as a public health issue

Given the epidemic nature over the last 20 years, the health burden of obesity and its impact on medical spending, it is reasonable that this problem should be addressed as a public health issue. Recently, New York has led the way into legislative interventions that seek to reduce the drivers of obesity. Steps have included bans on the use of trans fats and requirements for menu labelling (Mello 2009). Although promising, the benefit of this strategy remains undefined.

Future developments

Mechanistic developments are likely to centre on the contribution of adipokines, inflammation, and fatty acids.

Fat is an active endocrine organ and various signalling pathways may be manipulated to control obesity. Adiponectin is particularly promising from this standpoint, this agent is reduced by obesity, and associated with endothelial health. CRP production is driven by cytokines from adipose tissue. The inflammatory process may be an important contributor to atherogenesis. Fatty acids have an important toxic effect, and the obese state is associated with reduction of insulin's suppression of free fatty acids.

On the clinical front, while it is already clear that weight loss offers substantial health benefits, there are no randomized data to show outcome benefits. The LookAHEAD trial will report next year on the ability of moderate weight loss and exercise to improve survival.

References

Allison DB, Fontaine KR, Manson JE, et al. Annual deaths attributable to obesity in the United States. JAMA 1999;**282**:1530–8.

Australian Institute of Health and Welfare. The relationship between overweight, obesity and cardiovascular disease. Cardiovascular Disease series #24, 2004. http://www.aihw.gov.au/publications/cvd/rboocvd/rboocvd.pdf, accessed 9/5/09.

Flegal KM, Carroll MD, Ogden CL, Johnson CL. Prevalence and trends in obesity among US adults. JAMA 2002;**288**:1723–7.

Kenchaiah S, Evans J, Levy D et al. Obesity and the risk of heart failure. N Engl J Med 2002;**347**:305–13.

Mello MM. New York city's war on fat. N Engl J Med 2009;**360**: 2015–20.

Poirier A, Giles TD, Bray GA, et al. Obesity and cardiovascular disease: pathophysiology, evaluation, and effect of weight loss. An Update of the 1997 American Heart Association Scientific Statement on Obesity and Heart Disease From the Obesity Committee of the Council on Nutrition, Physical Activity, and Metabolism. Circulation 2006;**113**:898–918.

Sattar N, McConnachie A, Ford I, et al. Serial metabolic measurements and conversion to type 2 diabetes in the West of Scotland coronary prevention study: Specific elevations in alanine aminotransferase and triglycerides suggest hepatic fat accumulation as a potential contributing factor. Diabetes 2007;**56**:984–91.

Wilson P, D'Agostino R, Sullivan L, et al. Overweight and obesity as determinants of cardiovascular risk. The Framingham experience. Arch Intern Med 2002;**162**:1867–72.

Wong C, Marwick TH. Obesity cardiomyopathy: Pathogenesis and pathophysiology. Nat Clin Pract Cardiovasc Dis 2007;**4**:436–43.

Websites

Australian obesity guidelines. http://www.health.gov.au/internet/main/publishing.nsf/Content/obesityguidelines-index.htm

NICE (UK) obesity guidelines. http://www.nice.org.uk/CG043

NIH obesity guidelines. http://www.nhlbi.nih.gov/guidelines/obesity/. Includes practical guide and BMI calculator.

Coronary heart disease and women

Cardiovascular disease (CVD) is the major cause of death in women in the developed and developing countries, accounting worldwide for a third of all deaths (Shaw et al. 2006). As CVD increases in prevalence with age, and as women live longer than men, in many countries more women than men die from CVD each year (Mosca et al. 2007).

- In the USA 38.2 million women (34%) are living with CVD
- In Europe CVD is the cause of death in 43% of men and 55% of women
- CVD in women causes more deaths than all cancers added together (Table 12.6.1).

Risk factors

The American Heart Association has reclassified CVD risk in women in 2007 (Table 12.6.2) (Mosca et al. 2007). The emphasis is on promoting a healthy lifestyle with a more aggressive approach as risk increases. Women's awareness of CVD risk is 62% in white and only 38% in black women with under 50% aware of a healthy level of risk factors (Mosca et al. 2006).

Cigarette smoking

Women <55 years of age have a sevenfold increase in relative risk due to smoking and the degree of risk is dose dependent (Figure 12.6.1) (Bolego et al. 2002). It is recommended that women should not smoke and should avoid passive smoking (Williams 2005).

Blood pressure

The evidence of benefit from treating hypertension has been demonstrated for men and women, with women well represented in the major studies (Williams 2005). With regard to preventing a CVD event, the recommendation is to lower the blood pressure using weight loss, diet, exercise, and sodium restriction with drug therapy initiated if ≥140/90, or ≥130/80 mmHg if diabetic, documented CVD or chronic renal disease (Mosca et al. 2006).

Hyperlipidaemia

In postmenopausal women as in men an elevated cholesterol increases CVD risk (LaRosa et al. 1990). In women prior to the menopause the risk is less clear except for familial hypercholesterolaemia. Women benefit as much as men from lipid-lowering therapy (Stramba-Badiale et al. 2006).

Lifestyle factors

In the UK 43% of men and 34% of women are overweight and 22% of men and 23% of women are obese. As body weight increases so does CVD risk (Stramba-Badiale et al. 2006). Weight reduction reduces CVD risk, blood pressure, LDL cholesterol and triglycerides and exercise raises HDL cholesterol. In the Women's Health Initiative (73 743 postmenopausal women aged 50–79 years) brisk walking for 30 minutes at least five times a week reduced CVD events by 30% over a 3-year follow-up period (Manson et al. 2002). Women need to exercise for 60–90 minutes if weight loss is needed. Alcohol in moderation (14 units a week or less) reduces coronary mortality, whereas binge drinking increases it.

Waist circumference in women should be 80 cm (31.5 inches) or less.

Diabetes and metabolic syndrome

Diabetes is more common in the UK in women (17.7%) than men (13.4%) and it increases in Asians. The risk of CVD is increased fourfold (Shaw 2006; Stramba-Badiale

Table 12.6.2 Classification of cardiovascular disease (CVD) risk in women

Risk status	Criteria
High risk	Established coronary heart disease
	Cerebrovascular disease
	Peripheral artery disease
	Abdominal aortic aneurysm
	End-stage or chronic renal disease
	Diabetes mellitus
	10-year Framingham global risk >20%[a]
At risk	≥1 major risk factors for CVD including:
	Cigarette smoking
	Poor diet
	Physical inactivity
	Obesity, especially central adiposity
	Family history of premature CVD (CVD at <55 years) of age in male relative and <65 years of age in female relative
	Hypertension
	Dyslipidaemia
	Evidence of subclinical vascular disease (e.g. coronary calcification)
	Metabolic syndrome
	Poor exercise capacity on treadmill test and/or abnormal heart rate recovery after stopping exercise
Optimal risk	Framingham global risk <10% and a healthy lifestyle, with no risk factors

[a]Or at high risk on the basis of another population adapted tool used to access global risk.

Table 12.6.1 Causes of death in men and women

Disease	Men (%)	Women (%)
CAD	21	23
Stroke	11	18
Other CVD	11	15
Cancer	21	18 (breast 3)
Respiratory	8	6
Injuries/poisoning	12	4
Other	16	16

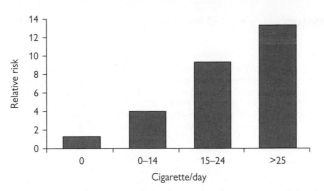

Fig. 12.6.1 The relationship between number of cigarettes smoked and myocardial infarction in women below the age of 55. Adapted from Bolego *et al.* 2002. With permission from Oxford University Press.

et al. 2006). The target for a diabetic is an HbA1c <7% with all risk factors aggressively addressed (Mosca *et al.* 2007).

Women with the metabolic syndrome have a 4-year relative risk of CVD increased twofold compared with those with a normal metabolic status (Stramba-Badiale *et al.* 2006). Depression is linked to the metabolic syndrome and the prevalence of depression in women of up to 70% is a concern as depression itself is a risk factor for CVD (Stramba-Badiale *et al.* 2006). All risk factors need addressing and specific antidepressant therapy instituted as needed.

Hormones

These have been covered in Chapter 12.10. Hormone replacement therapy (HRT) is not recommended for primary or secondary prevention of CVD (Mosca *et al.* 2007).

Aspirin

There is no evidence of benefit in primary prevention. Secondary prevention benefits have been established (Ridker *et al.* 2005).

Drug therapy

Women benefit from beta-blockers post myocardial infarction and/or when there is left ventricular dysfunction (Stramba-Badiale *et al.* 2006). They also benefit from angiotensin-converting enzyme (ACE) inhibitors where there is left ventricular dysfunction or heart failure but have an increased incidence of ACE-induced cough. They benefit similarly to men regarding lipid-lowering therapy with statins.

Presentation and management

Angina is a more common presenting symptom in women whereas sudden death and myocardial infarction are more common in men. However 40% of initial CVD events in women are fatal so being alert to symptoms is important. Women more often have atypical chest pain (at rest, during sleep, stress related, affecting jaw, teeth, arms, neck, shoulders, back, and abdomen) when younger (Douglas and Ginsburg 1996). Exercise testing (Chapter 1.3) is less accurate in women, whereas stress echocardiography has a sensitivity of 86% and specificity of 79% for CVD (Kwok *et al.* 1999; Redberg and Shaw 2003).

Women are older at presentation with an acute coronary syndrome (ACS) and have a higher prevalence of risk factors and more complex and diffuse coronary anatomy. In the presence of high risk an early invasive strategy benefits women as much as men (Glaser and Herrman 2002). Increased interventional or surgical risks are related to

small vessel size and disease extent as well as increased co-morbidities rather than gender *per se*.

Key points

- Cardiovascular disease is the greatest cause of morbidity and mortality in women.
- Women may present differently to men but should receive the same therapy as men.
- Risk factor management is essential, but HRT is not indicated for primary or secondary prevention.
- Gender bias in management is inexcusable.

References

Bolego C, Poli A, Paoletti R. Smoking and gender. *Cardiovasc Res* 2002;**53**:568–76.

Douglas PS, Ginsburg GS. The evaluation of chest pain in women. *N Engl J Med* 1996;**334**:1311–15.

Glaser R, Herrman HC, Murphy SA, *et al.* Benefit of an early invasive management strategy in women with acute coronary syndromes. *JAMA* 2002;**288**:3124–9.

Kwok Y, Kim C, Grady D, *et al.* Meta-analysis of exercise testing to detect coronary artery disease in women. *Am J Cardiol* 1999;**83**:660-6.

LaRosa JC, Hunninghake D, Bush D, *et al.* The cholesterol facts. A summary of the evidence relating dietary fats, serum cholesterol, and coronary heart disease. A joint statement by the American Heart Association and the National Heart, Lung and Blood Institute. The task force on cholesterol issues, American Heart Association. *Circulation* 1990;**81**:1721–33.

Manson JE, Greenland P, LaCroix AZ, *et al.* Walking compared with vigorous exercise for the prevention of cardiovascular events in women. *N Engl J Med* 2002;**347**:716–22.

Mosca L, Banka CL, Benjamin EJ, *et al.* Evidence-based guidelines for cardiovascular disease prevention in women: 2007 update. *Circulation* 2007;**115**:1481–501.

Mosca L, Mochari H, Christian A, *et al.* National study of women's awareness, preventive action and barriers to cardiovascular health. *Circulation* 2006;**113**:525–34.

Redberg RF, Shaw LJ. Diagnosis of coronary artery disease in women. *Prog Cardiovasc Dis* 2003;**46**:239–58.

Ridker PM, Cook NR, Lee IM, *et al.* A randomized trial of low-dose aspirin in the primary prevention of cardiovascular disease in women. *N Engl J Med* 2005;**352**:1293–304.

Shaw K-T. Epidemiology of coronary heart disease in women. *Heart* 2006;92(Suppl. III):iii2–4.

Stramba-Badiale M, Fox KM, Priori SG, *et al.* Cardiovascular disease in women: a statement from the policy conference of the European Society of Cardiology. *Eur Heart J* 2006;**27**:994–1005.

Williams B. Recent hypertension trials: implications and controversies. *J Am Coll Cardiol* 2005;**45**:813–27.

Cardiac tumours

Incidence

Primary cardiac tumours are rare. With an incidence of 0.0017% to 0.28% of autopsy series, they are far less common than metastatic tumours to the heart (Tazelaar et al. 1992). The relative incidence of cardiac tumours is influenced greatly by age at diagnosis, and to a lesser degree, the sex of the patient. In autopsy series, one-quarter to one-half of primary cardiac tumours are myxomas. The proportion of myxomas as the total number of cardiac tumours is much higher in surgical series, and is approximately 80%. Almost all primary cardiac malignancies are sarcomas and they are classified similarly to sarcomas of extracardiac soft tissue. Rare types of primary cardiac malignancies include lymphomas and malignant paragangliomas.

Classification

Cardiac masses range from benign lesions to high-grade malignancies and occur over a wide range of ages (Table 12.7.1). Cardiac masses discovered by imaging can be considered in three groups:

1 Benign tumours: this group includes both benign neoplasms and non-neoplastic masses. Treatment is generally surgical.
2 Malignancies: almost all primary cardiac malignancies are sarcomas but also include lymphomas and metastases. Sarcomas have a dismal prognosis regardless of treatment;

Table 12.7.1 Classification of cardiac tumours

Adult heart tumours	Paediatric heart tumours
Benign neoplasms	**Hamartomas**
Cardiac myxoma	Rhabdomyoma
Paraganglioma/phaeochromocytoma	Fibroma
Non-neoplastic masses	Purkinje cell hamartoma/histiocytoid cardiomyopathy
Mural thrombi	
Lipomatous hypertrophy, atrial septum	
Papillary fibroelastoma	**Germ cell tumours**
Malignant neoplasms	
Sarcomas	
Angiosarcoma (mostly right atrium/pericardium)	
Sarcomas with myofibroblastic differentiation (mostly left atrium)	
Undifferentiated/malignant fibrous histiocytoma	
Leiomyosarcoma	
Fibrosarcoma	
Osteosarcoma	
Rhabdomyosarcoma	
Synovial sarcoma	
Lymphomas	
Metastatic tumours	
Carcinomas	
Renal cell/hepatocellular, mostly intracavitary	
Sarcomas	
Melanoma	

optimal treatment awaits more sophisticated surgical techniques and chemotherapeutic regimens.
3 Paediatric tumours: primary cardiac tumours in children are extremely rare. This group is composed mainly of hamartomas including rhabdomyoma and fibroma. Paediatric tumours are associated in many cases with genetic syndromes.

Clinical findings

Symptoms

Cardiac tumours present with a variety of symptoms, including those related to obstruction of blood flow, embolic phenomena, pericardial involvement, cardiac failure, and elaboration of substances resulting in constitutional symptoms. The presenting symptom is generally related less to the tumour type than to the site in the heart and the friability of the lesion.

For example, tumours of the left atrium often present as mitral valve disease (mitral stenosis most commonly). Tumours in the right ventricle resulting in pulmonic stenosis can present with syncopal episodes. Tumours with luminal involvement, for example myxomas and papillary fibroelastomas, can present with systemic or pulmonary emboli, depending on the site of origin in the heart. Tumours with extensive myocardial involvement may result in congestive heart failure. If there is pericardial involvement, pericardial effusions and chest pain may dominate the clinical picture and the cardiac tumour may be diagnosed only after pericardiocentesis. Other than lymphomas, treatment of neoplasms is primarily surgical, with complete excision if possible.

Imaging of cardiac tumours

Echocardiography has the best spatial and temporal resolution of the cardiac imaging modalities, providing excellent anatomic and functional information. It is generally the only imaging modality required preoperatively, and is the preferred modality for imaging small masses (<1 cm) or masses arising from a valve. Magnetic resonance imaging (MRI) has the highest soft tissue contrast of the imaging modalities, which makes it the most sensitive modality for detection of tumour infiltration, and is more amenable to manipulation than other imaging modalities (Siripornpitak and Higgins 1997).

Computed tomography (CT) has better soft tissue contrast than echocardiography, and can be used to characterize fatty content and calcifications. The overall soft tissue contrast and ability to characterize tumour type and extent of infiltration is less than that of MRI (Tatli and Lipton 2005).

Tumours occurring primarily in the left atrium

Cardiac myxoma

Cardiac myxoma is an endocardial-based neoplasm of uncertain histogenesis with unique histopathological features not seen in extracardiac locations. In surgical series, cardiac myxomas account for the majority of heart tumours. The mean age at presentation is 50 years and approximately two-thirds of patients are women (Burke et al. 2004). Almost 90% of myxomas occur in the left atrium as polypoid lesions attached to the oval fossa (Figure 12.7.1). Histologically, the tumour is composed of 'myxoma' cells within a myxoid matrix.

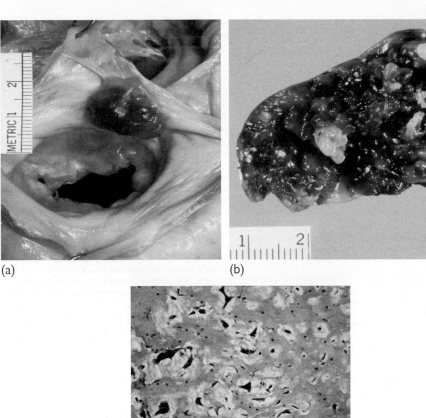

Fig. 12.7.1 Cardiac myxoma. (a) The majority of cardiac myxomas are located in the left atrium near the fossa ovalis. The mitral valve is intact and not obstructed by this small myxoma, which was an incidental finding at autopsy. (b) Cut surface of a different myxoma shows friable surface. One-third to one half of cardiac myxomas have a friable surface prone to embolize. (c) Histologically, myxoma cells are stellate, multinucleated and may form cords and rings.

Clinical

The clinical presentation of cardiac myxoma is more varied than any other cardiac tumour. Cardiac myxomas cause symptoms in three ways: by mass effect, embolization, and constitutional effects. Because cardiac myxoma is most often located in the left atrium, the most common presentation secondary to mass effect is that of mitral stenosis. The tumours are often friable and embolic phenomena occur in 30–40% of patients. Symptoms related to embolic phenomena include strokes, transient ischaemic attacks, claudication of the extremities, renal insufficiency, myocardial infarction, and pulmonary emboli (right-sided tumour). Constitutional symptoms include weakness, malaise, fevers, and are related to haematological abnormalities such as anaemia, hypergammaglobulinaemia, and increased sedimentation rate. Rarely, myxomas can become infected, leading to bacterial endocarditis.

Diagnosis and treatment

At echocardiography, cardiac myxomas typically appear as a mobile mass attached to the endocardial surface by a stalk, usually arising from the fossa ovalis.

The majority of patients are cured with surgical removal. Recurrence is seen in less than 1–2% of cases after excision (Larsson *et al.* 1989). Recurrences are generally at intracardiac sites distant from the original tumour.

Myxoma syndrome

In a small minority of patients, there is a familial constellation of abnormalities that include cardiac myxoma, spotty pigmentation, endocrine overactivity, and myxoid neurofibromas referred to as myxoma syndrome. These patients are much younger than patients with sporadic cardiac myxoma and usually become symptomatic by the third decade. In contrast to patients with sporadic tumours, about 10% of patients with familial myxomas either have recurrent tumours or develop another tumour in a different location.

Cardiac sarcomas

Primary sarcomas of the heart are rare, and constitute less than 25% of primary cardiac tumours and only 10% of surgically resected cardiac tumours. The left atrium is the site of 50% of cardiac sarcomas. There is no sex predilection and the mean age at presentation is 41 years. Virtually all types of sarcomas have been shown to arise within the cardiac muscle mass, demonstrating the pluripotentiality of the malignant mesenchymal cell. The histological types are essentially identical to those found in extracardiac soft tissue.

Classification

There are three categories of primary cardiac sarcomas.

1 Endomyocardial-based tumours, which usually have features of smooth muscle or fibroblastic differentiation. Sarcomas with myo- or fibroblastic differentiation are the most pathological diverse cardiac sarcomas and typically form endoluminal masses that are most frequently found in the left atrium. They have been subclassified as malignant fibrous histiocytoma (recently designated as undifferentiated pleomorphic sarcoma), osteosarcoma, leiomyosarcoma, and fibrosarcoma or myxofibrosarcoma.

2 Rhabdomyosarcomas (rare) are typically ventricular lesions in children or young adults.

3 Angiosarcoma is usually located in the right atrium and will be discussed below.

Clinical

The clinical presentation of any primary malignant tumour of the heart depends on its location. Because more than half of cardiac sarcomas are located in the left atrium, the most common presenting symptom is dyspnoea secondary to left ventricular inflow obstruction. Other modes of presentation include pericardial involvement embolic phenomena, chest pain, syncope, fever of unknown origin, and peripheral oedema. Distant metastases commonly develop in patients with primary sarcoma and are sometimes the presenting symptom. Metastatic sites are most commonly the lungs, followed by vertebrae, liver, brain, bowel, long bones, spleen, adrenals, and skull.

Diagnosis and treatment

Diagnosis is best made by echocardiography but invasion into adjacent atria or valves may sometimes be demonstrated by MRI or CT. The prognosis of cardiac sarcomas is poor and is generally measured in months. Pathological findings associated with increased survival include left-sided tumours, a low mitotic rate, and absence of necrosis. However, even with sarcomas of low mitotic rate lacking necrosis, the long term outlook is poor and few patients survive 5 years. Complete resection of malignant primary cardiac tumours can be achieved, but usually palliative surgery is performed because many patients present with mechanical obstruction. Adjunctive chemotherapy, radiation therapy, or both are sometimes used.

Tumours occurring primarily in the right atrium

Right-sided myxoma

Approximately 10% of cardiac myxomas occur in the right atrium. Because of location and smooth tumour surface, patients are often asymptomatic, although tricuspid obstruction and rarely pulmonary embolism can occur.

Lipomatous hypertrophy of the atrial septum

Lipomatous hypertrophy of the atrial septum is exclusively limited to the cardiac atria, especially the interatrial septum, and is probably hamartomatous in origin. Histologically there is a mixture of mature and brown fat, which ultrastructurally contains abundant mitochondria (Burke et al. 1996). It is a rare lesion but the true incidence is difficult to assess because most cases are incidental findings at autopsy. The typical imaging findings are those of a right sided mass with fat density on MRI. Lipomatous hypertrophy is removed incidentally during open-heart surgery for other causes or for relief of cardiac symptoms, such as supraventricular arrhythmias, congestive heart failure or vena caval obstruction.

Angiosarcoma

The most common differentiated cardiac sarcoma is angiosarcoma. Unlike other types of cardiac sarcoma, there is a marked right sided predominance. Sixty per cent or more of angiosarcomas occur in the right atrium, most often near the atrioventricular groove but it has been reported in the other three chambers as well as in the pericardium. The mean age at presentation is 40 years (range 36 months to 80 years) and there is a male predilection (2.5:1). There has been no documented relationship between cardiac angiosarcoma and occupational or toxic exposure. Overall, cardiac angiosarcomas have a poor prognosis because they typically present with metastasis, most frequently to the lung and liver. Angiosarcoma is treated by a combination of surgery and radiation with or without chemotherapy.

Mural thrombi

The majority of surgically excised atrial thrombi are right-sided, occur in patients without heart disease and are seen in patients with either documented or occult coagulation disorders. One of the more common coagulopathies diagnosed in patients with mural thrombi is the antiphospholipid syndrome, but a wide variety of conditions may be a predisposing factor including essential thrombocytosis, protein C or S deficiency, and Behcet's disease.

Tumours occurring on cardiac valves

Papillary fibroelastoma is a benign tumour composed of avascular papillary structures. This tumour may occur at any location on the valve, usually aortic or mitral valve, and achieves a large size. The true incidence is unknown because they can be easily overlooked at autopsy. Papillary fibroelastomas occur in adults of both sexes equally. The mean age at detection is approximately 60 years (Ngaage et al. 2005). Endocardial scarring secondary to radiation therapy, post-inflammatory valve disease, and other causes may predispose to the formation of papillary fibroelastoma. Because tumour mobility is an independent predictor of death or non-fatal embolization, asymptomatic patients with a mobile tumour may be treated surgically. Asymptomatic patients with non-mobile lesions can be followed closely with periodic clinical evaluation and echocardiography.

Paediatric tumours

Cardiac rhabdomyoma

Cardiac rhabdomyoma is the most common cardiac tumour in children. Patients with tuberous sclerosis have a 40–86% incidence of cardiac rhabdomyoma. They may occur in any location in the heart but are more common in the ventricles. At echocardiography, rhabdomyomas appear as homogeneous well-circumscribed echogenic masses in the ventricular myocardium possibly protruding into the ventricular myocardium. Surgery is recommended if there is significant outflow obstruction or if medical antiarrhythmic treatment is not successful. Rhabdomomas have a history of spontaneous regression.

Cardiac fibroma

Cardiac fibromas usually occur in the ventricular free wall or interventricular septum. Most cardiac fibromas are discovered in children before 1 year of age. At echocardiography, fibromas typically appear as a large well-circumscribed solitary mass in the septum or ventricular free wall and in some cases may be confused with hypertrophic cardiomyopathy (Araoz et al. 1999). Cardiac fibroma is benign but may cause conduction defects and arrhythmias. If the mass is too large for resection, heart transplantation may be considered.

Miscellaneous tumours

Cardiac lymphoma

The incidence of cardiac lymphoma has increased since the advent of iatrogenic immunosuppression in transplant patients as well as the acquired immune deficiency syndrome. However, In Immunocompetent patients, primary cardiac lymphoma is quite rare, accounting for 1.3% of primary cardiac tumours and 0.5% of extranodal lymphomas (Gowda and Khan 2003). The presenting symptoms vary according to the site in the heart, and may be related to conduction system disturbances, pericardial fluid accumulations, valvular obstruction, and congestive heart failure.

Early diagnosis with accurate imaging has been emphasized as important in the successful long-term outcome of patients with cardiac lymphoma. Lymphomas manifest as an ill-defined infiltrative mass and are typically best depicted with MRI because of its superior soft tissue contrast. Cardiac lymphomas are virtually all of B-cell origin and include follicular centre cell lymphomas, immunoblasic lymphomas, diffuse large cell lymphomas, and Burkitt's lymphoma. Treatment is not primarily surgical but includes chemotherapy and anti-CD20 treatment.

Metastatic cardiac tumours

In a series of 133 surgically resected cardiac tumours, 11% were metastases. They are typically right sided and represent either cavoatrial extensions from abdominal tumours such as renal cell carcinomas or hepatocellular carcinomas or haematogenous metastases that may present months or years after initial tumour excision. Malignancies metastatic to the heart include in order of incidence, carcinomas of the lung, lymphomas, carcinomas of the breast, leukaemia, carcinomas of the stomach, malignant melanoma, hepatocellular carcinoma, and colonic carcinomas. Currently, it is accepted practice to surgically remove metastatic deposits of relatively indolent tumours to improve cardiac function.

References

Araoz PA, Eklund HE, Welch TJ, et al. CT and MR imaging of primary cardiac malignancies. Radiographics 1999;**19**:1421–34.

Burke AP, Litovsky S, Virmani R. Lipomatous hypertrophy of the atrial septum presenting as right atrial mass. Am J Surg Pathol 1996;**20**:678–85.

Burke AP, Tazelaar H, Gomez-Roman JJ, et al. Benign tumors of pluripotent mesenchyme. In: Travis W (ed.) Tumours of the lung, thymus, pleura and heart. Lyon: Springer-Verlag, 2004: pp. 260–5.

Carney JA, Gordon H, Carpenter PC, et al. The complex of myxomas, spotty pigmentation, and endocrine overactivity. Medicine 1985;**64**:270–283.

Gowda RM, Khan IA. Clinical perspectives of primary cardiac lymphoma. Angiology 2003;**54**:599–604

Larsson S, Lepore V, Kennergren C. Atrial myxomas: results of 25 years' experience and review of the literature. Surgery 1989;**105**:695–698.

Ngaage DL, Mullany CJ, Daly RC, et al. Surgical treatment of cardiac papillary fibroelastoma; a single center experience with eighty-eight patients. Ann Thorac Surg 2005;**80**:1712–18.

Sirlpornpitak S, Higgins CB. MRI of primary malignant cardiovascular tumors. J Comput Assist Tomogr 1997;**21**:462–6.

Tatli S, Lipton MJ. CT for intracardiac thrombi and tumors. Int. J Cardiovasc Imaging 2005;**21**:115–31.

Tazelaar HD, Locke TJ, McGregor CG. Pathology of surgically excised primary cardiac tumors. Mayo Clin Proc 1992;**67**:957–65.

Adverse cardiac effects of drugs

Adverse drug reactions (ADRs) affect a minority of treated patients but are numerically commonplace due to the global prevalence of prescribed drug treatments. The negative impact of any adverse event (including iatrogenic death) may be offset by net beneficial effects of treatment of illness. Adverse events are not necessarily avoidable and some are inevitable consequences of treatment. Most are a product of dose and duration of treatment and generally interact with concomitant illness or other treatments. Generalized hypersensitivity reactions are not reliable ADRs and are non-specific and can occur with placebo therapy. The risk–benefit relationship in cases of ADRs are individually dependent on the disease, the treatment, and the relative risks and benefits of alternatives.

Indirect cardiac adverse drug effects

This section does not deal with drug-related hypotensive or hypertensive effects that can indirectly affect the heart, cardiac function rhythm, or coronary structure. These are often predictable, commonly asymptomatic, and non-specifically seen with a huge range of medicines (e.g. iodinated contrast, iron preparations, intravenous anaesthetics, lidocaine). Moreover, a range of cardiac adverse events involve indirect drug effects on other systems associated with homeostasis, including the stability of arterial pressure, e.g. methotrexate (causing lung fibrosis) meglitinides (causing rapid shifts in glycaemia), and adrenaline (epinephrine) (affecting perfusion and cardiac rhythm). Some agents cause minor peripheral side-effects mistaken as cardiogenic in origin, e.g. peripheral vasogenic oedema following calcium antagonists, dopamine agonists, or glitazones. In addition, major adverse reactions that are directly or indirectly a product of drug effect, e.g. Jarish–Herxheimer reaction, proarrhythmic effects of antiarrhythmic drugs, thrombosis with oestrogens, or serum oestrogen receptor modulating drugs (tamoxifen, raloxifene), are not considered here.

Drugs prescribed for cardiac disease have direct impact on the heart via concentration-dependent effects in keeping with their known pharmacology or pharmacokinetics during routine dosing or in overdose, e.g. arrhythmia following digoxin use or due to a well-known idiosyncratic reaction on chronic dosing, e.g. pulmonary fibrosis following amiodarone use. In this section the adverse cardiac effects of primary cardiac treatment given in therapeutic doses (or overdose) or due to pharmacogenetic individual patient sensitivity are not considered.

Although the majority of cardiac adverse effects represent minor, self-limiting symptoms and predictable target organ effects, some cardiac ADRs can generate major injury, and/or result in hospitalization and death. The general features of cardiac ADRs are best considered in the broad context of which aspect of cardiac structure or function is affected.

In general the effects of any drug treatment on cardiac function are dependent on drug concentration and the susceptibility of the individual heart to drug effect. In this regard ADRs generally maintain a preserved concentration effect relationship, although the effect may be non-linear

in situations of overdose. Within this relationship a great many drugs exert adverse effects on the heart in overdose. A much smaller number exert effects on cardiac function in a proportion of patients within their normal therapeutic window. These effects are generally only recognized on population exposure in large (sometimes very large) numbers of patients. Most adverse cardiac effects are exacerbated in the structurally abnormal heart (affected by pre-existent disease) regardless of the site of

---

Mechanisms of cardiac adverse drug reactions

Concentration-dependent (dosing and duration sensitive) organ response (most primary cardiac drugs) can be due to concomitant pharmacokinetic interaction.

Idiosyncratic systemic reaction involving the heart in systemic response (hypotension; hypertension; induced arrhythmia; *is situ* thrombosis and embolism resulting in vascular occlusion).

Non-cardiac therapy with a known or unknown cardiac effects.

---

adverse effect, e.g. coronary perfusion, cardiac myocyte, etc. Most have some interaction with co-prescribed cardiac treatments that make interpretations and unequivocal linkage complex.

Defining adverse drug effects on the heart

Post-marketing pharmacovigilance is a complex area and is not well coordinated globally. Much is left to national prescribing and regulatory authorities to coordinate ADR data and potentially collate new interactions and or patterns of illness that might be linked to the use of a new medicine or of a combination of medicines in a specific vulnerable population. Individual prescribers are to some extent in most systems tasked with central notification. Some countries encourage submission by pharmacists and other paramedical staff and there is strong reason to believe that in the current environment under-reporting in this system remains an issue. Reporting by members of the treated public has been considered but is not widely employed.

Population linkage of anonymous adverse events that may be drug related is a somewhat insensitive technique but has defined worthwhile unknown effects of licensed treatments. A certain amount of post-marketing safety data is collated by the manufacturer, but these mostly relate to issue that are known during the clinical trials development of new drugs. These do not reliably indicate the likelihood or planned definition of an unpredicted drug-related injury and may be influenced by commercial conflicts of interest that are difficult to reconcile.

Patients with cardiac illness and concomitant cardiac therapy are at heightened risk not only of adverse effects on the heart from their prescribed treatment and concentration dependent drug effects as above but also of adverse effects on their heart of non-cardiac drug therapies.

General management

Major suspected adverse cardiac reactions require discontinuation of therapy; consideration of active elimination of drug (by activated charcoal; controlled emesis if safe); haemofiltration (if relevant and possible); and supportive cardiac care (including ventilation support and invasive blood pressure monitoring) rhythm control measures and mechanical arterial pressure support (aortic counter-pulsation) if required.

The duration of such therapies will be guided by the kinetics of elimination of the drug in question and the pre-existent disease burden of the patient.

All fatal adverse events should be subject to post event round table discussion and centralized notification.

Formal notification of even a known adverse event and regardless of outcome is always a useful step.

Further reading

Anton C, Cox AR, Ferner RE. Improving follow up rates in spontaneous adverse drug reaction reporting effectiveness of a targeted letter used by a regional centre in the UK. *Drug Safety* 2009;**32**:1135–40.

Aronson JK. *Meyler's side effects of cardiovascular drugs*. Amsterdam: Elsevier, 2009: pp. 1–829.

Howick J, Glasziou P, Aronson JK. The evolution of evidence hierarchies: what can Bradford Hill's guidelines for causation contribute? *J Roy Soc Med* 2009;**102**:186–94.

Martin RM, Kapoor KV, Wilton LV, Mann RD. Under reporting of suspected adverse drug reactions to newly marketed drugs in general practice: observational study. *Br Med J* 1998;**317**:119–20.

Noren NG, Edwards IR. Modern methods of pharmacovigilance: detecting adverse effects of drugs. *Clin Med* 2009;**9**:486–9.

Specific cardiac effects of drugs

A very large spectrum of drug treatments have direct and indirect concentration-dependent effects on different aspects of cardiac function. Adverse effects can be subdivided into the primary aspect of cardiac function that may be affected.

Drugs having adverse effects on coronary vascular tone or coronary disease

Coronary vasospasm

Drugs may directly induce coronary spasm in susceptible individuals: agents having a cholinomimetic effect in patients with endothelial dysfunction, e.g. muscarinic antagonists, direct coronary vasospastic agents, paradoxical vasospasm with non-selective beta-adrenergic blocking drugs, drugs such as noradrenaline (norepinephrine) give a direct constriction of coronary tone; drugs with indirect effect on the 5HT3 receptor such as sumatriptan; zolmitriptan and cogeners (although these rarely appear to cause vasospasm in the absence of underlying coronary plaque). Drugs used in migraine prophylaxis such as pizotifen. Inappropriate high-dose ionic calcium infusion. Ergot alkaloids particularly in overdose but in some patients with an exaggerated response to therapeutic doses can cause arterial spasm in the coronary circulation and induce myocardial infarction. This effect extends to methysergide. Asian subjects may be predisposed to these arterial spasm effects to ergot preparations.

Spasm induced by cocaine in a structurally normal coronary circulation is well recognized but the frequency of this is over-diagnosed among the many cardiac symptoms presented by cocaine users. Myocardial infarction is rare and confirmation of ischaemia among cocaine users is much lower than matched controls (1.4 versus 9.4%). Accelerated atherosclerosis and aortic dissection are recorded. More obvious catecholaminergic stimulants such as amphetamines rarely cause much problem in defining their impact on coronary tone.

Sibutramine neuronal reuptake inhibition affecting both norepinephrine and serotonin commonly increases diastolic pressure marginally on population use. Concerns over cardiac toxicity proarrhythmia; infarction (with or without epicardial coronary occlusion) are such that a specific trial is ongoing to define cardiac safety (Sibutramine Cardiac OUtcomes Trial) in terms of the known impact of consistent impact on blood pressure and heart rate.

Both flucytosine and 5-fluorouracil (5-FU) (particularly during intravenous infusion) cause a drug- or metabolite-related increase in coronary vasomotor tone and propensity to spasm and myocardial ischaemia (in up to 10% of patients receiving 5-FU infusions). Sudden death has been recorded. These effects appear unrelated to patient demography, age, gender, etc., and are not influenced by concomitant cardiac disease. Some reports suggest concomitant vasodilator therapy and drug discontinuation may offset the impact of this adverse effect.

Desmopressin use is associated with systemic prothrombotic effects, including thrombotic occlusion and spontaneous myocardial infarction. The infusion of more powerful vasoconstrictor analogue of vasopressin, terlipressin has been known to induce myocardial ischaemia.

COX-2 inhibition and coronary disease

COX-2 inhibitors and non-specific inhibitors of both cyclo-oxygenase within the non-steroidal anti-inflammatory class (NSAID) class have complex effects in small numbers of patients with documented coronary artery disease, particularly those with prior surgical revascularization. Pooled analyses of individual patient data across all exposures to rofecoxib versus placebo; non-selective NSAIDS or naproxen provided no evidence of an excess of cardiovascular events for rofecoxib to placebo or some non-selective NSAIDs. Previous suggested differences between rofecoxib and placebo (in the VIGOR meta-analysis) in fact show naproxen to have a small protective effect. The exact mechanism of action whereby COX-2 inhibitors produce this relative rise in infarction is unclear, but a small impact on thrombotic vascular events is suggested. The exact mediator or genetic predisposition to this adverse drug reaction are unclear. Although highlighted for some COX-2 inhibitors such as rofecoxib, valdecoxib, and celecoxib, it is clear that this effect is not limited to selective COX-2 inhibitors but is also present to a small degree with unselective NSAIDs such a diclofenac. Naproxen's 'protective' effect remains an enigma.

Drugs linked to accelerating coronary atherosclerosis

Biguanide oral antidiabetic agents (e.g. metformin) are linked to an odds ratio of death due to ischaemic heart disease of 1.63 (1.27–2.09) when used as monotherapy in diabetic patients compared with other strategies in diabetes care.

A 4.8-fold increase in acute myocardial infarction is linked to recent (<1 hour) cannabinoid intake (in the Determinants of Acute Myocardial Infarction Study) as smoking marijuana. The mechanism and association of this population linkage to acute or chronic intake is less clear.

Long-term glucocorticoid use is linked to a wide range of adverse acute and chronic cardiovascular adverse effects in particular to accelerating coronary atherosclerosis but in addition exacerbating the sequelae of transmural infarction such as cardiac rupture.

Granulocyte colony-stimulating factor (GCSF) use is linked to accelerated recurrence of in stent restenosis in intracoronary infusion with or without stem cell treatments. Molgramostim (granulocyte macrophage colony-stimulating factor; GM-CSF) use in myelodysplasia is linked with non-haematological side-effects and induction of myocardial infarction.

Dipyridamole used particularly as a pharmacological stressor in thallium imaging is known to induce myocardial ischaemia and stroke following induction infusions. Similarly acute infarction and cardiac rupture have been linked to dobutamine stress in similar circumstances. These linkages are confounded by the exposure in this patient group.

Pseudoephedrine use has been linked to acute myocardial infarction in the context of angiographically normal coronary arteries and thus presumed acute coronary spasm.

Acute treatment with rituximab for the management of lymphoma has been linked to provocation of acute coronary syndromes most probably due to abrupt cytokine release.

A hyperadrenergic state induced by intravenous beta-sympathomimetic agents such as salbutamol, etc., has been linked to provocation of acute myocardial infarction by predictable positive inotropic and chronotropic effects and redistribution of coronary blood flow. These effects are not seen with distinct ipratropium/tiotropium-based inhaled bronchodilators.

Incautious introduction of thyroxine replacement by use of high doses or abruptly up titrating therapy in patients with long standing hypothyroidism is well noted to be linked to acute myocardial infarction. This can occur without underlying coronary artery disease.

Notwithstanding the known linkage of depressive illness to high rates of myocardial infarction, most tricyclic antidepressants (TCAs) (with the possible exception of dothepin) are associated with a 2.2-fold relative increase in cardiac event rates (95% CI 1.3–2.7). This is not seen with selective serotonin reuptake inhibitor (SSRI) use. TCAs are avoided in all depressed patients with known cardiovascular disease or significant risk factors for atherosclerosis.

Vinca alkaloids such as vincristine, vinblastine, and vinorelbine by infusion with or without the addition of other drugs having adverse cardiac effects (such as etoposide; bleomycin, and platinum analogues) is linked to acute ischaemia, electrocardiogram (ECG) changes, and ischaemic pulmonary oedema. Whether these acute events relate to spasm or not is uncertain. This confusion is based mostly on speculation over the structural similarity of these agents to ergot alkaloids that are clearly vasospastic.

Management
Standard methods of defining and managing myocardial ischaemia apply. Asymptomatic changes in stable patients should follow coherent review of the importance of the primary therapy and the possibilities for alternative treatments. Specific treatments for spasm may be applicable, such as high-dose nitrovasodilators given to avoid tachyphyllaxis or calcium channel blocking drugs.

Drugs having adverse effects on myocyte composition and function
Impact on cardiac contraction can be direct or indirect. The fundamentals are effects mediated by cumulative myocyte toxicity or a profibrotic impact on supporting cardiac connective tissue.

Anthracycline dilating cardiomyopathy
The most well-known myocyte toxins are the anthracycline antibiotics used in cancer chemotherapy (doxorubicin/adriamycin, daunorubicin, and epirubicin) affecting a significant minority of treated patients. This effect may be preventable. The response may be pharmacogenetic. A class effect is seen but the impact in individual cases may be variable between agents. Anthracyclines and related compounds induce late-onset cumulative lifetime dose, dilated cardiomyopathy, and replacement fibrosis worsened by increased age, pre-existent cardiac disease, or concomitant radiotherapy. The effects are irreversible but are thought to be responsive to conventional treatment including orthotopic transplantation that has been successfully deployed.

Traztuzumab dilating cardiomyopathy
Traztuzumab cardiotoxicity is a well-known and major side-effect of this adjuvant treatment of breast cancer subtypes. It is particularly evident with concomitant anthracycline use (~25%) but also its incidence is also accelerated when used when traztuzumab is used alongside either cyclophosphamide or paclitaxel (~13%). Impairment of left ventricular (LV) function can be severe and life-threatening but thankfully responds to discontinuation of treatment and standard antifailure therapy. The mechanism of this reaction is unclear but baseline MUGA scanning of all treated patients is routinely recommended.

Immunosuppressive therapy
Imatinib therapy for myeloid leukaemia appears to induce LV systolic dysfunction in a small proportion (0.04%) of treated patients, particularly in those with pre-existent cardiac disease. This rate is much lower than that attributable to the alternative therapy with cytosine arabinoside and interferon.

Interferon-α use in viral hepatitis is associated with rare but significant falls in left ventricular ejection fraction (LVEF) even without prior history of cardiac disease. These are reversible on discontinuation of treatment and appear to be dose related.

Among commonly used neuroleptic drugs the atypical antipsychotic drug clozapine has the highest prevalence of cardiac side-effects at 4.5/10 000 patients (exposure unclear) with pan-myocarditis and dilated cardiomyopathy (0.01–0.19%) being a rare but well recognized problem. This effect may be linked to the treatment of psychotic patients with coincidental selenium deficiency.

Long-term glucocorticoid use has been linked to cardiomyocyte hypertrophy in addition to its indirect impact on fluid retention and raising arterial pressure. The effects are dose and duration dependent and reversible.

Precipitation of decompensation of known left ventricular systolic dysfunction (LVSD) by concomitant use of NSAID and diuretics is well recognized (RRR 1.8 95% CI 1.4–2.4) and may account for as much as 20% of admissions for decompensation in elderly patients with LVSD.

Imatinib an effective therapy for inflammatory bowel disease was tested without obvious benefit in LVSD; in fact LVSD worsens when it is given in higher doses.

Management
In some instances, e.g. traztuzumab, the prevalence of cardiomyopathy is so severe and the consequences so detrimental that specific screening of baseline ventricular contractility is recommended. In most cases, presentation of unexplained and confirmed pulmonary oedema or symptoms of ventricular dysfunction should provoke a search for an aetiology. Drug-related toxicity is generally a common pathway. Drug discontinuation even in the setting of cancer therapies is generally mandatory and the full range of supportive antifailure strategies can be implemented with effect in most instances.

Drugs having adverse effects on cardiac connective tissue and valvular structure or function
Drugs with known direct effects on cardiac connective tissue structure are rare.

Anorexogens and other drugs affecting valve structure
The use of fenfluramine or dexfenfluramine (alone or with phentermine; FenPhen) in the Hypertension Genetic Epidemiology Network Study was clearly associated with valvular aortic regurgitation. This can occur distinct from

any effects on pulmonary artery hypertension (below). The prevalence of both left and right-sided valvular regurgitation with anorexigens such as these is not clearly related to dose or duration of use. It is not consistently reversed by drug withdrawal and for a period most patients are asymptomatic. On balance screening echocardiography is not recommended. These effects do not appear to extend to more modern non amphetamine agents such as sibutramine.

Methysergide can induce both valvular stenosis and fibrosis but can more rarely extend to more generalized endomyocardial fibrosis or pericardial fibrosis.

The antineoplastic agent busulfan is linked to idiosyncratic pericardial and endomyocardial fibrosis.

Serosal reactions pericarditis: pericardial effusions

Clozapine has been linked to serositis and pericarditis with pleural effusion.

High-dose cytarabine induces pericardial effusion and acute pericarditis responsive to glucocorticoid and treatment cessation.

Pericarditis has been reported following interferon-α.

The ergot derived dopamine agonist drug pergolide is well recognized to induce restrictive changes in cardiac valve structure. This appears to be dose related and predominantly affects the mitral valve. Restrictive valve pathology is only partially reversible by drug discontinuation. The prevalence of this problem led to the downgrading of this dopamine agonist in anti-parkinsonian treatment.

Management

Quantification of effects by appropriate quantitative echocardiography and where necessary cardiac catheter studies or magnetic resonance imaging (MRI) is feasible. Transvenous cardiac biopsy of affected tissue for microscopy and EM is possible if myocardial involvement is suspected but changes are generally non-specific. Drug withdrawal in these cases may not be greatly effective and progressive fibrosis and fixed changes in cardiac structure are potential outcomes despite prompt action.

Drugs adversely affecting cardiac conduction and arrhythmia patterns.

Pharmacogenetic interactions most notably with the HERG-2 potassium rectifier current channelopathies are in part behind many of the QT prolongation effects and potential torsade de pointes (tdp) arrhythmia and sudden death cases.

QTc (rate corrected QT interval) interval prolongation and torsade de pointes VT

Anti-psychotic drugs

Most but not all antipsychotic drugs prolong rate corrected QTc. QTc prolongation is not a class effect. The atypical antipsychotic agent olanzapine in particular seems to have little effect on QTc. Impact on QT dispersion is a separate issue. Both have a complex linkage to spontaneous ventricular tachycardia (VT) (in this case a specific pattern of tdp, which in turn is separate from linked sudden death).

The linkage of QTc prolongation to malignant proarrhythmia (ventricular torsade de pointes tachycardia) in individual cases is complex. Dose, duration and concomitant therapies (particularly tricyclic antidepressants), increasing age and the presence of structural heart disease are key to the latter adverse events.

It has been suggested that the antidepressant venlafaxine while producing definable dose-related QTc prolongation does not facilitate tdp VT even in overdose. On the other hand, haloperidol, droperidol, thioridazine, mesoridazine, sulpiride, and pimozide all provide variable QTc prolongation but are particularly linked with tdp and sudden death. These agents should not be used in patients with structural heart disease. The impact of thioridazine may be due in part to a documented poor elimination phenotype (in part characterized by debrisoquine elimination).

Haloperidol in intravenous use has a particular propensity to tdp and can cause malignant VT without obvious impact on QTc. These effects are evident notwithstanding concomitant use of drugs known to prolong QT interval but are worsened by the polypharmacy necessary in major psychosis. Citalopram and ecitalopram both prolong QTc in routine doses but tdp is less clearly problematic.

Ziprasidone an atypical antipsychotic has a greater capacity to produce QTc prolongarution than other antipsychotic drugs although its impact on tdp is not clear.

Macrolide antibiotics (erythromycin, azithromycin, clarithromycin, roxithromycin) appear to be the most sensitive to QTc prolongation and tdp is documented and linkage of recent erythromycin use to sudden death was seen in the Tennessee Medicaid cohort in 1476 cases of adult sudden death.

Methadone in high doses, common in opiate dependency management, is powerfully associated with QTc prolongation and tdp despite the multiple confounding drug use (including agents such as cocaine that inhibit the hepatic clearance of methadone) and difficulties in establishing dose relationships. Additional effects on QRS widening and bradycardia are well accepted.

Quinolone antibiotics such as ciprofloxacin orfloxacin, enoxacin, levofloxacin and norfloxacin all induce dose and duration related QTc prolongation. The rate of tdp is lower for ciprofloxacin (0.3 cases per 10 million prescriptions). Some drugs in this class have proven so cardiotoxic they have been withdrawn outright, e.g. grepafloxacin.

Prolongation of QTc and tdp is a class effect of the antifungal azoles such as fluconazole and ketoconazole. These changes occur on monotherapy.

Probucol has been shown to induce QTc prolongation and tdp is documented.

The administration of intravenous pentamidine is linked to induction of ventricular tachycardia. It may be acutely preceded by QT interval prolongation and tdp has been described. Because of its long half-life and slow elimination, arrhythmia can occur many days after treatment.

In general SSRIs do not share the prolongation of QTc common across the TCA group; however, there are isolated reports of QTc prolongation, atrial arrhythmias, and dose-dependent bradycardia following fluoxetine and paroxetine.

Non QTc prolongation effects on cardiac rhythm

Antiepileptic and anti-Alzheimer drugs

Phenytoin and carbamazepine induce symptomatic bradyarrhythmia almost exclusively on intravenous dosing. Ventricular standstill and death are recorded. Effects are more prevalent in pre-existent conduction disease and may be response to topiramate.

In addition to well recognized effects on increasing syncope due to carotid sinus syndrome; sinus node dysfunction

(SND) and atrioventricular (AV) block. Donepezil also induces ventricular tachycardia which in patients with impaired ventricular contraction is linked to increased mortality. No mortality effect is seen in treated patients with normal left ventricular contraction.

Antidepressants

TCAs are highly concentrated in myocardium and consistently induce by both central and peripheral means an observable sinus tachycardia. Conduction delay distal to the AV node is common and can cause AV block and fascicular block. The linkage of these changes to observed rates of sudden death in TCA users is much less clear and plasma concentrations are unhelpful given the extensive tissue distribution of drugs in this class.

Although lithium commonly causes surface ECG changes such a pseudo-infarct patterns and non-specific ST and T wave changes, the most commonly seen adverse effect is sinus node dysfunction and bradyarrhythmia. These normally resolve with drug discontinuation but this is not a universal observation. The first patients ever treated with therapeutic lithium for mania developed symptomatic bradycardia following trial dose escalation.

Antineoplastic agents

The antineoplastic drugs paclitaxel and docetaxel are both linked to asymptomatic sinus bradycardia, which can occur in 10–20% of treated patients. The mechanism of this adverse effect on sinus node function is unclear. Higher grade AV block is documented but rare and caution is generally only required where pre-existent conduction disease is evident.

Platinum-containing cytostatic drugs such as cisplatin and carboplatin create a dose-related but reversible sinus bradycardia in intravenous infusion.

Intravenous high-dose chloroquine is linked to variable levels of sinus node and AV block including cardiac arrest.

Prolonged oral use in rheumatoid disease is linked to emergent complete heart block.

Anaesthetics such as halothane and isoflurane produce acute bradycardia and conduction block and additionally ventricular arrhythmia during maintenance anaesthesia. These are unrelated to other effects on lowering blood pressure.

Orphenadrine has anticholinergic effects that will aggravate established relatively begin arrhythmias such as atrial fibrillation and can precipitate non sustained VT.

In addition to its potential for fatal cardiovascular collapse and depression of cardiac contraction on induction the intravenous anaesthetic agent propofol also has the ability to induce bradyarrhythmia due to sympathetic blockade.

Quinine and more obviously its diastereoisomer quinidine can both provoke ventricular tachycardia and tdp arrhythmia.

Management

Management of arrhythmia is an evolving emergency that is dependent on patients' stability. Continuous monitoring, non invasive supportive measures; confirmation or reversal of standard electrolyte deficiencies and facilitated drug elimination if possible is critical. Securing underlying stable cardiac output while the offending drug is eliminated can be problematic. Even relatively simple techniques such as temporary pacing support by transvenous routes can be hazardous in irritable myocardium and take a relatively stable if symptomatic bradyarrhythmic patients to an arrest situation. Use of binding antibodies where concomitant digoxin toxicity may be aggravating rhythm is always useful. Overdrive pacing or emergent (rapid, planned but without syncope) or repeated direct current cardioversion may be necessary.

Postmenopausal hormone therapy and cardiovascular diseases

Introduction

Cardiovascular disease (CVD) is the leading cause of death in women after the age of 50 years in industrialized countries and since the mid-1980s more women than men die each year because of CVD (Reunanen et al. 1985; Lerner and Kannel 1986; Colditz et al. 1987; Tunstall-Pedoe et al. 1999). Furthermore, after the menopause, CVD claims more deaths than all other causes of disease together. In Europe, more than two in three women after the age of 50 years die from CVD (Tunstall-Pedoe et al. 1999).

The lower incidence of CVD and cerebrovascular disease in menstruating women than in men of similar age and their rapid increase after the menopause has led to speculation that ovarian hormones may play a key role in protecting women from CVD. Several epidemiological findings suggest the role of ovarian hormone deficiency in the development of CVD in women as cardiovascular risk increases after the menopause and, at any age, postmenopausal women have a significantly higher incidence of CVD than normo-menstruating women (Kannel et al. 1976). The increased incidence of CVD in women is a recent phenomenon that is consequent to the increased life expectancy and the increase in the population of postmenopausal women. In fact, only from the 1920s onwards has the life expectancy of women living in industrialized countries exceeded menopausal age, which had remained stable around the age of 51 for the past centuries. Therefore, only when the population of postmenopausal women grew did CVD become an important epidemiological disease. The postmenopausal increase in CVD observed after the menopause is matched by an increased incidence of other diseases, such as osteoporosis and dementia, which are influenced by oestrogen deficiency and that were also uncommon in women until a few decades ago.

Since the late 1970s and until the publication of the Women's Health Initiative (WHI), oestrogen and oestrogen–progestin replacement therapy (ERT and HRT) have been widely prescribed in early postmenopausal women for the relief of menopausal symptoms. In the 1990s, their use was extended, in particular in the USA, to several years after menopause with the understanding that both replacement regimens might reduce the occurrence of CVD (Bush et al. 1987; Gruchow et al. 1988; McFarland et al. 1989; Henderson et al. 1991; Stampfer and Colditz 1991; Grodstein and Stampfer 1995; Grodstein et al. 1997). This belief was supported by the large body of evidence demonstrating a favourable effect of ovarian hormones on lipid profile, cardiovascular risk, progression of atherosclerosis and vascular functions (PEPI 1995; WHI 2002). However, despite the beneficial effect of oestrogens and oestrogen progestin associations on cardiovascular functions and surrogate cardiovascular end-points, the biological plausibility of a positive effect of ERT and HRT on cardiovascular events and, despite the strong suggestions of a significant cardiovascular benefit of hormone replacement therapy from several observational studies (Bush et al. 1987; Gruchow et al. 1988; McFarland et al. 1989; Henderson et al. 1991; Stampfer and Colditz 1991; Grodstein and Stampfer 1995; Grodstein et al. 1997), results of recent randomized trials conducted with a fixed HRT formulation in populations of predominantly elderly postmenopausal

women failed to show a cardioprotective effect of ERT/HRT (Hulley et al. 1998; WHI 2002). The publication of the WHI (2002) caused scepticism on the effect of ERT/HRT both in doctors and in women. However, fuelling the confusion on the effect of ERT/HRT on CVD were not the results of the WHI but their misinterpretation.

Hormone replacement therapy and cardiovascular risk

In the late 1980s and in the 1990s a large body of evidence supported the belief that ERT and HRT might reduce the occurrence of cardiovascular disease as several studies demonstrated a favourable effect of ovarian hormones on surrogate end-points of cardiovascular disease and a significant reduction in CV events (Bush et al. 1987; Gruchow et al. 1988; McFarland et al. 1989; Henderson et al. 1991; Stampfer and Colditz 1991; Grodstein and Stampfer 1995; Grodstein et al. 1997). Because of the benefit found in primary prevention in early postmenopausal women by observational studies it has been hypothesized that hormone replacement therapy might be beneficial in postmenopausal women with coronary artery disease. However, the HERS study (Hulley et al. 1998) failed to show any protective effect of HRT in late postmenopausal women with proven coronary artery disease. The study has also suggested a potential initial harm of HRT when started in late postmenopausal women with proven cardiovascular disease. This initial risk, however, was completely abolished in those women who were taking statins at the initiation of the study.

More recently the results of the WHI (2002) added to the confusion regarding the cardiovascular effect of hormone replacement therapy in postmenopausal women. The WHI was a NIH-sponsored study aimed at evaluating the effect of ERT/HRT with a single combination of conjugated equine oestrogens and medroxyprogesterone acetate and other preventative strategies on several outcomes in late postmenopausal women free of menopausal symptoms, a population not usually prescribed with HRT. The oestrogen–progestin arm of the study was discontinued because of a supposed increase in the Global Index, an index of cumulative events that has never been validated. The study failed to show any effect of diet on cardiovascular end-points, found a number of results concordant with those of the observational studies, but instead of documenting a protective effect of HRT against CHD, set a warning on a possible increase in CVD risk induced by such therapy in late postmenopausal women (WHI 2002). The initial findings of the possible increase in cardiovascular risk suggested by the oestrogen–progestin arm of the study have not been confirmed by the oestrogen-only arm of the study (Hsia et al. 2006).

Overall, the WHI showed that ERT and HRT do not reduce cardiovascular events in late postmenopausal women. However, the study has shown that in early postmenopausal women, those within 10 years since menopause, initiation of ERT or HRT may reduce CVD (Rossouw et al. 2007). A recent combining analysis of the two arms of the study suggested a reduction in total mortality in early postmenopausal women receiving ERT (Rossouw et al. 2007). This analysis also found that in early postmenopausal women—women very similar to those included in the observational studies—ERT reduces cardiovascular risk by an extent similar to that suggested by the observational studies.

The results of the WHI study on cardiovascular outcomes suggest that two factors, time to initiation of hormone replacement therapy since menopause, and oestrogen–progestin associations, are of importance to explain the widely divergent findings on the cardiovascular effects of observational studies and randomized controlled studies.

Time since menopause and CV effect of oestrogens

Clinical and experimental evidence suggests that most of the cardioprotective and anti-atherogenic effects of ovarian hormones are receptor mediated and endothelium dependent. Both oestrogen receptors and endothelial function are markedly influenced by time of oestrogen deprivation. The significant, age-related increase in methylation of the promoter region of the oestrogen receptors, as well as the progressive decrease in density of oestrogen receptors with time since menopause suggest that oestrogen receptor expression and function in the arterial wall diminishes sharply with time after menopause (Losordo et al. 1994; Post et al. 1999; Hodgin et al. 2001; Mendelsohn and Karas 2005; Nakamura et al. 2005). Thus, women who have been postmenopausal for several years have a longer period of oestrogen deprivation, which leads to reduced number and activity of vascular oestrogen receptors. Experimental studies conducted in monkeys have shown that oestrogen administration delays the progression of atherosclerosis progression if administered early after oophorectomy but that this effect disappears when ERT/HRT is introduced late (several years) after surgical menopause (Clarkson and Appt 2005). In accordance with the above findings, there is evidence of a time-dependent effect of ERT/HRT on the cardiovascular system (Hodis et al. 2001; Manson et al. 2007; Vitale et al. 2008). It has been shown that the time since menopause influences vascular response to oestrogens and in women aging more than 60 years ERT/HRT may increase the vascular inflammatory response (Vitale et al. 2008). In these women the vascular response to oestrogens is significantly reduced compared with the early postmenopause. Therefore, the administration of ERT/HRT within a short time since menopause is associated with significant vascular and endothelial responses that overwhelm the increased prothrombotic effects of oestrogens. On the other hand, the administration of ERT/HRT late after menopause does not have a significant effect on the endothelium and on the vasculature and cannot counterbalance the prothrombotic effect of ovarian hormones leading to an increased risk of thrombotic events.

Therefore, time of initiation of ERT/HRT explains the divergent results of observational studies and those of WHI on CVD. Indeed, women included in the observational studies chose to take ovarian hormones because of menopausal symptoms; in contrast, in the randomized trials the absence of menopausal symptoms was a prerequisite for inclusion in the study. In order to include women without menopausal symptoms, the WHI included a population of predominantly late postmenopausal women. Women included in the randomized studies were significantly older than those who started ERT/HRT in the observational studies and this difference explains the differences in results. Furthermore, the lack of symptoms

indicates a physiological adaptation to ovarian hormone deprivation, due to a slow decline in oestrogen levels and/or to the long time lapsed from menopause, and corresponds to the development of a new homeostasis. However, the analysis of results of the WHI according to age groups supports the timing hypothesis as women 50–59 included in the study showed a reduction in CVD similar to that reported by the observational studies. Recent meta-analyses of randomized studies with ERT/HRT on CVD support the timing hypothesis for the cardioprotective effect of ERT/HRT, as they have shown that initiation of therapy before the age of 60 years is associated with a significant reduction in CVD whereas initiation of such therapy after the age of 60 years is not associated with any cardiovascular protective effect and may increase the risk of stroke (Salpeter et al. 2004, 2006).

Hormone regimen

As a consequence of the different results of the ERT and HRT arms of the WHI, it appears manifest the importance of hormone regimen and in particular of progestins in enhancing or counteracting the beneficial cardiovascular effect of oestrogens. The unfavourable effect of the oestrogen/progestin combination used in the randomized studies appears to be related not to the hormone preparation per se but to the use of that hormone regimen in the less receptive group of women.

The WHI investigators acknowledged that in women aged 50–59 years ERT/HRT may reduce the overall mortality and ERT may also decrease CV events. This statement represents a U turn in the analysis of the WHI and moves towards a more balanced interpretation of the effect of ERT/HRT on CVD. Therefore, the critical analysis of the WHI data supports the concept that ERT/HRT, introduced early after the appearance of menopausal symptoms, may be continued with a cardioprotective objective. One important point regarding the effect of ERT/HRT on the cardiovascular system is represented by the effect of this replacement therapy on blood pressure. Women recruited in the WHI had a high incidence of uncontrolled risk factors such as arterial hypertension and obesity compared with women included in the observational studies. This condition may have reduced the effectiveness of the cardioprotective effect of oestrogens and increased the negative effects of progestins related to their mineralocorticoid-like effects. The effect of HRT upon blood pressure is a very relevant issue since the changes in systolic blood pressure observed in individuals randomized to such treatment in WHI are likely to explain the small increase in stroke observed in the study. Women included in the WHI had often uncontrolled arterial hypertension; this circumstance may have been worsened by the mineralocorticoid effect of medroxyprogesterone.

The mineralocorticoid effect of progestins may be enhanced by the effect of oestrogens on the production of angiotensinogen, which in turn may increase the production of angiotensin and aldosterone. Therefore progestins with anti-mineralocorticoid and anti-aldosterone effects such as progesterone, dihydrogesterone, and drospirenone should be preferred in the treatment of postmenopausal women, especially if they have a family history of arterial hypertension or if they report increase in arterial blood pressure, weight gain, or bloating with other oestrogen/progestin combinations.

Conclusion

HRT prescription must take into account the specific risk–benefit ratio for each woman, and patients should be informed and counselled about advantages and disadvantages of the therapy and supported in making an aware decision. In fact, clinical judgement and choice of the right oestrogen–progestin combination are of pivotal importance to maximize the beneficial effect of ERT HRT, especially if given within a reasonable time after the menopause to the women that need the therapy for the relief of menopausal symptoms. In conclusion, observational and randomized studies have suggested that HRT is protective in early postmenopausal women. Conversely, ageing, time since menopause and presence of CV risk factors or CV disease may increase the risk of CVD. The results of the WHI in women aging <60 years suggest that ERT/HRT may be prescribed without fear and foreseeing a CV benefit.

References

Bush TL, Barrett-Connor E, Cowan LD, et al. Cardiovascular mortality and noncontraceptive use of estrogen in women: results from the Lipid Research Clinics Program Follow-up Study. *Circulation* 1987;**75**:1102–9.

Clarkson TB, Appt SE. Controversies about HRT—lessons from monkey models. *Maturitas* 2005;**51**:64–74.

Colditz GA, Willett WC, Stampfer MJ, et al. Menopause and the risk of coronary heart disease in women. *N Engl J Med* 1987;**316**:1105–10.

Grodstein F, Stampfer M. The epidemiology of coronary heart disease and estrogen replacement in postmenopausal women. *Prog Cardiovasc Dis* 1995;**38**:199–210.

Grodstein F, Stampfer MJ, Colditz GA, et al. Postmenopausal hormone therapy and mortality. *N Engl J Med* 1997;**336**:1769-75.

Gruchow HW, Anderson AJ, Barboriak JJ, Sobocinski KA. Postmenopausal use of estrogen and occlusion of coronary arteries. *Am Heart J* 1988; **115**:954–63.

Henderson BE, Paganini-Hill A, Ross RK. Decreased mortality in users of estrogen replacement therapy. *Arch Intern Med* 1991;**151**:75–8.

Hodgin JB, Krege JH, Reddick RL, et al. Estrogen receptor alpha is a major mediator of 17beta-estradiol's atheroprotective effects on lesion size in Apoe-/- mice. *J Clin Invest* 2001;**107**:333–40.

Hodis HN, Mack WJ, Lobo RA, et al. Estrogen in the prevention of atherosclerosis. *A randomized, double-blind, placebo-controlled trial. Ann Intern Med* 2001;**135**:939–53.

Hsia J, Langer RD, Manson JE, et al., Women's Health Initiative Investigators. Conjugated equine estrogens and coronary heart disease: the Women's Health Initiative. *Arch Intern Med* 2006;**166**:357–65.

Hulley S, Grady D, Bush T, et al. Randomized trial of estrogen plus progestin for secondary prevention of coronary heart disease in postmenopausal women. *Heart and Estrogen/progestin Replacement Study (HERS) Research Group. JAMA* 1998;**280**:605–13.

Kannel WB, Hjortland MC, McNamara PM, Gordon T. Menopause and risk of cardiovascular disease: the Framingham study. *Ann Intern Med* 1976;**85**:447–52.

Lerner DJ, Kannel WB. Patterns of coronary heart disease morbidity and mortality in the sexes: a 26-year follow-up of the Framingham population. *Am Heart J* 1986;**111**:383–90.

Losordo DW, Kearney M, Kim EA, et al. Variable expression of the estrogen receptor in normal and atherosclerotic coronary arteries of premenopausal women. *Circulation* 1994;**89**:1501–10.

Manson JE, Allison MA, Rossouw JE, et al., WHI and WHI-CACS Investigators. Estrogen therapy and coronary-artery calcification. *N Engl J Med* 2007;**356**:2591–602.

McFarland KF, Boniface ME, Hornung CA, et al. Risk factors and noncontraceptive estrogen use in women with and without coronary disease. *Am Heart J* 1989;**117**:1209–14.

Mendelsohn ME, Karas RH. The protective effects of estrogen on the cardiovascular system. *N Engl J Med* 1999;**340**:1801–11.

Mendelsohn ME, Karas RH. Molecular and cellular basis of cardiovascular gender differences. *Science* 2005;**308**:1583–7.

Nakamura, Y, Suzuki T, Sasano H. Estrogen actions and in situ synthesis in smooth muscle cells and their correlation with atherosclerosis. *J Steroid Biochem Mol Biol* 2005;**93**:263–8.

PEPI. The writing group for the PEPI trial. Effects of Estrogen or Estrogen/Progestin regimens on Heart Disease risk factors in postmenopausal Women. *JAMA* 1995;**273**:199-208.

Post WS, Goldschmidt-Clermont PJ, Wilhide CC, et al. Methylation of the estrogen receptor gene is associated with aging and atherosclerosis in the cardiovascular system. *Cardiovasc Res* 1999;**43**:985–91.

Reunanen A, Suhonen O, Aromaa A, et al. Incidence of different manifestations of coronary heart disease in middle-aged Finnish men and women. *Acta Med Scand* 1985;**218**:19–26.

Rossouw, JE, Prentice RL, Manson et al. Postmenopausal hormone therapy and risk of cardiovascular disease by age and years since menopause. *JAMA* 2007;**297**:1465–77.

Salpeter SR, Walsh JM, Greyber E, et al. Mortality associated with hormone replacement therapy in younger and older women: a meta-analysis. *J Gen Intern Med* 2004;**19**:791–804.

Salpeter SR, Walsh JM, Greyber E, Salpeter EE. Coronary heart disease events associated with hormone therapy in younger and older women. *A meta-analysis. J Gen Intern Med* 2006;**21**:363–6.

Stampfer MJ, Colditz GA. Estrogen replacement therapy and coronary heart disease: a quantitative assessment of the epidemiologic evidence. *Prev Med* 1991;**20**:47–63.

Tunstall-Pedoe H, Kuulasmaa K, Mahonen M, et al. Contribution of trends in survival and coronary-event rates to changes in coronary heart disease mortality: 10-year results from 37 WHO MONICA project populations. Monitoring trends and determinants in cardiovascular disease. *Lancet* 1999;**353**:1547–57.

Vitale C, Mercuro G, Cerquetani E, et al. Time since menopause influences the acute and chronic effect of estrogens on endothelial function. *Arterioscler Thromb Vasc Biol* 2008;**28**:348–52.

WHI. Writing Group for the Women's Health Initiative Investigators. Risks and benefits of estrogen plus progestin in healthy postmenopausal women: principal results from the Women's Health Initiative randomized controlled trial. *JAMA* 2002;**288**:321–333.

Stroke and cardiovascular diseases

Embolism from a cardiac or aortic source accounts for 15–20% of all ischaemic strokes. In addition, cardiac embolism may account for a sizeable proportion of those strokes that have no apparent explanation ('cryptogenic strokes'), in which the identification of an embolic source may allow a more rational strategy for the prevention of recurrent events. The principal cardiac and aortic conditions associated with an increased stroke risk are described below.

Atrial fibrillation

Atrial fibrillation increases the risk of ischaemic stroke by three to fourfold (up to 17-fold in cases of associated rheumatic mitral disease). Overall incidence of first stroke is 2–4% per year, but is drastically increased by the presence of associated conditions (see below). The proportion of strokes attributable to atrial fibrillation increases with age, and is over 20% in patients over the age of 80 years. Atrial fibrillation is associated with increased stroke risk even when paroxysmal, not only when persistent.

Diagnostic studies

The presence of thrombus or spontaneous echocontrast (indicative of stagnant blood flow) in the left atrium increases the risk of embolization to the brain. Their presence can be investigated by transoesophageal echocardiography (TEE) in cases in which antiplatelet treatment is considered instead of systemic anticoagulation (see below), or to shorten the time of anticoagulation prior to electrical or pharmacological cardioversion. TEE allows the visualization of thrombus in the left atrial appendage, the most frequent location of thrombus formation in atrial fibrillation.

Therapy

According to current ACC/AHA/ESC guidelines, anticoagulation with warfarin (target international normalization ratio (INR) 2–3) is recommended in patients with any of the following:

- Previous stroke, transient ischaemic attack (TIA), or embolism
- Mitral stenosis
- Prosthetic heart valve (INR >2.5)

or with at least two of the following:

- Age ≥75 years
- Hypertension
- Heart failure
- Left ventricular ejection fraction ≤35%
- Diabetes mellitus.

In the absence of the above indications, either aspirin (81–325 mg/day) or warfarin can be chosen. A TEE positive for thrombus or spontaneous echocontrast indicates the need for anticoagulation.

Left ventricular dysfunction

A decreased left ventricular (LV) systolic function, especially when severe, increases the risk of thromboembolic events, including stroke, because of the possibility of blood stasis and consequent thrombus formation. An increased incidence of stroke (with annual rates of up to 3.5%) has been reported in patients with chronic heart failure, although the frequent co-existence of atrial fibrillation may contribute to this finding. The stroke risk appears to increase in parallel with the severity of reduction in LV systolic function.

Diagnostic studies

Transthoracic echocardiography can quantify the degree of LV dysfunction, and assess for the presence of mural thrombus, both elements that can drive the decision to start anticoagulation with warfarin.

Therapy

The role of anticoagulation with warfarin is established in patients with heart failure and atrial fibrillation, but is more controversial in those in sinus rhythm. In the WATCH trial, conducted in patients with LV ejection fraction ≤35% and in sinus rhythm, treatment with warfarin decreased the stroke incidence compared with treatments with aspirin or clopidogrel; however, the total number of strokes in that study was small, and the benefit of warfarin was offset by a higher frequency of cerebral haemorrhagic complications. In the absence of definitive data to date, anticoagulation with warfarin appears definitely indicated in patients in atrial fibrillation. For patients in sinus rhythm, anticoagulation appears indicated when there is evidence of left ventricular thrombus, a history of prior embolic events (especially stroke), and possibly in case of very low LV ejection fraction (<20%). Given the increased risk of major bleeding from anticoagulation, the risk–benefit ratio of this treatment must be assessed individually.

An increased risk of stroke exists in patients with acute myocardial infarction (MI).

- In the first month after the MI, the frequency of ischaemic stroke is 1–2%, with half of the events occurring in the first 5 days after the MI. The risk of stroke remains higher than in the general population at least to 1 year
- Stroke risk increases in cases of LV dysfunction, atrial fibrillation, hypertension, prior stroke
- Anterior MI, especially when involving the LV apex, is more frequently associated with embolic events, especially when an apical aneurysm is present.

Patients with atrial fibrillation, mural thrombus or akinetic/dyskinetic LV segment on echocardiogram should receive moderate-intensity (INR 2–3) warfarin therapy in addition to aspirin (75–162 mg), the latter needed for secondary prevention of MI. Duration of anticoagulation depends on the underlying source of embolism. Anticoagulation should be lifelong in patients with atrial fibrillation. In patients in sinus rhythm with documented LV thrombus, at least 3 months of anticoagulation are recommended, after which the continuation of treatment should be based on follow-up echocardiogram findings (resolution or persistence of the LV thrombus).

Infective endocarditis

Infective endocarditis is associated with a high risk of embolic stroke. It is estimated that approximately one in five patients with acute infective endocarditis and documented valvular vegetation will suffer a stroke early in the course of the disease. Regarding the risk of stroke and other embolic events, the following should be noted:

- The embolic risk is highest in the first 7–10 days.
- The risk is related to vegetation size (higher over 1 cm), extension to more than one valve/leaflet, mobility and consistency.
- The risk decreases drastically after 2 weeks of effective antibiotic treatment.

Diagnostic studies

TEE is the test of choice to detect vegetations and evaluate their size, extension, and mobility. Transthoracic echocardiography has high specificity but far lower sensitivity than TEE for the diagnosis of endocarditis, and may miss small valvular vegetations.

Therapy

Blood culture-guided antibiotic treatment is the mainstay of treatment, but early surgery, when feasible, is associated with a drastic reduction in the risk of stroke. Main indications for early surgery are haemodynamic instability, uncontrolled infection, or repeated embolic episodes while on antibiotic treatment. Early surgery is also recommended in prosthetic valve endocarditis.

Cardiac tumours

Approximately 75% of all cardiac tumours are benign, and 50% of them are myxomas. Myxomas can occur anywhere in the heart, but most commonly in the left side of the atrial septum, hence their potential for embolization to the brain. It is estimated that 30–40% of myxomas will eventually embolize, to the brain in over 50% of cases. Papillary fibroelastomas are the second most common source of cerebral embolization, and mostly occur on cardiac valves. For both types of tumours, embolization can occur from tumour fragments, or superimposed thrombus.

Diagnostic studies

Echocardiography, and especially TEE, are the mainstay for the diagnosis of cardiac tumours. Cardiac MRI may be useful in case of diagnostic uncertainty.

Therapy

Surgical excision of the tumour is the treatment of choice to prevent cerebral embolization. The role of anticoagulation in cases in which surgery is contraindicated is uncertain.

Patent foramen ovale

The presence of a patent foramen ovale (PFO) is associated with an increased risk of ischaemic stroke, especially cryptogenic. The prevalence of PFO is significantly higher in patients with cryptogenic stroke than in controls of the same sex and age. The stroke mechanism is believed to be paradoxical embolization, secondary to right-to-left shunting across the PFO of thrombotic material originating in the venous circulation. Therefore, the co-existence of a deep venous thrombosis or of a hypercoagulable state may increase the likelihood of embolization to the brain. Treatment is aimed at reducing the risk of recurrent events in stroke patients, while no treatment is indicated in asymptomatic patients with a PFO, given the high prevalence (approximately 25%) of this condition and the apparently low risk of events in the general population.

An atrial septal aneurysm (ASA), a protrusion of a redundant interatrial septum towards either atrial chamber, has also been associated with an increased stroke risk. This may be secondary to the frequent coexistence of a PFO in patients with ASA (60–70% of patients with an ASA).

Diagnostic studies

The presence of a PFO can be ascertained by transthoracic echocardiography (with aerated saline injection as a contrast material). TEE, however, allows a better visualization of the PFO and associated shunt, which may be especially useful when PFO closure is considered.

A hypercoagulability workup (including factor V Leiden and prothrombin G20210A mutation) should be obtained to evaluate the need for anticoagulation. Doppler ultrasound may be useful when venous thrombosis is suspected.

Therapy

Antithrombotic treatments have been shown to be effective in decreasing the risk of recurrent events in stroke patients with a PFO. In the Patent Foramen Ovale In Cryptogenic Stroke (PICSS) study, in which stroke patients were randomized to treatment with warfarin or aspirin, no significant difference in the risk of recurrent stroke and death at 2 years was found in patients with or without a PFO. Recently, transcatheter PFO closure has also been proven effective in reducing the risk of recurrent events. There are currently no data from randomized studies comparing the efficacy of medical treatment with transcatheter PFO closure. According to current AHA/ASA guidelines, the following treatment is recommended:
* Antiplatelet agents should be used in most patients with a stroke and a PFO
* Warfarin treatment is a reasonable choice in patients with a hypercoagulable state or evidence of venous thrombosis
* PFO closure may be considered for patients with recurrent cryptogenic stroke despite medical therapy.

Atherosclerosis of the proximal aorta

The presence of atherosclerotic plaques in the aortic arch is a risk factor for ischaemic stroke, and is especially relevant in patients over the age of 60 years. High-risk plaques can be diagnosed by TEE (see below). Plaque characteristics that increase the risk of embolization to the brain are the following:
* Thickness ≥4 mm
* Presence of complex features (ulcerations, superimposed mobile thrombus)
* Hypoechoic appearance, no calcification.

High-risk plaques are associated with a three- to fourfold increase in stroke risk. The annual incidence of embolic events in patients with large or complex plaques has been reported to be approximately 14%. Unsuspected atherosclerosis of the aorta is an important cause of stroke after cardiac surgery (due to embolization of plaque fragments during cannulation of the aorta) or after diagnostic tests involving the aorta (for example left heart catheterization).

Diagnostic studies

TEE is the most sensitive and widely used diagnostic test for aortic plaque detection. MRI can be considered when TEE is contraindicated.

Therapy

The best preventive treatment in patients with stroke and aortic plaques is controversial. Since the stroke mechanism is considered to be thromboembolic, antithrombotic treatment appears reasonable, but evidence-based data on its efficacy are scant. In a recent study published from the PICSS cohort, large plaques (≥4 mm in thickness) remained associated with a twofold increase in the risk of stroke and death at 2 years despite treatment with warfarin or aspirin. Complex plaque morphology (ulcerations, mobile components) further added to the risk. At the current stage of knowledge, warfarin treatment appears indicated when mobile components (most commonly representing superimposed thrombus) are present on the plaque. In other cases, antiplatelet agents are often prescribed as part of the secondary prevention of stroke. The role of warfarin or other antithrombotic treatments in patients with large but non-complex plaques needs further investigation. Statins appear as a promising preventive treatment and are usually prescribed in stroke patients, but evidence-based data on their effect on the risk of recurrent events in patients with arch plaques are not yet available.

Further reading

Di Tullio MR, Russo C, Jin Z, Sacco RL, Mohr JP, Homma S Aortic arch plaques and risk of recurrent stroke and death. *Circulation* 2009;**119**:2376–82.

Fuster V, Ryden LE, Cannom DS, *et al.*, ACC/AHA/ESC 2006 Guidelines for the Management of Patients with Atrial Fibrillation: a report of the American College of Cardiology/American Heart Association Task Force on Practice Guidelines and the European Society of Cardiology Committee for Practice Guidelines (Writing Committee to Revise the 2001 Guidelines for the Management of Patients With Atrial Fibrillation): developed in collaboration with the European Heart Rhythm Association and the Heart Rhythm Society. *Circulation* 2006;**114**:e257–e354.

Massie BM, Collins JF, Ammon SE, *et al.* Randomized trial of warfarin, aspirin, and clopidogrel in patients with chronic heart failure: the Warfarin and Antiplatelet Therapy in Chronic Heart Failure (WATCH) trial. *Circulation* 2009;**119**:1616–24.

Murdoch DR, Corey GR, Hoen B, *et al.* Clinical presentation, etiology, and outcome of infective endocarditis in the 21st century: the International Collaboration on Endocarditis-Prospective Cohort Study. *Arch Intern Med* 2009;**169**:463–73.

Sacco RL, Adams R, Albers G, *et al.* Guidelines for prevention of stroke in patients with ischemic stroke or transient ischemic attack: a statement for healthcare professionals from the American Heart Association/American Stroke Association Council on Stroke: co-sponsored by the Council on Cardiovascular Radiology and Intervention: the American Academy of Neurology affirms the value of this guideline. *Stroke* 2006;**37**:577–617.

Connective tissue disease

Systemic connective diseases can affect the cardiovascular system. Cardiologist could be the first to examine a patient with a connective disease and recognize the immunological underlying problem (Table 12.12.1).

Rheumatoid arthritis

This common polyarthritis is associated with an increased cardiovascular mortality, thought to be due to ischaemic heart disease.

The increased risk may be due to accelerated atherosclerosis, which is probably multifactorial. Traditional risk factors may only contribute partially, and may be augmented or aggravated by rheumatoid inflammatory pathways.

Other cardiovascular complications include pericardial effusion, pericarditis, and vasculitis. Chronic pericardial effusion is more common than acute pericarditis. Non-steroidal anti-inflammatory drugs, systemic immunosuppressive treatment, or pericardiocentesis comprise the recommended therapy.

Rheumatoid arthritis is not usually complicated with a clinical myocarditis, but the incidence of congestive heart failure is increased.

Table 12.12.1 Clinical presentation, diagnosis and treatment of main connective tissue diseases

Disease	Clinical presentation	Diagnosis	Treatment
Rheumatoid arthritis	Symmetrical polyarthritis, that progresses from the periphery to more proximal joints, may lead to destruction of joints due to erosion of cartilage and bone Stiffness after any prolonged period of inactivity	It is based upon the aggregation of characteristic symptoms, signs, laboratory data, and radiologic findings (polyarthritis, morning stiffness, rheumatoid nodules, anti-CCP antibodies, acute phase reactants, erosions of cartilage and bone)	Treatment options include medications (disease-modifying antirheumatic drugs), reduction of joint stress, physical and occupational therapy, and in some occasions surgical intervention
Rheumatoid factor-negative spondyloarthropathies	It is a group of disorders that share a predilection to cause enthesitis (inflammation in the site of ligament insertion into bone) and an association with the human leukocyte antigen HLA-B27	Enthesitis The prevalence of HLA-B27 in patients with reactive arthritis is generally less than 50 percent	NSAIDs, corticosteroids and sulfasalazine are useful to reduce pain secondary to inflammation and systemic symptoms. TNF-α antagonists have potential as disease-modifying agents
Systemic lupus erythematosus	It is a chronic inflammatory disease of unknown cause which can affect the skin, joints, kidneys, lungs, nervous system, serous membranes and/or other organs of the body	Eleven criteria were established by the American Rheumatism Association. Patients with ≥4 of these criteria, the diagnosis is strongly suggested	The goal of treatment is to relieve symptoms (NSAIDs, corticosteroids, antimalarial drugs), and protect organs by decreasing inflammation and/or the level of autoimmune activity in the body (immunosuppressive drugs)
Antiphospholipid antibody syndrome	It is defined by two major components: the occurrence of vascular event or pregnancy morbidity, and the presence of at least one type of autoantibody known as an antiphospholipid antibody	The presence of lupus anticoagulant, anticardiolipin antibodies or antibodies to β2-glycoprotein-I	The risk of thrombotic recurrence is relatively high for both arterial and venous events. So, patients are generally started on long-term (even life-long) oral anticoagulation
Systemic scleroderma	Skin involvement, Raynaud phenomenon, pulmonary artery hypertension	It is based on clinical suspicion and Anti-Scl-70 and anticentromere antibodies	Treatment and management focus on relieving symptoms and limiting damage
Polymyositis and dermatomyositis	Symmetric proximal muscle weakness, heliotrope rash	Elevated serum muscle enzymes, myopathic changes on electromyography, characteristic muscle biopsy abnormalities and the absence of histopathological signs of other myopathies	Both are treated with high doses of corticosteroids. Immunosuppressive drugs are considered in those patients without clinical improvement after corticosteroids

Vasculitis
  Churg–Strauss syndrome
  Polyarteritis nodosa
  Takayasu arteritis
  Kawasaki disease
  Giant cell arteritis
	The clinical presentation may vary, depending on the size of the vessel involved. Palpable purpura is a common finding	The diagnosis of vasculitis is difficult and usually requires a biopsy of an involved organ	Corticosteroids and NSAIDs are the drugs more frequently used. But occasionally immunosuppressive drugs are required

Anti-CCP antibodies, antibodies to cyclic citrullinated peptides.

Rheumatoid factor-negative spondyloarthropathies

These include ankylosing spondylitis, psoriatic arthritis, inflammatory bowel disease associated arthritis and post-infectious reactive arthritis. Many of them have the HLA-B27 gene. The hypothetic increased risk of ischaemic heart disease has not extensively been studied. But patients with psoriatic arthritis are at increased risk of cardiovascular morbidities, mainly myocardial infarction and hypertension.

Aortic root disease is a common finding in ankylosing spondylitis; it produces aortic root dilation and valve regurgitation. Cardiac conduction disease is observed in these diseases, mainly AV node block. Atrial fibrillation frequency is also increased. Pericarditis is not characteristic in these diseases.

Systemic lupus erythematosus

Pericarditis is the most common complication in this condition. Ischaemic heart disease is increased and different factors have been identified to accelerate atherosclerotic disease. Myocardial dysfunction is usually related to ischaemic disease and hypertension. Cardiac valvular disease is common in lupus, and classically non-bacterial vegetative endocarditis can be observed (Libman–Sacks).

Systemic embolism can be observed, mainly related to antiphospholid antibody syndrome.

The treatment of cardiac manifestation in systemic lupus erythematosus should be focused to control the systemic disease.

Antiphospholipid antibody syndrome

Cardiac manifestations are related to the increased risk of thrombosis, i.e. ischaemic heart disease and cardiac chamber thrombosis. The presence of vegetations in cardiac valve is frequent. Recommended therapy is high-dose anticoagulation.

Systemic scleroderma

Pericardial effusion is a frequent finding, but usually asymptomatic. Ischaemic heart disease is more frequently related to microvascular occlusion. Severe pulmonary hypertension can be observed, and is the main clinical problem, besides renal failure.

Polymyositis and dermatomyositis

Infrequently pericarditis and ischaemic heart disease is presented. In occasions, systolic dysfunction is shown in echocardiographic studies.

There are no controlled studies, but systemic disease therapy is recommended.

Vasculitis

Churg–Strauss syndrome

Several cardiac manifestations are observed, mainly pericarditis, myocarditis, and heart failure. They are the main cause of death in this disease. The treatment of the systemic disease is recommended.

Polyarteritis nodosa

Cardiac involvement is less frequent, i.e. pericarditis, heart failure and ischaemic heart disease. Although subclinical disease is more frequent.

Takayasu arteritis

Arterial stenosis and aneurysms are observed. Aortic valve disease can occur. Hypertension is frequently developed. Peripheral arterial disease confers a limited functional situation in these patients.

Kawasaki disease

Cardiac manifestations are quite various, i.e. pericardial effusion, myocarditis, heart valve disease, aortitis, and arrhythmias. The most classical finding is the presence of coronary aneurysms.

Giant cell arteritis

A higher incidence of aortitis and aortic aneurysms are observed. Prednisone and aspirin are recommended.

Summary

Connective diseases frequently show cardiac manifestations. Mainly pericarditis and pericardial effusion, increased incidence of ischaemic heart disease, and myocarditis. Although heart failure is not common, asymptomatic systolic dysfunction is a relative frequent finding.

Treatment of cardiac manifestations is usually pointed to the systemic disease.

Cardiology in the developing world

Cardiologists and public health officials, responsible for the medical care of patients living in developing regions of the world, are faced with the unique challenge of a wide spectrum of cardiac diseases: valvular and heart muscle diseases of infectious aetiology and chronic degenerative diseases such as hypertensive and coronary heart diseases. Therefore, knowledge about cardiac diseases affecting developing countries should include epidemiological explanations for their heterogeneity as well as the distinctive characteristics of individual cardiac diseases.

Epidemiological transition of cardiac diseases

According to the World Bank, countries with a gross national income per capita lower than US$9200 are considered low- and middle-income countries. These countries are located in six regions of the world: East Asia and the Pacific, Central Asia and Europe, South Asia, Middle East and North Africa, Sub-Saharan Africa and Latin America and the Caribbean.

Cardiovascular diseases and cardiovascular mortality have decreased progressively in the last decades in most high-income countries. However, low- and middle-income countries show just the opposite tendencies. More than two-thirds of the world cardiovascular deaths occur in these countries, the prevalence of risk factors is also increasing and cardiovascular diseases are the leading causes of death. Cardiovascular deaths affect the population at the peak of their working age and the benefits of secondary prevention are not readily available to all patients (Joshi et al. 2008). These obvious differences, with developed countries are probably due to the stage of epidemiological transition. Low- and middle-income countries are undergoing or have partially experienced the epidemiological transition from the ages of pestilence–famine and receding epidemics to the age of degenerative and man-made diseases (Gaziano 2007).

The prevalence of certain cardiac diseases is closely related to the degree of economic development and social organization. Thus, malnutrition and infectious diseases lead to rheumatic heart disease and its long-term effects on heart valves. These cardiac diseases are most prevalent in sub-Saharan Africa, rural areas of Latin America, South Asia, and in the indigenous populations of Australia and New Zealand. Chagas' disease, which mainly affects heart muscle and is particularly related to housing conditions, is endemically present in Latin America. However, migration of infected individuals has now extended this endemic disease to high-income countries. Industrialization, improved nutrition, and control of infections have allowed for the transition to the next two stages: receding pandemics and degenerative and man-made diseases. Chronic diseases such as hypertension and its disabling consequence (i.e. ischaemic stroke) are now present. Risk factors for coronary artery disease (cigarette smoking, diabetes mellitus, and obesity) show a marked tendency to increase (Gaziano 2007; Bestetti et al. 2008).

- Deaths because of cardiovascular diseases were estimated worldwide, by the year 2005, at 17.5 million.
- Eighty per cent of all cardiovascular deaths occur in low- and middle-income countries.
- Cardiovascular diseases are the main causes of death in persons of all ages, in developing countries.
- One-half of all cardiovascular deaths affect the population under 70 years of age.
- Loss of economic production from heart disease, stroke and diabetes, by the year 2015, has been estimated in US$84 billion.

Malnutrition and infectious cardiac diseases in geographical regions of the developing world

Twenty million people living in South America have Chagas' disease due to infection by *Trypanosoma cruzi*. Recent surveys among blood donors indicate that in some regions up 3.4 percent of the population have positive serological tests. In the early stages of this disease, myocardial damage is localized and progresses to a diffuse form of a congestive cardiomyopathy, which is a common cause of hospitalization for congestive heart failure. Compared with congestive heart failure of other aetiologies, Chagas' cardiomyopathy is considered to be the main prognostic factor of mortality. However, when chagasic patients with congestive heart failure are given the same non-specific treatment strategy, based on beta-adrenergic blockers, mortality is similar to that of patients with non-chagasic heart failure (Bestetti et al. 2008).

Rheumatic heart disease affects about 15.6 million people worldwide. It is estimated that every year about 300 000 individuals develop rheumatic heart disease. The incidence of acute rheumatic fever in children from developing countries is four to five times higher than in high-income countries. Indigenous populations of Australia and New Zealand have an incidence of 80% per 100 000 children, whereas the non-indigenous population of these two same countries is less than 10% per 100.000 children (Carapetis et al. 2005). The prevalence of rheumatic heart disease is also heterogeneous and related to the diagnostic strategies used for diagnosis (Marijon et al. 2007). Thus, in countries like Cambodia and Mozambique, systematic screening with echocardiography has shown a much higher prevalence than clinical screening (21.5 cases per 1000 children versus 2.2 cases per 1000 children. Different prevalences, notwithstanding the current controversy (changing virulence of group A streptococci versus changing living conditions), are now present in countries like China, where hospitalizations due to rheumatic heart disease have declined from 50% in 1948–57 to 2% in 2000–5 (Cheng 2009).

Natural history of Chagas' disease

Acute phase

- Self-limited febrile illness, usually diagnosed in about 5% of infected individuals.

Indeterminate phase

- Asymptomatic stage, with normal cardiac findings. Very low morbidity and good prognosis. Fifty per cent of the patients will progress to a chronic cardiac or digestive form (Brazil).

Arrhythmic and congestive phases

- Cardiac rhythm and conduction abnormalities. Symptoms and signs of congestive heart failure.

Clinical and serological diagnosis

- Two positive serologic tests (indirect immunofluorescence, indirect haemagglutination, or enzyme-linked immunosorbent assay (ELISA)) and evidence of cardiomyopathy.

Independent predictors of mortality
- Impaired left ventricular function, New York Heart Association functional classes III/IV, cardiomegaly, non-sustained ventricular tachycardia, and no treatment with beta-adrenergic blockers.

Treatment
Specific treatment with benznidazol is currently indicated only in patients with unequivocal evidences of, or at high risk for, acute infection by *Trypanosoma cruzi* (organ transplant and immunosuppression). Cardiac arrhythmias and congestive symptoms should be treated as in non-chagasic heart diseases.
- 15 million cases of rheumatic heart disease are found in developing countries.
- Rheumatic heart disease is present in 1–2% of Latin American children.
- The prevalence of rheumatic heart disease increases with age, reaching its peak by age 25–34 years.
- Mitral regurgitation is the dominant lesion, but stenosis becomes more common with increasing age.

Degenerative and man-made diseases in geographical regions of the developing world
Risk factors for coronary artery disease and stroke
Risk factors for coronary artery disease and stroke are on the rise in most low- and middle-income countries. At the present time, diabetes affects more than 150 million people of the entire world population. By the year 2025, the rate of increase will be 170% in low- and middle-income countries compared to 42% in high-income countries. The population affected is between 45 and 65 years of age, and as in developed countries it is detected in subjects over 65. Concerning tobacco use, about 1 billion people are smokers and more than two-thirds of them reside in developing countries. The prevalence of smoking among adult men in Russia has increased from 57% to 62%. In contrast, Australia decreased its prevalence from 28% to 25%. Quit rates are very low and range from 5% to 2% in countries like China and India respectively (Gaziano 2007; Joshi et al. 2008).

Average blood pressure levels, for all ages, are highest in Eastern Europe, Russia, Middle East, North Africa and sub-Saharan Africa. Prospective studies carried out in white and Asian populations have demonstrated a direct continuous association of usual levels of systolic and diastolic blood pressure with the risk of coronary heart disease and stroke. The prevalence of these risk factors in Latin America has similar patterns (Cubillos-Garzón et al. 2004; Perkovic et al. 2007).

Heart failure as the final and common pathway for all cardiac diseases
Myocardial damage induces, regardless of the underlying aetiology, maladaptative and compensatory mechanisms that ultimately lead to heart failure. Earlier investigations in low-income countries attributed heart failure to cardiomyopathy and valvular heart disease. However, more recent studies in Africa and Latin America clearly indicate that, in the developing world, the most common causes of congestive heart failure are hypertension and coronary artery disease (Cubillos-Garzón et al. 2004; Stewart et al. 2008). In other words, epidemiological transition is also modifying the spectrum of heart diseases responsible for heart failure.

- Stroke-related deaths in certain developing countries among people age 15–59 years is three to eight times than in high-income countries.
- Less than one-fifth of those patients with past medical history of cardiovascular disease have access to secondary prevention treatment.
- WHO budget: $7.50 is spent per communicable disease death, only $0.50 is spent per death from chronic disease.
- In Latin American countries, the ratio of deaths from cardiac diseases to deaths from infectious diseases will rise from 1.1 to 4.75.
- Prevalence of hypertension in urban populations of Latin American countries: 14.1 in Colombia to 32.0 in Mexico.
- Prevalence of obesity in urban populations of Latin American countries: 6.9 in Brazil to 25.7 in Paraguay.
- Prevalence of diabetes in urban populations of Latin American countries: 4.0 in Chile to 8.5 in Argentina.

Contribution of different regions of the world to scientific research
The vast majority of scientific articles published between 1995 and 2002 originated from Western Europe (39.4%) and the USA (37.1%). The USA, Oceania, and Canada had the highest mean impact factor. The number of scientific articles from Eastern Europe, Latin America and the Caribbean, and Asia was much smaller. Although, the contribution of Africa was very low, the rate of increase in the number of published articles was higher than in developed countries. This promising trend will surely provide new knowledge and therapeutic strategies to reduce the growing burden of cardiovascular diseases on the developing world.

References
Bestetti RB, Tatiana AD, Theodoropoulos TAD, *et al.* Treatment of chronic systolic heart failure secondary to Chagas heart disease in the current era of heart failure therapy. *Am Heart J* 2008;**156**:422–30.

Carapetis JR, McDonald M, Wilson NJ. Acute rheumatic fever. *Lancet* 2005;**366**:155–168.

Cheng TO. Editorial How much of the recent decline in rheumatic heart disease in China can be explained by changes in cardiovascular risk factors?. *Int J Cardiol* 2009;**132**:300–2.

Cubillos-Garzón LA, Casas JP, Morillo CA, Bautista LE. Congestive heart failure in Latin America: The next epidemic. *Am Heart J* 2004;**147**:412–17.

Gaziano TA. Reducing the global burden of cardiovascular disease in the developing world. *Health Affairs* 2007;**26**:13–24.

Joshi R, Jan S, Wu Y, MacMahon S. Global inequalities in access to cardiovascular health care. *J Am Coll Cardiol* 2008;**52**:1877–25.

Marijon E, Ou P, Celermajer DS, *et al.* Prevalence of rheumatic heart disease detected by echocardiographic screening. *N Engl J Med* 2007;**357**:470–6.

Perkovic V, Huxley R, Wu Y, *et al.* The burden of blood pressure-related: A neglected priority for global health. *Hypertension* 2007;**50**:991–7.

Rosmarakis ES, Vergidis PI, Soteriades ES, *et al.* Estimates of global production in cardiovascular diseases research. *Int J Cardiol* 2005;**100**:443–9.

Stewart S, Wilkinson D, Hansen C. Predominance of Heart Failure in the Heart of Soweto Study Cohort: Emerging Challenges for Urban African Communities. *Circulation* 2008;**118**:2360–7.

Stem cell and gene therapy for heart disease

Coronary artery disease remains the major cause of morbidity and mortality worldwide. Despite recent advances in reperfusion therapy for acute myocardial infarction (MI) and pharmacotherapy for post MI left ventricular (LV) remodelling, an increasing trend of incidence and mortality is observed. In this regard, stem cell and gene therapies have emerged as potential novel therapies for patients with acute MI, heart failure, and chronic myocardial ischaemia.

Stem cell therapies

Mechanism of action

- Stem cell-based therapy relies on the belief that exogenous cells or mobilized endogenous cells can transdifferentiate into mature cardiomyocytes (CMs) and integrates both electrically and mechanically with host CMs to improvement of cardiac function.
- In addition, data have demonstrated that cellular mediated paracrine effects also played an important role for the improvement in LV function by secreting proangiogenic cytokines to enhance neovascularization.
- The paracrine factors secreted from the transplanted cells exert anti-apoptotic effects, alter the restoration of extracellular matrix and recruit endogenous stem cells.

Different type of cell source

- Various types of stem or progenitor cells, including bone marrow (BM)-derived cells, placental/cord blood-derived cells, adipose tissue-derived cells, resident cardiac progenitor cells, embryonic stem cells and induced pluripotent stem cells, have been investigated for cardiac repair. Their advantages and disadvantages are shown in Table 12.14.1.

Mode of cell delivery

- One of the greatest challenges in stem cell therapy is optimal delivery, engraftment, and survival of transplanted cells.
- The homing and engraftment of stem or progenitor cells after administration relies on the method of cell delivery, the characteristics of transplanted cells, and the host environment.
- In addition to direct cell delivery, mobilization of endogenous stem cell can be achieved by administration of cytokines or growth factors.
- Potential application of different methods of cell delivery is shown in Table 12.14.2.
- In the setting of acute MI, stem cells can be delivered by intravenous or intracoronary routes after coronary revascularization. The intravenous infusion is the simplest approach, but have a low efficacy for cellular engraftment (<1%) due to the cell trapping in the other organs. However, both intravenous and intracoronary routes are not suitable for patients with an occluded artery and for delivery of stem cells of larger size or limited migration ability, such as skeletal myoblasts due to risk of microembolization.
- For patients with chronic myocardial ischaemia, direct intramyocardial injection via either surgical epicardial or transcatheter endocardial approaches is needed for optimal cell delivery. These techniques allow direct cell delivery into the targeted regions even in patients with occluded artery and with the use of certain larger cell types.
- Finally, in patients with post-MI heart failure due to large area of infarcted and non-viable myocardium, direct

Table 12.14.1 Different types of stem cells for cardiovascular diseases

Celltypes	Advantage	Disadvantage
Embryonic stem cells	Pluripotent. Unlimited supply Autologous transplantation possible via therapeutic cloning	Social and ethical concerns Risk of rejection and required immunosuppression for allogenic transplant Risk of tumour formation Proarrhythmic risk
Induced pluripotent stem cells	Same as embryonic stem cells	Risk of tumour formation Risk of viral vector Proarrhythmic risk
Skeletal myoblast	Autologous transplantation High yield Resistant to fatigue and ischaemia	Cannot differentiate into cardiomyocyte Lack of integration with host cardiomyocyte with arrhythmogenic potential
Bone marrow stem cells	Autologous transplantation Can induce angiogenesis, possible pluripotent	Limited ability to differentiate into cardiomyocyte Limited supply and need for *in vitro* expansion Difficult to isolate and propagate in culture
Mesenchymal stem cells	Autologous transplantation Can induce angiogenesis and possible pluripotent Lower risk of rejection	Limited ability to differentiate into cardiomyocyte Limited supply and need for *in vitro* expansion Difficult to isolate and propagate in culture
Adult cardiac stem cells	Cardiomyocyte phenotype with no need for differentiation Can integrate with host cardiomyocyte Autologous transplantation	Very limited supply Difficult to isolate and propagate in culture Proarrhythmic risk

Table 12.14.2 Potential clinical strategies for stem cell delivery

Strategies	Advantage	Disadvantage
Intravenous	Easily available and avoid the risk of any invasive procedure	Low efficacy of cell delivery Not applicable to patients with occluded artery Risk of systemic administration unclear
Intracoronary	Possible wide use in catheterization laboratory Limited risk of systemic administration	Uncertain efficacy of cell delivery Not applicable to patients with a occluded artery Not applicable for stem cell with large cells
Catheter-based direct intramyocardial injection	Higher efficacy of cell delivery Short-term safety proven	Need for specialized catheters and imaging technology to guide the procedure
Open heart direct epicardial injection	Applicable to patients who need open heart surgery Allow direct visualization of the site of injection	Risk of mortality and morbidity of open heart surgery
Direct epicardial patch	Applicable to patients who need open heart surgery Avoid uneven distribution of cell in the myocardium Allow direct delivery of a large amount of cell	Need tissue engineering to create cellular patch Risk of mortality and morbidity of open heart surgery

injection of stem cells into myocardium scar will result in low graft survival and differentiation. Therefore, the use of bioengineering approaches, such as cardiac patches and injectable delivery matrices may be needed to improve cell retention, survival, and differentiation. Nevertheless, the safety and efficacy of this approach has not been tested in clinical trials due to the lack of optimal technique to create three-dimensional viable cellular patches.

Clinical applications
Acute myocardial infarction
- In patients with acute MI, the majority of randomized controlled clinical trials are focused on the use of intracoronary administration of autologous BM cells in patients who had undergone successful percutaneous coronary intervention of infarcted related artery.
- These studies yielded mixed results on the effect of intracoronary administration of BM cells due to relative small patients sample size (<200), differences in the study population, the dosage, preparation and types of cells, timing of cell transfer, and the methodology of functional assessment. Nevertheless, none of these studies showed major adverse effects.
- Trials have demonstrated a modest (~3–4%) but significant improvement in left ventricular ejection fraction and a small reduction in infarct scar size and left ventricular dimension (Siu *et al.* 2010).
- Clinical efficacy of intracoronary BM cells therapy, the optimal timing and dosage of cell administration required several larger ongoing trials to address.

Congestive heart failure
- There are only two randomized controlled clinical trials on the use autologous BM or skeletal myoblast in patients with congestive heart failure after MI (Siu *et al.* 2010).
- Patients received intracoronary BM cell transplantation but not circulating progenitor cells showed a modest but significant improvement in LV ejection fraction (2.9%) at 3 months compared with controls. However, there was no difference in LV dimension after cell transplantation.
- The Myoblast Autologous Grafting in Ischemic Cardiomyopathy (MAGIC) trial investigated the safety and efficacy of low dose (400×10^6) or high-dose (800×10^6) autologous skeletal myoblasts versus placebo in patients with ischaemic cardiomyopathy and indication for coronary artery bypass grafting. Because of the safety concern of proarrhythmia in the early pilot studies, all patients were treated with implantable cardioverter-defibrillators before transplantation. At 6 months there were no significant differences in regional or global LV function as determined by echocardiogram and arrhythmia events among these three groups. However, patients receiving the highest dose of cells had a significant decrease in LV end-diastolic and end-systolic volume as compared with control, suggesting the possibility of reverse remodelling.

Chronic myocardial ischaemia/infarction
- In contrast to acute MI, there are only a few small randomized controlled clinical trials on stem cell therapy for treatment of refractory angina due to chronic myocardial ischaemia.
- These trials mainly focused on the use of intramyocardial injections of BM cells into chronic ischemic myocardium which are not amenable to conventional coronary revascularization (Siu *et al.* 2010).
- In these studies, cell transplantation was performed by three-dimensional electromechanical mapping guided catheter-based intramyocardial injection into the ischaemic myocardium as described previously. Use in chronic ischaemic myocardium not amendable to conventional coronary revascularization.
- An improvement in clinical status, angina frequency, exercise capacity, and left ventricular ejection fraction has been demonstrated in these trials.
- No significant adverse events including cardiac arrhythmias have been reported.

Gene therapy
Gene therapy is a potential new treatment of cardiovascular disease and may provide a novel approach to treat patients with both genetic disorders and acquired pathophysiologies such as arteriosclerosis, heart failure, and arrhythmias. Recombinant DNA technology and the sequencing of the human genome have identified many candidate therapeutic genes available for cardiovascular diseases. However, the major challenge in the field of gene therapy for cardiovascular disease is to develop effective and safe gene delivery systems for localizing gene therapy to specific sites to optimize transgene expression and efficacy.

- Several pathological alterations that occur during heart failure have been targets for gene therapy, but main focus has been emphasized on restoring Ca^{2+} transport using gene therapy, including *SERCA2a*, phospholamban (*PLB*), ryanodine receptor (*RyR2*), and the sodium–calcium exchanger (*NCX*).
- Among them, SERCA has proven a very promising candidate for gene transfer because its expression and activity are decreased in a wide variety of pathologic conditions in heart failure.
- One phase I clinical trial (CUPID trial: Calcium Up-Regulation by Percutaneous Administration of Gene Therapy in Cardiac Disease) using *SERCA2* gene transfer (AAV1-*SERCA2a*, Mydicar; Celladon Corporation, La Jolla, CA) in patients with congestive heart failure has been completed. Seven of nine patients treated showed improvements over 6 months in several areas: symptomatic (five patients), functional (four patients), biomarker (two patients) and left ventricular function/remodelling

(six patients). Two patients with pre-existing antibodies to the viral vector delivery system did not show improvements. Importantly, the approach was shown to have an acceptable safety profile. Currently, Phase II CUPID trial is ongoing.
- Furthermore, another phase I study using AAV6-*SERCA2a* to evaluate efficacy and safety in ischemic patients undergoing left ventricular assist placement is also planned.

Further reading

Gnecchi M, Zhang Z, Ni A, *et al.* Paracrine mechanisms in adult stem cell signaling and therapy. *Circ Res* 2008;**103**:1204–19.

Habib M, Caspi O, Gepstein L. Human embryonic stem cells for cardiomyogenesis. *J Mol Cell Cardiol* 2008;**45**:462–74.

Menasche P. Stem cells for clinical use in cardiovascular medicine: current limitations and future perspectives. *Thromb Haemost* 2005;**94**:697–701.

Siu CW, Liao SY, Liu Y, *et al.* Stem cells for myocardial repair. *Thromb Haemost* 2010;**104**:6–12.

Index

Note: figures are in bold, and tables are in italics.